AN ESSENTIAL GUIDE TO HEARING AND BALANCE DISORDERS

AN ESSENTIAL GUIDE TO HEARING AND BALANCE DISORDERS

Edited by

R. Steven Ackley
Gallaudet University
University of Colorado

T. Newell Decker
University of Nebraska-Lincoln

Charles J. Limb
Johns Hopkins Hospital
Johns Hopkins University School of Medicine

LEA LAWRENCE ERLBAUM ASSOCIATES, PUBLISHERS
2007   Mahwah, New Jersey   London

MW

Senior Acquisitions Editor: Cathleen Petree
Senior Editorial Assistant: Karin Wittig-Bates
Cover Design: Tomai Maridou
Full-Service Compositor: MidAtlantic Books and Journals, Inc.

This book was typeset in 10/12 pt. Times Roman, Italic, Bold, and Bold Italic.

Lawrence Erlbaum Associates, Inc., Publishers
10 Industrial Avenue
Mahwah, New Jersey 07430
www.erlbaum.com

CIP information for this volume can be obtained by contacting the Library of Congress.

ISBN 978-0-8058-5893-8—0-8058-5893-8 (case)
ISBN 978-0-8058-5894-5—0-8058-5894-6 (paper)
ISBN 978-1-4106-1775-0—1-4106-1775-0 (ebook)

Books published by Lawrence Erlbaum Associates are printed on
acid-free paper, and their bindings are chosen for strength and durability.

Printed in the United States of America

10   9   8   7   6   5   4   3   2   1

6/15/09

This book is dedicated with gratitude to our patients, teachers, mentors, students, and families.

Contents

Preface

The theme of this book is hearing/balance disorders. Essential aspects of the topic from cause and diagnosis to treatment and cure are described. Each chapter details a specific topic area along the continuum of how medical personnel diagnose disorders of hearing/balance to how surgical implantation and rehabilitation can remedy various conditions. The pathway through this process begins with the case history in chapter 1, followed by detailed descriptions of current knowledge regarding fundamental causes of hearing loss and balance disorder, and then providing thorough description of objective assessment. Chapters 8–11 offer specialized treatment and rehabilitative options for the various disorders, and the remaining chapters cover special topics and conclude with pertinent case studies. The reader will learn the most sophisticated methods of diagnosis and treatment of hearing and balance disorders from experts in various subspecialties of this broad topic. As the title implies, this resource will be an 'essential guide' to the topic and in a concise format. The information is critical to hearing/balance related disciplines including audiology, otolaryngology, general medicine and rehabilitation oriented allied health care professions.

Editors and Contributors

R. Steven Ackley, PhD
Professor and Director of Audiology
Hearing, Speech and Language Sciences
Gallaudet University
Washington, DC 20002
  and
Research Associate
University of Colorado
Boulder, CO 80309

Iee Ching W. Anderson, MD
Johns Hopkins University School of
  Medicine/Johns Hopkins Hospital
Department of Otolaryngology-
  Head and Neck Surgery
Baltimore, MD 21287

Scott J. Bally, Ph.D.
Department of Hearing Speech and
  Language Sciences
Gallaudet University
Washington, DC 20002

Kathryn Laudin Beauchaine, MA
Boys Town National Research Hospital
Omaha, NE 68131

Stephen Boney, PhD
University of Nebraska
Lincoln, NE 68583

Carmen C. Brewer, PhD
Otolaryngology Branch
National Institute on Deafness and
  Other Communication Disorders
National Institutes of Health
Bethesda, Maryland 20892

Kathleen C. M. Campbell, PhD
Professor & Director of Audiology
  Research
Southern Illinois University School
  of Medicine
Springfield, IL 62794-9629

T. Newell Decker, PhD
Professor and Graduate Chair
Department of Special Education &
  Communication Disorders
University of Nebraska-Lincoln
Lincoln, NE 68583

Brian Dunham, MD
The Listening Center
Johns Hopkins Hospital
Department of Otolaryngology—
    Head & Neck Surgery
Baltimore, MD 21287

Marc D. Eisen, MD, PhD
Otology, Neurotology, and Skull Base
    Surgery
Department of Otolaryngology—
    Head & Neck Surgery
Johns Hopkins University
Baltimore, Maryland 21287

Leisha R. Eiten, MA
Boys Town National Research Hospital
Omaha, NE 68131

John A. Ferraro, PhD
University of Kansas Medical Center
Kansas City, KS 66160

Robert Folsom, PhD
University of Washington
Seattle, WA 98105

Annette Hurley, PhD
Louisiana State University Health
    Sciences Center
New Orleans, LA 70112

Danielle Inverso, AuD
Gallaudet University
Washington, DC 20002

Benjamin L. Judson, MD
Resident
Dept of Otolaryngology-HNS
Georgetown University Medical Center
3800 Reservoir Rd, NW
Washington, DC 20007

H. Jeffrey Kim, MD
Associate Professor
Dept of Otolaryngology-HNS
Georgetown University Medical
    Center
3800 Reservoir Rd, NW
Washington, DC 20007
    and
Senior Staff Clinician
Otolaryngology Branch
National Institute on Deafness and
    Other Communication Disorders
National Institutes of Health

Charles J. Limb, MD
Assistant Professor of Otology,
    Neurotology, and Skull Base Surgery
Department of Otolaryngology—
    Head & Neck Surgery
Johns Hopkins Hospital
Johns Hopkins University School of
    Medicine
Baltimore, Maryland 21287

Lisa R. Mancl, MS
University of Washington
Seattle, WA 98105

Annette Mazevski, AuD
Gallaudet University
Washington, DC 20002

Kerri S. McDill, MS
Wyoming Otolaryngology
940 E 3rd St Ste 215
Casper, WY 82601

Deanna K. Meinke, PhD
Assistant Professor-Audiology
University of Northern Colorado
Greeley, CO 80639

Michael J. Metz, Ph.D.
Audiology Associates, P.C.,
    Irvine California
University of California-Irvine,
    Irvine California
EPIC Hearing Health Care
Industry, California 91748

Robin Moorhouse, AuD
Louisiana State University Health
    Sciences Center
New Orleans, LA 70112

Walter E. Nance, MD, PhD
Department of Human Genetics
Virginia Commonwealth
    University
Richmond, VA 23298

Jodell Newman-Ryan, PhD
Northern Illinois University
Department of Communication
    Disorders
Dekalb, IL 60115-2899

Janet L. Pray, PhD
Department of Social Work
Gallaudet University
Washington, DC 20002

Jennifer Ratigan, AuD
Phoenix Ear Associates
Phoenix, AZ 85034

Neil T. Shepherd, PhD
Department of Special Education
    & Communication Disorders
University of Nebraska Lincoln
Lincoln, NE 68583
    and
Boys Town National Research Hospital
Omaha, NE 68131

Jeffrey Simmons, MA
Boys Town National Research Hospital
Omaha, NE 68131

Mark R. Stephenson, PhD
Senior Research Audiologist
Centers for Disease Control and
    Prevention
National Institute for Occupational
    Safety and Health
Atlanta, GA 30333

James W. Thelin, PhD
University of Tennessee
Knoxville, TN 37996

Robert M. Traynor, EdD, MBA
President, Audiology Associates of
    Greeley, Inc.
Greeley, Colorado 80635

Erik H. Waldman, MD
Department of Otolaryngology—
    Head & Neck Surgery
Johns Hopkins University School of
    Medicine
Baltimore, Maryland 21287

AN ESSENTIAL GUIDE TO HEARING AND BALANCE DISORDERS

CHAPTER 1

Case History

Charles J. Limb
Johns Hopkins Medical Center

R. Steven Ackley
Gallaudet University

The case history is generally regarded in medicine as the "first test." An accurate and thorough case history, when interpreted correctly, directs all necessary testing, which in turn helps to narrow the differential diagnosis. Clinical acumen, knowledge, and experience are essential to forming an accurate initial diagnostic interpretation of a patient's condition. Although inexperienced clinicians are unlikely to misdiagnose cerumen impaction, they may fail to recognize, for example, that a patient who describes a Tullio phenomenon (sound-induced oscillopsia) may have a less common condition, such as superior semicircular canal dehiscence syndrome. Thus, although there is no fixed formula for obtaining a patient's history that applies to all cases, a comprehensive and systematic approach to patient history-taking will greatly assist the clinician. The goal of the case history is to efficiently yet thoroughly extract the relevant patient background and details of his or her complaints in such a way that they can be appropriately interpreted. The background knowledge and clinical experience required to successfully diagnose the majority of pathologies on the basis of case history information are acquired through years of study and clinical practice. Therefore, this chapter is intended to outline several guidelines that can be used as part of a thorough approach to the patient case history. This chapter provides a format for encapsulating the process of gaining accurate information from patients and then synthesizing that information into a meaningful conclusion.

ELEMENTS OF THE CASE HISTORY

Demographic and Identifying Information

The information that is used to identify the patient within the clinic must be general enough to be interpreted by other clinics while maintaining necessary confidentiality. In addition to the patient's legal name, other names used by this patient previously should be noted, including maiden names or aliases. Although a medical office or hospital will nearly always acquire social security identifiers for every patient, this information should be kept confidential and not be routinely included on all paperwork (the medical record number is more appropriate). Other identifying information that is required is straightforward: address, phone/TTY number, e-mail address, date of birth, medical insurance, and emergency contact information. In addition, information regarding the patient's referral source is necessary so that medical correspondence can be sent to the referring source.

Chief Complaint

The principal symptom or complaint motivating the patient's visit should be described by the patient with minimal prompting from the clinician or other caregivers, if possible. When appropriate, the chief presenting complaint is written verbatim. The chief complaint describes the single most compelling factor(s) that prompted the individual to seek medical evaluation. The chief complaint frames the patient's concerns hierarchically, in that it is this complaint that the patient wishes to have explicitly addressed during the visit, rather than numerous other, less pressing complaints. Questions can be asked to clarify a symptom, such as, *Is it only your right ear that is "ringing"?*, but introducing possible related symptoms should be avoided in this section of the case history, to avoid unduly influencing patients (this is especially relevant for potential malingerers). As in most human interactions, there is a wide range of variability in how patients respond to the questioning of their chief complaint, and this inherent variability requires flexibility on the examiner's part.

Onset

The timing of onset of symptoms is a critical piece of information for all cases; ideally, a screening process should provide a method by which relative emergencies (such as sudden sensorineural hearing loss) may be identified and promptly evaluated. Often the timing of onset alone may not reveal the seriousness of the pathology, if taken out of context, such as a sudden hearing loss that occurs without any apparent reason, in comparison with the sudden conductive hearing loss that can occur after bathing, if cerumen becomes waterlogged and subsequently impacted; therefore, it is imperative to determine not only the timing of onset, but any contextual factors that may be relevant. The general question format for this topic is, *When did you first notice the problem?* This simple question can lead to a complex answer. For example, in cases of delayed endolymphatic hydrops, the patient might report that hearing loss was first noticed a decade earlier, but that vertigo or other vestibular symptoms began quite recently within the past month. More commonly, patients with presbycusis or noise-induced hearing loss might report that they have not really noticed a problem at all, but that a family member insists that a hearing loss is present and recommends a hearing test. Also, when questioning patients regarding symptom onset, it is important to identify each germane symptom, as they can indicate widely differing pathologies. This symptom list includes (but is not limited to) discussions hearing loss, vertigo, imbalance, tinnitus, otalgia, aural pressure, facial weakness, and headache.

Time Course of Symptoms

It is crucial to document whether or not multiple symptoms are occurring either together or in sequence. For example, tinnitus may be high-pitched, constant, and nonlocalized in elderly patients who are experiencing insidious hearing loss, whereas Menière's patients may describe low-pitched, intermittent, and unilateral tinnitus with bouts of sudden hearing loss and vertigo. Documenting the course of the symptoms is vital. A change in one's tinnitus to a more pronounced intensity on one side with increased distortion might signal a progressive retrocochlear problem, such as a cerebellopontine angle tumor. Increasing duration or frequency of vertigo episodes for the patient with Menière's disease might be associated with concurrent accelerated hearing deterioration. Every attempt should be made to confirm symptoms with objective measures. Tinnitus matching procedures can determine the approximate frequency and intensity of the symptom. Videonystagmography or traditional electronystagmography can record nystagmus in response to sound (Tullio phenomenon) or ear canal pressure change (known as Hennebert's sign or a positive fistula test response). Acoustic reflex procedures can document middle-ear muscle spasm (tonic tensor tympani phenomenon) or absent stapedius muscle contraction in the case of otosclerosis.

Laterality of Symptoms

Hearing loss and tinnitus that are unilateral often (but not always) suggest a need for surgical treatment more frequently than bilateral conditions, with the exception of bilateral profound sensorineural hearing loss that is amenable to cochlear implantation or due to advanced neurofibromatosis type 2. Although challenging, imbalance and vertigo of peripheral origin can generally be attributed to an offending ear, especially in straightforward cases such as benign positional vertigo or uncomplicated Menière's disease. Additional lateralizing symptoms, such as ear fullness or pressure, may help narrow the differential diagnosis as well as identify the side of vestibular loss. Mild symptoms should not necessarily be ignored. For example, unilateral tinnitus without significant hearing loss may not be alarming, but it can also be the presenting symptom of acoustic neuroma (more properly known as vestibular schwannoma).

Otologic Health History

Documentation of ear infections, otalgia, otorrhea, and otologic surgical history should include as much detail as possible. The number and frequency of confirmed bouts of otitis media with effusion (OME) can determine the need for pressure equalization tubes. If the hearing fluctuates, it is important to note what factors cause it to improve or worsen. Chronic tympanic membrane perforation, sometimes reported as otalgia and hearing loss during showering, as well as a history of chronic otorrhea, may require surgical treatment. Ear surgical history has implications for interpretation of test results and rehabilitation. Tympanoplasty with mastoidectomy may close an existing air-bone gap but will also lead to an enlarged mastoid cavity that results in abnormal physical volume test results and requires special consideration during earmold impression acquisition and hearing aid adjustment, given the subsequent changes in resonance that result from a mastoid defect.

General Health History

General medical history is important for several reasons. It is vital to identify broader health disorders that might affect hearing, such as diabetes or autoimmune disease. The clinician might introduce this area of questioning by asking "How is your overall health?" and allowing for a brief narrative in the patient's words. In addition, specific questions regarding currently taken prescription and over-the-counter medications and known drug allergies should be listed. Immunizations given within the past five years should be documented. Mental health status and history of mental illness should be reported. History of hospitalization for any reason should be reiterated in this section where there is no apparent link to hospitalization for reasons related to hearing. The question *Have others observed a change in your health recently?* might offer a way of extracting this information. It is crucial to record pharmaceutical treatments that could damage hair cells, including treatment for certain cancers, tuberculosis, and life-threatening infections (see chapter 5). History of allergies may have implications for ear infections or vertigo attacks. Head injury can affect hearing in complicated ways, including concussion presenting as noise-induced hearing loss; perilymphatic fistula; ossicular damage; and facial, vestibular, or auditory nerve damage (see chap. 8). A complete review of systems, typically acquired by physicians, is a thorough and systematic way to review non-otologic health issues that may be pertinent.

Vestibular History

For the dizzy patient, a separate case history as an addendum to the primary case history is often necessary, given the exhaustive detail that is typically required. It is important to remember that dizzy patients are often quite debilitated, frustrated, and depressed, lending a quality of despair to many of their interactions. In this context, it is critically important to acquire an accurate, thorough history, as the history alone will often rule out many causes of dizziness. The initial goals of the audiologist and otolaryngologist in the evaluation of dizziness are to identify any neurological emergencies (e.g., stroke) that might warrant prompt evaluation; such cases are typically accompanied by other neurologic deficits and can be quite obvious, whereas other neurologic deficits can be more subtle (e.g., in the case of a posterior inferior cerebellar artery stroke, or Wallenberg's stroke), particularly early in the course of disease. The next step is the separation between central nervous system causes of dizziness and peripheral otologic causes of dizziness. This distinction is crucial, because it will determine the proper treatment course for the patient in most cases. Otologic causes of dizziness can be unilateral (e.g., benign positional vertigo, Menière's disease), bilateral (e.g., severe Menière's disease, bilateral vestibular hypofunction) and frequently are difficult to diagnose without follow-up testing (e.g., superior semicircular dehiscence syndrome). Standard vestibular testing may include electronystagmography or videonystagmography, posturography, rotary chair testing, and vestibular evoked myogenic potential tests. Imaging studies, particularly magnetic resonance imaging tests, are often helpful as well. History acquisition should focus on the character of the symptoms (to differentiate vertigo from disequilibrium), the time course of episodes of dizziness (how long they last and how frequently they occur), inciting factors (such as dietary factors, positional changes, or loud sound), relieving factors (such as medication, resting), and previous treatments attempted. As mentioned earlier, other localizing nonvestibular symptoms (e.g., hearing loss, fullness, tinnitus, headache) can be helpful in identifying the problematic ear in unilateral cases or cases of vestibular migraine.

Headache

Headaches, particularly those of a migrainous nature, are commonly associated with dizziness. Hence, questions related to location and progression of the pain, duration, severity, and constancy may help to show a possible connection between migraine headaches and vestibular symptoms, if present. Aggravating stimuli such as dietary factors (e.g., caffeine, chocolate) and bright lights should be identified; it is well known that dietary modification alone can result in significant improvement in the majority of migraine-induced vestibulopathy. It is significant that not all migraine vestibulopathy has classic migraine headache symptoms, and that dizziness itself may be the most obvious symptom to the patient of underlying pathophysiology that is likely to be migrainous in nature.

Neurological Symptoms

To help determine whether a central neurological rather than peripheral origin to the complaint is suspected, a series of less obvious (to the patient) questions should be included. These should cover such topics as mood (depression/anxiety/despair), memory or concentration losses, history of seizures, speech and swallowing changes, history of sleep disorder, reduced energy level, muscle weakness, change in dexterity, and "tingling" sensations that may be indicative of neuropathies. Referral to a neurologist is clearly indicated when such symptoms are present.

Dietary Factors

The most common associations between diet and imbalance are those of Menière's disease and migraine-induced vestibular dysfunction. In the case of Menière's disease, a high salt intake is known to be a trigger for episodes of aural fullness, dizziness, or hearing loss. A patient suspected of Menière's disease should have sodium levels estimated as accurately as possible, so that control over salt intake can proceed in a systematic fashion (<1500 mg/day of sodium is recommended for patients with Menière's disease). In cases of migraine-induced vestibular dysfunction, there is a long and detailed list of dietary factors possibly associated with migraine headaches and, in some patients, dizziness or disequilibrium. It is important to assess whether a patient's diet contains high levels of any known triggers (e.g., caffeine, chocolate), so that early identification of relevant dietary factors can be achieved. During treatment, patients will typically be asked to eliminate nearly all known migraine factors from their diet in order to determine whether a dietary trigger exists. Although compliance with this recommendation varies, it is essential to proper management and care of the patient with migraine vestibular dysfunction.

Genetic Hearing Loss

Like the vestibular questionnaire, this section may constitute an addendum to the primary case history. Alternatively, if a family history of hearing loss is evident, it is in the best interest of the patient and family to seek a genetic counselor for appropriate genetic testing. Such testing goes beyond mere curiosity, as it may be crucial in order to predict the likelihood of trait heritability in future offspring. This information can be initially screened with a series of questions such as: *What family members have hearing loss? What is thought to have caused their hearing loss? At what age was their hearing loss noticed? How severe is their hearing loss? How was/is their hearing loss treated (hearing aids, etc.)?* and the obvious question: *Has genetic testing been done?*

Amplification

Use of hearing aids or assistive technology and history of this use need to be detailed, including specific make/models and success with the various devices. This information has an obvious purpose of helping to determine further rehabilitative planning, but it also gives an accounting of hearing loss progression, which can indicate a need for an additional site of lesion testing.

Occupational/Military Hearing History

Aging and noise exposure are the two most common causes of permanent sensorineural hearing loss. Hearing loss caused by aging, or presbycusis (or presbyacusis), is suspected if the patient is in the sixth decade of life or older. Various conditions can cause premature presbycusis, such as diabetes and a variety of genetic factors. Noise exposure may confuse a diagnosis of presbycusis in a patient who is in his or her fifties. Similarly, degree of noise-induced hearing loss (NIHL) may be difficult to determine in elderly patients. Arriving at an accurate diagnosis for compensation cases and others, though difficult, is typically achieved by way of a noise history. Nonetheless, a thorough noise history will not define a degree of NIHL risk, because of variability of noise susceptibility across the human population. Eighty-five dBA exposure for an eight-hour work shift, which now serves as an "action level" for Occupational Safety and Health Administration (OSHA) purposes, does not protect 100% of the workforce from NIHL. As such, it represents a compromise between OSHA and private industry protecting most employees from NIHL if measures are taken when this action level is reached. Nonetheless, no action is mandated for workers exposed to 84 dBA, and a certain percentage will incur hearing loss with this exposure level. Therefore, detailed logging of noise history may have little or no bearing on the diagnosis in some cases, but in most cases extensive history of noise exposure will support the diagnosis of NIHL, as will a characteristic audiogram with 4-kHz "notch" configuration. However, the 4-kHz notch may also occur at 3 kHz or 6 kHz, and the notch can disappear entirely when exposure duration occurs over a lifetime.

Pediatric Case History

As in the genetic hearing loss and vestibular case histories, the pediatric questions are usually organized as a separate form or addendum to the original case history. Questions unique to this form include such topics as neonatal hearing screening results, changes in behavior, developmental delays/changes, pregnancy/birth history, and (pre)school performance. Most infants born in the United States have their hearing screened shortly after birth by an otoacoustic emissions test. If the infant fails the screening, a second screening is conducted. If the infant fails that test, a more thorough test, such as auditory brainstem response (ABR) testing, is required. Questions about follow-up testing should be asked when it is determined that screening tests were failed. Delayed speech and language development in an infant is a common reason for a hearing test referral. However, relative regression of speech and language production that was initially progressing according to schedule at an earlier age is also suggestive of (delayed onset) hearing loss. Behavioral changes might include the profile of a child who was once outgoing and cooperative and is now reticent or withdrawn, or perhaps a child who is now hyperactive and uncontrollable. Extreme behaviors in infants and children may indicate hearing loss or the more difficult to diagnose auditory processing disorder (APD). Birth history information may suggest a possible etiology, but can also indicate a need to test for an APD. For example, a newborn with hyperbilirubinemia or Rh incompatibility may pass initial newborn hearing tests but may fail APD testing in early childhood. A history of complications or maternal diseases during pregnancy can provide information about etiology (e.g., rubella), but may also have implications for subsequent pregnancies (e.g., cytomegalovirus infection). Last, below-average pre-school and school performance is a common indication for testing to rule out abnormal hearing testing or to identify the presence of an APD.

Miscellaneous Information

There is a wide variety of information that does not fall neatly into the above-listed categories, but it may be relevant to a diagnosis of hearing loss or imbalance. For example, in addition to a family history of hearing loss, a family history of craniofacial anomalies is important to identify, as it may suggest an underlying genetic etiology that the patient may not recognize. Similarly, a phenotypic severe pinna deformity may not necessarily be related to genetic causes or to branchial cleft developmental anomaly, as in the case of perinatal trauma (e.g., during delivery or other complications of pregnancy), yet such information may determine whether a patient requires genetic counseling. It is also important to recognize when contextual information may be less relevant to a patient's case. For example, the ability to localize sound sources in three-dimensional space is a relatively sophisticated and learned response that is difficult to evaluate in infants younger than 6 months. Thus, the apparent inability of a 3-month-old infant to localize sound sources should not be interpreted as cause for concern. On the other hand, inability to sound field localize at age 2 years when other hearing milestones have been reached might suggest unilateral hearing loss.

Similarly, assessment of hearing in the presence of background noise can be an indicator of bilateral high-frequency sensorineural hearing loss. Conversely, when hearing seems to improve in the presence of background noise, paracusis willisi (willisiana) is noted, and stapes fixation or conductive hearing loss due to other mechanisms may be suspected. History of tuberculosis treatment was once a common issue on the case history questionnaire, because of the use of streptomycin (or dihydrostreptomycin) as an ototoxic treatment of the disease. More broadly, treatment with ototoxic medications, especially aminoglycosides, should be noted; these agents are used commonly today for systemic infection as well as vestibule-ablative agents (e.g., chemical labyrinthectomy via intratympanic injection of gentamicin). Other illnesses, such as Lyme disease and chronic fatigue syndrome, may provide possible explanations and neural links to symptoms of imbalance or disequilibrium. If the patient has traveled abroad, there may have been exposure to malaria. Quinine, when used either as an anti-malarial or to cut heroine addiction, may cause (reversible) hearing loss and tinnitus. Rheumatoid arthritis may not directly cause hearing loss, but excessive aspirin ingestion may cause (reversible) hearing loss and tinnitus. A more sensitive area of questioning relates to one's social habits and should therefore be openly but delicately approached, without judgment. A history of sexually transmitted diseases might reveal a herpes virus infection (possible Ramsey Hunt syndrome) or history of syphilis, which can cause hearing loss or imbalance, as well as treatment for human immunodeficiency virus (HIV) disease, which may also cause disequilibrium. Other childhood illnesses may be covered under this category or elsewhere on the form. This line of questioning should include information regarding any history of mumps, whether or not it was contracted in childhood. In fact, there is higher risk of unilateral SNHL if mumps is contracted in later childhood or early adulthood than in early childhood. Likewise, CMV or toxoplasmosis may have been contracted in adulthood, which would have no bearing on hearing status but might have implications for a pregnancy in the family and the developing fetus.

Cranial Nerves

The majority of the 12 cranial nerves have functional relevance for hearing and/or balance. Cranial nerve I (olfactory) provides the sense of smell, which is intrinsically linked to the neural limbic systems and may affect general states of awareness and alertness, particularly in the presence of aversive stimuli. The cranial nerve II (optic) is a crucial part of the balance system that enables visual input to be integrated centrally during head movements. Cranial nerves III (oculomotor), IV (trochlear), and VI (abducens) are responsible for coordinated eye movement and are thereby linked to the facet of the vestibular system that allows ocular target fixation. Cranial nerve V (trigeminal), in addition to detection of facial sensation, serves the tensor tympani and tensor veli palatini muscles and may be important in Eustachian tube dysfunction. Cranial nerve VII (facial) serves the stapedius muscle as well as the chorda tympani nerve branch, in addition to facial movement. Given the intimate anatomic relationship between the facial nerve and the temporal bone, many otologic conditions affect facial function, and the consequences of facial paralysis are devastating. Cranial nerve VIII (vestibulocochlear) provides input from both the cochlear and vestibular portions of the inner ear to the brainstem. Cranial nerve IX (glossopharyngeal) is less obviously important for hearing, but can be affected in cases of retrocochlear pathology (e.g., glomus jugulare). Cranial nerve X (vagus) serves Arnold's branch in the ear canal and explains the occasional coughing reflex that occurs when the ear canal is stimulated. In addition, the vagus nerve gives rise to the recurrent laryngeal nerves, which are responsible for vocal function; hoarseness is often a presenting symptom in large lesions of the skull base. Cranial nerve XI (accessory) controls sternocleidomastoid muscle and trapezius muscle movement. These muscle groups are especially relevant to evaluation of vestibular-evoked myogenic potentials. Cranial nerve XII (hypoglossal) provides for ipsilateral tongue motion, which is not clearly required for proper hearing or balance. In cases of facial paralysis, the hypoglossal nerve may be used as a conduit (cranial nerve VII to XII crossover anastomosis) to reinnervate the facial nerve.

Cranial nerve evaluation can be accomplished with a variety of procedures. First, olfaction (I) is not often tested in hearing or balance cases. Vision (II) and pupil dilation are grossly measured, as is peripheral vision to determine possible tunnel vision, which develops in retinitis pigmentosa and Usher's syndrome. Oculomotion (III, IV, VI) is tested by having the patient look in all directions (e.g., following a finger) and tracking appropriately when the head is moved from side to side (keeping the eyes on target with horizontal head movement). Sensation to a cotton ball at the three divisions of the trigeminal (V) nerve on each side of the face will give an estimate of this function; further use of sharp or dull stimuli provides further information. Testing contraction of the tensor tympani muscle as an immittance procedure will help with this determination. Facial symmetry on grimacing, bilateral eye hydration, and bilateral salivation will give evidence of facial (VI) nerve function. Audition (VIII) is tested crudely with whisper, finger rubbing, and tuning fork tests. Balance (VIII) can be grossly assessed with finger-to-nose pointing, standing heel-to-toe (eyes open and closed), and station and gait observations. Vocal quality, gag reflex (bilateral), centered uvula, salivation, and pharyngeal arch position are maintained by the glossopharyngeal (IX) and vagus (X) nerves. Sternocleidomastoid (SCM) can be roughly assessed with head turn to right and left, which gives some measure of the spinal accessory (XI) nerve. Finally, hypoglossal (XII) function can be screened with tongue centering and extension movements.

OVERVIEW OF BASIC HEARING/BALANCE ASSESSMENT PROCEDURES

Otoscopic Examination

Examining the ear canals and visualizing the tympanic membranes must precede all other procedures. Observation of cerumen or other ear canal debris should be noted, even when it does not result in impaction or blockage. A small amount of wax or debris may not affect hearing but can affect testing, such as air-caloric irrigation procedures during electronystagmography (ENG) or videonystagmography (VNG) assessment. Osteomas and exostoses may be evident also without the patient's knowledge or any hearing impairment. A normal "light reflex" generally means a healthy eardrum and middle ear, but observation of scar tissue, monomeric condition, or vasculature may be noted despite this normal finding. Suspected perforation is confirmed with pneumatic procedures, including tympanometry. Water-caloric irrigations should be excluded from the ENG/VNG test sequence when tympanic membrane perforation is found, or when a perforation has recently been repaired with tympanoplasty techniques.

Audiometric Evaluation

If the case history is the "first test," then the audiometric evaluation is the second test. Although much of what is found during the case history will determine which tests are necessary, in the majority of cases a complete hearing test is advised. Obviously, if cerumen impaction is seen during otoscopic examination, removal of the obstruction should precede other procedures, but additional disorders (such as mild high-frequency hearing loss) will be found only if a complete audiogram is taken. However, the patient may elect to have only the wax removed, in which case the case history information (e.g., "plugged ear during showering") determines the diagnosis and treatment. The basic audiometric evaluation should consist of the following procedures: pure tone air conduction threshold (125–8 kHz octave frequencies); pure tone bone conduction thresholds (250–6 kHz, or where hearing loss occurs); speech recognition (reception) threshold (SRT); word recognition score (WRS); tympanogram; acoustic reflex thresholds (.5k, 1k, 2k), and reflex decay. This is somewhat "thorough"; however, it is also limiting. For example, pure tone testing spans only frequencies of speech production, and so the full range of normal hearing (20–20 kHz) is never tested. Subtle lesions (e.g., small tumor) on the auditory nerve may affect only ultra-audiometric frequencies, and the "comprehensive audiometric evaluation" would not identify this disorder. Bone conduction testing is limited in its frequency band as well as its calibration stability, making this the least reliable of the procedures. Speech and word testing are routinely conducted with the use of "monitored live voice" (MLV), which adds speaker/tester variability to the procedure. Recorded versions of speech and word tests are time consuming to administer, but have greater cross-clinic validity. Still, they are not routinely used in busy clinics. The tympanogram is an objective measure, but not all instruments are capable of reliably testing infants who require a higher frequency probe tone for accurate measurement of eardrum mobility. Measurement of the acoustic reflex, also an objective procedure, can require some interpretation to determine threshold as well as degree of decay. Nonetheless, the audiometric evaluation, when understood in the context of these limitations, gives sufficient "second test" information to determine need for the next level of testing.

Vestibular Testing

The basic vestibular assessment should include ENG or VNG, vestibular evoked myogenic potential (VEMP), a test for perilymphatic fistula, and an auditory brainstem response (ABR) test. To be sure, many clinics will include posturography and a rotary chair. Most clinics do not routinely include the VEMP procedure because they lack the CPT code, although an electromyogenic (EMG) code would satisfy this requirement. Furthermore, standardization of the VEMP protocol is still somewhat under revision, making this an experimental procedure in many clinics. Some clinics may require electrocochleography (ECoG), especially when cochlear hydrops or classical Menière's is suspected. Including the ABR test as part of the vestibular work-up is in order to identify the small percentage of imbalance cases that are secondary to tumor or neurological disease. ABR may provide a sufficient screening procedure to determine the need for further (radiologic) work-up. In addition, the ABR provides a physiology study, which should always supplement the anatomical result provided by MRI or CT scan. It is often reasoned that an MRI is necessary for surgical purposes, so additional information the ABR test may provide is debatable, or when it is used to screen for tumors, if positive, the MRI will be ordered anyway. However, the physiological information gleaned from the ABR test may indeed help in the diagnosis. For example, in rare cases of a seventh nerve internal auditory canal tumor that is not growing or impinging on the eighth cranial nerve bundle, ABR would be negative, whereas MRI might suggest acoustic neuroma. More detailed MRI study might then give the more accurate diagnosis of a facial nerve tumor. It might then be advisable to "monitor" the mass periodically with ABR, and should baseline measures (interpeak latencies; latency shift with rapid stimulus rate) change, MRI would be repeated.

CONCLUSION

In summary, the elements of the case history form provide an organized guide and format by which information can be acquired. A thorough and accurate recording of case history information by a skilled diagnostician will lead to a relevant differential diagnosis and suggest further tests that will narrow the diagnosis. The astute clinician should be aware that multiple pathologies may coexist in a single patient, and that simple solutions are not always the most appropriate or effective. Hence, the case history is the critical foundation upon which appropriate medical care can be based. As such, the case history should form the cornerstone of all interactions between patients and care providers.

CHAPTER 2

Medical Diseases and Disorders of the Ear

Erik H. Waldman
Johns Hopkins University School of Medicine

Carmen C. Brewer
National Institutes of Health

When a patient presents with hearing loss, tinnitus, vertigo, or other otologic symptoms, determination of the underlying etiology is typically the first goal. Diagnosis is the key element guiding (1) medical management of underlying disease, (2) prognosis, (3) referral to other specialists, and (4) rehabilitation. Differential diagnosis is the process of determining which of several probable diseases or disorders account for the patient's signs and symptoms. Fundamental to the differential strategy is a thorough knowledge of the prevalence, presentation, and important diagnostic features of the myriad causes of hearing loss and related symptoms. Efficiency is achieved with clinical algorithms, or triage, in which an orderly sequence of data-driven decisions leads to diagnosis and management. The diagnostic evaluation begins with a detailed patient history and physical examination (H&P) (see chap. 1). Based on the findings of the H&P, treatment may ensue immediately, or a series of diagnostic tests may be ordered. These include auditory and vestibular assessments, medical laboratory tests, imaging studies, and other electrophysiological measures. Findings on the initial tests may quickly lead to diagnosis or may indicate the need for additional testing. In some cases, response or lack of response to treatment may contribute to the diagnostic process.

Auditory and vestibular signs and symptoms can be caused by or occur in conjunction with a variety of diseases and disorders. Table 2–1 provides an overview of the major causes of otopathologic conditions affecting the outer, middle, and inner ear as well as the central auditory pathways. Some of these causes are addressed individually in other chapters (aging, noise induced hearing loss, ototoxicity, genetics, Ménière's disease). This chapter provides an overview of infectious, inflammatory/immune mediated, traumatic, neoplastic, and idiopathic

TABLE 2-1
Major Categories of Otologic Diseases and Disorders

Cause	Examples
Congenital/Hereditary	Enlarged vestibular aqueduct
	Syndromic hearing loss
Infectious	Otitis media and related sequelae
	Chronic suppurative otitis media
Inflammatory/Immune mediated	Autoimmune inner ear disease
	Cogan's syndrome
Traumatic	Temporal bone fracture
	Noise induced hearing loss
Neoplastic	Vestibular schwannoma
	Squamous cell carcinoma
Idiopathic	Bell's Palsy
	Meniere's disease

causes of otologic diseases and disorders. Presenting signs and symptoms, pertinent laboratory and imaging findings, audiologic results, and medical management are reviewed. Table 2–1 identifies major categories of otologic disease with examples.

DIAGNOSTIC TESTS

Imaging Studies

Since the first observation of the x-ray by Wilhelm Roentgen in 1895, the ability to image the human body has progressed from that of a gross image to one of exquisite and precise detail (Novelline, 2004). Plain x-rays have limited use in modern otology. The advent of computerized tomography (CT) in the 1980s and magnetic resonance imaging (MRI) in the early 1990s revolutionized the ability to examine the small and complex structures of the ear. CT is the method of choice for imaging bony structures and MRI is best for viewing soft tissue and fluid. Together, these methods complement each other, allowing visualization of normal anatomy and pathologic processes.

CT uses a highly focused x-ray beam that is rotated around the body in a spiral configuration. This beam is differentially absorbed by air, water, soft tissue, and bone. On CT images, dense structures such as bone appear white, less dense tissues are darker, and air is black (Novelline, 2004). Computerized algorithms generate two-dimensional slice images based on absorption values. Routine temporal bone CT uses a slice thickness of 0.5 to 1.5 mm and is conducted in both the axial (horizontal) and coronal (frontal) planes of section. Bone algorithms, which provide the sharpest bone margins, are most useful for examining the temporal bone. Intravenous (IV) iodinated contrast media can be used to delineate blood vessels and enhance vascular tumors; however, contrast is not routine for most temporal bone studies. CT is most useful for delineating anatomic changes,

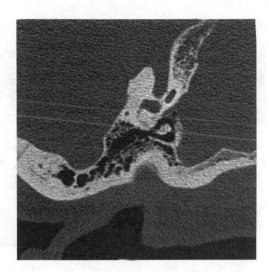

FIGURE 2–1.   Normal CT appearance of temporal bone.

whether they are related to conductive hearing loss (CHL), inflammatory or
metastatic bone destruction, or trauma (Tucci & Gray, 2000; Butman, Patronis,
& Kim, 2006).

MRI does not involve x-ray radiation at all. Instead the patient is placed in the
bore of a very strong magnet. The MR scanner presents a series of pulsed radio
waves and measures responding radio waves emitted by various tissues. The emitted signals result from the interaction of hydrogen nuclei (protons) with these radiofrequency pulses. The intensity of the resultant MR signal is dependent on the
number of free protons in the tissue being imaged and on the magnetic relaxation
times, T_1 and T_2 (Novelline, 2004). T_1- and T_2-weighted images provide a different appearance to the same tissue. On a T_1-weighted image, fluid is dark, fat is
bright, and tissues have an intermediate signal. On a T_2-weighted image, fluid is
brighter than fat, and white matter is darker than gray matter. Pathological
processes may alter the number of free protons, causing the lesion to look different from normal tissue. Images obtained with a T_1 weighting can be enhanced with
a contrast agent such as gadolinium. Planes of section on MRI include axial, coronal, and sagittal. MRI is most useful in evaluating sensorineural hearing loss, per-
ineural invasion, and intracranial extension of disease (Tucci & Gray, 2000;
Butman, Patronis, & Kim, 2006).

Angiography, a technique in which the vascular system is imaged by intravenous injection of iodinated agents, may be used as a supplemental diagnostic
study or to preoperatively examine the blood supply to a tumor. Angiography is
most often used when there is a highly vascular lesion. Newer technology is allowing CT and MR to effectively image the vascular structures. These algorithms
are called CT angiography (CTA) and MR angiography/venography (MRA/
MRV). Nuclear imaging measures, such as positron emission tomography (PET)
and nuclear scintigraphy (i.e., bone scans), are not often used in otologic diagno-

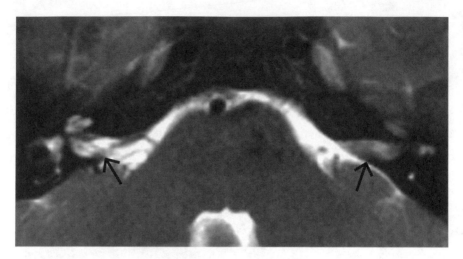

FIGURE 2–2.   Normal appearance of auditory, vestibular, and facial nerves in the internal auditory canal (arrow).

sis. However, they can be useful in the diagnosis of osteomyelitis of the skull base/temporal bone or in evaluating a patient in whom there is suspicion of tumor recurrence or metastasis.

Laboratory Tests

Laboratory tests of blood and urine can provide additional insight into the etiology of hearing loss. The most commonly used tests are listed in Table 2–2. These tests are selected based on patient history and physician suspicion of underlying metabolic, hematologic, infectious, and immune system disorders. When a genetic origin is suspected, testing for specific mutations (e.g., Connexin-26 mutations, Pendred syndrome gene mutations) can be carried out. Further description of genetic testing is presented in Chapter 4.

INFECTIOUS CAUSES OF OTOLOGIC DISEASE

The term *infection* refers to localized or systemic invasion and multiplication of microorganisms in body tissues. Infectious diseases are caused by microbes (bacteria, viruses, and parasites) and large organisms (fungi and flukes). Infections of the outer, middle, and inner ear among the most frequent problems seen by the otologist. Treatment is directed at eliminating the offending microbe. Initial antimicrobial agents are selected based on their efficacy against the most common infecting organisms. When an infection is unresponsive (refractory) to treatment, laboratory culture of fluid or tissue to identify the causative microbe will allow specific antimicrobial therapy to be used.

External Ear

Acute otitis externa, referred to as "swimmer's ear" in cases of recreational water exposure, is the most common external ear infection. This bacterial infection occurs most often in warm, humid climates and may be precipitated by accumulation of moisture, local trauma, and bacterial exposure. Early signs and symptoms include external auditory canal (EAC) edema and pruritis (itching). As the infectious process progresses, the epithelium of the EAC becomes erythematous (reddened because of capillary congestion) and stenotic or completely swollen shut. Otorrhea (drainage from the ear) can range from clear and odorless to seropurulent secretions. The patient complains of characteristic pain on tragal manipulation that ranges from mild to intense. Hearing is affected when the ear canal becomes stenotic. The most common pathogens cultured from the EAC are *Pseudomonas aeruginosa*, Peptostreptococcus species, and *Staphylococcus aureus*. Medical management includes control of infection with topical or systemic antibiotics and avoidance of precipitating conditions (Balkany and Ress, 1998).

Chronic otitis externa is a persistent low-grade inflammatory process characterized by atrophic or excoriated skin in the EAC and lack of cerumen. The chief complaint of patients with this condition is intense pruritis. Treatment for chronic otitis externa consists of removal of EAC debris and steroid drops (Balkany and Ress, 1998).

Necrotizing otitis externa, also known as malignant otitis externa, is a rapidly progressive and potentially lethal form of external otitis. The disease usually man-

TABLE 2–2
Common Laboratory Tests for the Diagnosis of Otopathologic Conditions

Test Name	Purpose
Complete blood count (CBC)	Evaluate for anemia, leukemia, infection and other blood related disorders
Erythocyte sedimentation rate (ESR)	Evaluate for inflammation or infection
C-reactive protein	Evaluate for inflammation or infection
Antinuclear antibodies (ANA)	Evaluate for lupus and other autoimmune disorders
Rheumatoid factor	Evaluate for rheumatoid arthritis and other autoimmune disorders
Lipid panel	Evaluate for elevated triglycerides and cholesterol
Vitamin B12	Evaluate for neuropathy
Hemoglobin A1C	Evaluate for diabetes mellitus
Thyroid function tests (TSH, T3, T4)	Evaluate for thyroid disease
Blood urea nitrogen (BUN) and creatinine; supplement with urinalysis	Evaluate for kidney disease
Virus titers (cytomegalovirus, rubella, herpes simplex, HIV)	Evaluate for viruses associated with hearing loss
Fluorescent treponemal antibody absorption (FTA-ABS)	Evaluate for syphilis
Lyme titer	Evaluate for Lyme disease
Genetic Tests	Evaluate for specific gene mutations in connexin–26 (GJB2) or the Pendred Syndrome gene (PDS)

ifests in those with compromised immune systems (diabetics, cancer patients, etc.). The classic presentation consists of persistent and disproportionate otalgia (ear pain) that is worse at night and granulation tissue on the floor of the EAC at the bony cartilaginous junction. As the infection spreads beyond the soft tissues of the EAC, there is resultant osteomyelitis of the bony canal and surrounding skull base, with eventual extension into the central skull base and even the contralateral temporal bone. Signs of progression along the skull base include trismus (lockjaw), facial nerve paralysis, and involvement of cranial nerves IX, X, and XI (glossopharyngeal, vagus, and accessory nerves). Imaging studies such as nuclear bone scans may confirm the diagnosis. High-resolution CT is helpful in evaluating the extent of disease extension and the success of therapeutic intervention. The most common pathogen cultured from this infection is *P. aeruginosa*. Treatment with oral and/or intravenous antibiotics can be intense and long-term, based on the extent of the infection (Parisier, Kimmelman, & Hanson, 1997; Balkany & Ress, 1998).

Otomycosis is a fungal ear infection. Patients experience intense pruritis and may also complain of aural discomfort, hearing loss, tinnitus, or otorrhea. The appearance on otoscopic examination includes fungal bodies when *Aspergillus* is the causative agent or copious white, soft cheesy material seen with *Candida* infections. Treatment includes thorough, repeated cleaning, acidification of the ear canal, and topical antifungal medications (Balkany & Ress, 1998).

Ramsay-Hunt syndrome is caused by the herpes zoster virus and is a variant of herpes zoster oticus. The clinical presentation is rapid onset of facial paralysis associated with eruption of skin vesicles in the concha and lateral EAC and along the sensory course of the facial nerve. Auditory symptoms include subjective hearing loss, hyperacusis, and tinnitus. Sensorineural hearing loss (SNHL) and/or vertigo resulting from involvement of the vestibular and/or cochlear branches of the auditory nerve occur in 75% (Peitersen, 2002). Audiometric presentation can include normal hearing, high-frequency SNHL, or, less often, severe to profound SNHL. Hearing thresholds improve in most cases, with a greater prognosis of recovery in those with losses limited to the high frequencies (Wayman, Pham, Byl, & Adour, 1990). Spontaneous recovery of facial palsy occurs in only 21–31% (Peitersen, 1992). Treatment regimens include systemic antiviral therapy and corticosteroids (Rubinstein & Gantz, 1997).

Middle Ear and Mastoid

Otitis media is an infection, or inflammation, of the middle ear, usually with fluid (effusion) behind an intact tympanic membrane (Gates, 1997). Acute otitis media (AOM) occurs frequently in children and is the most common infection for which antibacterial agents are prescribed in the United States (American Academy of Pediatrics Subcommittee on Management of Acute Otitis Media, 2004). When treated successfully with medications or surgery, it is cured or controlled, but complications of the disease may spread to involve intracranial or intratemporal structures. Otitis media terminology can be confusing. Table 2–3 summarizes the common definitions associated with this disease.

TABLE 2–3
Terminology for Otitis Media

Otitis media without effusion	Infection or inflammation of middle ear mucosa/tympanic membrane without middle ear effusion.
Acute otitis media	Purulent infection and inflammation of the middle ear space, usually with rapid onset. Also known as acute suppurative or purulent otitis media.
Otitis media with effusion	Middle ear effusion without evidence of purulence or other signs of infection. Also known as secretory, nonsuppurative, or serous otitis media.
Chronic otitis media with effusion	Accumulation of inflammatory fluid in the middle ear without other signs of inflammation, usually >6 weeks, >30 days.
Chronic suppurative otitis media with or without cholesteatoma	Chronic middle ear and mastoid infection often associated with otorrhea through a TM perforation or tympanostomy tube. May or may not be associated with cholesteatoma. Also known as chronic suppurative otitis media and mastoiditis, chronic purulent otitis media, chronic otomastoiditis

Acute Otitis Media

The certain diagnosis of AOM requires all of the following: (1) acute onset, (2) middle ear effusion (MEE), and (3) signs and symptoms of middle ear inflammation. Symptoms of AOM include pain that is often disruptive to sleep, irritability, otorrhea, and/or fever. MEE appears as fullness or bulging of the tympanic membrane (TM), reduced TM mobility, air-fluid level behind an intact TM, or purulent otorrhea through a TM perforation or tympanostomy tube. Inflammation may appear as erythema of the TM or in some cases as bluish-red blisters on the TM. When blisters are present, the ailment is termed bullous myringitis. Tympanometry may be used to corroborate the diagnosis, but pneumatic otoscopy is often sufficient (Bluestone, 1998, American Academy of Pediatrics Subcommittee on Management of Acute Otitis Media, 2004).

The seasonal incidence of AOM parallels that of upper respiratory infections (URI), occurring least during the summer months. AOM occurs most often in infants (Bluestone, 1998). By 3 years of age, almost 50% of children have experienced three or more episodes of AOM and 16% have had 6 or more episodes (Teele, Klein, & Rosner, 1989). There are a number of well-known risk factors for AOM, including male gender, premature birth, genetic predisposition, and Native American or Inuit ethnicity. Individuals with anatomic defects involving craniofacial structures, such as cleft palate, are at increased risk, as are those with congenital or acquired immune system deficiencies. Household situations such as greater number of siblings, passive smoke exposure, family history of recurrent OM, day-care attendance, and even supine bottle feeding may be associated with a higher risk of AOM. In addition, low socioeconomic groups where living conditions include crowding and poor sanitation are at increased risk (American Academy of Pediatrics Subcommittee on Management of Acute Otitis Media, 2004).

Management of AOM begins with controlling pain (otalgia) with analgesics. Antibiotics are routinely prescribed for children less than 6 months of age, whether the AOM diagnosis is certain or uncertain, and for children 6 months to 2 years of age when the diagnosis is certain (American Academy of Pediatrics Subcommittee on Management of Acute Otitis Media, 2004). A bacteriologic diagnosis may be necessary in rare cases, especially if the illness is refractory to initial treatment. This involves sampling the fluid from the middle ear, a process known as tympanocentesis. TM rupture may also produce material suitable for laboratory analysis.

The most common pathogens in AOM are *Streptococcus pneumoniae, Haemophilus influenzae*, and *Moraxella catarrhalis* (Klein, 1994). Typically, a middle ear effusion will persist after the proper treatment of AOM. Effusions vary in duration, lasting 2 weeks in 60–70%, 4 weeks in 40%, and 8 weeks in 10–25 % of cases (Teele, Klein, & Rosner, 1989). The best therapy, however, is prevention, which involves controlling risk factors when possible, proper vaccinations, and occasional surgical management. Surgical management is necessary and is indicated when infection has gone beyond the borders of the middle ear (brain, facial nerve, labyrinth) and usually begins with myringotomy (cutting a hole in the eardrum) with tympanostomy tube insertion.

Otitis Media with Effusion

OME indicates a situation where the middle ear is filled with fluid, but typically without signs or symptoms of acute ear infection other than hearing loss. The TM may be dull in appearance, with distinctly impaired mobility evident on pneumatic otoscopy, or an air-fluid meniscus (and sometimes obvious air bubbles) may be visible through the intact TM. TM erythema is not a common finding in OME and is seen in only 5% of cases. Pneumatic otoscopy should be the primary diagnostic method for OME, and it should be distinguished from AOM. Pneumatic otoscopy has a sensitivity of 94% and a specificity of 80% compared with tympanometry, which has a sensitivity of 81% and a specificity of 74% (Bluestone, 2003). Still, in some cases proper diagnosis is provided only by myringotomy with direct examination of the middle ear contents.

Symptoms of OME in infants may be masked by upper respiratory infection or teething, but may include mild, intermittent ear pain, which involves ear rubbing, excessive irritability, and sleep disturbances in this population. Failure of the infant to respond appropriately to voices or environmental sounds generally indicates hearing loss that accompanies recurrent AOM with persistent MEE between episodes. In older children, problems with school performance, balance problems, unexplained clumsiness, and/or delayed speech language development are other signs of the process (American Academy of Family Physicians; American Academy of Otolaryngology—Head and Neck Surgery; American Academy of Pediatrics Subcommittee on Otitis Media with Effusion, 2004).

A child who is not at risk for developmental delay should be managed with watchful waiting for 3 months from the date of effusion onset (if known) or diagnosis (if onset is unknown). In cases of bilateral effusion, however, hearing loss can be very significant, and the potential impact of this loss on language development prompts more immediate treatment measures. OME is usually self-limited; 75–90% of effusions resolve spontaneously within 3 months. OME of greater than 3 months' duration resolves spontaneously in 30% over the next 6–12 months (Bluestone, 2003; American Academy of Family Physicians; American Academy of Otolaryngology—Head and Neck Surgery; American Academy of Pediatrics Subcommittee on Acute Otitis Media with Effusion, 2004). Hearing testing is recommended when OME persists for 3 months or longer or any time language delay, learning problems, or a significant hearing loss is suspected in a child with OME. Language testing should be conducted on children with identified hearing loss. Hearing thresholds with OME range from 0 to 55 dB HL, with the 50th percentile at ~25 dB HL and 20% exceeding 35 dB HL (Fria, Cantekin, & Eichler, 1985).

Risk factors that decrease the chance of spontaneous resolution include OME onset in summer or fall, hearing loss greater than 30 dB HL in the better ear, history of prior tympanostomy tubes, and not having had adenoidectomy. Surgical treatment for OME is myringotomy with tympanostomy tube insertion. It is the most common surgical procedure in the western world. Tympanostomy tube insertion is often based on hearing status, with otalgia, unexplained sleep disturbance, recurrent AOM, and developmental delay as relative indicators (American Academy of Family Physicians; American Academy of Otolaryngology—Head and Neck Surgery; American Academy of Pediatrics Subcommittee on Acute Otitis Media with Effusion, 2004).

Chronic Suppurative Otitis Media

Chronic middle ear and mastoid infection with otorrhea through a TM perforation or tympanostomy tube is termed chronic suppurative otitis media. It often occurs in the setting of a cholesteatoma, which is an inclusion of keratinizing squamous epithelium that proliferates within the temporal bone. *Cholesteatoma* is a misnomer, as it is not made of cholesterol and it is not a tumor. It essentially represents skin growing in the wrong place. It is significant in that it may erode bone and can be highly aggressive and destructive. Growth can be stimulated by infection, inflammation, or pressure from retained keratin (Parisier, Kimmelman, & Hanson, 1997).

Cholesteatomas are classified into types based on their origin (Table 2–4). A congenital cholesteatoma grows behind an intact tympanic membrane, arising from an aberrant embryonic inclusion of squamous epithelium in the middle ear. By the strictest of definitions, there should be a negative history of otitis media or other factors associated with acquired cholesteatomas. Congenital cholesteatomas occur more often in males (3:1), with a mean age at presentation of 4.5 years. On otoscopic inspection, a pearly white mass is observed behind an intact tympanic membrane, most often in the anterosuperior mesotympanum (Friedberg, 1998).

TABLE 2–4
Types of Cholesteatomas

Type	Mechanism	Preceding event
Congenital	Embryonic inclusion of undifferentiated squamous epithelium in middle ear	Embryonic cell deposit
Primary acquired	Invagination of the tympanic membrane to form an epithelial lined cyst that accumulates keratin	Eustachian tube dysfunction and persistent negative middle ear pressure
Secondary acquired	Ingrowth of keratinizing squamous epithelium through a tympanic membrane perforation	Tympanic membrane perforation
Iatrogenic	Inadvertent deposit of squamous epithelium in middle ear space	Surgical procedure

Primary acquired cholesteatoma, the most common type, occurs secondary to chronic eustachian tube dysfunction and the resultant persistent negative middle ear pressure. The tympanic membrane retracts and eventually folds in on itself to form a pocket in which keratin debris is trapped and an epithelial lined cyst forms. Secondary acquired cholesteatoma arises as the result of ingrowth of keratinizing epithelium through a tympanic membrane perforation. Iatrogenic cholesteatoma can occur as the result of a surgical procedure, such as a myringotomy, in which squamous epithelium is unintentionally deposited in the middle ear space (Parisier, Kimmelman, & Hanson, 1997).

The most common complication of cholesteatoma is conductive hearing loss. This may be caused by ossicular erosion, or the obstructive effect of the cholesteatoma mass blocking transmission of sound. When cholesteatoma extends to the otic capsule, mixed or sensorineural hearing loss and/or vertigo may occur. Additional and serious complications include facial nerve paralysis and intracranial infections resulting from erosion of the mastoid or middle ear tegmen (Chole & Choo, 1998). Left untreated, cholesteatomas can lead to epidural abscess, meningitis, and even death.

Clinical diagnosis of cholesteatoma is often made on otoscopic and otomicroscopic inspection. Patients with acquired cholesteatomas typically present with a history of recurrent foul-smelling otorrhea and hearing loss. There is often accumulation of granulation tissue or aural polyps in a tympanic membrane perforation or retraction site. CT scans allow visualization of bone erosion. Mastoid surgery is the means by which cholesteatoma is eradicated. The primary surgical goal is to rid the ear of the cholesteatoma itself. Secondarily, reconstruction of the tympanic membrane and /or ossicles may be necessary to preserve or improve hearing.

Inner Ear

The inner ear is that part of the hearing mechanism that incorporates the cochlea and vestibular structures into what is known as the labyrinth. As such, it is responsible for sensorineural hearing (cochlea) and responding to linear and angular acceleration

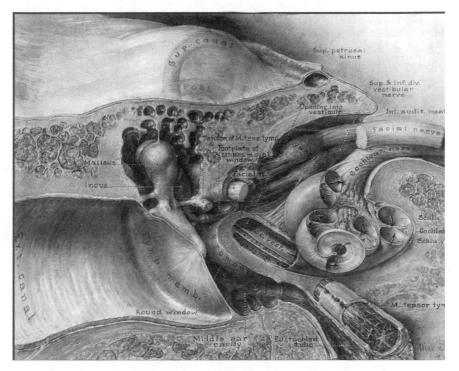

FIGURE 2–3.   Cross-sectional view through the ear, showing the external, middle, and inner ear anatomy, in addition to the neural structures leading to/from the brainstem (Drawing supplied courtesy of the Max Brödel Archives at the Department of Art Applied to Medicine, Johns Hopkins School of Medicine, Baltimore, MD).

(vestibule/semicircular canals). Infections affecting the inner ear are most commonly caused by direct extension from the middle ear; that is, as a complication of acute otitis media or chronic suppurative otitis media with cholesteatoma. Congenitally acquired illnesses and complications of meningitis may also affect the inner ear. These infections are generally caused by viruses, bacteria, or protozoa. They are quite worrisome, as they often cause significant and even permanent sensorineural hearing loss and vertigo, or may lead to meningitis, brain abscess, or death.

Acquired Inner Ear Infection

Labyrinthitis (acute inner ear infection) as a direct extension from the middle ear is the most worrisome of the intratemporal complications of otitis media. It has a high association with hearing loss and intracranial complications. Serous labyrinthitis is caused by the diffusion of toxins from the middle ear into the inner ear. Vestibular symptoms (vertigo) tend to be pronounced. Treatment involves antibiotic agents aimed at typical bacterial agents for AOM, possible myringotomy with or without tympanostomy tube placement, and close observation for development of suppurative labyrinthitis.

Suppurative labyrinthitis is caused by frank purulence within the labyrinth and implies bacterial invasion. Sudden onset of severe vertigo, disequilibrium, deep-seated pain, nausea, vomiting, and sensorineural hearing loss are the telltale signs. Meningitis can be a result of such a condition. MRI and CT imaging can aid in the diagnosis. Treatment involves immediate tympanocentesis and myringotomy with tympanostomy tube insertion, intravenous antibiotics, close observation in the hospital, and treatment and/or prevention of meningitis (Eisele & McQuone, 2000).

Labyrinthitis ossificans, usually an end result of meningitis, involves fibrous replacement or new bone formation in part, or in the entire labyrinth. The end result is labyrinthine dysfunction, and usually sensorineural hearing loss. Steroid therapy given in a timely fashion may prevent this unfortunate progression, but treatment of meningitis usually focuses on bacterial control, and steroids can decrease immunocompetence (Hartnick, Kim, Chute, & Parisier, 2001). Early cochlear implantation may be necessary to avoid complete ossification of the labyrinth and inability to implant the ear.

In the United States, most children are effectively vaccinated against measles and mumps. However, these illnesses may still cause devastating infections. Mumps is associated with a unilateral profound SNHL occurring without vestibular symptoms. Measles and mumps may cause meningoencephalitis leading to inner ear ossification and sensorineural hearing loss similar to that caused by bacterial meningitis. Treatment for actively infected cases involves supportive care. Prevention through vaccination is key.

Congenital Inner Ear Infection

Congenital inner ear infections are those acquired by the fetus either in utero or at the time of birth. Cytomegalovirus is the main etiologic agent; *Toxoplasma gondii* (a protozoan), *Treponema pallidum* (the agent responsible for syphilis), rubella virus, and herpes simplex virus are the other main causative agents. Cytomegalovirus is the most common nongenetic cause of early-onset SNHL in infants and children (Bluestone, 2003); it affects approximately 1% of live newborns in the United States. Symptoms range from asymptomatic to classic inclusion disease, which may include mental retardation, severe to profound hearing loss, ocular problems, language or learning difficulties, and/or jaundice. Extensive inclusion disease is seen in about 10% of infected neonates. The other 90% of patients may go on to develop significant disabilities, including delayed-onset, progressive SNHL. Isolation of CMV from a newborn's urine is the gold standard for confirming infection. Treatment and prevention have been slow to develop, but active research is ongoing. Periodic audiologic screening is necessary, as the hearing loss may not become evident immediately and is usually progressive.

Congenital *Toxoplasma gondii* infection is also acquired transplacentally. Cats are the natural reservoir of the protozoa. It infects mothers as they ingest *Toxoplasma* cysts in undercooked meat or oocysts in food contaminated with cat feces. Identifying antibodies against the organism provides confirmation of the diagnosis. Spiramycin (antibiotic) therapy is given to actively infected mothers, and long-term treatment with multiple agents is recommended for infected neonates. Neonates infected are at risk for SNHL, chorioretinitis, central nervous system involvement, and even encephalitis and death.

Congenital syphilis is caused by *Treponema pallidum* infection acquired transplacentally. Classical congenital symptoms include SNHL, interstitial keratitis, notched incisors, and nasal septal perforation. Penicillin remains the treatment of choice, with systemic steroids for hearing stabilization as needed. Specific laboratory tests (FTA-ABS and the Western blot assay) assist in diagnosis. Congenital rubella viral infection, on the other hand, produces a triad of cataracts, heart defects, and congenital hearing loss that can be progressive in nature. Widespread administration of rubella vaccine has all but eradicated the disease from developed nations.

Systemic Infection

Lyme disease is a multisystem tick-borne infection caused by the spirochete *Borellia burgdorferi*. Early localized infection is characterized by a distinctive, expanding bull's-eye erythematous rash at the site of inoculation known as erythema migrans. The early disseminated stage results from hematologic or lymphatic spread to other organ systems with resultant neurologic, rheumatologic, and cardiac involvement. The third stage, chronic disseminated disease, can occur months to years after infection and may cause chronic arthritis; peripheral neuropathies; and memory, concentration, and sleep disturbances (Steere, 1989; Moscatello, Worden, Nadelman, Wormser, & Lucente, 1991).

Otologic manifestations of Lyme disease include acute facial palsy, vestibular symptoms ranging from positional vertigo to Ménière's-like attacks, otalgia, and tinnitus. Hearing loss has been described in 1.5–44% (Logigian, Kaplan, and Steere, 1990; Quinn, Boucher, and Booth, 1997). Diagnosis of Lyme disease is based on clinical presentation and history and is confirmed by serologic antibody testing for *B. burgdorferi*. Antibiotics and steroids are used for treatment (Nadol & Merchant, 1998).

Acquired syphilis is caused by the spirochete *Treponema pallidum*. It is contracted through sexual contact and may affect the outer, middle, or inner ear, usually in its late stages (Klemm & Wollina, 2004). Osteitis and destructive larger lesions, known as gummas, may result in TM perforation, chronic otitis media, and conductive hearing loss. Inner ear involvement results probably from induction of endolymphatic hydrops and may cause SNHL (Fayad & Linthicum, 1999). When endolymphatic hydrops is present, ocular deviation is seen with positive or negative pressure in the external auditory canal. This phenomenon is known as Hennebert's sign. Syphilis is diagnosed usually by high clinical suspicion, biopsy, and laboratory testing. Treatment consists of antibiotics with corticosteroids to manage SNHL.

INFLAMMATORY AND AUTOIMMUNE EAR DISEASE

Generalized inflammatory conditions and autoimmune illnesses occurring in the absence of infection may also affect the otologic system. These illnesses are relatively rare as causes of ear disease but extremely important to identify. They may affect the ear only, as in autoimmune inner ear disease (AIED), or have typical systemic symptoms, as exemplified by sarcoidosis, Wegener's granulomatosis, or polychondritis. Systemic lupus erythematosus, rheumatoid arthritis, Cogan syndrome, and generalized vasculitides may also affect the ear.

AIED is characterized by rapidly progressive (weeks to months) bilateral sensorineural hearing loss that responds to the administration of corticosteroids (Ruckenstein, 2004). It may initially present unilaterally and may be confused with sudden sensorineural hearing loss, and it may take months for the bilaterality to manifest. Half of affected patients experience vestibular symptoms that can be confused for Ménière's disease. Diagnosis obviously can be difficult. Tests of cellular immunity and detection of a specific antibody directed against a 68-kDa antigen are thought to be helpful, but not completely specific. Therapy consists of high-dose systemic corticosteroids, with the possibility of cochlear implantation for those patients who develop profound bilateral hearing loss.

Cogan syndrome involves labyrinthine and ocular manifestations and is thought to be autoimmune as well. The presence of nonsyphilitic interstitial keratitis, SNHL, vertigo, and tinnitus characterizes the symptom complex, which can be confused with Ménière's disease (especially if keratitis is not immediately present) (Cundiff, Kansal, Kumar, Goldsein, & Tessler, 2006). Prompt and early treatment is key to preventing permanent sequelae. Oral steroids are the mainstay of therapy. Wegener's granulomatosis is an autoimmune disease that affects multiple organ systems, typically involving the sinuses, respiratory tracts, and sometimes the renal system. Its effects on the otologic system usually involve middle ear disease, causing conductive hearing loss and recurrent otitis media, but it may also cause SNHL.

TRAUMATIC CAUSES OF OTOLOGIC DISEASE

Injury to the ear can occur as the result of head trauma incurred in motor vehicle accidents, falls, assaults, self-inflicted wounds, industrial and recreational accidents, and thermal incidents. Damage may be limited to a single part of the ear, or it can be more pervasive, involving the outer, middle, and inner ear as well as central structures. Injuries can be categorized as (1) trauma without fracture, (2) trauma with fracture, (3) compressive injuries, (4) penetrating injuries, and (5) thermal injuries (Huang & Lambert, 1997).

Blunt Trauma

The unprotected location of the auricle makes it particularly vulnerable to injury. A direct blow may result in an auricular hematoma, a localized collection of blood that typically occurs between and separates the perichondrium and cartilage. The patient initially presents with a soft mass on the outer surface and warmth in the pinna, as well as otalgia. Left untreated, cartilage necrosis, infection, and formation of new cartilage will occur, resulting in a thickened deformity of the pinna, known as cauliflower ear (Kinney, Kinney, & Vidimos, 1997). Blunt trauma fracture can cause soft tissue injury in the EAC, TM rupture, or ossicular chain disruption, all of which can cause CHL. Whereas the auricle is very exposed, the temporal bone is very dense, and minor blows rarely produce significant injury. Direct hair cell damage, rupture of the membranous labyrinth, and cochlear concussion can cause SNHL. Cochlear concussion without fracture may be seen as high-signal intensity (brightness) on unenhanced T_1-weighted MRI.

Compressive Injuries

Barotrauma or aerotitis occurs when the eustachian tube does not open and equalize middle ear pressure during rapid changes in atmospheric pressure. This causes inflammation of the middle ear and mastoid mucosa, and the patient experiences extreme otalgia. In some cases there is also TM rupture. Common precipitating situations are descent from flying and ascent from deep-water diving. The hearing loss associated with barotrauma is most often conductive. However, cochlear and vestibular damage, including perilymphatic fistula, inner ear hemorrhage, or labyrinthine membrane tears, can occur because of the implosive and explosive forces of barotraumas (Talmi, Finkelstein, & Zohar, 1991). The resultant SNHL ranges from mild to profound, may fluctuate, and may be accompanied by vertigo. The diagnosis is based on patient history and onset of symptoms within several hours of a precipitating event. Treatment includes recommendation of situational avoidance, especially for those with known eustachian tube dysfunction. When there is SNHL, surgical fistula repair may be indicated. Other compressive injuries, such as the implosive force of being struck or slapped on the side of the head, can cause tympanic membrane ruptures. Blasts and bomb explosions can cause more severe compressive damage involving both the TM and cochlea.

Penetrating Injuries

Self-cleaning or probing the ear canal with a foreign body, such as a cotton swab, is a frequent cause of ear canal lacerations. Presenting complaints include otalgia and bloody otorrhea. Untreated canal wounds may lead to infection or canal stenosis. TM ruptures, ossicular discontinuity, and inner ear injuries may also occur because of probing. Audiologic evaluation may be useful in evaluating the status of the middle ear and inner ear (Kinney, 1998). Survivors of gunshot wounds to the ear and temporal bone will have varied and considerable injury, depending on the type of weapon; the mass, angle, and trajectory of the bullet; and the entrance point and anatomic course of the bullet. Hearing loss can result directly from physical and acoustic damage to the ear, or indirectly from compromise of vital neurovascular structures. Concomitant facial nerve damage occurs in about half of those with gunshot wound injuries to the ear or temporal bone.

Thermal Injuries

Frostbite can cause localized injury to the pinna, with resultant tissue loss and vascular disruption. Burns may cause tissue damage, with resultant scarring of the auricle and external canal stenosis. Localized burns of the ear canal and perforations of the tympanic membrane are often seen in welders when molten slag enters the ear canal. These injuries require aggressive and long-term medical attention (Parisier, Kimmelman, & Hanson, 1997). High-voltage electrical injuries to the ear, including lightning strikes, can cause SNHL, vertigo, facial nerve paralysis, and/or chronic otorrhea.

Temporal Bone Fractures

Skull fractures occur in 23–66% of patients with head injury (Steadman & Graham, 1970; Nosan, Benecke, & Murr, 1997; Ishman & Friedland, 2004). Of these, 18–22% involve the temporal bone (Cannon & Jahrsdoerfer, 1983). Although temporal bone fractures most commonly occur following blunt trauma sustained in motor vehicle accidents, falls, or assaults, they can also result from penetrating injuries such as gunshot wounds. They occur more frequently in males than females, with a ratio of 3:1 to 4:1, and are bilateral in 10–17% (Brodie & Thompson, 1997).

Longitudinal fractures are the most common type, occurring in 70–90% of temporal bone fractures. This type of fracture most often occurs as the result of a temporal or parietal blow to the head. Longitudinal fractures run parallel to the long axis of the petrous pyramid and involve the squamous portion of the temporal bone, mastoid air cells, posterior-superior wall of the EAC, tympanic membrane, and roof of the middle ear. The fracture typically occurs anterior to and spares the labyrinthine capsule. Presenting signs and symptoms include laceration and/or collapse of the EAC, tympanic membrane laceration, bloody otorrhea, protruding ossicles, CHL, and Battle's sign (bluish discoloration behind the ear). When the fracture involves the mastoid rather than the EAC, there may be hemotympanum without a tympanic membrane fracture (Cannon & Jahrsdoerfer, 1983).

Transverse fractures are much less common, comprising 10–30% of temporal bone fractures (Ishman & Friedland, 2004). They typically result from an occipital or parietal blow to the head. Transverse fractures run perpendicular to the long axis of the petrous pyramid and cross the petrous pyramid, extending through the internal auditory canal and/or labyrinthine capsule. These fractures do not typically affect the ossicular chain or EAC. Clinical signs and symptoms include hemotympanum with or without EAC or TM disruption, profound SNHL, and vertigo.

As many as 50–75% of temporal bone fractures are mixed in their axis of orientation, meaning that there is both a longitudinal and a transverse component.(Huang & Lambert, 1997). Alternative nomenclature for temporal bone fractures has been proposed, including "otic capsule sparing" versus "otic capsule violating" and "petrous" versus "nonpetrous"(Brodie & Thompson, 1997; Ishman & Friedland, 2004). These classification schemes may more accurately

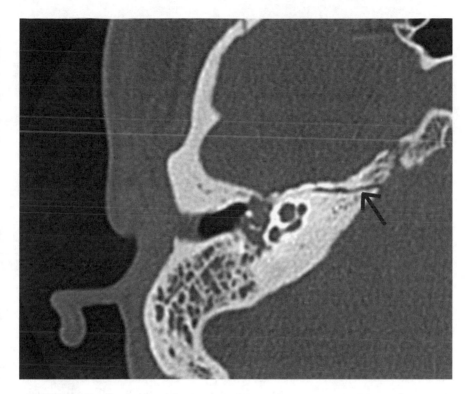

FIGURE 2–4.   Temporal bone fracture (arrow).

reflect findings on high-resolution CT and better predict clinical sequelae and outcomes.

Complications of temporal bone fractures occur as the result of damage to structures housed in or coursing through the temporal bone and include hearing loss, facial nerve paralysis, vertigo, cerebrospinal fluid (CSF) leakage, and secondary meningitis. Diagnosis of temporal bone fractures is confirmed with high-resolution CT. The subsequent evaluation is focused on assessing complications and determining need for interventions.

NEOPLASMS OF THE EAR AND TEMPORAL BONE

Benign and malignant tumors of the ear and temporal bone are fairly rare (Myers, 2003). They make up a wide variety of pathologies and occur in the region from the external auricle to the internal auditory canal of the cerebellopontine angle. In general, tumors may originate in the ear and temporal bone proper, may be extensions from nearby structures, or may represent metastasis from distant primary tumors. These tumors often present in a subtle manner and therefore may evade diagnosis, making definitive care more difficult.

External Ear

Exostoses and Osteomas.   Exostoses and osteomas are benign, nonneo-plastic bony growths that develop in the EAC. Exostoses grow in the medial (bony) portion of the EAC and are typically multiple and bilateral. They frequently result from periosteal activation caused by chronic cold-water exposure and are often seen in swimmers and divers. Osteomas occur on the lateral walls of the EAC at the bony cartilaginous junction and are usually unilateral and singular. They occur most often in children and young adults. Both exostoses and osteomas may remain undetected prior to an incidental otoscopic examination. The potential for symptoms occurs when the growths (1) become large enough to occlude the EAC or encroach on the TM, causing CHL, or (2) trap debris and moisture with resultant otitis externa. Surgical excision may be required to alleviate these sequellae (Parisier, Kimmelman, & Hanson, 1997).

Epidermal Carcinomas.   Malignant lesions of the auricle and external auditory canal are uncommon and are most often epidermal carcinomas. Hearing loss may be associated with these lesions as they become obstructive or invasive. Squamous cell carcinoma is the most common malignant tumor of the EAC and appears as a meaty or polyp-like mass. Patients typically present with a history of CHL, otorrhea, and inordinate and persistent otalgia that has not responded to topical or oral antibiotics. Undiagnosed and untreated, these tumors can extend into the temporal bone, causing SNHL, facial nerve paralysis, and other cranial neuropathies (Pensak & Friedman, 1997). Although less common, squamous cell carcinoma can occur on the auricle and typically presents as an indurated (hardened) plaque or nodule with ulceration and bleeding (Kinney, Kinney, & Vidimos, 1997). Basal cell carcinomas, typically associated with long-term sun exposure, occur more commonly on the auricle. Initially, they appear as painless papules or ulcers with scaly patches. As the tumor extends, chronic external ear infection may occur.

Other External Ear Tumors.   There are several rare, glandular tumors of the EAC that are referred to collectively as ceruminomas. Benign ceruminomas include ceruminous adenomas, pleomorphic adenomas, and cylindromas. Malignant ceruminomas comprise adenoid cystic carcinomas, ceruminous adenocarcinomas, and mucoepidermoid carcinomas (Lustig & Jackler, 1997). Secondary malignancies can develop in the EAC either by direct extension from proximal tissues such as the parotid gland, or metastatic spread from remote sites.

Middle Ear

Glomus Tumors (Paragangliomas).   Paraganglioimas, also known as glomus tumors, are the most common neoplasm of the middle ear and the second most common tumor of the temporal bone in adults (Spector, Maisel, & Ogura, 1973). In the tympanic cavity and skull base, these tumors arise from glomus bodies along Jacobson's nerve (tympanic branch of the glossopharyngeal nerve) or, more rarely,

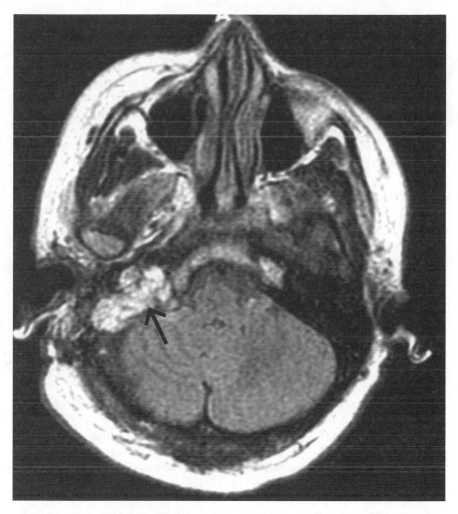

FIGURE 2–5.   MRI of glomus jugulare.

along Arnold's nerve (auricular branch of the vagus nerve). Paragangliomas that arise from the jugular fossa are termed glomus jugulare. Those arising from Jacobson's nerve within the promontory of the middle ear cleft are termed glomus tympanicum, and those arising from Arnold's nerve are termed glomus vagale (Baguley, Irving, Hardy, Harada, & Moffat, 1994). Classification systems for glomus tympanicum and glomus jugulare tumors are based on the anatomic location and extension of these tumors (Oldring & Fisch, 1979; Jackson, Glasscock, & Harris, 1982). Paragangliomas occur more often in females than males (5:1). They typically present clinically in the fifth and sixth decades of life, but have been reported in all age groups (Spector, Maisel, & Ogura, 1973; Jackson, Glasscock, & Harris, 1982). Most are sporadic and solitary, with multiple tumors occurring in only 10% (Balatsouras, Eliopoulos, & Economou, 1992). Seven to nine percent are familial with an unusual genomic imprinting mode of inheritance; 30% of those with the heritable paragangliomas have multiple tumors (van der Mey, Frijns, Cornelisse, Brons, van Dulken, Terpstra, & Schmidt, 1992). A small number (1–3%) of these tumors produce catecholamines and put the patient at risk for life-threatening intraoperative hypertension (Gulya, 1993). Most paragangliomas are benign, with a reported 4% incidence of malignancy (Jackson, 2001).

The most frequent initial symptom of a glomus tympanicum tumor is pulsatile tinnitus (50–76%), followed by hearing loss (30–74%). Additional symptoms include aural fullness (4–18%), otalgia (7%), vertigo/dizziness (9%), EAC bleeding (7%), and headache (4%) (O'Leary, Shelton, Giddings, Kwartler, & Brackmann, 1991; Woods, Strasnick, & Jackson, 1993). On otoscopic examination, a glomus tympanicum appears as a red-blue mass behind or involving the tympanic membrane. Brown's sign, blanching of the tumor with positive pressure, occurs in one-third of cases (Forest, Jackson, & McGrew, 2001). Conductive hearing loss is the most common audiometric finding occurring in up to 52% as the result of reduced ossicular mobility or destruction. As the tumor grows medially, there is cochlear involvement, resulting in a mixed hearing loss in 17% and sensorineural loss in 5% (Woods, Strasnick, & Jackson, 1993).

A glomus jugulare tumor may remain asymptomatic for many years, and a patient may not seek treatment until there is cranial nerve involvement or the tumor has expanded into the middle ear space, causing symptoms similar to those experienced with a glomus tympanicum tumor (Lustig & Jackler, 1997). The most common presenting symptoms are pulsatile tinnitus (78–98%) and hearing loss (61–63%) (Green, Brackmann, Nguyen, Arriaga, Telischi, & De la Cruz, 1994). Additional ear-related symptoms include aural fullness (32%), otalgia (12–13%), and dizziness/vertigo (14–21%). Signs and symptoms related to cranial nerve involvement from a glomus jugulare tumor include hoarseness (12–28%), dysphagia (8–17%), decreased gag reflex (23%), vocal cord paralysis (34%), tongue deviation (20%), and facial numbness (14–15%). Middle ear masses are observed in 72–94%, and EAC masses occur in 6–7%.

In the case of a suspected paraganglioma, the differential diagnosis includes aberrant internal carotid artery, facial neuroma, high riding jugular bulb, persistent stapedial artery, hemangiomas, an arterial venous malformation, aural polyps, and cholesterol granulomas (Cheng & Niparko, 1997; Forest, Jackson, & McGrew, 2001). Imaging studies are a critical part of the diagnostic process. CT scans are the best imaging method for differentiating glomus jugulare from glomus tympanicum tumors and show the degree of bony erosion as well as the tumor's relationship to surrounding structures. MRI with contrast enhancement is important in evaluating the extent of intracranial involvement and assessing regional neurovascular anatomy. Angiography is typically performed in the perioperative period to define blood supplies to the tumor, for examination of the relationship of the tumor to the internal carotid artery, and for presurgical embolization (Jackson, 2001).

Surgical excision is the treatment of choice unless it is contraindicated by patient medical condition or tumor location and biology. Radiation therapy is an alternative management that can be used to control tumor growth.

Rhabdomyosarcoma.   Rhabdomyosarcomas are soft tissue tumors that occur most often in children and account for 5–15% of childhood neoplasms. The ear is the third most common head and neck site for this malignant tumor. Originating sites include the muscles of the eustachian tube, middle ear, and auricle. Clinical presentation includes aural polyps, bloody otorrhea, otalgia, conductive hearing loss, and occasional facial paralysis. The diagnostic evaluation includes a CT scan and MRI. Diagnosis is confirmed by surgical biopsy. Treatment regimens include multi-agent chemotherapy, radiation therapy, and surgical resection (Doyle, 1998).

Inner Ear

Neoplasms originating in the inner ear are rare. Endolymphatic sac tumors are aggressive, but benign tumors that arise from the endolymphatic sac or duct in the posterior petrous bone. Vestibulocochlear symptoms include sensorineural hearing loss, tinnitus, vertigo or dysequilibirum, and aural fullness. Hearing loss is either sudden in onset or stepwise in its progression. These tumors have been associated with Von Hippel-Lindau disease, an autosomal dominant neoplastic disorder (Kim, Butman, Brewer, Zalewski, Vortmeyer, Glenn, Oldfield, and Lonser, 2005). In its early stages, erosion of the aqueduct walls may be detectable by CT. In some cases, labyrinthine enhancement on MRI due to intralabyrinthine hemorrhage may be the initial manifestation (Butman, Patronis, & Kim, 2006). Surgical resection with the goal of preventing audiovestibular morbidity is indicated for small tumors. Large tumors associated with profound hearing loss should be resected when there are signs of neurolologic compromise or compression.

Internal Auditory Canal and Cerebellopontine Angle Lesions

Acoustic Neuroma (Vestibular Schwannoma).   The cerebellopontine angle is the region formed by the junction of the brainstem and the cerebellum, at the level of the pons. The internal auditory canal is the bony canal carrying the facial and vestibulocochlear nerves as they course from the brainstem to the lateral temporal bone. The CPA is a common location for intracranial tumors, especially the acoustic neuroma (more properly known as vestibular schwannoma), which accounts for 80% of tumors in this location. Vestibular schwannomas make up almost 10% of all intracranial tumors. They most commonly arise from the vestibular portion of the eighth cranial nerve and are benign schwann cell tumors by histology.

Ninety-five percent occur sporadically, and the other 5% are associated with a genetic disorder known as neurofibromatosis type 2 (NF 2). Patients with NF 2 usually manifest with bilateral vestibular schwannomas and have family members with the disease. Because these tumors arise in an area near many vital structures (facial nerve, brainstem, etc.), increased growth usually causes a stepwise advancement in symptoms. Patients typically develop unilateral SNHL with poor speech discrimination, tinnitus, and vertigo initially. As the tumor slowly grows, it

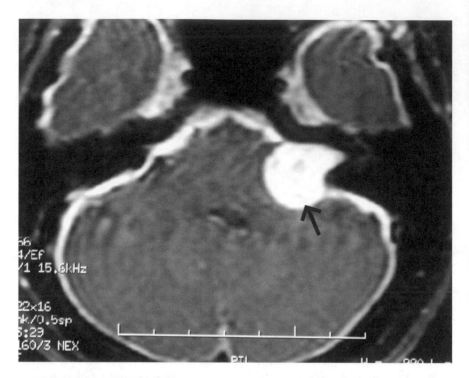

FIGURE 2–6.   MRI of acoustic neuroma.

is possible to compress other cranial nerves at the brainstem, causing midface numbness, facial weakness or spasm, and narrowing of the brain's fourth ventricle. Critical enlargement causes obstructive hydrocephalus, leading to increased intracranial pressure, with resultant nausea, vomiting, changes in mental status, and even death.

MRI with gadolinium contrast is the gold standard for diagnosis and may detect small tumors. Audiometric evaluation usually shows an asymmetric, downsloping, high-frequency SNHL with word recognition scores lower than predicted by the pure tone thresholds. Auditory brainstem response (ABR) testing and CT can be used, but they do not match the sensitivity and specificity of MRI; of the two, ABR is significantly more useful in the diagnosis of possible vestibular schwannoma, although it provides little information about tumor size, the neuroanatomical structures involved, or treatment implications. Not all tumors require treatment secondary to their slow growth. In fact, observation is recommended when the lifespan of the patient is likely to be less than that required to cause problems from the tumor (Rutherford & King, 2005). Often, repeating the MRI 6 months after initial presentation will allow one to assess the growth rate of the tumor and make recommendations accordingly.

When treatment is indicated, options include surgical resection to remove the tumor or highly focused radiation therapy (stereotactic radiation therapy, or "gamma knife") to halt the tumor's growth. Surgery is performed by a multidisciplinary team utilizing one or more surgical approaches, depending on the characteristics, size, and location of the tumor. The translabyrinthine approach may be used for tumors of any size, gives good visualization of the facial nerve during surgery and thereby allows excellent facial nerve preservation, but destroys all hearing on the operated side. The retrosigmoid approach (or suboccipital approach) allows for hearing preservation, but is often accompanied by persistent postoperative headache. A third approach through the middle cranial fossa also allows hearing preservation and is often used for smaller tumors that occupy the IAC.

Complications of surgical therapy include spinal fluid leak, meningitis, facial nerve paresis or paralysis, and loss of hearing. Outcome depends mainly upon original tumor size and location. Radiation therapy may also result in facial nerve dysfunction and fifth cranial nerve neuropathy and makes surgery much more difficult if the treatment fails (Limb, Long, & Niparko, 2005).

Up to 10% of CPA tumors are meningiomas, which arise from the cells lining the arachnoid villae (Brackmann & Arriaga, 2005). These tumors can be hard to distinguish from vestibular schwannomas, but on imaging have a broad dural base and are eccentric to the internal auditory canal. They are also benign tumors, but they can be locally aggressive. The signs and symptoms are similar to those seen with vestibular schwannoma in that small tumors cause hearing loss, tinnitus, and imbalance, whereas larger tumors affect other cranial nerves and may cause brainstem compression. Surgical treatment is the mainstay of therapy.

Epidermoids, nonacoustic neuromas such as facial neuromas, arachnoid cysts, metastases, and many other rare entities may affect the CPA or IAC. These tumors may be confused for vestibular schwannomas and often present with similar signs and symptoms. Because of their rarity, they are not covered here.

IDIOPATHIC FACIAL PALSY (BELL'S PALSY)

Bell's palsy is the most common cause of acute facial nerve weakness and accounts for as many as 70% of facial palsies (Adour, Byl, Hilsinger, Kahn, & Sheldon, 1978). This condition is characterized by rapid onset of unilateral facial palsy over a 24–72-hour period and involves all muscle groups innervated by the facial nerve. Additional presenting signs and symptoms may include pain or paresthesias around the ear, reduced or altered taste on the anterior two-thirds of the tongue, excessive tearing or dry eye, and hyperacusis on the affected side. Notably absent are associated hearing loss, vertigo, and signs of CNS or CPA disease.

Paralysis is partial in 30% and complete in 70% of patients (Peitersen, 2002). Bilateral paralysis is rare, occurring in only 0.3% of cases (Adour, Byl, Hilsinger, Kahn, & Sheldon, 1978). The annual incidence of Bell's palsy is 17–32 per 100,000 population per year. It occurs in all age groups, but more often in those older than 60 years of age. There is a family history of Bell's palsy in 4–8% and a history of previous paralysis in 7–9%. Bell's palsy occurs equally often in males and females and on the right and left sides. Risk factors include pregnancy and diabetes mellitus. Although commonly referred to as "idiopathic facial palsy," recent evidence strongly

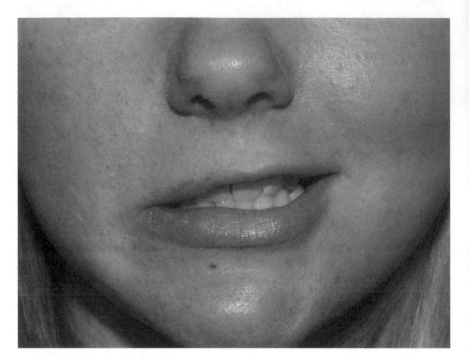

FIGURE 2–7.   Photo of patient with unilateral facial paralysis.

implicates that the herpes simplex virus is the causative agent in Bell's palsy, although controversy regarding etiology still remains (Linder, Bossart, & Bodmer, 2005). Unilateral facial palsy can be caused by a diverse variety of lesions, and the diagnosis of Bell's palsy is largely one of exclusion. The differential diagnosis includes trauma, Ramsay-Hunt syndrome, local infection, tumors, CNS disease, otitis media, Lyme disease, diabetes mellitus, cranial polyneuritis, sarcoidosis, and congenital anomalies (May & Klein, 1991; Berg, Jonsson, and Engstrom, 2004). The history and physical examination provide significant insight in ruling out many of these causes. Partial facial nerve paralysis, involvement of other cranial nerves, facial rash or vesicular lesions, an enlarged parotid gland, and auditory and/or vestibular symptoms are indicators of a diagnosis other than Bell's palsy. High-resolution CT and gadolinium-enhanced T_1-weighted MRI are used to rule out these other causes and identify sites of inflammation along the course of the facial nerve (Schwaber, Larson, & Zealer, 1990). Supplemental blood tests may be used to evaluate for potential infectious causes, as well as underlying systemic disease such as diabetes.

While hearing loss is not a typical manifestation of Bell's palsy, audiology evaluation provides information regarding the functional status of the middle ear muscle reflex (MEMR), which is absent in up to 46–71% of cases (Peitersen, 1992). Those patients with absent MEMRs are more likely to experience hyperacusis. In addition, 65% of those with absent MEMRs have a significant decline of 41% or greater in word recognition at high intensity levels (PB rollover) (Mc-Candless and Schumacher, 1979). Several cases with a delayed I-V interval and abnormal interaural latency difference for wave V have been reported (Rosenhall, Edstrom, Hanner, Badr, & Vahlne, 1983).

Grading of facial nerve function, using a system such as the House-Brackmann Scale (Table 2–5), provides a standardized method for documenting the extent of dysfunction and clinical outcome (House and Brackmann, 1985). Most patients with Bell's palsy have spontaneous recovery to good facial function by 3 to 6 months. Prognosis is best for those with a House-Brackmann grade V or less, signs of recovery by 2 months, young age, present middle ear muscle reflex, electromyography (EMG) evidence of voluntary activity, and/or electroneuronography (ENoG) evidence of <90% degeneration at two weeks post-onset (Rubinstein and Gantz, 1997). Eye care and protection is very important for those who cannot readily close their eyes (House-Brackmann grade III or worse). Pharmaceutical management with corticosteroids and antivirals is recommended by some. Surgical management by means of facial nerve decompression is controversial but may be conservatively applied to those patients with total paralysis who are seen within

TABLE 2–5
House-Brackmann Scale of Facial Nerve Function

Grade	Interpretation	Gross	At rest	Motion
I	Normal			
II	Mild	Slight weakness observed on close inspection	Normal symmetry and tone	Forehead—moderate to good
				Eye—complete closure with minimum effort
				Mouth—slight asymmetry
III	Moderate	Obvious, but not disfiguring asymmetry, may have hemifacial spasm	Normal symmetry and tone	Forehead—slight to moderate movement
				Eye—complete closure with effort
				Mouth—slightly weak with maximum effort
IV	Moderately severe	Obvious weakness and/or disfiguring asymmetry	Normal symmetry and tone	Forehead—no movement
				Eyes—incomplete closure
				Mouth—asymmetric with maximum effort
V	Severe	Only barely perceptible motion	Asymmetry	Forehead—no movement
				Eye—incomplete closure
				Mouth—slight movement
VI	Total paralysis	No movement		

two weeks of symptom of onset, 90% or greater degeneration on ENoG, and no voluntary EMG activity (Rubinstein & Gantz, 1997).

CONCLUSION

A systematic, thorough approach is required to properly diagnose and manage medical disorders and disease of the ear. A clear understanding of temporal bone anatomy, particularly the middle ear and mastoid structures, is essential in understanding the pathologic mechanisms behind these conditions. Because of the proximity of the intracranial cavity to the temporal bone, the consequences of a seemingly innocuous presentation can be severe. Furthermore, because many systemic conditions have otologic manifestations, a broad-based approach is needed to establish a proper differential diagnosis. Fortunately, when identified promptly, almost all medical conditions of the ear can be successfully treated or controlled.

REFERENCES

American Academy of Pediatrics Subcomittee on Management of Acute Otitis Media. (2004). Diagnosis and management of acute otitis media. *Pediatrics, 113*(5), 1451–1465.

American Academy of Family Physicians; American Academy of Otolaryngology—Head and Neck Surgery; American Academy of Pediatrics Subcommittee on Otitis Media with Effusion. (2004). Otitis media with effusion. *Pediatrics, 113*(5), 1412–1429.

Adour, K. K., Byl, F. M., Hilsinger, R. L., Kahn, Z. M., & Sheldon, M. I. (1978). The true nature of Bell's palsy: analysis of 1,000 consecutive patients. *Laryngoscope, 88*(5), 787–801.

Baguley, D. M., Irving, R. M., Hardy, D. G., Harada, T., & Moffat, D. A. (1994). Audiological findings in glomus tumours. *British Journal of Audiology, 28*(6), 291–297.

Balatsouras, D. G., Eliopoulos, P. N., & Economou, C. N. (1992). Multiple glomus tumours. *Journal of Laryngology and Otology, 106*(6), 538–543.

Balkany, T. J., & Ress, B. D. (1998). Infections of the external ear. In C. W. Cummings, J. M. Fredrickson, L. A. Harker et al. (Eds.), *Otolaryngology: Head and neck surgery* (Vol. 4, pp. 2979–2986). St. Louis: Mosby-Yearbook.

Berg, T., Jonsson, L., & Engstrom, M. (2004). Agreement between the Sunnybrook, House-Brackmann, and Yanagihara facial nerve grading systems in Bell's palsy. *Otolology and Neurotology, 25*(6), 1020–1026.

Bluestone, C. D. (1998). Otitis media: A spectrum of diseases. In A. K. Lalwani and K. M. Grundfast (Eds.), *Pediatric otology and neurotology* (p. 728). Philadelphia: Lippincott-Raven.

Bluestone, C. D. (2003). *Pediatric otolaryngology*. Philadelphia: Saunders.

Brackmann, D. E., & Arriaga, M. A. (2005). Extra-axial neoplasms of the posterior fossa. In C. W. Cummings, J. M. Fredrickson, L. A. Harker et al. (Eds.), *Otolaryngology: Head and neck surgery*. St. Louis: Mosby-Yearbook.

Brodie, H. A., & Thompson, T. C. (1997). Management of complications from 820 temporal bone fractures. *American Journal of Otology, 18*(2), 188–197.

Butman, J., Patronis, N., & Kim, H. J. (2006). Imaging of the temporal bone. In B. J. Bailey, J. T. Johnson, S. D. Newlands, et al. (Eds.), *Head and neck surgery—Otolaryngology* (Vol. 2, p. 3024). Philadelphia: Lippincott, Williams & Wilkins.

Cannon, C. R., & Jahrsdoerfer, R. A. (1983). Temporal bone fractures. Review of 90 cases. *Archives of Otolaryngology, 109*(5), 285–288.

Cheng, A., & Niparko, J. K. (1997). Imaging quiz case 2. Glomus tympanicum tumor of the temporal bone. *Archives of Otolaryngology—Head and Neck Surgery, 123*(5), 549, 551–552.

Chole, R. A., & Choo, M. (1998). Chronic otitis media, mastoiditis, and petrositis. In C. W. Cummings, J. M. Fredrickson, L. A. Harker, et al. (Eds.), *Otolaryngology: Head and neck surgery* (Vol. 4, pp. 3026–3046). St. Louis: Mosby-Yearbook.

Cundiff, J., Kansal, S., Kumar, A., Goldstein, D. A., & Tessler, H. H. (2006). Cogan's syndrome: A cause of progressive hearing deafness. *American Journal of Otolaryngology, 27*(1), 68–70.

Doyle, K. J. (1998). Tumors of the temporal bone. In A. K. Lalwani & K. M. Grundfast (Eds.), *Pediatric otology and neurotology* (p. 728). Philadelphia: Lippincott-Raven.

Eisele, D., & McQuone, S. (2000). *Emergencies of the head and neck.* St. Louis: Mosby-Yearbook.

Fayad, J. N., & Linthicum, F. H., Jr. (1999). Temporal bone histopathology case of the month: Otosyphilis. *American Journal of Otology, 20*(2), 259–260.

Forest, J. A., III, Jackson, C. G., & McGrew, B. M. (2001). Long-term control of surgically treated glomus tympanicum tumors. *Otology & Neurotology, 22*(2), 232–236.

Fria, T. J., Cantekin, E. I., & Eichler, J. A. (1985). Hearing acuity of children with otitis media with effusion. *Archives of Otolaryngology, 111*(1), 10–16.

Friedberg, J. (1998). Congenital cholesteatoma. In A. K. Lalwani and K. M. Grundfast (Eds.), *Pediatric otology and neurotology* (p. 628). Philadelphia: Lippincott-Raven.

Gates, G. A. (1997). Otitis media with effusion. In G. B. Hughes & M. L. Pensak (Eds.), *Clinical otology* (pp. 205–213). New York: Thieme Medical.

Green, J. D., Jr., Brackmann, D. E., Nguyen, C. D., Arriaga, M. A., Telischi, F. F., & De la Cruz, A. (1994). Surgical management of previously untreated glomus jugulare tumors. *Laryngoscope, 104*(8 Pt 1), 917–921.

Gulya, A. J. (1993). The glomus tumor and its biology. *Laryngoscope, 103*(11 Pt 2, Suppl. 60), 7–15.

Hartnick, C. J., Kim, H. H., Chute, P. M., & Parisier, S. C. (2001). Preventing labyrinthitis ossificans: The role of steroids. *Archives of Otolaryngology—Head. and Neck Surgery, 127*(2), 180–183.

House, J. W., & Brackmann, D. E. (1985). Facial nerve grading system. *Otolaryngology—Head and Neck Surgery, 93*(2), 146–147.

Huang, M. Y., & Lambert, P. R. (1997). Temporal bone trauma. In G. B. Hughes & M. L. Pensak (Eds.), *Clinical otology* (pp. 251–267). New York: Thieme Medical.

Ishman, S. L., & Friedland, D. R. (2004). Temporal bone fractures: Traditional classification and clinical relevance. *Laryngoscope, 114*(10), 1734–1741.

Jackson, C. G. (2001). Glomus tympanicum and glomus jugulare tumors. *Otolaryngologic Clinics of North America, 34*(5), 941–970, vii.

Jackson, C. G., Glasscock, M. E., & Harris, P. F. (1982). Glomus tumors. Diagnosis, classification, and management of large lesions. *Archives of Otolaryngology, 108*(7), 401–410.

Kim, H. J., Butman, J. A., Brewer, C., Zalewski, C., Vortmeyer, A. O., Glenn, G., Oldfield, E. H., & Lonser, R. R. (2005). Tumors of the endolymphatic sac in patients with von Hippel-Lindau disease: Implications for their natural history, diagnosis, and treatment. *Journal of Neurosurgery, 102*(3), 503–512.

Kinney, S. E. (1998). Trauma to the middle ear and temporal bone. In C. W. Cummings, J. M. Fredrickson, L. A. Harker et al. (Eds.), *Otolaryngology: Head and neck surgery* (Vol. 4, pp. 3076–3087). St. Louis: Mosby-Yearbook.

Kinney, W. C., Kinney, S. E., & Vidimos, A. T. (1997). Disorders of the auricle. In G. B. Hughes & M. L. Pensak (Eds.), *Clinical otology* (pp. 177–189). New York: Thieme Medical.

Klein, J. O. (1994). Otitis media. *Clinical Infectious Diseases, 19*(5), 823–833.

Klemm, E., & Wollina, U. (2004). Otosyphilis: Report on six cases. *Journal of the European Academy of Dermatology and Venereology, 18*(4), 429–434.

Limb, C. J., Long, D. M., & Niparko, J. K. (2005). Acoustic neuromas after failed radiation therapy: Challenges of surgical salvage. *Laryngoscope, 115*(1), 93–98.

Linder, T., Bossart, W., & Bodmer (2005). Bell's palsy and Herpes simplex virus: Fact or mystery? *Otology and Neurotology, 26*(1), 109–113.

Logigian, E. L., Kaplan, R. F., & Steere, C. A. (1990). Chronic neurologic manifestations of Lyme disease. *New England Journal of Medicine, 323*(21), 1438–1444.

Lustig, L. R., & Jackler, R. K. (1997). Benign tumors of the temporal bone. In G. B. Hughes and M. L. Pensak (Eds.), *Clinical otology* (pp. 313–333). New York: Thieme Medical.

May, M., & Klein, S. R. (1991). Differential diagnosis of facial nerve palsy. *Otolaryngology Clinics of North America, 24*(3), 613–645.

McCandless, G. A., & Schumacher, M. H. (1979). Auditory dysfunction with facial paralysis. *Archives of Otolaryngology, 105*(5), 271–274.

Moscatello, A. L., Worden, D. L., Nadelman, R. B., Wormser, G., & Lucente, F. (1991). Otolaryngologic aspects of Lyme disease. *Laryngoscope, 101*(6 Pt 1), 592–595.

Myers, E. (2003). *Cancer of the head and neck*. Philadelphia: Saunders.

Nadol, J., & Merchant, S. (1998). Systemic disease manifestations in the middle ear and temporal bone. In C. W. Cummings, J. M. Fredrickson, L. A. Harker et al. (Eds.), *Otolaryngology: Head and neck surgery* (Vol. 4, pp. 3088–3107). St. Louis: Mosby-Yearbook.

Nosan, D. K., Benecke, J. E., Jr., & Murr, A. H. (1997). Current perspective on temporal bone trauma. *Otolaryngology—Head & Neck Surgery, 117*(1), 67–71.

Novelline, R. A. (2004). *Squire's fundamentals of radiology*. Boston: Harvard University Press.

O'Leary, M. J., Shelton, C., Giddings, N. A., Kwartler, J., & Brackmann, D. E. (1991). Glomus tympanicum tumors: A clinical perspective. *Laryngoscope, 101*(10), 1038–1043.

Oldring, D., & Fisch, U. (1979). Glomus tumors of the temporal region: Surgical therapy. *American Journal of Otology, 1*(1), 7–18.

Parisier, S. C., Kimmelman, C. P., & Hanson, M. B. (1997). Diseases of the external auditory canal. In G. B. Hughes & M. L. Pensak (Eds.), *Clinical otology* (pp. 191–203). New York: Thieme Medical.

Peitersen, E. (1992). Natural history of Bell's palsy. *Acta Otolaryngologica Supplement, 492*, 122–124.

Peitersen, E. (2002). Bell's palsy: The spontaneous course of 2,500 peripheral facial nerve palsies of different etiologies. *Acta Otolaryngolica Supplement,* (549), 4–30.

Pensak, M. L., & Friedman, R. A. (1997). Malignant tumors of the temporal bone. In G. B. Hughes & M. L. Pensak (Eds.), *Clinical otology* (pp. 335–343). New York: Thieme Medical.

Quinn, S. J., Boucher, B. J., & Booth, J. B. (1997). Reversible sensorineural hearing loss in Lyme disease. *Journal of Laryngology & Otology, 111*(6), 562–564.

Rosenhall, U., Edstrom, S., Hanner, P., Badr, G., & Vahlne, A. (1983). Auditory brain stem response abnormalities in patients with Bell's palsy. *Otolaryngology—Head & Neck Surgery, 91*(4), 412–416.

Rubinstein, J. T., & B. J. Gantz. (1997). Facial nerve disorders. In G. B. Hughes & M. L. Pensak (Eds.), *Clinical otology* (pp. 367–379). New York: Thieme Medical.

Ruckenstein, M. J. (2004). Autoimmune inner ear disease. *Current Opinion in Otolaryngology and Head & Neck Surgery, 12*(5), 426–430.

Rutherford, S. A., & King, A. T. (2005). Vestibular schwannoma management: What is the "best" option? *British Journal of Neurosurgery, 19*(4), 309–316.

Schwaber, M. K., Larson, T., & Zealear, D. (1990). MRI in evaluation of facial paralysis. *Otolaryngology—Head & Neck Surgery, 103*(4), 672.

Spector, G. J., Maisel, R. H., & Ogura, J. H. (1973). Glomus tumors in the middle ear. I. An analysis of 46 patients. *Laryngoscope, 83*(10), 1652–1672.

Steadman, J. H., & Graham, J. G. (1970). Head injuries: An analysis and follow-up study. *Proceedings of the Royal Society of Medicine, 63*(1), 23–28.

Steere, A. C. (1989). Lyme disease. *New England Journal of Medicine, 321*(9), 586–596.

Talmi, Y. P., Finkelstein, Y., & Zohar, Y. (1991). Barotrauma-induced hearing loss. *Scandinavian Audiology, 20*(1), 1–9.

Teele, D. W., Klein, J. O., & Rosner, B. (1989). Epidemiology of otitis media during the first seven years of life in children in greater Boston: A prospective, cohort study. *Journal of Infectious Disease, 160*(1), 83–94.

Tucci, D. L., & L. Gray (2000). Radiographic imaging in otologic disease. In R. J. Roeser, M. Valente, & H. Hosford-Dunn (Eds.), *Audiology diagnosis* (p. 640). New York: Thieme.

van der Mey, A. G., Frijns, J. H., Cornelisse, C. J., Brons, E. N., van Dulken, H., Terpstra, H. L., & Schmidt, P. H. (1992). Does intervention improve the natural course of glomus tumors? A series of 108 patients seen in a 32-year period. *Annals of Otology, Rhinology, & Laryngology, 101*(8), 635–642.

Wayman, D. M., Pham, H. N., Byl, F. M., & Adour, K. K. (1990). Audiological manifestations of Ramsay Hunt syndrome. *Journal of Laryngology & Otology 104*(2), 104–108.

Woods, C. I., Strasnick, B., & Jackson, C. G. (1993). Surgery for glomus tumors: The Otology Group experience. *Laryngoscope, 103*(11 Pt 2, Suppl. 60), 65–70.

CHAPTER 3

The Vestibular System: Basic Principles and Clinical Disorders

Marc D. Eisen
Charles J. Limb
Johns Hopkins University

The vestibular system acts to sense and control the head's orientation in space with respect to linear and rotational motion. The purposes of the vestibular system are to maintain one's orientation in space, postural stability, and gaze stability. Motion of the human body is typically a combination of turning, twisting, and leaning that can be complex to describe in three-dimensional space. Every complex motion in three-dimensional space, however, can be depicted as the vector sum of much simpler two-dimensional motions in the three orthogonal planes. As we will discuss, the normally functioning vestibular system utilizes such a strategy of reducing complex motion of the head in space into three orthogonal planes. This task is accomplished with two sets of vestibular sensory organs, one set on each side of the head; the two sides cooperate in a harmony of push-pull responses like children on a seesaw. As a result, disorders that cause an acute unilateral hypo- or hyper-function undermine this cooperation and cause the sensation of motion despite its absence (i.e., vertigo). This chapter uses as its foundation the basic cellular and neural anatomy of the vestibular system in order to describe its normal physiology. A description of the common vestibular disorders and their diagnosis and treatment is then presented based on how this normal vestibular function is altered.

ANATOMY

The Sensory Hair Cell

The peripheral vestibular organ and the cochlea have a common evolutionary origin. Given their common ancestry, it should come as no surprise that they utilize the same basic mechanotransducer—the sensory hair cell (Fig. 3–1). Common to

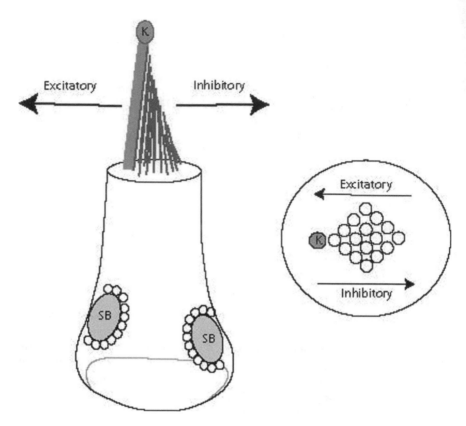

FIGURE 3–1.   Vestibular hair cell. The vestibular hair cell is polarized, with an apical end containing a tuft of sensory stereocilia and a basolateral surface in contact with the postsynaptic dendrites. The synaptic body (SB) is a presynaptic density surrounded by neurotransmitter vesicles and likely involved in the graded release of neurotransmitter. A feature of the vestibular hair cell that differentiates it from the auditory hair cell is the kinocilium (K), a true cilia located at the helm of the sensory hair bundle. Deflection of the sensory hairs in the direction of the kinocilium results in the release of neurotransmitter, and deflection of the hairs away from the kinocilium results in the decrease of neurotransmitter release.

hair cells of the auditory and vestibular system are several basic anatomic features: a tuft of microvilli, or sensory hairs, arranged in a gradation of heights protruding from the cell's apical end and housing the mechanosensory transduction channels, and a specialized ribbon-type synapse with dendrites of the cochleovestibular nerve at the cell's basolateral aspect. Unlike cochlear hair cells, however, the vestibular hair cells have a kinocilium, a true microtubule-containing cilium, at the vertex of the hair bundle (Engstrom & Wersall, 1958). Deflection of the hair bundle toward the kinocilium depolarizes the cell and results in increased neurotransmitter release, whereas deflection away from the kinocilium hyperpolarizes the cell and results in decreased neurotransmitter release (Hudspeth & Jacobs, 1979). Thus each hair cell acts as a graded one-dimensional motion detector, with sensitivity to motion along a single axis. Motion that is not along this axis of sensitivity results in no changes in the hair cell potential.

Vestibular hair cells have been classified into two distinct types, based on their anatomic relationship to the apposing afferent ending. The afferent endings of type I hair cells form a chalice around the basolateral portion of the cell and are appropriately termed *calyx* endings. The afferent endings of type II hair cells have smaller bouton-like endings, and numerous endings synapse with single hair cells. All of the vestibular end-organs consist of some combination of these two hair cell types (Engstrom, 1961). Understanding the orientation of the hair cells within the vestibular end organs and how they are stimulated can simplify the otherwise complex mechanism of vestibular signal transduction.

The Vestibular End Organs

The sensory hair cells in the vestibular periphery are housed in two sets (left and right) of three semicircular canals, which detect angular acceleration, and two sets of otolith organs (utricle and saccule), which detect linear acceleration—all contained within the petrous portion of the temporal bone. The hair cells in a semicircular canal are embedded in a narrow sheet of epithelium, the crista ampullaris, with their hair bundles aligned all in the same direction (Fig. 3–2). Above and in contact with the hair bundles is a gelatinous mass called the cupula. Motion of the fluid within the duct displaces the cupula. Displacement of the cupula then results in hair bundle deflections in the common axis of sensitivity. Deflection in

FIGURE 3–2. Crista ampullaris. The ampullated end of a semicircular canal contains the crista ampullaris (Cr), with its surface protruding into the lumen of the semicircular canal and bathed in endolymph. Endolymph flows around the toroid of the semicircular canal The surface epithelium of the crista contains hair cells with their hair bundles oriented in the same direction, depicted here as one hair bundle atop the crista. The cupula (Cu) is a gelatinous mass suspended from the ceiling of the ampulla down to the level of the hair bundles. The inset demonstrates the entire semicircular canal. Head motion, represented by black arrows, results in fluid flow around the toroid of the canal (gray arrows) in the direction opposite that of the head motion. Fluid flow deflects the cupula and along with it the hair bundles. Fluid flow in the direction of the kinocilium results in hair cell depolarization (+), and flow in the opposite direction results in hair cell hyperpolarization (−).

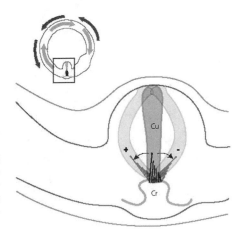

one direction is excitatory to the hair cells, and in the opposite direction, it is inhibitory.

The fluid bathing the hair bundles is endolymph, with a high-K^+, low-Na^+ composition similar to that of intracellular fluid. Surrounding the endolymph-containing duct is a compartment containing fluid high in Na^+ and low in K^+, known as perilymph. The adjacent location of the perilymph and endolymph compartments establishes the electrical potential gradient that drives cations into the hair cell during hair bundle deflections. The ducts containing endolymph and perilymph protrude from the crista parallel to the hair cells' axis of sensitivity in a nearly circular toroid (doughnut)-shaped duct that gives the organ its name of "semicircular" canal. This membranous portion of the semicircular canal is housed in the petrous portion of the temporal bone. The bone widens as the toroidal portion enters the space containing the cristae. The widened space in the bone is the ampulla of the semicircular canal. When the temporal bone, which is yoked to the head, moves with angular head movements in the plane of the canal, the endolymphatic fluid is "left behind" because of inertia. This results in relative motion of the fluid with respect to the head and displacement of the cupula in the direction opposite that of the head motion (Fig. 3–2). Hair bundle deflections and subsequent changes in the afferent vestibular nerve fiber firing rate follow. Afferent vestibular nerve fibers maintain spontaneous activity with rates as high as 100 spikes/second. The hair cell–afferent fiber synapse functions to modulate that rate either up with hair cell excitation or down with hair cell inhibition.

The three semicircular canals on each side of the head are arranged in three approximately orthogonal planes as shown in Fig. 3–3. One canal is positioned in a plane about 30% up from horizontal, one anterolateral to posteromedial, and one posterolateral to anteromedial. These canals have somewhat misleading common names: lateral (there is no medial), superior (there is no inferior), and posterior

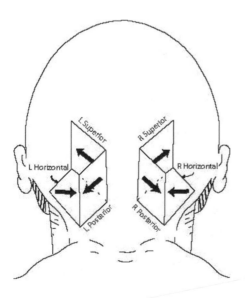

FIGURE 3–3.   Orientation of the semicircular canals in the head. The semicircular canals are oriented in orthogonal planes, as demonstrated by the arrows. In this schematic, the complementary pairs of semicircular canals can be observed from above and behind the head as being coplanar. The coplanar pairs are the left superior/right posterior canals, the left posterior/right superior canals, and the right and left horizontal canals.

(there is no anterior), respectively. With the canals in this formation, pairs of canals respond to angular accelerations in the same plane. These coplanar pairs are the right and left horizontal canals, the left superior and right posterior canals, and the left posterior and right superior canals (Della Santina, Potyagaylo, Migliaccio, Minor, & Carey, 2005). Angular accelerations in the horizontal plane toward the left excite the left lateral canal and inhibit the right lateral canal (Keller, 1976); bringing the chin down toward one shoulder excites the ipsilateral superior canal and inhibits the contralateral posterior canal; and throwing the head back over one shoulder excites the ipsilateral posterior canal and inhibits the contralateral superior canal.

There are two otolith organs on each side of the head. The *utricle* has its epithelium of hair cells arranged primarily in the horizontal plane, and those in the other organ, the *saccule*, are arranged in the vertical plane. The hair bundles contact a gelatinous layer overlying the hair cell surface. This gelatinous layer contains crystalline calcium carbonate particles called otoconia and is referred to as the otolithic membrane. Displacement of the otolithic membrane with gravity or other linear acceleration forces leads to hair bundle displacement, depolarization or hyperpolarization of hair cells, and release of hair cell neurotransmitter onto the dendrites of the utricular or saccular nerve fibers. The otolith organs are thus linear accelerometers for the head.

Blood Supply and Innervation

Blood supply to the vestibular periphery comes from the labyrinthine artery, which usually arises from the anterior inferior cerebellar artery (AICA). The labyrinthine artery has several branches to the membranous labyrinth that demonstrate anatomic variability. The first branch is usually to the utricle and anterior portions of the lateral and superior semicircular canals. Two other branches of the labyrinthine artery include one feeding primarily the saccule, posterior semicircular canal, and basal turn of the cochlea (the vestibulocochlear artery) and the other feeding the middle and apical turns of the cochlea (the cochlear artery) (Anson & Bast, 1960). The neural innervation of the vestibular periphery comes from the vestibular division of the eighth cranial nerve. In the internal auditory canal, through which the eighth cranial nerve travels from the brainstem to the inner ear, the vestibular portion of the eighth nerve occupies the posterior aspect of the canal. Further lateral in the canal toward the fundus, the vestibular portion divides into two parts, the inferior and superior vestibular nerves. The superior portion carries fibers bound for the ampullae of the lateral and superior semicircular canals and the maculae of the utricle and saccule. The inferior portion carries fibers to a posterior ampullary nerve (the singular nerve) and a saccular nerve. Cell bodies of the vestibular nerve fibers are consolidated at the vestibule into the vestibular (Scarpa's) ganglion.

Unstimulated primary vestibular afferent nerves maintain steady rates of spontaneous activity. Head motion toward the side of the afferent fiber's origin is excitatory, resulting in increased neural firing rates, and motion in the opposite direction is inhibitory, resulting in decreased neural firing rates (Keller, 1976). The code that the normally functioning vestibular periphery provides to the central nervous system is therefore the modulation of a baseline firing rate either up or down, depending on the direction of head motion.

Central Neural Pathways

From Scarpa's ganglion, which contains the cell bodies of the vestibular nerve, the nerve runs medially through the posterior aspect of the internal auditory canal and enters the cerebellopontine angle. As the vestibular nerve enters the brainstem at the lateral pontomedullary junction, the afferent fibers course dorsally and medially to terminate on the vestibular nuclei of the brainstem. In addition to ipsilateral vestibular nerve afferents, input to the vestibular nuclei is extensive, including sources as diverse as contralateral vestibular, brainstem, and cerebellar nuclei. The implication of such an extensive synaptic relay station is that the vestibular nuclei coordinate movements between the different motor and sensory systems.

The VOR Pathway

The vestibulo-ocular reflex (VOR) is only one of the movement coordination reflexes mediated by the peripheral vestibular apparatus, but it is the most clinically relevant because it lends itself to easily accessible clinical testing and manipulation. The function of the VOR is to maintain visual images on the retina during head movements. In order to accomplish this mission, angular motion of the head must stimulate equal and opposite angular motion of the eyes. The neural pathway mediating the VOR is very well understood. The structures involved are the semicircular canals; the vestibular nuclei; the oculomotor, abducens, and trochlear cranial nerve nuclei; the medial longitudinal fasciculus (MLF); and the extraocular eye muscles (Fig. 3–4). The neural reflex arc begins with the vestibular afferents that originate from the cristae of the semicircular canals and then synapse on brainstem vestibular nuclei. The vestibular nuclei send both inhibitory and excitatory interneurons to oculomotor nuclei. Excitatory neurons are sent to both ipsilateral and contralateral (via the MLF) oculomotor nuclei to stimulate eye movements in one direction, and inhibitory neurons are sent to complementary ipsilateral and contralateral (again through MLF) oculomotor nuclei to inhibit eye movements in the opposite direction.

The orientation of the extraocular muscles themselves in the orbit is such that the superior and inferior rectus muscles are coplanar with the ipsilateral superior semicircular canal and contralateral posterior semicircular canal; the superior and inferior oblique muscles are coplanar with the ipsilateral posterior canal and contralateral superior canal; the medial and lateral rectus muscles are coplanar with the horizontal canals. A consequence of the orientation of the extraocular muscles and the crossed brainstem VOR pathways is that pairs of extraocular muscles move the eyes in the plane of the coplanar semicircular canals depicted in Fig. 3–3.

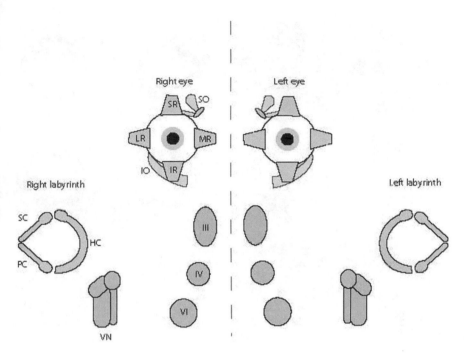

FIGURE 3–4. Anatomic structures involved in the VOR. The elements of the VOR are the semi-circular canals (HC, horizontal canal; SC, superior canal; PC, posterior canal), the vestibular nuclei (VN); the oculomotor (III), trochlear (IV), and abducens (VI) nuclei; and the extraocular muscles (IO, inferior oblique m.; SO, superior oblique m.; IR, inferior rectus m.; SR, superior rectus m.; MR, medial rectus m.; LR, lateral rectus m.

Figure 3–5 demonstrates the eye movements driven by the VOR in response to stimulation of individual semicircular canals. For the speed range of typical head motion (about 1 to 4 Hz) the normally functioning VOR matches all angular head motion with equal and opposite eye movements, and the visual field remains unaltered on the retina.

Normally, the VOR dictates that the eyes maintain the target on the fovea while the head is moving. When the eyes moving within the orbit reach a point sufficiently far from the center, another reflex arc engages, one driven by the optokinetic reflex. The eyes will then undergo a high-velocity counter-motion to reset their position within the orbit. This quick response is termed a saccade. Its high velocity blurs the image on the retina during its motion. *Nystagmus* is the term for repetitive cycles of slow VOR-mediated eye motion followed by resetting saccades, which appears as a jerky to-and-fro beating of the eyes. Inasmuch as the fast phase of this repetitive beating is easier to observe clinically than the slow phase of the eye movements, the convention is to name the nystagmus by the direction of the fast component, even though the eye movement induced by the vestibular afferent and the VOR is the slow component. Continued stimulation of one semicircular canal's vestibular afferent as shown in Fig. 3–5 would result in nystagmus in the plane of

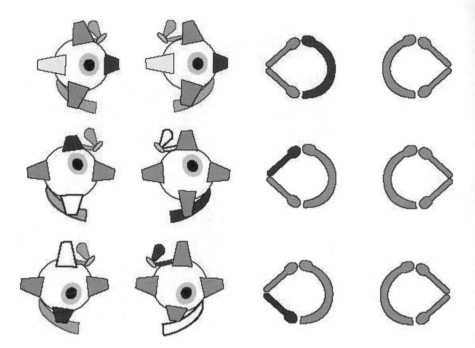

FIGURE 3–5. Individual canals and resulting eye movements. Eye movements driven by the VOR are shown for the case of individual canal stimulation (from top to bottom right horizontal, right superior, and right posterior canal). The eyes and canals are oriented as if looking at the patient. The stimulated canal is black. Inhibited muscles are white, and stimulated muscles are black.

the canal of origin, alternating with saccades toward the side of stimulation in the plane of the canal. The fast component thus "beats" toward the side of stimulation. A final concept to keep in mind when considering the clinical implications of the VOR is that *hyper*function of one canal's afferents and *hypo*function of the contralateral coplanar paired canal (i.e., superior canal one side and contralateral posterior canal, or horizontal canals) will both result in VOR slow phase nystagmus away from—and clinical signs of beating toward—the side of higher neural activity. This is due to the spontaneous activity of vestibular afferents and its modulation up or down during stimulation and inhibition, respectively. Discriminating one side's hypofunction from the other side's hyperfunction thus requires further information about the function of individual semicircular canals.

VESTIBULAR PHYSIOLOGY

Asymmetry of Vestibular Nerve Afferent Responses

Vestibular afferent fibers have a resting spontaneous level of activity even in the absence of motion, and excitatory and inhibitory stimulation modulates the spontaneous rate. The degree of afferent nerve fiber inhibition is limited in that the spontaneous rate cannot be reduced to less than zero spikes per unit time. Excitation, however, does not have such an apparent rate constraint and has a manyfold larger dynamic range of stimulation frequency. Thus whereas decreases in afferent firing rate with inhibition and increases with excitation are symmetric at low angular velocities of head motion, as the velocity of head motion increases, the degree of inhibition will plateau, while the degree of excitation continues to increase. An asymmetry between the excitatory and inhibitory directions emerges, with the excitatory direction eliciting a greater response than the inhibitory. This asymmetry at high angular head velocity can be exploited in clinical testing to differentiate the function of the right from the left labyrinth.

Central Control of VOR

Central connections to and from the vestibular nuclei are extensive, and central nervous system structures have control over several aspects of the VOR that have significant physiological and clinical implications. Central control over the VOR is able to suppress the VOR and change the calibration of eye movements with respect to head movements, referred to as the "gain" of the VOR. The CNS also monitors the eye movement velocity as a function of time in order to "keep track" of the position of the eyes in the orbit so that the image maintains the same retinal position both before and after saccades. This central function is termed the "velocity storage" or "neural integrator." Saccades that overshoot or undershoot their target are thus a sign of central nervous system dysfunction.

Otolith Organ and Eye Movements

The relationship between stimulation of the otolith organs (i.e., the utricle and saccule) and eye movements is not as straightforward as that with the semicircular canals. The utricle responds to linear accelerations of any direction in the horizontal plane, and the saccule responds to changes in head position with respect to the vertical force of gravity. Gross stimulation of the entire utricular nerve causes torsional eye movement, with intorsion and elevation of the ipsilateral eye and extorsion and depression of the contralateral eye. Loss of utricular function on one side creates the same sensation as tilting the head toward the contralateral side.

EVALUATION OF THE DIZZY PATIENT

Dizziness is one of the most common complaints of patients, especially in the elderly population, and the differential diagnosis for causes of dizziness is vast. Patient history, however, can narrow the diagnosis more efficiently than any test and is the most powerful tool of the vestibular diagnostician. Critical information that the history provides includes the nature of the dizziness, that is, whether or not it is characterized by lightheadedness, imbalance, or true vertigo (defined as illusory sense of motion); the duration of episodes; changes in auditory function; concomitant medical conditions and medications; history of ear disease; whether the symptoms recur or are isolated; any history of head trauma; inciting factors (e.g., dietary, positional); and family history of migraine.

Balance Function Testing

Unlike the auditory system, which can be objectively and effectively tested by audiogram, the vestibular system has no single primary objective test with which single diagnoses can be made. Rather, a cadre of tests are available that are used in different combinations to yield a vestibular evaluation and help reach a diagnosis. The most common tests are discussed here; these include electronystagmography (ENG), caloric irrigation, rotary chair, posturography, and the vestibular evoked myogenic potential (VEMP).

Electronystagmography

ENG records eye movements with the use of either changes in the direction of the corneo-retinal potential with electrodes or infrared video monitoring of the eyes themselves. Eye movements are first recorded and evaluated during saccades, pursuit, and optokinetic nystagmus. Abnormalities in saccadic eye movements such as over- or undershooting the target suggest central pathology but can also be due to pathological states of the extraocular musculature or oculomotor neurons. Similarly, an inability to perform smooth pursuit also suggests cerebellar or brainstem pathology.

Gaze-evoked nystagmus is then pursued with the eyes centered, then up, down, and to both sides. With peripheral lesions, gaze-evoked nystagmus maintains a single direction that has both horizontal and torsional components, regardless of eye position. Nystagmus due to peripheral lesions can also be reduced with fixation. Furthermore, positioning the eyes in the direction of the fast component of nystagmus increases the nystagmus magnitude (Alexander's law). With central lesions, however, gaze-evoked nystagmus may not suppress with fixation, may change direction with gaze, or can be purely vertical. Nystagmus is then evaluated in response to different head positions and movements that isolate individual semicircular canals.

Caloric Testing

Cool and warm irrigation of the external canal can be used to stimulate and suppress the ampullary nerve of the horizontal canal. The power of caloric testing is that it can be used to isolate the response of the labyrinth on one side from that of the other side. Caloric testing is based on the principle that cooling the external auditory canal establishes a temperature gradient in the horizontal semicircular canal and that this gradient results in convective endolymphatic flow away from the cupula and suppression of the vestibular nerve firing rate. Warm water has the opposite effect, resulting in an increase in the vestibular nerve firing rate. In a normally functioning patient, cool irrigation will thus yield nystagmus beating away from the side of irrigation, whereas warm irrigation yields nystagmus beating toward the side of irrigation (COWS; cold = opposite, warm = same).

In order to quantify the results of caloric irrigation on both right and left sides, eye movements are recorded during the irrigation, and the maximum slow phase velocity of induced nystagmus is used as the measure of canal responsiveness. Four measurements of maximum slow phase velocity are thus made—cool irrigation on the right (R_{cool}), warm on the right (R_{warm}), and cool and warm on the left (L_{cool} and L_{warm}, respectively). From these values the unilateral weakness is calculated, which simply compares the strength of the vestibular response between the right and left sides. Specifically, unilateral weakness is computed as $[(R_{cool} + R_{warm}) - (L_{cool} + L_{warm})]/(R_{cool} + R_{warm} + L_{cool} + L_{warm})$. A value of unilateral weakness greater than 20% compared with normal values of each laboratory is considered significant.

Unilateral hypofunction, manifested by a significant value of unilateral weakness, can occur with decreased function of the horizontal canal or ampullary nerve, even in cases where the weakness is well compensated centrally. Caloric responses are also used to monitor the titration of intratympanic gentamicin injections for Ménière's disease.

Rotary Chair

A disadvantage of caloric stimulation is that the caloric stimulus is not physiological, occurring in a clinically artificial context. The rotary chair overcomes this shortcoming by administering a physiological stimulus that can be quantified. Eye movements are recorded with electro-oculography while the patient sits in a sinusoidally oscillating chair with fixation removed. The patient's head is held 30% down from the horizontal in order to align the motion in the plane of the horizontal canal. Averaged, filtered, and fitted data are then used to compare the slow phase of nystagmus (VOR-driven) with the head velocity. Angular velocities between 0.01 Hz and 1.0 Hz can be tested with the rotary chair.

Several aspects of the VOR status can be gleaned from the rotary chair. Gain is the magnitude of the maximum slow phase eye velocity compared with that of the maximum head velocity. In a normally functioning vestibular system, the gain is one. Gains substantially less than one may be found in bilateral vestibular deficits. *Phase* refers to the time delay between the head movement and eye movement, which should normally be opposite (i.e., 180° phase difference, but by convention the sign of the eye velocity is reversed so that the ideal phase difference in the normal patient is zero). Asymmetries in the magnitude of the eye velocity response between left and right can indicate relative weakness of one side and recognize unilateral vestibular lesions. Rotatory chair testing is useful in patients who would not tolerate caloric testing, such as children.

Dynamic Posturography

Although the VOR lends itself well to a straightforward assessment of vestibular function, it does not address an important aspect of the vestibular system, which is control of the rest of the body in space, or postural control. Posturography is an attempt to objectively test the postural control aspect of the vestibular system. As the maintenance and manipulation of postural control relies on a complex integration of several sensory and motor systems, posturography is more a global assessment of balance than a diagnostic test of specific vestibular abnormalities. Nonetheless, in specific situations, posturography can be a useful addition to the vestibular testing battery.

The posturography testing procedure generally involves the patient standing on a platform that can rotate fore and aft, and a visual scene that can also be manipulated independently from the platform. The patient's weight symmetry between the two feet, the force distribution throughout the legs, latency of the patient's response to motion, ability to remain upright in the face of different stimuli, and adaptation to the stimuli are all measured. Basic posturographic paradigms emphasize either the motor or the sensory integration aspects of postural control. The sensory organization test, or SOT, assesses individual contributions of visual, somatosensory, and vestibular input to postural stability. The motor control test assesses the reflex control of posture to sudden changes in the patient's center of gravity.

The SOT monitors the degree of a patient's swaying back and forth on the platform as a means of computing the percentage of equilibrium compared with normal control subjects. Equilibrium is measured for each of six conditions of increasing difficulty. In the first condition (C1) the patient has eyes open with a stable platform and stable visual surround. The patient who can compensate for any deficits with one intact sensory component is expected to have normal equilibrium on this condition. In the second condition (C2) the eyes are closed, removing visual input as a cue for stability. In the third condition (C3) the visual surround is moving with the subjects' movement, which removes useful visual input to aid postural changes and forces the brain to disregard the unhelpful visual information in order to maintain balance. The fourth, fifth, and sixth conditions (C4, C5, and C6) are the same with respect to the visual input, but now the platform moves with the patient, which removes somatosensory input from the postural stability mechanism. C5 and C6 thus rely on vestibular input only to maintain stability. Patients with uncompensated unilateral vestibular lesions or bilateral vestibular weakness as isolated problems are expected to have significant deficits in postural stability with C5 and C6, but other conditions may be minimally affected (Baloh, Jacobson, Beykirch, & Honrubia, 1998).

The motor control test administers sudden movements to the platform while measuring the symmetry of weight distribution, delay (latency) of the response, and magnitude of the response. Delays in response and failure scale of the response magnitude to the magnitude of the platform's movement are signs of deficits along the reflex pathways controlling posture.

Posturography is better at detecting general balance control deficits than defining specific etiologies of vertigo (Goebel & Paige, 1989). Its utility is greatest in several clinical situations: in defining the functional severity of balance disorders, evaluating dizziness in the elderly (Baloh, Spain, Socotch, Jacobson, & Bell, 1995), monitoring progress with vestibular rehabilitation, assessing pre- and post-vestibular ablative procedures, and especially in identifying patients who may be malingering or have non-organic contributions to their balance complaints (Black, 2001).

Vestibular Evoked Myogenic Potentials

Normally, a loud acoustic click results in an inhibitory myogenic potential in the ipsilateral sternocleidomastoid muscle. The circuit responsible for this reflex appears to involve excitation of the saccule and conduction along the inferior vestibular nerve (Townsend & Cody, 1971). Vestibular evoked myogenic potentials (VEMPs) are measured by administering 0.1-ms impulse stimuli via headphones and measuring the ipsilateral sternocleidomastoid muscle potential electromyographically. The inhibitory muscle potential has a positive potential at about 12 ms followed by a negative potential. Threshold of the VEMP in normal subjects is about 85 dB (Colebatch, Halmagyi, & Skuse, 1994). The VEMP has clinical utility in three situations. First, in unilateral vestibular loss due to vestibular schwannoma or vestibular neuritis, the VEMP can be helpful in determining the extent of the inferior vestibular nerve. The VEMP may be more sensitive than caloric testing in these patients (Murofushi, Matsuzaki, & Mizuno, 1998). Second, in superior canal dehiscence syndrome, the "third window" that the dehiscent superior canal creates is the source of decreased resistance to inner ear fluid flow. As a result of this decreased resistance, VEMP thresholds are lowered in superior canal dehiscence syndrome (Streubel, Cremer, Carey, Weg, & Minor, 2001). Last, decreased or absent VEMP responses may indicate endolymphatic hydrops specifically of the saccule, helping to make the diagnosis of Ménière's disease (Murofushi, Shimizu, Takegoshi, & Cheng, 2001).

PERIPHERAL VESTIBULAR DISORDERS

The peripheral vestibular system, which refers to the labyrinth and vestibular nerves, provides the central nervous system (CNS) with a balance of signal input from the right and left sides. When functioning normally, angular head motion is conveyed to the CNS with an increase in the spontaneous firing rate from the stimulated side and decrease from the inhibited side. Pathological processes of the vestibular periphery result in changes to the input signals delivered to the CNS. When a pathological process affects only one ear, the balance of input to the CNS is disrupted. The CNS can compensate for chronic changes in peripheral sensitivity—but only if these changes are static. Acute changes in the peripheral sensitivity of one ear, however, create the sensation of motion despite the absence of movement, which is the definition of vertigo. Not all vertigo, however, can be attributed to alterations in the vestibular periphery. The diagnostician of vestibular disorders has as a primary challenge the task of "localizing the lesion." Especially for peripheral vestibular disorders, the duration of the vertigo may be the best clue to its etiology that a patient's history can provide. These disorders tend to fall into three durations of vertigo: seconds, minutes to hours, and days. The more common of these disorders are discussed in further detail here.

Benign Paroxysmal Positional Vertigo

Patients with benign paroxysmal positional vertigo (BPPV) present with episodes of vertigo lasting for several seconds, typically elicited by specific changes in head position. Nonspecific dizziness can persist after the true vertigo has subsided. Several episodes can occur in short succession and then be very infrequent. The proposed etiology of BPPV is the displacement of otoconia from the utricle into a semicircular canal, most commonly the posterior canal, irritating the cupula and stimulating the vestibular nerve. This displacement of otoconia into the canal is termed canalolithiasis. The natural history, diagnosis, and treatment of BPPV are explained so well by canalolithiasis that it is the accepted pathophysiology of the disorder (Epley, 2001).

The diagnosis of BPPV begins with the patient's history, which can strongly suggest BPPV. Aside from the character and timing of the vertiginous episodes (i.e., spinning vertigo arising suddenly after head movement and lasting for seconds), a history of closed head injury may also accompany the symptoms. The diagnosis can then be confirmed if the symptoms of BPPV can be elicited with a maneuver credited to Dix and Hallpike used to purposefully displace particles in the utricle into the posterior semicircular canal with the help of gravity (Dix & Hallpike, 1952). The Dix-Hallpike maneuver is performed by having the patient turn the head 45 degrees toward the presumed affected side and then rapidly bringing the patient from an upright to supine position with his or her head hanging off the top of the examining table. In this position the posterior canal is held vertical, with the cupula in the most dependent position. After a delay of a few seconds while the particles drift into the posterior canal and down toward the cupula, nystagmus ensues. The nystagmus follows the vertical-torsional pattern expected for posterior canal irritative lesions (see Fig. 3–5): the fast phase has both a vertical component and a rotatory (or tosional) component, such that the superior pole of the iris beats toward the side of the lesion. In the Dix-Hallpike position, this is toward the lower (affected) ear. The nystagmus elicited with this maneuver typically has its onset within 10 seconds of the head positioning and fatigues in about 30 seconds. The patient is then returned to the upright position, whereupon nystagmus in the opposite direction can ensue as the otoconia fall away from the cupula.

Treatment of BPPV is founded on the premise that removing the otoconia from the posterior canal will alleviate the symptoms. Epley described this "canalith repositioning" maneuver, which has proved particularly effective (Epley, 1992). The patient is positioned with the head turned toward the affected side and hanging similar to the Dix-Hallpike maneuver until the nystagmus has subsided. The head is then turned 180° such that the affected ear is then facing toward the ceiling before the patient is returned to the upright position.

Ménière's Disease

Ménière's disease is defined by a symptom complex consisting of recurring attacks of vertigo lasting minutes to hours, sensorineural hearing loss, tinnitus, and aural fullness (Monsell, 1995). The vertigo tends to be severe and is worsened by head movement. It is frequently accompanied by nausea, vomiting, and sweating. Although the attacks subside within minutes to hours, the hearing loss tends to accumulate over the course of the disease.

The exact etiology of Ménière's disease is not known. The pathological hallmark of the disease, however, is distension of the endolymphatic compartments of the inner ear, referred to as endolymphatic hydrops. However, not all patients with endolymphatic hydrops are symptomatic (Rauch, Marchant, & Thedinger, 1989). This suggests that hydrops is an epiphenomenon, that is, an associated finding rather than a causative mechanism. Ménière's disease is more likely caused by an alteration in the homeostatic mechanisms responsible for maintaining the endocochlear potential between endolymph and perilymph. Candidate molecular structures include ion channels, Na^+/K^+ ATPase, and intercellular junction proteins.

The hallmark of Ménière's disease is the recurrent attacks of vertigo accompanied by hearing loss. The attacks are typically preceded by an "aura" of aural fullness, tinnitus, and a decreased sensation of hearing. The clinical course is highly variable. Attacks can be frequent or sparse and may remit completely after years with the disease. Symptoms become bilateral in about half of the patients followed long-term (Kitahara, 1991). The disease can be psychologically disabling, at times out of proportion to the actual physical disability brought on by the disease.

The attacks are usually not active by the time a patient sees a physician, and thus the patient history yields the most important data for making the diagnosis. Other tests that can be helpful in diagnosing Ménière's disease include ENG, which can reveal weakness of the involved side after caloric irrigation, and audiogram, which typically shows low-frequency sensorineural hearing loss with a decrease in speech discrimination on the affected side. A glycerol challenge test can also be used, which is based on the theory that dehydrating the endolymph compartment should improve the hearing loss. The glycerol is an osmotic load that theoretically draws fluid out of the endolymph. Several times during the hours following the glycerol load, the audiogram is measured. In some patients with Ménière's disease the audiogram will show improvement in pure tone threshold and discrimination, supporting the diagnosis of Ménière's. Additionally, electrocochleography can reveal findings suggestive of Ménière's disease. Electrocochleography monitors three components of sound-evoked auditory potentials: the summating potential, which is the steady-state potential offset attributed to an inequality of excitation over inhibition of hair cell stimulation, the compound action potential of the auditory nerve, and the cochlear microphonic from the outer hair cells. In Ménière's disease the ratio of the summating potential to the compound cochlear nerve action potential (i.e., the SP to AP ratio) is elevated.

The natural history of Ménière's disease can take several courses. A portion of patients will have a remission of the vertiginous episodes of their disease without developing symptoms from the contralateral ear. The hearing loss tends to persist. A second portion of patients will have persistent unilateral disease, and another portion of patients will develop contralateral disease. First-line treatments for Ménière's disease are intended to prevent or lessen the severity of attacks based on the rationale of decreasing the volume of endolymph. Medical approaches to decreasing endolymph volume consist primarily of a low-salt diet and diuretics, although the efficacy of treatment may not be better than that of a placebo (van Deelen & Huizing, 1986). Surgical approaches to endolymph decompression consist of opening the endolymphatic sac through a transmastoid approach and possibly permanently shunting the sac open. The advantage of both medical and surgical approaches to endolymph decompression is its low morbidity. Efficacy, however, is variable and difficult to demonstrate as superior to placebo in controlled studies (Thomsen, Bretlau, Tos, & Johnsen, 1981a, 1981b). For those in whom more conservative treatment fails to curb the attacks, several options are available.

At least 10% of patients will have persistent vertigo despite medical and conservative therapy (Glasscock, Gulya, Pensak, & Black, 1984). More aggressive procedures for these patients focus on ablating the vestibular function of the involved side for unilateral disease. The most effective procedure for unilateral vestibular ablation is the vestibular nerve section. Vestibular neurectomy, however, is an intracranial procedure that carries the risks of facial nerve damage, hearing loss, leak of spinal fluid, and headaches (Glasscock, Thedinger, Cueva, & Jackson, 1991). Surgical labyrinthectomy, while a less invasive transmastoid procedure with lower surgical risks, is unlikely to conserve hearing and may be less effective at controlling symptoms.

Because of the risks associated with ablative surgical procedures to control vertigo in Ménière's disease, chemical ablation with ototoxic agents (aminoglycosides in particular) of the vestibular end-organ has increasingly gained favor. Aminoglycoside antibiotics enter sensory hair cells through the transduction channels in the apical cell surface and cause their death, leading eventually to the extrusion of the apical portion of the cell (Li, Nevill, & Forge, 1995). The concept of using intratympanic vestibulotoxic antibiotics to destroy the vestibular hair cells was introduced by Schuknecht in 1956 (Schuknecht, 1956) but fell out of favor because of the cochleotoxic (i.e., hearing loss) effects of the medication. Manipulating the dosing schedule of intratympanic administration of medication has lowered the rate of hearing loss, and the technique has again come to the forefront of the armamentarium used to treat Ménière's disease. Streptomycin has been replaced by gentamicin. Streptomycin is an effective anti-tuberculosis antibiotic that is kept under tight control by the CDC because of the potential for developing tuberculosis resistance with overuse (Meacci et al., 2005). Streptomycin is therefore rarely used in Ménière's treatment because of the difficulty of obtaining the medication. Vertigo control rates with gentamicin are reported as being nearly 90% of patients, with significant hearing loss occurring in an average of 26% over the studies evaluated (Diamond, O'Connell, Hornig, & Liu, 2003). Titration methods focus on titrating the number of gentamicin doses to an endpoint of either ablation of caloric response or a predetermined amount of hearing loss measured with serial audiograms. Intratympanic administration of dexamethasone is also a recently introduced therapy that shows great promise in the treatment of Meniere's disease, although further data are needed to establish its efficacy.

Superior Semicircular Canal Dehiscence

The bone of the middle fossa overlying the superior semicircular canal can be very thin or dehiscent. With this bony weakness a "third window" (i.e., in addition to the oval and round windows) ensues in the labyrinthine system that results in increased compliance of the endolymph-containing compartment. The clinical presentation of this entity is called superior semicircular canal dehiscence (SCD) syndrome, and although it is rare, it has been well described (Minor, 2000). Patients typically present with vertigo precipitated by loud sounds or straining. On examination, loud sound or pressure to the external ear can produce nystagmus in the plane of the affected superior canal, with the slow phase eye movement directed upward and away from the affected side. *Tullio's phenomenon* refers to vestibular activation in response to auditory stimulation (Tullio, 1929), and *Hennebert's sign* refers to conjugate slow horizontal eye movements induced by external auditory canal pressurization, with a reversed direction once the pressure is releaved (Hennebert, 1911). Both can be seen in SCD (Minor, Solomon, Zinreich, & Zee, 1998). Patients may have a conductive hearing loss on the affected side due to the increased compliance of the inner ear fluid. This type of conductive loss will manifest as a lateralization of the Weber tuning fork test to the affected side and an increase in the air conduction threshold with intact stapedius reflex on audiometric evaluation. As stapedius reflexes are intact and no ossicular chain abnormality is present, the hearing loss is classified as "cochlear conductive." Because Tullio's phenomenon is the activation of vestibulospinal reflexes with loud sound (Ishizaki, Pyykko, Aalto, & Starck, 1991), vestibular-evoked myogenic potentials (VEMPs) can be used as an objective assessment of Tullio's phenomenon and help with the diagnosis. In patients with dehiscence of the semicircular canal, a "third window" results in easier stimulation of the sacculus with loud sounds. Patients with superior canal dehiscence thus have a lower VEMP threshold on the side of the affected ear (Streubel et al., 2001). Diagnosis is then confirmed with CT scan with extra fine resolution (0.5-mm cuts) coplanar to the superior semicircular canal (Minor, 2005). Defects in the bone overlying the superior semicircular canal indicate SCD.

Treatment of SCD is to repair the inciting dehiscence in the middle fossa plate through the middle fossa approach with either resurfacing or plugging of the canal. Intraoperative image guidance techniques have aided in identifying the weakness in the superior canal bone. This technique has resulted in resolution of symptoms in the majority of patients treated (Minor, 2005).

Vestibular Neuritis

Vestibular neuritis is characterized by sudden-onset, severe vertigo that does not remit for hours or days. Patients typically report preceding symptoms consistent with viral illness, which aids the diagnosis. On exam, nystagmus, if present, is consistent with that expected for acute unilateral vestibular nerve hypofunction, which is horizontal and torsional, such that the superior pole of the iris moves away from the involved side during the slow phase of the VOR and then the fast phase beats toward the involved side. Bilateral involvement, although rare, is possible. The illness tends to be self-limited, and recovery of vestibular nerve function is expected. Treatment is therefore supportive, with vestibular suppressants as needed. Early activity aids central compensation of the vestibular dysfunction and can speed recovery. Mild imbalance, however, may be protracted for weeks to months following the illness.

CENTRAL VESTIBULAR DISORDERS

Vertebrobasilar Insufficiency

Vertebrobasilar insufficiency refers to decreased blood flow in the vertebral and basilar artery system that results in episodic transient hypoxia of the vessels supplying several components of the vestibular system. Imbalance and lightheadedness are more common than true vertigo with vertebrobasilar insufficiency. The entity is more common in elderly patients. Diagnosis is made primarily by patient history, although angiography can confirm the diagnosis when decreases in the caliber of these vessels are observed. Management of vertebrobasilar insufficiency consists of controlling the risk factors for vascular disease, such as diabetes, hypertension, and hyperlipidemia.

Vestibular Migraine

Classic migraine begins with an aura foreshadowing the onset of a severe headache and is considered to have a vascular origin. Basilar migraine consists of an aura with more than one brainstem symptom. Migraine can be associated with a multitude of neurological symptoms, including vestibular symptoms such as imbalance and true vertigo. Recently an entity has been recognized that can present with no aura, minimal headache, and only vestibular episodes, but it responds well only to anti-migraine medication (Dieterich & Brandt, 1999). Because the symptoms are limited to vestibular complaints only, this entity does not meet the classic definition of migraine, but is more properly considered as migraine-induced vestibular dysfunction, or vestibular migraine. Attacks of vertigo in these patients can have variable durations, from minutes to hours to even days, and can be exacerbated with head movement. Because of these similarities with other peripheral vestibular disorders, vestibular migraine should be considered in the differential diagnosis of episodic vertigo. Treatment is complex, but it relies primarily on dietary modification and administration of centrally acting agents (e.g., neurontin, antidepressants) or vasoactive agents (e.g., calcium channel blockers).

Brainstem and Cerebellar Infarction

Ischemia and infarction of the brainstem or cerebellum can involve structures vital to the vestibular system, and patients can present with sudden onset persistent vertigo. Other neurologic sequelae are typically associated. Several more common syndromes result from injury to a combination of brainstem structures that have a common blood supply. The lateral medullary syndrome (Wallenberg's syndrome) follows from injury to the dorsolateral medulla via occlusion of either the vertebral artery or the posterior inferior cerebellar artery. The involved structures include the spinothalamic tract, the lateral cuneate nucleus, the vestibular nuclei, the cranial nerve V nucleus and tract, and cerebellar connections. Injury to these structures results in loss of pain/temperature sensation to the contralateral body, Horner's syndrome, vertigo with nausea/vomiting, ipsilateral facial numbness, and limb ataxia. Diagnosis is made with imaging. Cerebellar infarction can result in vertigo and vomiting without brainstem symptoms, and this picture can resemble peripheral labyrinthine dysfunction. Discriminating cerebellar infarct from a more benign peripheral vestibular disorder relies on testing cerebellar function. Ataxia and dysmetria are cerebellar signs that raise significant suspicion of cerebellar lesions.

Tumor

Vestibular schwannoma is the most common neoplasm of the cerebellopontine angle. These tumors are slow-growing, benign masses that begin in the internal auditory canal and can grow medially to compress the brainstem. Vestibular schwannomas rarely present with vertigo, because of the slow growth of the tumor and gradual loss of vestibular nerve function. The CNS has time to compensate for this gradual loss of vestibular nerve function. Patients may complain of vague imbalance without true vertigo. Despite a lack of vestibular symptoms, patients who present with asymmetric hearing loss can benefit from vestibular testing and possible neuroimaging studies. In patients whose tumors have progressed in size and in whom vestibular function on the involved side is absent or diminished, head thrust test, calorics, and rotational chair testing can reveal unilateral vestibular weakness associated with the tumor. MRI with gadolinium (T1 weighted images in particular) confirms the diagnosis of vestibular schwannoma. Treatment for these tumors is performed via surgery, radiation therapy, or, in some cases (e.g., elderly, sick), observation.

SURGICAL PROCEDURES FOR VESTIBULAR DISORDERS

This section briefly describes the more common surgeries for vestibular disorders. Repair or resurfacing of superior canal dehiscence has already been described here and is not addressed in this section.

Labyrinthectomy

The labyrinthectomy involves destruction of the vestibular sensory apparatus. Transcanal labyrinthectomy can be performed, but with this approach complete removal of the vestibular sensory epithelium is difficult. More complete labyrinthectomy is accomplished through a transmastoid approach. The semicircular canals are exposed following a cortical mastoidectomy and opened with the drill. Once the bony labyrinth is obliterated, any remaining soft tissue of the membranous labyrinth is removed. Complete hearing loss is expected.

Endolymphatic Shunt

The endolymphatic sac is identified though a transmastoid approach. The sac is located just anterior to the sigmoid sinus, superior to the jugular bulb, inferior to the posterior semicircular canal, and medial to the facial nerve. Once encountered, the sac is opened and stented, opened, or excised. The advantages of the endolymphatic shunt are that it is outpatient surgery with minimal morbidity and a low complication rate. Steroids can be directly administered to the endolymphatic sac if desired.

Vestibular Nerve Section

Selective vestibular nerve section for intractable vertigo is intended to section the superior and inferior vestibular nerves while preserving the cochlear portion of the nerve and the facial nerve, all of which run in the internal auditory meatus. Vestibular nerve section can be accomplished through several approaches. The middle fossa approach entails a craniotomy in front of and superior to the external ear, with retraction of the temporal lobe of the brain medially and superiorly. The internal auditory meatus is therefore approached from above. The bone of the middle fossa plate is drilled, the dura opened, and the vestibular nerve sectioned within the lateral portion of the internal auditory canal. In the retrosigmoid approach, a craniectomy or craniotomy is made posterior to the sigmoid sinus. The cerebellum is retracted medially, revealing the posterior aspect of the internal auditory canal. The dura is opened, the facial nerve identified and preserved, and the vestibular nerve sectioned. The complications associated with these intracranial procedures are cerebrospinal fluid leak, headache, facial nerve injury, and meningitis. The control of vertigo in Ménière's disease, however, approaches 90% of cases (Silverstein, Wanamaker, Flanzer, & Rosenberg, 1992).

CONCLUSIONS

Despite its complexity, the basic anatomy and physiology of the peripheral vestibular system are well understood. This understanding of vestibular anatomy and physiology has led to the development of several useful tests of vestibular function. Also as a result of this understanding, the diagnosis and treatment of a few vestibular disorders have been solidly founded on basic scientific principles, such as benign paroxysmal positional vertigo and superior canal dehiscence syndrome. Other aspects of the vestibular system, however, are poorly understood, and clinical entities whose symptom complex is very well described remain pathologically unclear, such as Ménière's disease and vestibular migraine. Future scientific progress in these areas is required in order to improve diagnosis and treatment of these challenging disorders.

REFERENCES

Anson, B. J., & Bast, T. H. (1960). The surgical significance of stapedial and labyrinthine anatomy. *Archives Otolaryngology, 71*, 188.

Baloh, R. W., Jacobson, K. M., Beykirch, K., & Honrubia, V. (1998). Static and dynamic posturography in patients with vestibular and cerebellar lesions. *Archives Neurology, 55*(5), 649–654.

Baloh, R. W., Spain, S., Socotch, T. M., Jacobson, K. M., & Bell, T. (1995). Posturography and balance problems in older people. *Journal of the American Geriatric Society, 43*(6), 638–644.

Black, F. O. (2001). What can posturography tell us about vestibular function? *Annals of the New York Academy of Sciences, 942*, 446–464.

Colebatch, J. G., Halmagyi, G. M., & Skuse, N. F. (1994). Myogenic potentials generated by a click-evoked vestibulocollic reflex. *Journal of Neurology Neurosurgery and Psychiatry, 57*(2), 190–197.

Della Santina, C. C., Potyagaylo, V., Migliaccio, A. A., Minor, L. B., & Carey, J. P. (2005). Orientation of human semicircular canals measured by three-dimensional multiplanar CT reconstruction. *Journal of the Association for Research in Otolaryngology*, 1–16.

Diamond, C., O'Connell, D. A., Hornig, J. D., & Liu, R. (2003). Systematic review of intratympanic gentamicin in Meniere's disease. *Journal of Otolaryngology, 32*(6), 351–361.

Dieterich, M., & Brandt, T. (1999). Episodic vertigo related to migraine (90 cases): Vestibular migraine? *Journal of Neurology, 246*, 883–892.

Dix, M. R., & Hallpike, C. S. (1952). Pathology, symptomatology and diagnosis of certain disorders of the vestibular system. *Proceedings of the Royal Society of Medicine, 45*, 341.

Engstrom, H. (1961). The innervation of the vestibular sensory cells. *Acta Otolaryngologica Supplement, 163*, 30–40.

Engstrom, H., & Wersall, J. (1958). Structure and innervation of the inner ear sensory epithelia. *International Reviews of Cytology, 7*, 535–585.

Epley, J. M. (1992). The canalith repositioning positioning procedure: For treatment of benign paroxysmal positional vertigo. *Otolaryngology Head & Neck Surgery, 107*, 399.

Epley, J. M. (2001). Human experience with canalith repositioning maneuvers. *Annals of the New York Academy of Sciences, 942*, 179–191.

Glasscock, M. E., 3rd, Gulya, A. J., Pensak, M. L., & Black, J. N., Jr. (1984). Medical and surgical management of Meniere's disease. *American Journal of Otology, 5*(6), 536–542.

Glasscock, M. E., III, Thedinger, B. A., Cueva, R. A., & Jackson, C. G. (1991). An analysis of the retrolabyrinthine vs. the retrosigmoid vestibular nerve section. *Otolaryngology Head & Neck Surgery, 104*(1), 88–95.

Goebel, J. A., & Paige, G. D. (1989). Dynamic posturography and caloric test results in patients with and without vertigo. *Otolaryngology Head & Neck Surgery, 100*(6), 553–558.

Hennebert, C. (1911). A new syndrome in hereditary syphilis of the labyrinth. *Presse Med Melge Bussels, 63*, 467–470.

Hudspeth, A. J., & Jacobs, R. (1979). Stereocilia mediate transduction in vertebrate hair cells (auditory system/cilium/vestibular system). *Proceedings of the National Academy of Sciences, 76*(3), 1506–1509.

Ishizaki, H., Pyykko, I., Aalto, H., & Starck, J. (1991). Tullio phenomenon and postural stability: experimental study in normal subjects and patients with vertigo. *Annals of Otology Rhinology and Laryngology, 100*(12), 976–983.

Keller, E. L. (1976). Behavior of horizontal semicircular canal afferents in alert monkey during vestibular and optokinetic stimulation. *Experimental Brain Research, 24*(5), 459–471.

Kitahara, M. (1991). Bilateral aspects of Meniere's disease. *Acta Otolaryngologica Supplement, 485,* 74.

Li, L., Nevill, G., & Forge, A. (1995). Two modes of hair cell loss from the vestibular sensory epithelia of the guinea pig inner ear. *Journal of Comparitive Neurology, 355*(3), 405–417.

Meacci, F., Orrù, G., Iona, E., Giannoni, F., Piersimoni, C., Pozzi, G., et al. (2005). Drug resistance evolution of a mycobacterium tuberculosis strain from a noncompliant patient. *Journal of Clinical Microbiology, 43*, 3114–3120.

Minor, L. B. (2000). Superior canal dehiscence syndrome. *American Journal of Otology, 21*, 9–19.

Minor, L. B. (2005). Clinical manifestations of superior semicircular canal dehiscence. *Laryngoscope, 115*, 1717–1727.

Minor, L. B., Solomon, D., Zinreich, J. S., & Zee, D. S. (1998). Sound- and/or pressure-induced vertigo due to bone dehiscence of the superior semicircular canal. *Archives of Otolaryngology, 124*, 249–258.

Monsell, E. M. (1995). New and revised reporting guidelines from the Committee on Hearing and Equilibrium. American Academy of Otolaryngology-Head and Neck Surgery Foundation, Inc. *Otolaryngology. Head Neck Surgery., 113*(3), 176–178.

Murofushi, T., Matsuzaki, M., & Mizuno, M. (1998). Vestibular evoked myogenic potentials in patients with acoustic neuromas. *Archives of Otolaryngology, 124*(5), 509–512.

Murofushi, T., Shimizu, K., Takegoshi, H., & Cheng, P. W. (2001). Diagnostic value of prolonged latencies in the vestibular evoked myogenic potential. *Archives of Otolaryngology, 127*(9), 1069–1072.

Rauch, S. D., Marchant, S. N., & Thedinger, B. A. (1989). Meniere's syndrome and endolymphatic hydrops: A double-blind temporal bone study. *Annals of Otology, Rhinology, and Laryngology, 98*, 873.

Schuknecht, H. F. (1956). Ablation therapy for the relief of Meniere's disease. *Laryngoscope, 66*, 859–870.

Silverstein, H., Wanamaker, H., Flanzer, J., & Rosenberg, S. (1992). Vestibular neurectomy in the United States—1990. *American Journal of Otology, 13*(1), 23–30.

Streubel, S. O., Cremer, P. D., Carey, J. P., Weg, N., & Minor, L. B. (2001). Vestibular-evoked myogenic potentials in the diagnosis of superior canal dehiscence syndrome. *Acta Otolaryngology Supplement, 545*, 41–49.

Thomsen, J., Bretlau, P., Tos, M., & Johnsen, N. J. (1981a). Meniere's disease: Endolymphatic sac decompression compared with sham (placebo) decompression. *Annals of the New York of Sciences, 374*, 820–830.

Thomsen, J., Bretlau, P., Tos, M., & Johnsen, N. J. (1981b). Placebo effect in surgery for Meniere's disease. A double-blind, placebo-controlled study on endolymphatic sac shunt surgery. *Archives of Otolaryngology, 107*(5), 271–277.

Townsend, G. L., & Cody, D. T. (1971). The averaged inion response evoked by acoustic stimulation: its relation to the saccule. *Annals of Otology, Rhinology, and Laryngology, 80*(1), 121–131.

Tullio, P. (1929). *Das Ohr und die Entstehung der Sprache und Schrift*. Berlin: Urban & Schwarzenberg.

van Deelen, G. W., & Huizing, E. H. (1986). Use of a diuretic (Dyazide) in the treatment of Meniere's disease. A double-blind cross-over placebo-controlled study. *ORL Journal of Otorhinolaryngology and its Related Specialties, 48*(5), 287–292.

CHAPTER 4

The Genetics of Deafness

Walter E. Nance
Virginia Commonwealth University

Astonishing success has been achieved during the past decade in identifying genes for deafness, so that any current account of this research must be regarded as a "work in progress." For the first half of the twentieth century, geneticists argued about whether two, three, or perhaps four genes could explain the inheritance of deafness, and whether they were dominant or recessive. Now, more than 120 independent genes have been identified that can be the cause of hearing loss, and it now seems likely that this number may rise to include 1% of all human genes, or about 300. The goal of this review is to highlight some of the results and significance of this rapidly expanding body of knowledge and to suggest some of the directions that future research may take.

GENETIC EPIDEMIOLOGY OF DEAFNESS

Deafness has many recognized genetic and environmental causes. In this country, profound hearing loss occurs in about 0.8–1.0 per 1000 births, but the incidence is known to vary with time and place. Many previous studies have suggested that about 50% of profound deafness is genetic in etiology. However, during the last rubella pandemic in 1964, the estimated proportion of genetic cases fell to about 10%. Estimates of this type are obtained by the collection and analysis of the distribution of affected relatives in the families of deaf probands, or index cases. The method of analysis involves the reasonable assumption that all nuclear families with more than one affected individual ("multiplex cases") are genetic in origin. The task then becomes to estimate what proportion of the "simplex cases" with only one affected individual are also genetically determined. We know that simplex cases could represent true sporadic cases of environmentally caused deafness in which the chance of another affected child is very low. Alternatively, they could represent "chance isolated genetic cases" in which by chance there is only one affected child. The process of analysis is analogous to estimating the size of an iceberg from the part that is above water and knowledge of the density of ice and water. If only families with two or more affected children are considered to be genetic, the true proportion will be underestimated. On the other hand, assuming that all simplex cases of deafness are caused by sporadic, nongenetic factors would lead to the absurd conclusion that all deaf children in one-child families have nongenetic hearing loss. Data emerging from newborn hearing screening programs suggest that for every child with profound hearing loss, 1 to 2 are born with lesser but clinically significant degrees of hearing loss. Much less is known about the contribution of genetic factors to this latter group of patients, and systematic studies of these cases are badly needed. Although the genes that ultimately cause a child to be deaf are present from the time of conception, not all forms of genetic deafness are necessarily expressed at birth. Many families in which the hearing loss appears to have been delayed in onset have been observed, as have others in which there is a variable rate of progression. Genetic hearing loss can be classified in many ways, including the mode of inheritance, the age of onset, audiologic characteristics, presence or absence of vestibular dysfunction, and the location and/or identity of the causal gene(s). Analysis of large collections of family data have suggested that among genetic cases, approximately 77–88% are transmitted as autosomal recessive traits, 10–20% as dominants, and 1–2% as X-linked traits (Rose, Conneally, & Nance, 1977). The frequency of mitochondrial deafness is quite variable and can range from less than 1% to more than 20% in some populations. Some forms of genetic deafness are associated with distinctive audiologic findings, including conductive, low, mid-tone or high-frequency hearing losses or evidence of vestibular dysfunction. Finally, in 20–30% of cases, there may be other associated clinical findings that permit the diagnosis of a specific form of syndromic deafness.

CLASSIFICATION OF GENETIC DEAFNESS

Syndromic Deafness

Nearly 400 forms of deafness have been identified in which the presence of associated clinical findings permits the diagnosis of a specific form of syndromic deafness. In many of these syndromes, the hearing loss is a mild or inconstant feature. Some other syndromes are quite rare. However, there are several well-characterized entities in which hearing loss is a frequent or constant, and often the most clinically significant, feature. A few instructive examples of the latter group are described below. More comprehensive reviews and up-to-date information on several Internet sites are available elsewhere (Gorlin, Toriello, & Cohen, 1995; Keats, Popper, & Fay, 2002; Hereditary Hearing Loss Homepage, 2007; Online Mendelian Inheritance in Man, 2007).

The Branchio-Oto-Renal Syndrome.   The branchio-oto-renal (BOR) syndrome refers to the association of sensori-neural or mixed hearing loss with persistent branchial cleft fistulas, prehelical pits, malformations of the pinna, deformities of the inner ear (which may include the Mondini malformation and stapes fixation), along with renal anomalies, including dysplasia or adysplasia, polycystic kidneys, and malformations of the calyces (Melnick, Bixler, Nance, Silk, & Yune, 1976). About 80% of gene carriers have some degree of hearing loss, which can have a delayed onset. The trait was mapped to band 13.3 on the long (q) arm of chromosome 8 (i.e., 8q13.3) and later shown to result from mutations involving the EYA1 gene (Abdelhak et al., 1997). This gene is homologous to the Eya gene in Drosophila, which is required for the normal formation of its compound eye by the activation of downstream targets. These findings prompted a closer examination of the eyes of human subjects with EYA1 missense mutations, which revealed cataracts and anterior segment anomalies in some cases. It is remarkable that knowledge of the phenotype produced by Eya in the fruit fly led to the description of previously unrecognized clinical findings in humans. The BOR syndrome is transmitted as a dominant trait such that an affected individual has a 50% chance of transmitting the trait to each child.

Waardenburg Syndromes.   These disorders account for at least 1–2% of individuals with profound hearing loss. Bilateral or unilateral hearing loss of variable severity occurs in association with defects in tissues and structures derived from neural crest cells. The most conspicuous findings are pigmentary abnormalities, which can include brilliant blue eyes, complete or segmental heterochromia, lateral displacement of the inner canthi of the eyes, a pinched nose, synophorys, and variable patches of cutaneous hyper- or hypopigmentation (Waardenburg, 1951). Gastrointestinal symptoms such as chronic constipation are common, and some patients report symptoms of gastrointestinal dyskinesia or a history of Hirschsprung disease. The incidence of neural tube defects is increased, and limb defects may be seen. The disorder is genetically heterogeneous, and mutations involving at least eight loci can contribute to the phenotype. Waardenburg syndrome Type 1 (WS1) can result from any one of more than 50 different mutations involving the PAX3 gene on 2q35. The PAX3 gene produces a DNA-binding protein that regulates the MITF locus on 3q12, among other downstream targets. Mutations in MITF, in turn, give rise to WS2A, which is distinguished clinically from WS1 primarily by the absence or less frequent occurrence of the eyelid anomaly dystopia canthorum, and a higher frequency of deafness and heterochromia (Hughes, Newton, Liu, & Read, 1994; Liu, Newton, & Read, 1995). Some WS2A patients exhibit generalized hypopigmentation (albinoidism) with or without freckling. This phenotypic variant has been termed Tietz syndrome. Additional dominantly inherited WS2 variants have been localized to chromosomes 1p21–p13.3 (WS2B) and 8p23 (WS2C). Mutations involving the vasoactive peptide endothelin–3 (END3) on 20q13.2 or its receptor, ENDRB on 13q22, can also cause the features of WS, commonly in association with Hirschsprung disease (McCallion & Chakravarti, 2001). Homozygotes exhibit the full syndrome, whereas heterozygotes may only develop Hirschsprung disease. Single mutations involving the DNA-binding SOX10 locus on 22q13 can also lead to this combination of features. These phenotypic variants have been designated WS4 or the Shah-Waardenburg syndrome. Finally, homozygous carriers of deletions involving the SLUG transcription factor on 8q11 have a form of WS2 that shows recessive transmission (Sanchez-Martin et al., 2002). The gene product of MITF is also a DNA-binding regulatory protein, and its downstream targets include SLUG and the tyrosinase gene (TYR), which codes for the enzyme required for normal pigment formation that is deficient in one form of generalized albinism (Tachibana et al., 1994). Families have been reported in which the digenic interaction between a mutation at the MITF locus with a mild abnormality at the TYR locus resulted in the features of WS2 along with ocular albinism (Morell et al., 1997). These important observations show how pigment abnormalities are incorporated as a component of WS and illustrate how phenotypic variation in a syndrome can result from the effects of modifier genes at other loci. It is tempting to speculate that interactions of this type could explain in part why only about 20–30% of those who carry a PAX3 mutation develop profound bilateral hearing loss (Pandya et al., 1996). WS3 refers to the presence of limb defects in association with other features of WS. It can result from homozygosity for two PAX3 mutations; from particular PAX3 mutations in single dose; or from small chromosomal deletions involving the PAX3 locus. In the cochlea, neural crest cells are known to contribute to the intermediate layer of the stria vascularis, and it thus seems likely that the cause of deafness in WS may be related to a defect in the ability of the stria to maintain the critical endocochlear potential that is required for the hair cells to function normally. The successful cloning of PAX3 illustrates three powerful and complementary techniques that have been used to map human genes. First, the gene was localized to the long arm of chromosome 2 by testing of Waardenburg families for highly variable genetic marker genes located throughout the genome. The goal was to identify markers located close to the WS locus in which a particular allele at the markers was always transmitted in the families along with the WS1 trait. Markers in the 2q35 region met this criterion, and by invoking what might be characterized as "guilt by association," the approximate chromosomal location of the WS1 gene could be inferred. The next important clue was the description of a rare case of WS1 in a Japanese boy who was found to have a small inverted segment on the long arm of chromosome 2. This knowledge effectively localized the gene to one of the two break points of the inversion. Finally, the recognition that a coat color mutation in the mouse, known as "Splotch," mapped to the homologous region of the mouse genome served to focus attention on the human homolog of Splotch as a candidate gene for WS1. The discovery that pathologic mutations in PAX3 cosegregated with the WS in many but not all families confirmed the fact that PAX3 mutations can cause WS, and provided the first clear indication that mutations at other loci might also cause similar syndromes. The information that is emerging about the intricate hierarchy of genes that determine the Waardenburg syndromes is providing a dazzling glimpse of the interacting network of genes that control the development and function of the ear.

Usher Syndromes.   This eponym refers to the syndromic association of deafness with retinitis pigmentosa (RP), a progressive degeneration of the retina that leads to loss of night vision, restriction of the visual fields, and, ultimately, blindness. The incidence in this country has been estimated to be 4.4 per 100,000 (Boughman, Vernon, & Shaver, 1983), but the syndrome accounts for 2–4% of all cases of profound deafness and 50% of the deaf–blind population. Usher syndrome is both phenotypically and genetically heterogeneous. Approximately 40% of affected patients show a profound congenital hearing loss, with vestibular dysfunction and an early onset of RP, often within the first decade of life, that is characteristic of Usher syndrome Type 1 (USH1); 57% with USH2 have a less severe hearing loss, with a later onset of RP, and can usually communicate orally; in the remaining 3% with USH3, the severity of the hearing loss is variable and can be progressive (Rosenberg, Haim, Hauch, & Parving, 1997). To date, six genes for USH1 have been mapped (USH1A-G), and of these, four have been identified, as has one of three USH2 loci and one USH3 locus. Mutations involving the MYO7A gene have been shown to be the cause of USH1B. However, two forms of nonsyndromic deafness (NSD), the dominantly inherited DFNA11 and the recessive DFNB2, also map to the same region, 11q13.5, and have been shown to result from other alleles at the MYO7A locus. Another recessive form of NSD, DFNB18, maps to 11p15.1, the same location as USH1C, which codes for the protein harmonin. In this case, molecular studies have provided an interesting explanation for the differences between the mutations that cause USH1C and those that only cause deafness (i.e., DFNB18). Although genes are composed of linear sequences of nucleotides at a particular site on a given chromosome, typically the sequences are not continuous. Instead, the coding sequence, which specifies the amino acid sequence of the protein product, is normally interrupted by noncoding sequences known as introns. After the genetic message has been transcribed, these introns must be spliced out to form the mature messenger RNA. Expression of the enzymes required for this process can vary from tissue to tissue, such that some exons (as well as introns) may also be spliced out in some tissues but not in others. The coding sequence is not altered, but the message can be drastically edited to skip specific exons in particular tissues, resulting in the synthesis of proteins that can differ in length. It is as if each article in a scientific journal had a different editor who used different rules about whether an abstract, acknowledgments, footnotes, references, figures, or tables should be included in the published version. This feature of gene expression greatly expands the different ways in which a single gene can be expressed in different tissues or times during development. Returning to the phenotypic differences in harmonin mutations, in at least one subject with isolated hearing loss (i.e., DFNB18), the mutation occurs in an exon of the gene that is normally spliced out and not expressed in the retina (Ouyang et al., 2002). Any patient who is homozygous or even a compound heterozygote for a mutation of this type would be expected to show deafness without RP, providing a satisfying explanation for at least some of the striking phenotypic differences that can be seen between different mutations involving the same gene.

Jervell, Lang-Neilsen Syndromes (JLNS).   This syndrome refers to the association of sensori-neural deafness and prolongation of the QT interval on the electrocardiogram, reflecting a defect in cardiac repolarization. This in turn can lead to recurrent attacks of syncope, ventricular arrhythmia, and sudden death. In some cases, syncopal attacks have been precipitated by fright. The syndrome is a rare recessive trait accounting for perhaps one per thousand children with profound deafness. However, when informed about this entity, many superintendants of schools for the deaf can recall having had students in their schools who died suddenly of unexplained causes. Patients with JLNS should be under the care of a knowledgeable cardiologist, because treatment with beta-adrenergic blockers or other drugs is effective in most cases. In a second, much more frequent condition, the Ward-Romano syndrome, prolongation of the QT interval, recurrent syncope, and sudden death can be seen in the absence of hearing loss. It has been shown that in at least some cases, Ward-Romano patients are heterozygous for genes that cause JLNS when present in the homozygous state. Thus, the parents and other hearing relatives in the extended family of a JLNS patient may be at risk for syncope and sudden death. Mapping studies have shown that the gene (KVLQT1), which causes JLNS1 and the Ward-Romano syndrome, is a member of a large family of potassium channel genes, a discovery that has provided a profound insight into the physiology of hearing (Neyroud et al., 1997). The transduction of sound waves into a neural signal is initiated by the physical deflection of the hair cells of the cochlea, which mechanically opens ion channels in the hair cells and allows the passive inward flow of potassium ions from the high-potassium environment of the surrounding endolymphatic fluid. The high potassium concentration is in turn maintained by active transport through potassium channels such as those involved in the JLNS syndromes that are located in the stria vascularis at the outer periphery of the coiled cochlear duct. Like a battery, this system stores potential energy in the high potassium concentration of the endolymph for use by the hair cells during sound transduction (Davis, 1965). One possible reason for this evolutionary adaptation may be to avoid the need for active potassium transport in the cilia. Decreasing the energy requirements of the hair cells may dramatically increase their sensitivity to external sounds by allowing them to function in a microenvironment that is devoid of turbulent blood flow. Imagine the cacophony that would be produced if a capillary bed were required in the basal membrane that supports the hair cells, in order to provide the energy required for active potassium transport in the cillia! In addition to the JLNS1 locus on chromosome 11p15.5, recessive mutations involving another potassium channel gene, KCNE1, at the JLN2 locus on chromosome 21q22.1 can produce an identical phenotype. The expression of another potassium channel gene, KCNQ4, is limited to the outer hair cells. Although it does not contribute to homeostasis of the endolymph, mutations in the gene can cause a relatively common dominant form of progressive hearing loss (DFNA2) that typically begins in the first two decades of life, initially involves the high frequencies, and progresses to become a profound loss within about a decade.

Biotinidase Deficiency.   This autosomal recessive trait results from the deficiency of an enzyme that is required for the normal recycling of the vitamin biotin. Infants with severe deficiency are therefore entirely dependent on dietary sources of the vitamin for their nutritional requirements and typically develop skin rashes, seizures, hair loss, hypotonia, vomiting, and acidosis within the first few months of life, which may progress to coma and death. If untreated, 75% of affected infants develop hearing loss, which may be profound and persists despite the subsequent initiation of treatment (Wolf, Spencer, & Gleason, 2002). Because the symptoms of the disease, including the hearing loss, can be completely prevented by presymptomatic diagnosis and the administration of supplemental biotin, this disease has been included in many newborn screening programs throughout the world. The resulting data have shown that the incidence of affected homozygotes with severe enzyme deficiency is about is about 1 in 60,000. Biotinidase deficiency is an example of a completely preventable form of genetic deafness. Some treatments for hearing loss, such as hearing aides or cochlear implants, are generally effective for a wide range of affected individuals regardless of the etiology of their hearing loss. However, as illustrated by biotinidase deficiency, treatments that depend upon knowledge of the nature of the gene defect are likely to be very specific in their therapeutic relevance, even though they may be highly effective. Thus there is no indication that supplemental biotin would improve the hearing of anyone other than the 1–1.5% of hearing-impaired infants estimated to have biotinidase deficiency. This disease also illustrates another important strategy that has been particularly useful for mapping human genes for deafness. The term polymorphism refers to regions of the genome in which common sequence variations are found. Although some polymorphisms, such as the sickle cell gene, are maintained at high frequency in the population by the selective advantage they confer on heterozygous carriers, most polymorphisms have no detectable clinical effects, and many are not even located within the coding sequences of genes. These genetic markers have been useful for mapping genes, and some are so variable that it is unusual for an individual to be homozygous for exactly the same allele or variant. This feature has been used to map genes for rare recessive traits by "homozygosity mapping." We know that deaf individuals who are the offspring of consanguineous matings carry two alleles for deafness that must be identical because they are both copies of the same gene carried by one of the common ancestors. To localize a gene, therefore, all we need to do is type a sample of consanguineous probands for a large number of polymorphic markers and look for the chromosomal region where all of the affected individuals are homozygous or "identical by descent." In the case of biotinidase deficiency, the analysis of data from 18 consanguineous probands allowed the localization of the gene to a very small region on 3p25 that was only about 0.036% of the length of the entire genome (Blanton et al., 2000). Many rare forms of recessive NSD have only been observed in a single family, and homozygosity mapping has been of particular value for mapping these loci.

Pendred Syndrome.   This autosomal recessive disorder is characterized by neuorsensory deafness, goiter, and malformation of the inner ear. It is probably the commonest form of syndromic deafness and accounts for approximately 7.5% of all individuals with profound hearing loss (Fraser, 1965). The goiter results from a specific defect in the organification of iodine, which may be demonstrated by the abnormal release of radioactive iodine trapped by the thyroid after the administration of perchlorate. Unfortunately, this highly specific test is not widely available. The goiter may be delayed in onset and clinically unapparent and is usually not associated with hypothyroidism. A variety of malformations of the inner ear can be demonstrated radiographically in 86% of cases, including Mondini malformation and malformations of the vestibular canals, but the most characteristic finding is dilation of the vestibular acqueduct (Reardon, O'Mahoney, Trembath, Jan, & Phelps, 2000). The hearing loss is usually profound but can be variable in its onset, rapidly progressive, and even unilateral. The successful cloning of the gene for Pendred syndrome, SLC26A4, showed that it was a member of a family of genes involved in sulfate transport, but functional studies of pendrin, the protein product of the gene, suggest that it is primarily involved in the transport of iodine and chloride ions. As in the case of Usher syndrome, a form of nonsyndromic deafness, DFNB4 can also result from mutations in the Pendred gene. Cochlear abnormalities are also present in DFNB4, and it is not clear how many of these cases may have unapparent thyroid disease, since testing with the perchlorate discharge test has not been reported in these patients.

Congenital Fixation of the Stapes Footplate with Perilymphatic Gusher. Many examples of this association have been described, suggesting that it may be the commonest form of X-linked deafness. Affected males can have either a mixed or neurosensory deafness. In cases with a conductive component, a congenital fixation of the stapes footplate is found at the time of surgery, but attempts to mobilize the footplate typically lead to a profuse flow of endolymphatic fluid, which effectively prevents remediation (Nance et al., 1971). Computerized tomography shows dilation of the internal auditory meatus with an abnormal communication between the subarachnoid space and the cochlear endolymph, which accounts for the "gusher" at the time of stapes surgery. Carrier females may show a mild hearing loss and less severe abnormalities of the inner ear. After the locus was mapped to Xq21.1, affected males were found to carry mutations involving a DNA-binding regulatory gene, POU3F4 (de Kok et al., 1995). In many families, the mutation has been shown to be a deletion, which can vary greatly in size, and can sometimes involve nearby genes for mental retardation and choroideremia. In such cases, symptoms of two or all three diseases may be present in affected family members, a phenomenon known as a contiguous gene syndrome.

Alport Syndromes.   *Alport syndrome* refers to the association of neurosensory hearing loss with progressive nephritis. The latter begins with hematuria and can lead to progressive renal failure and death. About 50% of affected individuals develop a progressive bilateral hearing loss, which usually begins in the second decade of life, involves the high frequencies initially, and may become incapacitating. Ocular findings can include congenital cataracts, spherophakia, retinal flecks, and anterior lenticonus. The latter two findings are seen in about 85% and 25% of affected individuals and are highly characteristic of the syndrome. Renal biopsy shows irregular thickening of the glomerular basement membranes. The disease results from mutations involving one or the other of three tissue-specific polypeptide subunits of collagen that are encoded by the COL4A3, COL4A4, and COL4A5 genes. The latter is determined by an X-linked gene at Xq22, and the genes coding for the first two collagens are located adjacent to each other on 2q35. Typically males with the X-linked form of Alport syndrome are more severely affected than females, who may never develop end-stage renal disease. The three collagen subunits are expressed in the basilar membrane, spiral ligament, and basement membranes of the stria vascularis. However, interpretation of the molecular basis of the hearing loss is complicated by the fact that renal failure, dialysis, and ototoxic drugs that may be used for treatment can all contribute to hearing loss. The overall incidence of Alport syndrome is about 1 in 10,000, and the X-linked form is more common than both of the autosomal variants. About 8,000 individuals with glomerulonephritis progress to end-stage renal disease each year and make a substantial contribution to the 13,500 renal transplants that are performed each year.

Nonsyndromic Deafness

About 70–80% of genetic deafness is nonsyndromic. At least 58 recessive, 48 dominant, and 5 X-linked and one Y-linked locus have been mapped, and, among these, 45 of the causal genes have been identified. The dominant loci are identified by the symbol, and numbers DFNA1-54, the recessive loci are designated DFNB1-67, and DFN1-5 refers to the X-linked loci. A current listing of the mapped genes and identified loci, along with references, can be found at the Hereditary Hearing Loss homepage (http://webh01.ua.ac.be/hhh/). Several important examples of nonsyndromic deafness that have been identified to date are described in greater detail below.

Connexin Deafness.   In view of the large number of loci that have already been identified, the finding that most cases of genetic deafness are caused by mutations involving a single gene in many populations came as a surprise. The Connexins are a family of genes that code for the subunits of gap junction proteins. Gap junctions form when the hexameric hemi-connexons on the surface of two adjacent cells "dock" to form a complete gap junction. The resulting channels permit the flow of ions and small molecules between the cells. At least 14 mammalian Connexins have been identified and are designated by numbers that refer to their molecular size. Connexin 26 (also referred to as CX26 and GJB2), for example, has a molecular mass of 26,000 Daltons. The different Connexins vary in the tissues and developmental stages at which they are expressed. Furthermore, some are capable of forming heteromeric as well as homomeric connexons. Thus the clinical effects of a mutation may well depend on the degree of redundant expression of other Connexins as well as its pattern of expression within an organ or tissue. Seven of these genes are known to be the cause of human deafness or are expressed in the ear. More than 80 different mutations of the CX26 gene have been reported (The Connexin-Deafness Homepage, 2007). Many are "private" mutations, having been observed in only one or a few pedigrees, but examples of very common alleles have also been identified in several populations, including the 35delG mutation in Caucasians, the 167delT allele in Ashkenazi Jews, the 235delC allele in Asian populations, and the R143W mutation in Ghana. Most pathologic mutations are recessive, but at least six exhibit dominance. Similarly, Connexin deafness is usually not associated with other features, but characteristic dermatologic findings have been reported in association with specific mutations, including palmoplantar hyperkeratosis in association with the dominant G59A allele (Heathcoate, Syrris, Carter, Patton, 2000), mutilating keratoderma (Vorwinkle syndrome) in association with the D66H allele (Maestrini et al., 1999), and three dominant alleles associated with the keratoderma-ichytheosis-deafness (KID) syndrome (Richard et al., 2002). In addition, hearing loss occurs with dermatologic abnormalities in some mutations involving CX30 and CX31 and with neurologic abnormalities in X-linked Charcot-Marie–Tooth disease caused by the CX32 gene. In most large studies, deaf probands are encountered who are apparent CX26 heterozygotes. Since the reported frequency of heterozygotes in the general population has exceded 3% in some studies, the heterozygosity could be unrelated to the hearing loss. Alternatively, dominance or an unidentified second pathologic CX26 allele could be the explanation. Recently it was reported that a 342-kb deletion spanning the CX30 locus can interact with a single recessive CX26 mutation to cause deafness (del Castillo et al., 2002). The CX26 and CX30 genes are located within about 40 kb of each other on 13q11. Although the CX26 locus is not involved in the deletion, it is still not clear whether the deafness arises because the CX26 and CX30 proteins interact, or whether the deletion itself perturbs the expression of the adjacent normal CX26 gene. In Spain, this deletion accounted for two-thirds of 33 deaf probands who were apparent CX26 heterozygotes, whereas in the United States 17 of 625 (2.7%) deaf probands were found to carry the CX30 deletion, including one affected homozygote, and the deafness in 17.7% of deaf CX26 heterozygotes could be explained by this mechanism (Nance & Pandya, 2002).

Why mutations involving the Connexins are such a common cause of deafness is not clear. There is little to suggest that they have a high mutation rate or that there is a selective advantage for connexin carriers, as in the case of sickle cell disease. Population bottlenecks and founder effects can explain why some genes have a high prevalence and may contribute to the high frequency of the 167delT and R143W mutations among Ashkenazi Jews and in Ghana, but these effects are usually associated with small or relatively closed populations.

One interesting possibility is that the high frequency has resulted from the greatly improved social and economic circumstances of the deaf combined with intense assortative mating among the deaf. Both of these trends began with the introduction of sign language and the establishment of residential schools for the deaf about 300 years ago. An analysis of a large nationwide collection of pedigree data on deaf families collected 100–200 years ago, suggests that the relative frequency of Connexin deafness in the United States at that time cannot have been greater than about 17% (Nance & Pandya, 2002). Contemporary estimates suggest that this frequency may have doubled in the past 200 years. Marriages between individuals with precisely the same type of recessive deafness can only have deaf offspring, and are referred to as "noncomplementary matings." Since the frequency of these marriages is proportional to the fourth power of the respective gene frequency, only the commonest forms of deafness will make an appreciable contribution to these matings. Thus the combination of improved fertility (i.e., genetic fitness) and assortative mating is a mechanism that will selectively amplify the commonest form(s) of recessive deafness in the population, along with "modifier genes," such as the CX30 deletion, which can interact with the major gene (Nance & Pandya, 2002). In countries like India and Mongolia without a long tradition of sign language or intermarriage among the deaf, CX26 mutations are present, but Connexin deafness occurs at a very low frequency. The Bengkala village in Bali provides a striking contrast. The frequency of recessive DFNB3 deafness in the 2185 villagers is 2%; 17% of the hearing subjects are gene carriers, and all deaf by deaf matings are noncomplementary, as might be expected (Friedman et al., 1995). The dramatic increase in the frequency of this gene was accompanied by the development of an indigenous sign language, now learned by both the deaf and hearing villagers. In many primitive populations, the genetic fitness of the deaf is close to zero. Although "gene drift" undoubtedly played a role in the initial survival of the original DFNB3 mutation, it is difficult to escape the conclusion that the combination of improved fitness and assortative mating that followed the invention of a sign language must also have contributed to the dramatic increase in the frequency of deafness in the population. Clearly, this mechanism can increase the frequency of recessive genes for deafness other than the Connexins. It also seems likely that precisely the same forces led to the rapid fixation of genes for speech (Lai et al., 2001) when they first arose in the human species and subsequently contributed to the explosive evolution of the human brain that has occurred during the past 50,000–100,000 years. The evolutionary biologist Stephen Gould popularized the idea that during specific periods, the pace of evolution suddenly accelerated (Gould & Eldredge, 1977); the combination of intense assortative mating with improved fitness associated with the acquisition of speech may be the mechanism of at least one such event in human evolution, and computer simulation studies have confirmed the fact that this dual mechanism could have doubled the frequency of connexin deafness in the United States during the past 200 years (Nance & Kearsey, 2004).

Mitochondrial A1555G Mutation.   The A1555G mutation in the mitochondrial 12S ribosomal RNA gene was first shown to be a cause of deafness in a large Arab-Israeli pedigree with matrilineal transmission of a severe to profound hearing loss that typically began in infancy or early childhood (Jabber et al., 1992). Molecular testing revealed a homoplastic substitution in the 12S ribosomal RNA gene. Similar pedigrees with the same mutation have been reported from Spain, where the mutation appears to be a remarkably common cause of deafness (Estivill et al., 1998), and from Italy, but these families differ, in that the onset of hearing loss is later. In other countries such as the United States, China, South Africa, and Mongolia, A1555G deafness has been virtually confined to individuals who have been exposed to aminoglycoside antibiotics. The explanation for the great variation in the phenotypic expression of this mutation is not known with certainty, but the data support the idea that the risk and expression of hearing loss in subjects who carry the A1555G substitution can be strongly influenced either by other nuclear or mitochondrial genes or by environmental factors such as exposure to aminoglycosides. In the United States, where aminoglycosides are used selectively, but often in high doses, only about 15% of all patients whose hearing loss is attributed to aminoglycosides are found to carry the A1555G mutation (Fischel-Ghodsian et al., 1997). In contrast, in Mongolia, where aminoglycosides were widely used in the past, the A1555G mutation was the most common identifiable cause of deafness in a survey of students at the school for the deaf in Ulanbaatar in 1997 (Pandya et al., 1997). Other mutations in the same mitochondrial gene have been identified in patients with aminoglycoside ototoxicity who lack the A1555G substitution, including a delT961Cn mutation (Casano, Johnson, Bykhovskaya, Torricelli, Bigozzi, & Fischel-Ghodsian, 1999), but little is known about their prevalence. When a molecular diagnosis can be established, aminoglycoside ototoxicity is a trait in which there is a high potential for preventing the recurrence of deafness among matrilineal relatives. Whether all patients or perhaps all Hispanic patients admitted to neonatal intensive care units should be screened for relevant mitochondrial mutations before the administration of aminoglycosides is an issue that would depend critically on the population prevalence of the mutations. Unfortunately, these data represent an important gap in existing knowledge.

Dominantly Inherited Low-frequency Hearing Loss (DFNA6, 14 & 38).
Dominantly inherited low-frequency hearing loss was first reported in a large kindred whose impairment was confined largely to frequencies less than 2000 cps. A pseudolongitudinal analysis of the audiologic findings within the family provided little evidence for progression with age. Affected family members were not severely incapacitated, and the children responded well to preferential classroom placement (Vanderbilt University Hereditatry Deafness Study Group, 1968). The gene in this family was mapped to 4p16.3 (Lesperance et al., 1995). Two other forms of dominantly inherited heating loss, one of which exhibited progression, were subsequently mapped to the same region and designated DFNA14 and DFNA38. However, when DFNA6 was found to arise from mutations in

the Wolfram syndrome I gene (WFS1), DFNA14 and DFNA38 were shown to be the consequence of allelic mutations at the same locus (Bespalova et al., 2001). Mutations involving this locus are now thought to explain most cases of dominantly inherited low-frequency hearing loss. However, one additional gene, DFNA1, which led to a rapidly progressive hearing loss beginning in the low frequencies, was identified in a single large Costa Rican kindred, mapped to 5q31, and later shown to result from a mutation in the human homolog of the diaphanous gene in Drosophila (Lynch, Lee, Morrow, Welsch, Leon, & King, 1997). Wolfram syndrome is a complex recessive trait. The hallmarks are diabetes mellitus and insipidus, optic atrophy, and deafness, and a variety of neuropsychiatric symptoms can also be seen, including seizures, ataxia, retardation, depression, violent behavior, and suicide in some patient populations. Typically the hearing loss in affected homozygotes has been progressive, beginning with the high frequencies. Diabetes mellitus and hearing loss have been shown to occur with higher frequency in heterozygous carriers. Carrier status does not appear to be a major risk factor for psychiatric disease and suicide, but the possibility that some alleles have these effects has not been excluded (Crawford, Zielinski, Fisher, Sutherland, & Goldney, 2002).

MOLECULAR BASIS OF HEARING AND DEAFNESS

As new genes for deafness have been mapped and cloned, analysis of their base pair sequence has frequently allowed the structure and function of their protein products to be inferred. Molecular and histologic studies of messenger RNA (mRNA) synthesis have allowed the developmental stage, tissues, and cells in which these genes are expressed to be determined, resulting in an ever more detailed understanding of the molecular basis of hearing.

Transcription Factors

Several large classes of proteins are known that are typically required to initiate the transcription of mRNA. Some bind to specific sites within the promoter region of the gene, and others are involved in specific interactions with other proteins in the complete transcription complex. An abnormal phenotype can result from an abnormal base pair sequence in the promoter region or from a deficiency or abnormality in the transcription factor. Seven forms of deafness are known to result from mutations of transcription factors. Defects in PAX3, MITF, and SOX10 cause three forms of Waardenburg. Mutations involving the POU4F3 and POU3F4 genes cause a dominant form of progressive hearing loss (DFNA15) and the X-linked syndrome of congenital fixation of the stapes footplate, respectively. Finally, mutations involving the EYA1 and EYA4 genes are the cause of the Branchio-oto-renal syndrome and a dominantly inherited form of late onset hearing loss (DFNA10), respectively. Since these defective transcription factors act on both copies of a diploid target gene, all of these traits exhibit dominant transmission.

Intracellular Proteins

Atypical Myosins.   Mutations involving four different atypical myosins have been shown to be the cause of deafness. Different mutations in MYO7A can cause dominant or recessive NSD or Usher syndrome, type 1B. Mutations involving MYO6 and MYH9 lead to progressive forms of dominant hearing loss (DFNA22 & DFNA17), and MYO15 defects underlie a profound congenital form of recessive NSD (DFNB3).

Structural Proteins.   Two genes, DIAPH1 and STRC, are known to be highly expressed in the hair cells, where they act to promote actin polymerization in the hair cells, and the production of Sterocilin, a component of the microvillar proteins, respectively. Defects in the former result in the progressive dominantly inherited hearing loss of DFNA1 on 5q31, and the latter is associated with recessive deafness, DFNB16 on 15q15. The OTOF and TCOF1 are both intracellular proteins that are thought to be involved in the trafficking of intracellular organelles. Otoferlin is located in the cytoplasm and is anchored to the cell membrane, and the Treacle protein is involved in nuclear-cytoplasmic trafficking. TCOF1 is located on 5q31, and its mutations are the cause of Treacher Collins syndrome, and defects in OTOF cause a form of recessive NSD, DFNB9 on 2p23.

Transmembrane Proteins

Channelopathies.   Mutations involving at least three members of the Connexin family of gap junction proteins Cx26, Cx30, and Cx43 are known to cause hearing loss. Two potassium channel genes, KVLQT1 and KCNE1, are essential for maintaining the normal homeostasis of the cochlear endolymph. Defects in these genes cause two forms of the recessive Jervelle, Lange-Nielsen syndrome (JLN1 & 2). As noted previously, mutations in another potassium channel gene, KCNQ4, can cause DFNA2 but do not contribute to homeostasis of the endolymph. One other gene for deafness, SLC26A4, the cause of Pendred syndrome, is a membrane-bound protein that is involved in ion transport and the fixation of iodine in the thyroid gland. Prestin, the putative molecular motor protein of the outer hair cells, is a member of this same family of genes. A unique attribute of the outer hair cell is its ability to change its length in response to sound stimuli. This property is thought to greatly amplify and help resolve the transmission of sound waves along the basal membrane. Mutations in this gene have been identified in deaf probands, although the mode of inheritance is not yet clear (Liu et al., 2003).

Cell Adhesion.   Two genes for deafness are required for normal cell adhesion. CDH23, on 10q21, is a member of a calcium-dependent family of genes, the cadherins, which mediate cell adhesion. It is abnormal in USH1D as well as in families with recessive DFNB12. The claudins are another a large family of genes that form tight junctions that bind homologous as well as heterologous cells together. A mutation in CLDN14 on 21q22.3 is responsible for the recessive deafness in DFNB29.

Other Transmembrane Proteins.   The functions of the transmembrane USH3 and TMC1 proteins that are defective in USH3 on 3q21 and dominant or recessive forms of NSD (DFNB7/11, DFNBA36) on 9q13 are not as well established, but TMPRSS3, which causes a recessive form of NSD on 21q22.3, codes for a transmembrane protein with protease activity.

Extracellular Proteins

Mutations involving three collagen genes, COL2A1, COL11A2, and COL11A1, are the cause of the three recognized forms of Stickler syndrome, and mutations involving COL4A5, COL4A3, and COL4A4 cause the autosomal and sex-linked forms of Alport syndrome. The gene that causes USH2A codes for an extracellular matrix protein, and TECTA, the gene defective in DFNA8/12 on 11q22, codes for a component of the tectorial membrane. Otoancorin, the product of the OTOA gene, is thought to anchor the apical surface of the hair cells to the tectorial membrane and is defective in DFNB22 on16p12.2.

Energy Production

Both nuclear and cytoplasmic genes are active in the mitochondrion, which is the site of oxidative phosphorylation in the cell. Hearing loss can be a part of a large number of complex neurologic syndromes that involve deletions in the mitochondrial DNA or point mutations involving mitochondrial tRNA's. The A1555G substitution in the 12S mRNA gene and the A7445G substitution in the tRNA Ser(UNC) gene are examples of two mitochonrdial mutations that can lead to hearing loss alone. Finally, DDP, the Deafness/Dystonia peptide, is the product of a gene on Xq22 that is responsible for the deafness, blindness, retardation, and dystonia seen in Tranebjaerg syndrome. The protein product of this gene is normally transported into the mitochondria, but its precise function there has not been identified.

SOCIAL AND ETHICAL ASPECTS OF GENETIC DEAFNESS

Advances in human genetics have posed many ethical questions, related to such areas as privacy, autonomy, prenatal diagnosis, stem cell research, and the rights of children, that are just as applicable to deafness as they are to other genetic traits. In addition, however, there are issues that are particularly relevant if not unique to deafness.

Attitudes of the Deaf and Hearing Communities

The contrasting attitudes of the deaf and hearing communities about genetic issues have been highlighted in a number of recent surveys (Stern, Arnos, Murrelle, Welch, Nance, & Pandya, 2002; Middleton, Hewson, & Muellere, 1998). Many deaf individuals reject the medical model of deafness as a disability that needs to be "fixed." Most express no preference for hearing or deaf children; but many would prefer a deaf child and relatively few express a preference for hearing children. The attitudes of the deaf community toward genetic testing and the use of prenatal diagnosis, including the selective abortion of either deaf or hearing fetuses, tend to be more polarized than those of hearing parents. In contrast, the birth of a deaf child is often the supreme tragedy in the lives of hearing parents who would do anything to restore their hearing. There are few other human traits for which such divergent attitudes are held.

The Legacy of Alexander Graham Bell

Bell's involvement with the eugenics movement may have had a lasting influence on the attitudes of the deaf community toward genetics. Bell was an educator of the deaf who devoted most of his professional career to promoting the welfare of deaf children. In 1883, 17 years before the rediscovery of Mendel's work, he published a Memoir of the National Academy of Sciences in which he speculated that the continued intermarriage among the deaf might someday result in the formation of a deaf variety of the human race (Bell, 1883). Although some of Bell's genetic proposals cannot withstand modern criticism, his perceptions about the effect of the mating structure of the deaf population on the frequency of deafness may well have been correct. To avoid this effect, Bell advocated the closing of residential schools for the deaf in favor of what is now called mainstreaming. In this instance, he was actually advocating more random mating, as opposed to the selective breeding commonly associated with eugenics. Geneticists have generally discounted Bell's concerns about the mating structure of the deaf population because of the belief that the effect would be negligible in view of the large number of genes involved in deafness. However, it now appears that this mechanism may have contributed to an increase in the frequency of the most common form of recessive deafness during the last 200 years. Thus, Bell's prediction forces us to consider what attitude we should take toward the pattern of marriages that may have contributed to this increase. Assortative mating among the deaf is not the only example in which the marriage patterns of a population can have a profound influence on the frequency of specific genetic diseases. The frequencies of Tay-Sachs disease and sickle cell anemia in the United States are much higher than they would be if marriages occurred at random, and unless we are also prepared to abolish racial and ethnic homogamy, there would appear to be no rational genetic basis for prohibiting marriages among the deaf. It now seems likely that Bell's goal will be achieved not through the mainstreaming of deaf children, but because of the widespread use of cochlear implants. This development almost certainly represents a much greater threat to deaf culture than genetic testing. Deaf culture may well disappear in the United States by the end of this century. If that does occur, who among us can predict whether it will be viewed as one of the medical triumphs of the twenty-first century, or as an egregious example of cultural genocide?

Genetic Counseling

Genetic counselors are medical specialists who are especially skilled in the evaluation, diagnosis, and counseling of patients with genetic traits. In some cases, medical geneticists also become intimately involved in the treatment and long-term follow-up of patients with specific genetic diseases. In the case of hereditary deafness, geneticists can assist in the establishment of a specific etiologic diagnosis. In some cases, this may result in the diagnosis of a form of syndromic deafness for which specific treatments or diagnostic tests are indicated. The Jervelle, Lange-Neilsen syndromes, Usher syndromes, Branchio-oto-renal syndrome, and Alport syndromes are examples of genetic forms of deafness in which serious complications involving other organ systems may arise. Even when a diagnosis of nonsyndromic deafness is made, an increasing number of genetic tests are becoming available with which the diagnosis of a specific form of NSD can be made. These tests can be of particular value in confirming a genetic etiology in families where there is only one affected child and no other history of deafness in the family. Connexin testing has rapidly become the standard of care for the management of such cases. In the future, establishing a specific genetic etiology will become increasingly useful for providing prognostic information as to the natural history and possibly about specific therapy. Some forms of nonsyndromic deafness are progressive, and others are remarkably stable. Some have a conductive component that may be amenable to surgical treatment. Finally, reliable information about the chance that deafness will recur in the family or in the children of the proband can only be provided if the genetic form of deafness and its mode of inheritance are known. If this knowledge is provided in a way that can be understood and integrated by the patient, it can help dispel feelings of guilt and misconceptions and allow the parents to focus on planning for their child's future. For deaf adults, information about the cause of a trait that has had such an important influence on their lives can be empowering knowledge. In the past, deaf couples have never known how, why, or whether their children would be deaf, like they are, or hearing. For some, this uncertainty must be like not knowing what race your child will be. Increasingly, these questions can be answered prospectively for couples. Much is known about the genetics of profound deafness. In comparison, much less is known about the causes of lesser degrees of clinically significant hearing loss. Many of these children may have one or the other of the several hundred genetic syndromes that have been described in which hearing loss is a less conspicuous or inconstant feature. In many ways, these children are more in need of expertise in dysmorphology that a geneticist brings to the evaluation of such children than are those who have a clear-cut diagnosis. Finally, as more knowledge about genetics becomes incorporated into the training of audiologists, they should increasingly be able to recognize families who would benefit from genetic evaluation and counseling and to understand and reinforce information pro-vided to their patients during counseling.

FUTURE DIRECTIONS

In the recent past, the state of our knowledge was such that we lumped many forms of nonsyndromic deafness together; assumed that each form of syndromic deaf-ness was caused by a single gene; believed that dominance and recessivity were in-trinsic properties of genes; and had little insight into the heterogeneity of muta-tions and the molecular mechanisms involved in their effects. We used descriptive terms such as *reduced penetrance variable expressivity, multifactorial transmis-sion,* and *stochastic variation* to explain away examples of unexpected gene expression. We are now gaining a much more sophisticated understanding of ge-netic heterogeneity, the factors which influence the expression of genes, and their interactions with each other and with the environment. In the immediate future we can expect to see more of the same as additional genes for deafness are discovered and we listen to the incredible stories they have to tell. The coincident develop-ment of the newborn hearing movement during this new era of genetics provides an unparalleled opportunity for synergistic interactions between these two streams of medical and scientific progress. The time will come when the application of ex-isting "gene chip" technologies or other methods currently under development will make it possible to perform molecular genetic screening tests on blood samples from newborn infants at low cost for a virtually unlimited number of gene muta-tions that can cause deafness. The question then arises, what gene defects should we screen for and why? Would it be important to know that an infant has inher-ited a gene that may cause hearing loss when he or she is 50 years old? One pos-sible alternative would be to focus on forms of hearing loss that may not be ex-pressed at birth and could therefore be missed in current audiologic newborn screening programs. Another possible criterion would be to screen for very com-mon forms of deafness, or for forms that are associated with other serious and/or preventable clinical complications. Examples of the former might include hear-ing loss resulting from CMV infection or Pendred syndrome. Examples in the later group would include Connexin deafness, the mitochondrial A1555T mutation, genes for the JLN syndrome, and possibly one or more forms of Usher syndrome. Screening for a limited array of traits such as these could be performed with the newborn blood spots that are already collected for existing metabolic screening programs. If programs of this type are implemented in this country, it would be highly desirable to collect pilot data on the frequency of the traits and the sensi-tivity and specificity of the tests. In this way, it should be possible to incorporate the new tests in existing screening programs. Programs of this type should be viewed as a complement and not a substitute for existing newborn hearing screen-ing programs. They would identify additional high-risk infants who deserve close follow-up and accelerate an etiologic diagnosis in others. In view of the com-plexities surrounding the interpretation of even the simplest test results, it would not even be possible to contemplate a newborn molecular screening program without a preexisting audiologic screening program. For example, some deaf individuals are found to carry only a single Cx26 mutation. As noted previously, it is now known that many of these individuals also carry a deletion of the Cx30 gene. However, others are undoubtedly simply heterozygous carriers of a single Cx26 mutation. Without evidence that a newborn infant has normal hearing, it would be difficult to draw the conclusion that the test result merely indicated heterozygosity with any degree of certainty. In view of the rapidly expanding body of relevant genetic knowledge about genetic deafness, the American College of Medical Genetics has recommended that all infants with confirmed hearing losses who are identified in newborn screening programs should be referred to a human geneticist for clinical evaluation, the performance of indicated genetic tests, and counseling (Nance, Cunningham, & Davis, 2000) and has developed detailed practice guidelines for the evaluation of such infants (Genetic Evaluation of Congenital Hearing Loss Expert Panel, 2002). Unfortunately, although most states support genetic clinics and programs at their academic medical centers, these genetic programs have not in general been incorporated as an integral part of the newborn hearing screening movement, and the proportion of infants who are referred for evaluation is quite low. If all cases were referred, and if limited molecular screening programs were established, it would provide an unparalleled opportunity to collect population-based data on the prevalence and natural history of specific forms of both genetic and environmental deafness.

As noted previously, there are a very limited number of forms of genetic deafness for which specific therapy is currently available. It seems likely that many more preventive or curative treatments may someday be developed, but will only be applicable to specific forms of genetic deafness, thus emphasizing the importance of an accurate diagnosis. On the other hand, some forms of treatment such as hearing aids and cochlear implants are of benefit for hearing-impaired individuals with a wide range of genetic etiologies, and it is to be hoped that other therapeutic approaches such as the use of stem cell technology to replace hair cells may, in a similar manner, benefit a wider range of affected individuals. The prospects for new discoveries and improved treatments are bright, and it is an exciting time to be a geneticist who is interested in hearing loss.

ACKNOWLEDGMENTS

This work was supported in part by NIH grants R01-DC02530 and R01-DC04293. I am also grateful for the helpful suggestions of my colleague Dr. Arti Pandya.

REFERENCES

Abdelhak, S., Kalatzis, V., Heilig, R., Compain, S., Samson, D., Vincent, C., Levi-Acobas, F., Cruaud, C., Le, Merrer, M., Mathieu, M., Konig, R., Vigneron, J., Weissenbach, J., Petit, C., & Weil, D. (1997). Clustering of mutations responsible for branchiootorenal (BOR) syndrome in the eyes absent homologous region (eyaHR) of EYA1. *Human Molecular Genetics, 6,* 2247–2255.

Bell, A. G. (1883). Upon the formation of a deaf variety of the human race. *National Academy of Science Memoirs, 2,* 177–262.

Bespalova, I. N., Van Camp, G., Bom, S. J., Brown, D. J., Cryns, K., De Wan, A. T., Erson, A. E., Flothmann, K., Kunst, H. P., Kurnool, P., Sivakumaran, T. A., Cremers, C. W., Leal, S. M., Burmeister, M., & Lesperance, M. M. (2001). Mutations in the Wolfram syndrome 1 gene (WFS1) are a common cause of low frequency sensorineural hearing loss. *Human Molecular Genetics, 10,* 2501–2508.

Blanton, S. H., Pandya, A., Landa, B. L., Javaheri, R., Xia, X., Nance, W. E., Pomponio, R. J., Norrgard, K. J., Swango, K. L., Demirkol, M., Gulden, H., Coskun, T., Tokatli, A., Ozalp, I., & Wolf, B. (2000). Fine mapping of the human biotinidase gene and haplotype analysis of five common mutations. *Human Heredity, 50,* 102–111.

Boughman, J. A., Vernon, M., & Shaver, K. A. (1983). Usher syndrome: Definition and estimate of prevalence from two high-risk populations. *Journal of Chronic Diseases, 36,* 595–603.

Casano, R. A., Johnson, D. F., Bykhovskaya, Y., Torricelli, F., Bigozzi, M., & Fischel-Ghodsian, N. (1999). Inherited susceptibility to aminoglycoside ototoxicity: genetic heterogeneity and clinical implications. *American Journal of Otolaryngology., 20,* 151–156.

The Connexin-Deafness Homepage. (2007). http://davinci.crg.es/deafness/

Crawford, J., Zielinski, M. A., Fisher, L. J., Sutherland, G. R., & Goldney, R. D. (2002). Is there a relationship between Wolfram syndrome carrier status and suicide? *American Journal of Medical Genetics, 114,* 343–346.

Davis, H. (1965). A model for transducer action in the cochlea. *Cold Spring Harbor Symposium on Quantitative Biology, 30,* 181–190.

de Kok, Y. J., van der Maarel, S. M., Bitner-Glindzicz, M., Huber, I., Monaco, A. P., Malcolm, S., Pembrey, M. E., Ropers, H. H., & Cremers, F. P. (1995). Association between X-linked mixed deafness and mutations in the POU domain gene POU3F4. *Science, 267,* 685–688.

del Castillo, F. J., Rodriguez-Ballesteros, M., Alvarez, A., Hutchin, T., Leonardi, E., de Oliveira, C. A., Azaiez, H., Brownstein, Z., Avenarius, M. R., Marlin, S., Pandya, A., Shahin, H., Siemering, K. R., Weil, D., Wuyts, W., Aguirre, L. A., Martin, Y., Moreno-Pelayo, M. A., Villamar, M., Avraham, K. B., Dahl, H. H., Kanaan, M., Nance, W. E., Petit, C., Smith, R. J., Van, C. G., Sartorato, E. L., Murgia, A., Moreno, F., & del Castillo, I. (2005). A novel deletion involving the connexin-30 gene, del(GJB6-d13s1854), found in trans with mutations in the GJB2 gene (connexin-26) in subjects with DFNB1 nonsyndromic hearing impairment. *Journal of Medical Genetics, 42,* 588–594.

Estivill, X., Govea, N., Barcelo, E., Badenas, C., Romero, E., Moral, L., Scozzri, R., D'Urbano, L., Zeviani, M., & Torroni, A. (1998). Familial progressive sensorineural deafness is mainly due to the mtDNA A1555G mutation and is enhanced by treatment of aminoglycosides. *American Journal of Human Genetics, 62,* 27–35.

Fischel-Ghodsian, N., Prezant, T. R., Chaltraw, W. E., Wendt, K. A., Nelson, R. A., Arnos, K. S., & Falk, R. E. (1997). Mitochondrial gene mutation is a significant predisposing factor in aminoglycoside ototoxicity. *American Journal of Otolaryngology, 18,* 173–178.

Fraser, G. R. (1965). Association of congenital deafness with goiter (Pendred's syndrome): A study of 207 families. *Annuals of Human Genetics, 28,* 201–249.

Friedman, T. B., Liang, Y., Weber, J. L., Hinnant, J. T., Barber, T. D., Winata, S., Arhya, I. N., & Asher, J. H., Jr. (1995). A gene for congenital, recessive deafness DFNB3 maps to the pericentromeric region of chromosome 17. *Nature Genetics, 9,* 86–91.

Genetics Evaluation of Guidelines for the Etiologic Diagnosis of Congenital Hearing Loss. Genetic Evaluation of Congenital Hearing Loss Expert Panel. (2002). Genetics evaluation guidelines for the etiologic diagnosis of congenital hearing loss. *Genetics in Medicine, 4,* 162–171.

Gorlin, R. J., Toriello, H. V., & Cohen, M. M., (Eds.) (1995). *Hereditary hearing loss and its syndromes,* 1–457. New York: Oxford University Press.

Gould, S. J., & Eldredge, N. (1977). Punctuated equilibria: The tempo and mode of evolution reconsidered. *Paleobiology, 3,* 115–151.

Heathcote, K., Syrris, P., Carter, N. D., & Patton, M. A. (2000). A connexin 26 mutation causes a syndrome of sensorineural hearing loss and palmoplantar hyperkeratosis. *Journal of Medical Genetics, 37,* 50–51.

Hereditary Hearing Loss Homepage. (2007). http://webh01.ua.ac.be/hhh/

Hughes, A. E., Newton, V. E., Liu, X. Z., & Read, A. P. (1994). A gene for Waardenburg syndrome type 2 maps close to the human homologue of the mouse *microphthalmia* gene at chromosomal 3p12p14.1. *Nature Genetics, 7,* 509–512.

Jaber, L., Shohat, M., Bu, X., Fischel-Ghodsian, N., Yang, H. Y., Wang, S. J., & Rotter, J. I. (1992). Sensorineural deafness inherited as a tissue specific mitochondrial disorder. *Journal of Medical Genetics, 29,* 86–90.

Lai, C. S., Fisher, S. E., Hurst, J. A., Vargha-Khadem, F., & Monaco, A. P. (2001). A forkhead-domain gene is mutated in a severe speech and language disorder. *Nature, 413,* 519–523.

Lesperance, M. M., Hall, J. W., Bess, F. H., Fukushima, K., Jain, P. K., Ploplis, B., San Agustin, T. B., Skarka, H., Smith, R. J., & Wills, M. (1995). A gene for autosomal dominant nonsyndromic hereditary hearing impairment maps to 4p16.3. *Human Molecular Genetics, 4,* 1967–1972.

Liu, X.-Z., Newton, V. E., & Read, A. P. (1995). Waardenburg syndrome type II: Phenotypic findings and diagnostic criteria. *American Journal of Medical Genetics, 55,* 95–100.

Liu, X. Z., Ouyang, X. M., Xia, X. J., Zheng, J., Pandya, A., Li, F., Du, L. L., Welch, K. O., Petit, C., Smith, R. J., Webb, B. T., Yan, D., Arnos, K. S., Corey, D., Dallos, P., Nance, W. E., & Chen, Z. Y. (2003). Prestin, a cochlear motor protein, is defective in nonsyndromic hearing loss. *Human Molecular Genetics, 12,* 1155–1162.

Lynch, E. D., Lee, M. K., Morrow, J. E., Welcsh, P. L., Leon, P. E., & King, M. C. (1997). Nonsyndromic deafness DFNA1 associated with mutation of a human homolog of the Drosophila gene diaphanous. *Science, 278,* 1315–1318.

Maestrini, E., Korge, B. P., Ocana-Sierra, J., Calzolari, E., Cambiaghi, S., Scudder, P. M., Hovnanian, A., Monaco, A. P., & Munro, C. S. (1999). A missense mutation in connexin26, D66H, causes mutilating keratoderma with sensorineural deafness (Vohwinkel's syndrome) in three unrelated families. *Human Molecular Genetics, 8,* 1237–1243.

McCallion, A. S., & Chakravarti, A. (2001). EDNRB/EDN3 and Hirschsprung disease type II. *Pigment Cell Research, 14,* 161–169.

Melnick, M., Bixler, D., Nance, W. E., Silk, K., & Yune, H. (1976). Familial branchiootorenal dysplasia: A new addition to the branchial arch syndromes. *Clinical Genetics, 9,* 25–34.

Middleton, A., Hewson, J., & Muellere, R. F. (1998). Attitudes of deaf adults toward genetic testing for hereditary deafness. *American Journal Human Genetics, 63,* 1175–1180.

Morell, R., Spritz, R. A., Ho, L., Pierpont, J., Guo, W., Friedman, T. B., & Asher, J. H. J. (1997). Apparent digenic inheritance of Waardenburg syndrome type 2 (WS2) and autosomal recessive ocular albinism (AROA). *Human Molecular Genetics, 6,* 659–664.

Nance, W. E., Cunningham, G. C., Davis, J. G., Morton, C. C., Elsas, L. J., Finitzo, T., and Falk, R. E. (2000). Statement of the American College of Medical Genetics on universal newborn hearing screening. *Genetics in Medicine, 2,* 149–150.

Nance, W. E., & Kearsey, M. J. (2004). Relevance of connexin deafness (DFNB1) to human evolution. *American Journal of Human Genetics, 74,* 1081–1087.

Nance, W. E., & Pandya, A. (2002). Genetic epidemiology of deafness. In: B. J. B. Keats, A. N. Popper, & R. R. Fay (Eds.), *Genetics and Auditory Disorders,* 67–92. Springer Verlag, New York.

Nance, W. E., Setleff, R., McLeod, A., Sweeney, A., Cooper, C., & McConnell, F. (1971). X-linked mixed deafness with congenital fixation of the stapedial footplate and perilymphatic gusher. *Birth Defects Original Article Series, 7*(4), 64–69.

Nance, W. E., Xia, X., Gupta, V., Arnos, K. S., Welch, K. O., Landa, B. L., Dobrowlski, S., Blanton, S. H., & Pandya (2002). A Frequency of the Connexin 30 deletion (C×30del) in deaf probands from the U.S. and its occurrence in *cis* with Connexin 26 (C×26) mutations. *American Journal of Human Genetics, 71*(supplement), 510.

Neyroud, N., Tesson, F., Denjoy, I., Leibovici, M., Donger, C., Barhanin, J., Faure, S., Gary, F., Coumel, P., Petit, C., Schwartz, K., & Guicheney, P. (1997). A novel mutation in the potassium channel gene KVLQT1 causes the Jervell and Lange-Nielsen cardioauditory syndrome. *Nature Genetics, 15*, 186–189.

Online Mendelian Inheritance in Man OMIM . (2007). http://www.ncbi.nlm.nih.gov/omim/

Ouyang, X. M., Xia, X. J., Verpy, E., Du, L. L., Pandya, A., Petit, C., Balkany, T., Nance, W. E., & Liu, X. Z. (2002). Mutations in the alternatively spliced exons of USH1C cause non-syndromic recessive deafness. *Human Genetics, 111*, 26–30.

Pandya, A., Xia, X. J., Landa, B. L., Arnos, K. S., Israel, J., Lloyd, J., James, A. L., Diehl, S. R., Blanton, S. H., & Nance, W. E. (1996). Phenotypic variation in Waardenburg syndrome: mutational heterogeneity, modifier genes or polygenic background? *Human Molecular Genetics, 5*, 497–502.

Pandya, A., Xia, X., Radnaabazar, J., Batsuuri, J., Dangaansuren, B., Fischel-Ghodsian, N., & Nance, W. E. (1997). Mutation in the mitochondrial 12S rRNA gene in two families from Mongolia with matrilineal aminoglycoside ototoxicity. *Journal of Medical Genetics, 34*, 169–172.

Reardon, W., O'Mahoney, C. F., Trembath, R., Jan, H., & Phelps, P. D. (2000). Enlarged vestibular aqueduct: A radiological marker of Pendred syndrome, and mutation of the PDS gene. *Quarterly Journal of Medicine, 93*, 99–104.

Richard, G., Rouan, F., Willoughby, C. E., Brown, N., Chung, P., Ryynanen, M., Jabs, E. W., Bale, S. J., DiGiovanna, J. J., Uitto, J., & Russell, L. (2002). Missense mutations in GJB2 encoding connexin–26 cause the ectodermal dysplasia keratitis-ichthyosis-deafness syndrome. *American Journal Human Genetics, 70*, 1341–1348.

Rose, S. P., Conneally, P. M., & Nance, W. E. (1977). Genetic analysis of childhood deafness. In F. H. Bess (Ed.), *Childhood deafness* (pp. 19–35). New York: Grune & Stratton.

Rosenberg, T., Haim, M., Hauch, A. M., & Parving, A. (1997). The prevalence of Usher syndrome and other retinal dystrophy-hearing impairment associations. *Clinical Genetics, 51*, 314–321.

Sanchez-Martin, M., Rodriguez-Garcia, A., Perez-Lasoda, J., Sagrera, A., Read, A. P., & Sanchez-Garcia, I. (2002). SLUG (SNAI2) deletions in patients with Waardenburg disease. *Human Molecular Genetics, 11*, 3231–3236.

Stern, S. J., Arnos, K. S., Murrelle, L., Welch, K. O., Nance, W. E., & Pandya, A. (2002). Attitudes of deaf and hard of hearing subjects towards genetic testing and prenatal diagnosis of hearing loss. *Journal of Medical Genetics, 39*, 449–453.

Tachibana, M., Perez-Jurado, L. A., Nakayama, A., Hodgkinson, C. A., Li, X., Schneider, M., Miki, T., Fex, J., Francke, U., & Arnheiter, H. (1994). Cloning of MITF, the human homolog of the mouse microphthalmia gene and assignment to chromosome 3p14.1-p12.3. *Human Molecular Genetics, 3*, 553–557.

Vanderbilt University Hereditary Deafness Study Group. (1968). Dominantly inherited low-frequency hearing loss. *Archives of Otolaryngology, 88*, 242–250.

Waardenburg, P. J. (1951). A new syndrome combining developmental anomalies of the eyelids, eyebrows and nose root with pigmentary defects of the iris and head hair with congenital deafness. *American Journal of Human Genetics, 3*, 195–253.

Wolf, B., Spencer, R., & Gleason, T. (2002). Hearing loss is a common feature of symptomatic children with profound biotinidase deficiency. *Journal of Pediatrics, 140*, 242–246.

CHAPTER 5

Evaluation and Management of Pediatric Hearing Loss

Iee Ching W. Anderson and Charles J. Limb
*Johns Hopkins University School of Medicine
and Johns Hopkins Hospital*

The child's brain is striking in its abundant degree of neural plasticity. Much of this plasticity is devoted to the child's processing of environmental stimuli, and appropriate reception of such stimuli, in turn, is necessary for proper neural development. The ability to hear is critical for a child's speech and language acquisition, and his or her subsequent social and academic development. Major strides have been made in the past decade in broadening our understanding of the etiologic factors involved in childhood hearing loss, the pathophysiologic mechanisms underlying this condition, and methods of auditory rehabilitation for affected children. The ramifications of childhood hearing loss should not be underestimated. An estimated 5000 infants are born each year in the United States with moderate to profound bilateral permanent hearing loss (Thompson, McPhillips, Davis, Lieu, Homer, & Helfand, 2001). The overall prevalence of hearing impairment ranges from 1 to 6 per 1,000 (Connolly, Carron, & Roark, 2005; Maki-Torkko, Lindholm, Vayrynen, Leisti, & Sorri, 1998; Fortnum & Davis, 1997; Stein, 1999; Van Naarden, Decoufle, & Caldwell, 1999). Early detection and management are thus important for minimizing the adverse effects of hearing impairment on an affected child's cognitive and social development (Early identification of hearing impairment in infants and young children, 1993).

ANATOMY AND PHYSIOLOGY OF AUDITION

During normal hearing, sound waves travel through the air and, via the external auditory canal, generate tympanic membrane vibration and subsequent ossicular movement. Vibration of the middle ear ossicles, specifically the stapes footplate in the cochlear oval window, allows for sound pressure waves to be transmitted to the scala vestibuli portion of the cochlea. Pressure differences between the scala vestibuli and the scala tympani create a displacement wave along the basilar membrane. As a result of shear forces generated by basilar membrane movement, the stereocilia of inner hair cells in the organ of Corti are displaced, producing depolarizing receptor potentials that subsequently generate action potentials in auditory nerve fibers. These auditory nerve afferents then transmit acoustic information to the auditory cortex (Robles & Ruggero, 2001), thereby resulting in an auditory percept.

Hearing losses may be categorized as conductive, sensorineural, or mixed. Conductive hearing loss occurs when sound is poorly conducted through the external auditory canal, tympanic membrane, or middle ear space (including the ossicles), whereas sensorineural hearing loss (SNHL) refers to impairment resulting from the pathology of the cochlea (usually hair cell dysfunction) or auditory nerve afferent fibers. Mixed hearing loss has both conductive and sensorineural components. Although this is a somewhat simplistic method of categorization, it provides a nice framework within which the complex subject of pediatric hearing loss may be addressed.

ETIOLOGY

Elucidating the etiology of a patient's hearing loss is useful for optimizing management, predicting progression, and determining the risk of hearing impairment in family members and offspring. Approximately one-third of patients have hereditary hearing loss, one-third have acquired hearing loss, and the remaining one-third have hearing loss of unknown etiology (Fraser, 1974). Given the vast number of causes of hearing loss, an overview of those more commonly encountered in practice is presented in this chapter.

GENETIC CAUSES OF HEARING LOSS

Hereditary hearing loss can be divided into syndromic and nonsyndromic forms. Syndromic hereditary hearing loss is characterized by the presence of specific associated anomalies diagnostic of a known syndrome, whereas in nonsyndromic hereditary hearing loss, no such anomalies are present. Approximately 30% of hereditary hearing loss is considered syndromic, and there are over 400 such syndromes (Friedman, Schultz, Ben Yosef, Pryor, Lagziel, Fisher, Wilcox, Riazuddin, Ahmed, Belyantseva, & Griffith). Hereditary hearing loss can be also classified by genetic inheritance pattern, such as autosomal, X-linked, and mitochondrial patterns of inheritance.

SYNDROMIC HEREDITARY HEARING LOSS

Autosomal-Dominant Syndromic

Waardenburg Syndrome.   In 1951, Petrus J. Waardenburg described this syndrome, characterized by congenital SNHL, pigmentary abnormalities (such as white forelock, vitiligo, and heterochromia irides), and dystopia canthorum, or lateral displacement of the medial canthi (Waardenburg, 1951). The estimated prevalence is 1:10,000 to 20,000 (Newton, 2002), and it is found in 2–5% of congenitally deaf patients (Nayak & Isaacson, 2003). Waardenburg syndrome is classified into four types. The presence of dystopia canthorum is the distinguishing characteristic of WS1, as opposed to the lack of dystopic canthorum in WS2. WS3, also known as Klein-Waardenburg syndrome, includes upper-limb defects in addition to WS1 features. WS4, or Waardenburg-Shah syndrome, is characterized by an association with Hirschsprung's disease, or aganglionic megacolon. Mutations associated with Waardenburg syndrome are found on the genes *PAX3* (WS1, WS3), *MITF* (WS2), *END3* (WS4), and *ENDRB* (WS4) (Nance, 2003). Sensorineural hearing loss is thought to be caused by defective melanocyte migration into the stria vascularis (Hone & Smith, 2001a). Expressivity of the hearing impairment phenotype is variable, with hearing loss more commonly associated with WS2 than with WS1 (Liu, Newton, & Read, 1995). The temporal bone is often normal on imaging, although infrequently malformation of the semicircular canals or hypoplasia of the cochlea is seen (Oysu, Oysu, Aslan, & Tinaz, 2001).

Stickler Syndrome.   First recognized by Stickler in 1965, this syndrome includes progressive myopia, premature degenerative joint changes, joint hypermobility, cleft palate, and hearing loss (Nowak, 1998; Stickler, Hughes, & Houchin, 2001). Mutations in the genes COL2A1 and COL11A2, which encode for collagen proteins, are responsible for Stickler syndrome (Francomano, Liberfarb, Hirose, Maumenee, Streeten, Meyers, & Pyeritz, 1987; Nowak, 1998). Prevalence is estimated to be 1:10,000 (Nowak, 1998). Hearing loss is found in almost 50% of Stickler syndrome patients, and it can be conductive, sensorineural, or mixed. This hearing loss, however, is generally mild, with sensorineural loss more common in adults and conductive loss more common in children (Stickler, Hughes, & Houchin, 2001). Conductive loss is thought to be associated with middle-ear dysfunction from coexisting cleft palate or midfacial hypoplasia (Nowak, 1998). The pathophysiology underlying SNHL is not well understood but may involve alterations in pigmented inner ear epithelium (Weingeist, Hermsen, Hansen, Bumsted, Weinstein, & Olin, 1982) or structural changes in the labyrinth due to collagen abnormalities (Szymko-Bennett et al., 2001).

Branchio-Oto-Renal Syndrome.   Branchio-oto-renal (BOR) syndrome, described by Melnick in 1975, is characterized by branchial cleft fistulas or cysts, otologic abnormalities (including hearing loss, external ear malformations, and preauricular pits), and renal anomalies (Melnick, Hodes, Nance, Yune, & Sweeney, 1978). The estimated prevalence is 1:40,000 (Rodriguez, 2003), and BOR is found in 2% of patients with profound deafness (Fraser, Sproule, & Halal, 1980). Hearing loss is the most common phenotypic anomaly, found in 90% of patients (Smith & Schwartz, 1998). Onset of hearing loss varies from childhood to early adulthood (Hone & Smith, 2001b). The hearing loss associated with BOR can be sensorineural, conductive, or mixed; the last is the most common. Otologic abnormalities include ossicular malformations, semicircular dysplasia, cochlear hypoplasia, and internal auditory canal anomalies (Smith & Schwartz,

1998). BOR is caused by mutations in the gene EYA1 or in chromosome 1p31 (Hone & Smith, 2001b).

Treacher-Collins Syndrome. Characteristic features of Treacher-Collins syndrome, or mandibulofacial dysostosis, include bilateral symmetrical craniofacial abnormalities, including lower eyelid colobomas, down-slanting palpebral fissures, hypoplastic zygomatic arches, cleft palate, micrognathia, microtia, and ossicular malformations. The estimated prevalence is 1:50,000 (Marsh, Dixon, & Dixon, 1998). Treacher-Collins syndrome accounts for approximately 1% of patients with severe to profound deafness. Hearing loss is conductive because of a combination of pinna, external auditory canal, and ossicular malformations, but can be associated with a high-frequency sensorineural loss as well (Tekin, Arnos, & Pandya, 2001). Treacher-Collins syndrome is caused by mutations in the TCOF1 gene (Marszalek, Wojcicki, Kobus, & Trzeciak, 2002).

Autosomal-Recessive Syndromic

Pendred Syndrome. Pendred syndrome has features of hearing loss, thyroid goiter, and developmental abnormalities of the inner ear. The prevalence of Pendred syndrome is estimated to be 1:10,000 to 13,000 (Kopp, 2000), and it accounts for 5–10% of hereditary prelingual deafness (Gurtler & Lalwani, 2002b; Park et al., 2003). Hearing loss is usually bilateral, prelingual, sensorineural (or mixed, in rare instances), and severe to profound, but it may also be progressive, fluctuating (Friedman et al., 2003b), or unilateral (Nance, 2003). Goiter development occurs in childhood, but adult onset has been reported. The goiter is typically present despite clinical euthyroidism, although hypothyroidism has been reported as well (Gurtler & Lalwani, 2002b). Common inner-ear abnormalities in Pendred syndrome include enlarged vestibular aqueduct and Mondini (cochlear) dysplasia (Hone & Smith, 2002a; Phelps et al., 1998; Reardon, O'Mahoney, Trembath, Jan, & Phelps, 2000). Pendred syndrome is caused by mutations in the gene *SLC264A* (Everett, Glaser, Beck, Idol, Buchs, Heyman, Adawi, Hazani, Nassir, Baxevanis, Sheffield and Green, 1997), which encodes for the protein product *pendrin*, a chloride and iodide ion transporter (Kopp, 2000). Goiter is caused by defective organification of iodine in the thyroid (Nance, 2003). Hearing loss in Pendred syndrome is presumably related to disruption of chloride and iodide transport, but the exact pathophysiology of hearing loss remains unclear (Kopp, 2000).

Usher Syndrome. Characteristics of this clinically and genetically heterogeneous syndrome include bilateral SNHL, progressive visual loss caused by retinitis pigmentosa, and, in some variants, vestibular dysfunction. The estimated range of prevalence is 1:16,000 to 1:50,000 (Keats & Corey, 1999). Usher syndrome is found in 3–6% of patients with severe to profound deafness (Vernon, 1969). Three clinical types of Usher syndrome are recognized. Diagnostic criteria for Usher syndrome type I (USH1) include severe to profound hearing loss across all frequencies, absence of vestibular function, and childhood onset of retinitis pigmentosa. The hearing loss in Usher syndrome type II (USH2) is stable, with moderate loss at lower frequencies and more severe loss at high frequencies. Retinitis pigmentosa onset occurs during the teenage years, and vestibular function is normal. Usher syndrome type III (USH3) is characterized by progressive hearing loss, with variability in retinitis pigmentosa onset and extent of vestibular dysfunction (Keats & Savas, 2004). Sensorineural hearing loss results from defects in cochlear hair cell structure and function (Petit, 2001). Mutations associated with Usher syndrome have been found on several genes, including USH1A-G, USH2A-C, USH3, MYO7A, and CDH23 (Nance, 2003; Hone & Smith, 2001b).

Jervell and Lange-Nielsen Syndrome.   Features of this rare syndrome, described in 1957 by Jervell and Lange-Nielsen, are profound bilateral congenital SNHL, prolonged QT interval on the electrocardiogram, and syncope (Jervell & Lange-Nielsen, 1957). Jervell and Lange-Nielsen syndrome (JLNS) is inherited in an autosomal recessive fashion. The more common autosomal-dominant inherited prolonged QT interval syndrome is called Romano-Ward syndrome; it is not associated with sensorineural deafness (Towbin & Vatta, 2001). Prevalence varies with geographical location, ranging from 1:55,000 to 1:500,000 (Tranebjaerg, Bathen, Tyson, & Bitner-Glindzicz, 1999). JLNS is found in roughly 0.2% of patients with congenital deafness (Ocal, Imamoglu, Atalay, & Ercan, 1997). Mutations in the genes KCNQ1 and KCNE1, which encode for potassium channels found in both the stria vascularis and the heart, result in altered potassium channel function, leading to disruption of inner-ear endolymph homeostasis and hearing loss (Neyroud et al., 1999; Duggal et al., 1998; Liu, Newton, & Read, 1995; Chiang, 2004). Histopathologic findings in the deaf Kcnq1 knockout mouse, including atrophy of the stria vascularis, contraction of endolymphatic compartments, and organ of Corti degeneration, provide further support for KCNQ1 as a causative gene in JLNS (Lee et al., 2000; Rivas & Francis, 2005).

X-linked Syndromic

Alport Syndrome.   First recognized by Alport in 1927, this syndrome is characterized by nephropathy (manifested as hematuria, proteinuria, and progressive renal failure) and SNHL. X-linked inheritance occurs in approximately 85% of patients, with the remaining cases inherited in an autosomal dominant or autosomal recessive fashion. Mutations in the gene COL4A5 (which encodes for the α-5 chain of type IV collagen) are found in X-linked Alport syndrome, and mutations in the genes COL4A3 and COL4A4 (which encodes for the α-3 and α-4 chains of type IV collagen, respectively) are associated with autosomally inherited Alport syndrome (Hudson, Tryggvason, Sundaramoorthy, & Neilson, 2003). Prevalence is estimated at 1:5,000 to 1:10,000 (Rizk & Chapman, 2003). Onset of hearing loss usually occurs in late childhood, and the hearing loss is characteristically bilateral, symmetric, and progressive. Hearing loss is usually no greater than 70 dB, and patients often have good speech discrimination scores. Sensorineural hearing loss in Alport syndrome may be due to altered cochlear micromechanics as a result of structural abnormalities in the organ of Corti and organ of Corti cell basement membranes (Merchant et al., 2004).

Mitochondrial Syndromic

Because mitochondria are involved in cellular metabolism, mitochondrial diseases often affect energy-demanding tissues, such as the central nervous system, muscle, pancreas, and inner ear (Kornblum et al., 2005; Wallace, 1992). Sensorineural hearing loss is seen in 42–70% of patients with mutations in maternally inherited mitochondrial DNA (Schrijver, 2004). Hearing loss can be present in mitochondrial neuromuscular syndromes such as Kearns-Sayre syndrome (KSS); myoclonic epilepsy and ragged red fibers (MERRF); and mitochondrial encephalopathy, lactic acidosis, and stroke-like episodes (MELAS). Besides hearing loss, other features of KSS include progressive external ophthalmoplegia and pigmentary retinopathy before age 20, ataxia, and/or cardiac conduction defects (Mohri et al., 1998). MERRF is mainly characterized by myoclonic epilepsy, myopathy, and ataxia, but frequently optic atrophy, dementia, and hearing impairment are seen as well. MELAS, a progressive syndrome with childhood onset, can present with a variety of symptoms, including seizures, proximal limb weakness, stroke-like episodes, cortical blindness, short stature, and, in 30%, hearing impairment (van Camp & Smith, 2000). Another example of mitochondrial syndromic hearing loss is the syndrome maternally inherited diabetes and deafness (MIDD), which accounts for 0.5–2.8% of patients with type 2 diabetes mellitus (Guillausseau et al., 2001). Typically, hearing impairment in these mitochondrial inheritance syndromes is a progressive high-frequency sensorineural loss, with onset in childhood or early adulthood. Interestingly, hearing loss is thought to result from loss of cochlear outer hair cell function; the cochlear nerve seems to be unaffected. Mitochondrial mutations are rarely involved in prelingual deafness (Bitner-Glindzicz, 2002).

NONSYNDROMIC HEREDITARY HEARING LOSS

Most nonsyndromic hereditary hearing loss is sensorineural; approximately 15–20% is autosomal-dominant (gene locus nomenclature designated DFNA), 80% is autosomal-recessive (DFNB), 1% is X-linked, and at least 1% is mitochondrial in origin (Hereditary Hearing Loss Homepage, http://webhost.ua.ac.be/hhh/). Autosomal-dominant nonsyndromic SNHL tends to be postlingual (usually before age 20) and progressive, whereas autosomal-recessive nonsyndromic SNHL is almost always prelingual in onset (Schrijver, 2004). Mutations associated with nonsyndromic hereditary hearing loss have been found in genes that encode for cell membrane components, cytoskeletal components, extracellular matrix components, and transcription factor proteins. Involved genes encoding for cell membrane components include the connexin (gap junction protein) genes *GJB2* (loci DFNB1 and DFNA3), *GJB3* (DFNA3), and *GJB6* (DFNA2); the potassium channel gene *KCNQ4* (DFNA2); the chloride-iodide transporter gene *PDS* (DFNB4 as well as Pendred syndrome); and the tight junction protein gene *CLDN14* (DFNB29). Implicated genes encoding for cytoskeletal components include the myosin genes *MYO7A* (DFNB2 and DFNA11 as well as Usher syndrome type IB), *MYO15* (DFNB3), and *MYH9* (DFNA17); the cadherin gene *CDH23* (DFNB12); and the collagen protein gene *COL11A2* (DFNA13 as well as Stickler syndrome). Involved extracellular matrix genes include the gene *TECTA* (encoding for the tectorial membrane component a-tectorin; mutations found at loci DFNA8, DFNA12, and DFNB21) and the gene *COCH* (DFNA9). Genes for transcription factors involved in nonsyndromic hearing loss include *EYA4* (DFNA10), *POU4F3* (DFNA15), and *POU3F4* (DFN3) (Gurtler & Lalwani, 2002; Li & Friedman, 2002).

Autosomal-Dominant Nonsyndromic

Currently, 54 gene loci for autosomal-dominant nonsyndromic hearing loss have been mapped, and 18 genes identified (Hereditary Hearing Loss Homepage, http://webhost.ua.ac.be/hhh/). Characteristic phenotypic features can be used to distinguish among the various forms of autosomal-dominant nonsyndromic hearing loss. For example, onset of hearing loss can occur later (during the third and fourth decades) for mutations at loci DFNA4, DFNA9, and DFNA10. Low-frequency hearing loss is rapidly progressive in patients with mutations at loci DFNA1, whereas mildly progressive low-frequency loss is associated with mutations at loci DFNA6/14/38 (*WFS1* gene). Midfrequency hearing loss is seen with mutations at loci DFNA12 (*TECTA* gene), DFNA13 (*COL11A2* gene), and DFNA21 (Bitner-Glindzicz, 2002).

Autosomal-Recessive Nonsyndromic

To date, there are 46 known gene loci for autosomal-recessive nonsyndromic hearing loss, and 21 genes have been identified (Hereditary Hearing Loss Homepage, http://webhost.ua.ac.be/hhh/). Some forms of autosomal-recessive nonsyndromic hearing loss have distinguishing phenotypic characteristics. For example, although autosomal-recessive nonsyndromic hearing loss is characteristically prelingual in onset, postlingual onset of hearing loss may be seen in mutations at loci DFNB2 (*MYO7A* gene), DFNB8/10 (*TMPRSS3* gene), and DFNB16 (*STRC* gene). Vestibular symptoms can be seen with mutations at DFNB2 (*MYO7A* gene),

DFNB4 (*SLC26A4* gene), and DFNB12 (*CDH23* gene); DFNB4 may also be associated with enlargement of the vestibular aqueduct, a condition linked to both sensorineural hearing loss and occasionally disequilibrium.

Approximately 50% of autosomal-recessive nonsyndromic deafness is due to mutations in the *GJB2* gene, at the DFNB1 locus. The allele variant 35delG is the most common mutation seen in populations of European descent, whereas the allele variants 235delC and 167delT are most prevalent mutations in Japanese and Ashkenazi Jewish populations, respectively (Smith, 2004). The typical phenotype associated with *GJB2* mutations is a stable severe-to-profound congenital deafness, but there can be variation in the severity, stability, and onset (prelingual but not always congenital) of hearing loss. Patients with DFNB1 deafness have normal vestibular function and temporal bone imaging (Bitner-Glindzicz, 2002). The *GJB2* gene encodes for connexin 26, a gap junction protein involved in the recirculation of potassium ions back to the endolymph following hair cell stimulation. Mutations in *GJB2* lead to connexin 26 dysfunction and disruption of endolymph ionic homeostasis. Connexin 26 is expressed at multiple locations within the cochlea, including the stria vascularis, limbus, basement membrane, and spiral prominence (Gurtler & Lalwani, 2002; Schrijver, 2004).

X-linked Nonsyndromic

There are currently four known gene loci for X-linked nonsyndromic hearing loss, with one gene identified (Hereditary Hearing Loss Homepage, http://webhost.ua. ac.be/hhh/). The most common form of X-linked nonsyndromic hearing loss, found at locus DFN3, is caused by mutations in the transcription factor gene *POU3F4*. Deafness due to mutations in *POU3F4* is typically from mixed hearing loss, and this condition is associated with congenital stapes fixation and the development of a perilymphatic gusher during stapes surgery, thought to result from increased perilymphatic pressure (REF). Associated radiologic findings include abnormal dilation of the internal auditory canal and vestibule (de Kok et al., 1995).

Mitochondrial Nonsyndromic

Mitochondrial mutations have been implicated in nonsyndromic hearing loss, susceptibility to aminoglycoside ototoxicity, and presbycusis. The A1555G mutation in the mitochondrial 12S ribosomal RNA (12S-rRNA) is responsible for nonsydromic hearing loss as well as susceptibility to aminoglycoside-induced ototoxic hearing loss (Fischel-Ghodsian, 2003). Phenotypic variability in onset and severity of hearing loss associated with this mutation suggest that modifier genes may be involved, although none have been identified thus far (Finsterer & Fellinger, 2005). Mitochondrial DNA mutations may be involved in the development of presbycusis, or age-related hearing loss, as some studies have shown a greater number of mitochondrial mutations in cochlear tissue from individuals with presbycusis (Fischel-Ghodsian, 2003).

ACQUIRED ETIOLOGY

Prenatal Acquired Hearing Loss

In utero exposure to teratogens during the prenatal period can result in hearing loss. Maternal medical conditions associated with congenital hearing loss in the infant include infections from the TORCHS group of pathogens (toxoplasmosis, rubella, cytomegalovirus, herpes simplex, and syphilis), varicella zoster virus, and measles virus, as well as gestational diabetes and hypothyroidism. Prenatal exposure to chemical teratogens, such as alcohol, methyl mercury, retinoids, and ototoxic medications, can also lead to the development of hearing loss (Tharpe & Bess, 1999; Kim, Bothwell, & Backous, 2002; Roizen, 2003). The developing auditory system is most vulnerable to teratogenic exposure from weeks 3 to 12 of gestation (Rivas & Francis, 2005; Dyer, Strasnick, & Jacobson, 1998).

Cytomegalovirus.   Cytomegalovirus (CMV) is the most common cause of intrauterine infection, occurring in 0.4–2.3% of live births in the United States. Sensorineural hearing loss due to congenital CMV infection is found most often in patients with symptomatic disease, with clinical findings such as petechiae, intrauterine growth retardation, hepatosplenomegaly, and thrombocytopenia. While only 10–15% of infants with congenital CMV infection are symptomatic, approximately 50% of such patients will eventually develop hearing loss (Rivera et al., 2002). Delayed onset up to age 5 has been reported. In the majority of cases, hearing loss worsens over time, although the mechanisms of progressive loss are unclear (Roizen, 2003).

Syphilis.   Current statistics suggest that congenital syphilis infection affects approximately 11.2 per 100,000 live births in the United States (Woods, 2005). Hearing loss is a late manifestation of congenital syphilis, with age at presentation ranging from 10 to 40 years (Roizen, 2003). Classically, high-frequency loss occurs first, with subsequent progression to complete bilateral sensorineural hearing and vestibular loss. Conductive hearing loss can also be seen, which is due to ossicular fibrosis (Pletcher & Cheung, 2003).

Chemical Teratogens.   Maternal ingestion of the aminoglycosides streptomycin, gentamicin, and kanamycin, particularly during the period of fetal inner-ear development (gestational weeks 3 to 12), can result in sensorineural hearing loss in the infant. Aminoglycosides exert their ototoxic effects by damaging cochlear and vestibular hair cells. Aminoglycoside-associated hearing loss is typically bilateral, symmetric, and high-frequency in nature (Dyer, Strasnick, & Jacobson, 1998).

Prenatal exposure to alcohol has been implicated in both sensorineural and conductive hearing loss. Fetal alcohol syndrome (FAS) is characterized by growth retardation, neurologic and behavioral disorders, and craniofacial dysmorphic features, including microcephaly, midface hypoplasia, and cleft palate (Roizen, 2003; Dyer et al., 1998). In one small case series of 14 children with FAS referred for otolaryngologic evaluation, 93% had a clinically significant history of recurrent bilateral serous otitis media, and 29% also had bilateral sensorineural hearing loss (Church & Gerkin, 1988).

Perinatal Acquired Hearing Loss

Specific perinatal medical conditions, as well as medical conditions requiring neonatal intensive care, can lead to hearing loss. Hearing loss due to perinatal events is typically sensorineural and bilateral (Newton, 2001). According to the Joint Committee on Infant Hearing, one of the risk factors for hearing loss in neonates is an illness or condition necessitating a NICU stay of 48 hours or greater (2000). Some of the treatments commonly undertaken during the course of a NICU stay, such as mechanical ventilation and aminoglycoside and loop diuretic administration, have been linked to hearing loss. Higher rates of mechanical ventilation requirement have been found in infants with hearing loss compared with those with normal hearing. Treatment with aminoglycosides and loop diuretics, both of which have known ototoxicity, is more commonly seen in hearing-impaired infants as well (Cone-Wesson et al., 2000).

Hyperbilirubinemia during the neonatal period is a medical condition that has been implicated in hearing impairment. Neonates are particularly susceptible to hyperbilirubinemia because of the high rate of bilirubin production (due to high red blood cell turnover) coupled with a limited ability to eliminate bilirubin (Dennery, Seidman, & Stevenson, 2001). One theory suggests a hyperbilirubinemic state leads to deposition of bilirubin in the cochlear nuclei of the brainstem, with subsequent hearing loss (Newton, 2001). However, there is conflicting evidence in the medical literature for the role of hyperbilirubinemia in hearing loss. Although several small case series have found associations between elevated bilirubin levels and sensorineural hearing loss (Roizen, 2003), larger studies have failed to find a significant relationship between bilirubin level and the development of hearing loss (Van de Bor et al., 1992; Newman & Klebanoff, 1993).

Postnatal Acquired Hearing Loss

Causes for acquired hearing loss in infants and children can be infectious, traumatic, anatomic, iatrogenic, or associated with medical disease. Infectious causes of acquired hearing loss include otitis media, bacterial meningitis, parvovirus B–19 infection, otitis externa, and Lyme disease. Among the traumatic causes of hearing loss are temporal bone or labyrinthine injury, acoustic trauma, and foreign body injury to the tympanic membrane, middle ear, or inner ear. Examples of anatomic causes are external auditory canal stenosis (from surgery or otitis externa), erosion of the ossicular chain (from infection or cholesteatoma), and tympanic membrane perforation (from infection or trauma). Iatrogenic causes include radiation therapy, administration of ototoxic medications, and surgical trauma. Hearing loss can occur in association with hypothyroidism or autoimmune disorders such as type I diabetes, juvenile rheumatoid arthritis, and systemic lupus erythematosis. Neoplastic disease in the temporal bone or at the cerebellopontine angle may also have hearing loss as one of its manifestations (Kenna, 2004a).

Otitis Media with Effusion.   The most common cause of acquired hearing loss in children is otitis media with effusion (OME), defined as the presence of middle-ear fluid without evidence of acute infection. Fortunately, OME is generally self-limited, with resolution of symptoms within 3 months for the majority of patients (Rosenfeld & Kay, 2003). The presence of middle-ear fluid can result in a conductive hearing loss. Characteristically, conductive threshold levels are roughly 25 to 30 dB, but values can range from 0 to 50 dB. Hearing loss may be worse if OME is present bilaterally or for a period of several months (Lous et al., 2005). A few studies have suggested that persistent OME can lead to sensorineural hearing loss as well (Roberts et al., 2004). Asymmetric hearing loss due to unilateral OME may also have adverse effects on auditory processing skills such as binaural hearing, perception of speech in a noisy environment, and sound localization (American Academy of Family Physicians, American Academy of Otolaryngology—Head and Neck Surgery, American Academy of Pediatrics Subcommittee on Otitis Media with Effusion, 2004). Although there has been concern about the negative effect of OME-related hearing loss on the development of language skills, recent studies have found that effect to be minimal to none, particularly when confounding factors such as the quality of the home environment and socioeconomic status are taken into account (American Academy of Family Physicians, American Academy of Otolaryngology—Head and Neck Surgery, American Academy of Pediatrics Subcommittee on Otitis Media with Effusion, 2004; Roberts, Rosenfeld, & Zeisel, 2004; Robert Rosenfeld, & Zeisel, 2004b).

Bacterial Meningitis.   Bacterial meningitis is the most common cause of acquired sensorineural hearing loss in children, accounting for 6% of all pediatric SNHL cases. Younger children are disproportionately affected by bacterial meningitis, with 75% of patients under the age of 2 (Smith, Bale, & White, 2005). The most common pathogens involved in bacterial meningitis are *Haemophilus influenzae, Neisseria meningitidis,* and *Streptococcus pneumoniae* (Tunkel & Scheld, 1993), although the prevalence of *H. influenzae* is waning with the use of *H. influenzae* type B vaccination (Hone & Smith, 2002b). In neonatal meningitis, group B streptococcus species and *Escherichia coli* are the leading causative organisms (Heath, Nik Yusoff, & Baker, 2003). Hearing loss is reported to occur in 6–16% of bacterial meningitis cases (Francis et al., 2004). The hearing impairment is usually present early in the course of disease, with possible progression in severity (Kenna, 2004b). Bilateral hearing loss occurs in about 60% of cases, and, in many cases, such hearing loss is asymmetric in degree between the right and left ears (Hone & Smith, 2002).

EVALUATION OF THE PEDIATRIC PATIENT WITH HEARING LOSS

The pediatric patient with suspected hearing loss may present to medical attention in a variety of ways. Because of the adoption of mandatory newborn hearing screening programs in several states, hearing loss in infants may be identified through auditory brainstem response (ABR) or otoacoustic emission (OAE) testing. In cases of acquired hearing loss, delayed onset of congenital deafness, or lack of availability of newborn hearing screening, the hearing loss may not be suspected until difficulties in communication, language development, or school performance arise (Kenna, 2004). A thorough history, physical examination, audiologic assessment, and judicious laboratory and radiologic testing, as well as consultation with other medical specialties (such as genetics or ophthalmology) when appropriate, are recommended to determine the type and extent of the hearing loss, its etiology, and available management options.

History

A detailed history should begin by determining the clinical features of the hearing loss, including the suspected time of onset of hearing loss (congenital, infancy, early childhood, or late childhood), any progression of impairment, and the presence of any associated symptoms (such as vertigo, tinnitus, symptoms of systemic medical disease, or symptoms found in hearing loss syndromes). Prenatal history, perinatal history, other past medical history, and family history are all important in identifying the possible risk factors and etiologies for hearing loss, whether it be acquired or genetic, and syndromic or nonsyndromic.

Prenatal History.   The patient or guardian should be asked about maternal exposure to medications, alcohol, tobacco, illegal drugs, and other possible teratogenic substances during pregnancy. Any maternal medical conditions or infections during pregnancy should be noted, as well as any medical complications of the pregnancy itself.

Perinatal History.   The birth history should be elicited, including gestational age at delivery (pre-term or term), complications of delivery, and requirement for resuscitative efforts such as supplemental oxygen or endotracheal intubation. The patient or guardian should be asked whether NICU care was required, and, if so, about the medical conditions necessitating such care and medical treatments given during that NICU stay.

Past Medical History.   Medical history beyond the perinatal period can also provide valuable information in the evaluation of pediatric hearing loss. The patient or guardian should be asked about any history of pertinent infections, such as otitis media or bacterial meningitis, or systemic medical disease. Medication history should focus in particular on exposure to ototoxic medications, such as aminoglycosides, loop diuretics, chemotherapeutic agents, and retinoids. Any history of head trauma or ear trauma should be noted. The patient or guardian should also be asked about any history of symptoms that may be found in hearing loss syndromes, such as vision and balance problems (Usher syndrome), hematuria (Alport syndrome), and recurrent syncopal episodes (Jervell and Lange-Nielsen syndrome).

Family History.   A positive family history may suggest a hereditary form of hearing loss. First- and second-degree relatives with hearing loss, especially those with onset of impairment prior to 30 years of age, should be noted (Tomaski & Grundfast, 1999; Hone & Smith, 2002). The patient or guardian should be asked whether any family members have features associated with syndromic hereditary hearing loss, such as craniofacial abnormalities (Treacher-Collins syndrome, Waardenburg syndrome), renal abnormalities (branchio-oto-renal syndrome, Alport syndrome), visual problems (Usher syndrome), and early childhood cardiac arrhythmias (Jervell and Lange-Nielsen syndrome) (Doyle & Ray, 2003; Hone & Smith, 2002).

Physical Examination

Physical exam findings (with the exception of hearing tests) are normal in many cases of pediatric hearing loss. Physical abnormalities may be seen in association with syndromic hereditary hearing loss or congenital infection, but these abnormalities can be subtle in presentation (Tomaski & Grundfast, 1999; Hone & Smith, 2002b). A systematic approach to the physical exam is helpful in the detection of pertinent physical findings. The patient's general appearance and stature should be noted. Findings of interest in the craniofacial exam include abnormal skull or facial shape, facial asymmetry, hypoplasia, and other dysmorphic features. For the eye examination, the clinician should evaluate both visual acuity and the external appearance of the eyes, looking for any abnormalities in the palpebral fissure positions, intercanthal distance, iris color, cornea, or retina. Malformations of the external ear, such as preauricular pits, sinuses, skin tags, pinna abnormalities, microtia, and external auditory canal stenosis, should be noted. Otomicroscopic examination can be performed to look for impacted cerumen, presence of a foreign body, middle-ear fluid, cholesteatoma, vascular lesions, ossicular chain abnormalities, or mass lesions. Pneumatic otoscopy, which allows for evaluation tympanic membrane movement in response to positive and negative pressure, can provide information about the compliance of the tympanic membrane. Tympanic membrane compliance can be altered in the presence of middle-ear fluid or ossicular chain abnormalities. The oral cavity should be examined to check for cleft palate. In examining the neck, the clinician should check for neck masses, branchial abnormalities (cysts, pits, or sinuses), and thyroid goiter. The skin and extremities should be examined, in particular to note any abnormalities in the digits or skin pigmentation. A thorough neurological exam should be performed, including evaluation of the cranial nerves and vestibular function (Doyle & Ray, 2003; Hone & Smith, 2002; Tomaski & Grundfast, 1999). Table 5–1 lists pertinent physical findings in pediatric hearing loss patients and the hearing loss conditions with which these findings are associated.

TABLE 5–1
Physical Findings in Pediatric Hearing Loss

General	Tall stature	Stickler syndrome
	Dwarfism	Achondroplasia
Craniofacial	Hemifacial microsomia	Treacher Collins syndrome
	Small or hypoplastic midface	Fetal alcohol syndrome
Eye	Dystopia canthorum	Waardenburg syndrome
	Heterochromia irides	Waardenburg syndrome
	Downslanting palpebral fissures	Treacher Collins syndrome
	Lower eyelid coloboma	Treacher Collins syndrome
	Retinitis pigmentosa	Usher syndrome
	Hazy corneal discoloration	Congential syphilis infection
	Lens opacification	Congenital rubella infection
	Loss of visual acuity	Usher syndrome
		Stickler syndrome
		Norrie syndrome
Ear	Pinna malformation	Treacher Collins syndrome
		Goldenhar syndrome
		CHARGE syndrome
	Preauricular pits	Branchio-oto-renal syndrome
	External auditory canal stenosis	Down syndrome
Oral cavity	Cleft palate	CHARGE syndrome
		Isolated anomaly
Neck	Branchial cleft cyst or fistula	Branchio-oto-renal syndrome
	Thyroid goiter	Pendred syndrome
Skin/Extremities	Areas of skin hypopigmentation (including white forelock)	Waardenburg syndrome
	Fused digits	Apert syndrome
Neurologic exam	Vestibular hypofunction	Usher syndrome

Audiologic Assessment

There are several means of audiologic assessment that can be used in pediatric patients. Selection of the appropriate audiologic tests will depend on the age of the patient and the type of information being sought. Table 5–2 shows the categories of hearing impairment as defined by the levels of hearing threshold, or decibel hearing levels (dB HL). The type of hearing loss (conductive, sensorineural, or mixed) can be determined from audiogram results. Figure 5–1 presents examples of audiograms obtained from pure tone audiometry, as seen in different types of hearing loss. An audiogram from a patient with normal hearing is seen in panel A, showing thresholds less than 20 dB nHL (within the normal range) at all frequencies tested. The audiogram in panel B is representative of conductive hearing loss, in which air conduction thresholds are abnormally elevated but bone conduction thresholds are normal. In the panel C audiogram, representative of sensorineural hearing loss, the difference between air and bone conduction thresholds does not exceed 10 dB. Mixed hearing loss is characterized by bone conduc-

TABLE 5–2
Categories of Hearing Impairment

Normal	<25 dB HL
Mild	25–40 dB HL
Moderate	41–55 dB HL
Moderately severe	56–70 dB HL
Severe	71–90 dB HL
Profound	>90 dB HL

tion thresholds out of normal range and an air-bone conduction gap greater than 10 dB (Gregg, Wiorek, & Arvedson, 2004).

Auditory Brainstem Response. Auditory brainstem response (ABR) testing is commonly used to assess peripheral auditory function in infants, although this testing may be used in all age groups. In ABR testing (which is reviewed in detail in Chapter 6), scalp surface electrodes are used to detect a characteristic evoked electrophysiologic response that is seen within 20 ms of an auditory stimulus presentation. The ABR, generated from the eighth cranial nerve and auditory brainstem structures, is not affected by the subject's attention status, which allows for its use in sleeping or sedated patients. ABR testing can be done with air-conducted and bone-conducted auditory stimuli, to distinguish between conductive and sensorineural hearing loss. Auditory threshold levels as determined by ABR testing are within 10 to 15 dB of threshold levels obtained by behavioral audiometric testing (Hayes, 2003).

Otoacoustic Emissions. Otoacoustic emission (OAE) testing is also commonly used for testing of auditory function in infants, but is suitable for all ages as well. OAEs are acoustic signals generated from cochlear outer hair cells. These emissions are propagated from the cochlea back through the middle ear into the external auditory canal, where they are clinically detected by microphones. OAEs are thought to be the natural by-products of outer hair cell motility, which plays a role in the amplification of low-level auditory stimuli. Although OAEs can occur spontaneously or in response to an acoustic stimulus, the latter is better suited for clinical testing. Evoked OAEs in response to an acoustic transient (transient evoked otoacoustic emissions; TEOAEs) or tone pairs (distortion product otoacoustic emissions; DPOAEs) are used clinically to assess cochlear and middle-ear function. OAEs are abnormal in mild hearing loss, and they cannot be detected when hearing loss is greater than 30 dB. Although OAEs have limited utility in determining hearing threshold levels, they may useful in localizing the site responsible for hearing loss. For example, normal OAEs in the setting of abnormal or absent ABRs might indicate a retrocochlear locus of pathology responsible for hearing loss (Johnson, 2002; Sininger, 2003).

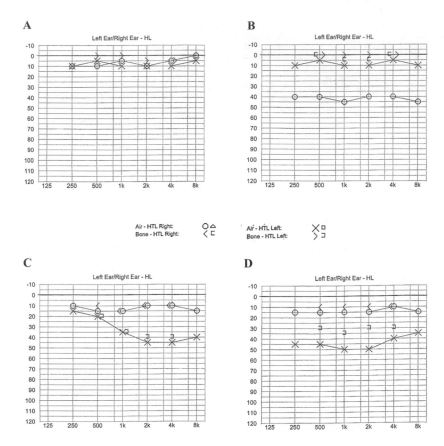

FIGURE 5–1. Examples of audiograms in (A) normal hearing, (B) conductive hearing loss, (C) sensorineural hearing loss, and (D) mixed hearing loss.

Behavioral Audiometry. In young infants up to 6 months of age, behavioral evaluation of hearing is limited to observation, looking for temporal correlation of gross behavioral changes in the infant with the presentation of auditory stimuli. With this method, the lack of conditioned, reproducible responses to an auditory stimulus makes it difficult to determine whether the infant is truly reacting in response to the intensity of the auditory stimulus, as opposed to its novelty, or lack thereof. From age 6 months to 2½ years, visual reinforcement audiometry (VRA) can be used. The child is conditioned to turn toward an auditory stimulus by visual reinforcement with an animated or illuminated toy. Once this behavior is established, the intensity of the auditory stimulus is lowered to determine the hearing threshold level. If insert earphones are used, ear-specific thresholds can be obtained. In children ages 2½ to 5, conditioned play audiometry (CPA) is used. After being taught to perform motor tasks in response to sound, children can be tested for ear-specific air- and bone-conduction hearing thresholds with the use of earphones or bone-conduction oscillators, respectively. After age 5, most children are developmentally capable of responding to pure tone audiometry tests and can be taught to signal when they perceive tones of varying frequencies and intensities that are presented, as adults do (Doyle & Smith, 2003; Johnson, 2002).

Tympanometry.   The assessment of middle-ear function provided by tympanometry can be useful in patients with suspected conductive hearing loss. In tympanometry, varying amounts of air pressure are applied to the external ear while a probe tone is presented. A tympanogram is generated by plotting the amount of acoustic energy reflected back from the tympanic membrane as a function of pressure. Tympanogram shapes can be classified as type A (normal middle-ear pressure, peak at 0 daPa), type B (flat, no peak), type C (negative pressure peak), and type D (notched pressure peak), as shown in Fig. 5–2 (Jerger, 1970; Liden, 1975). Typically, characteristic tympanometric patterns are associated with

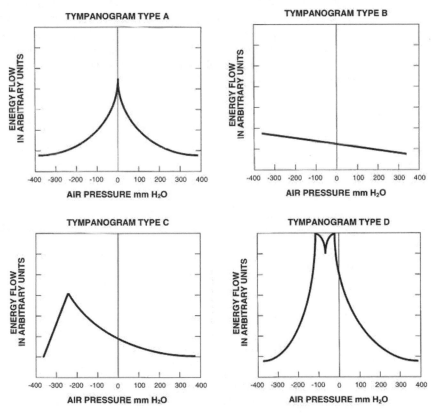

FIGURE 5–2.

different types of middle-ear pathology, such as tympanic membrane perforation (type B), middle-ear fluid (type B), or negative middle-ear pressure (type C) (Doyle & Smith, 2003; Johnson, 2002).

Laboratory Testing

The battery of laboratory tests required in the evaluation of a pediatric hearing loss patient will vary, depending on the differential diagnoses being considered. Recent studies examining the utility of routine laboratory studies in determining the etiology and management of unexplained hearing loss in children have found that the diagnostic yield is generally low (Ohlms, Chen, Stewart, & Franklin, 1999; Preciado et al., 2004; Mafong, Shin, & Lalwani, 2002). Appropriate laboratory tests should be ordered based on clinical suspicion, as directed by the history and physical findings. All children with bilateral severe to profound sensorineural hearing loss should have electrocardiograms (ECGs) performed to detect prolonged QT intervals, associated with Jervell and Lange-Nielsen syndrome (JNLS). Although low in diagnostic yield, the life-saving potential of the ECG in diagnosing JLNS justifies its broad use in this patient population (Preciado et al., 2004). For patients with a possible genetic etiology for hearing loss, screening is clinically available for three genes involved in hereditary hearing loss: *GJB2*, *SLC26A4*, and *WFS1* (Smith, 2004); see Chapter 4 for further detail. Table 5–3 presents laboratory tests that may be useful in determining the etiology of hearing loss (Smith, 2004; Mafong et al., 2002; Ohlms et al., 1999).

Radiologic Testing

In contrast to the low diagnostic yield of routine laboratory testing, the diagnostic utility of radiologic imaging in pediatric hearing loss patients is much

TABLE 5–3
Laboratory Tests in the Evaluation of Pediatric Hearing Loss

Test	Diagnosis
Complete blood count (CBC)	Leukemia
	Fechner syndrome (Alport syndrome variant)
Blood glucose	Diabetes
Thyroid function	Hypothyroidism
	Pendred syndrome
Urinalysis	Alport syndrome
Elecrocardiogram	Jervell and Lange-Nielsen syndrome
TORCHS titers	Congenital TORCHS infection
RPR	Syphilis
Genetic screening	*GJB2* mutation (connexin 26)
	SLC26A4 mutation (Pendred syndrome/dilated vestibular aqueduct)
	WFS1 mutation

higher, with reported diagnostic yields of 27–39% for high-resolution computed tomography (CT) imaging (Antonelli, Varela, & Mancuso, 1999; Mafong, Shin, & Lalwani, 2002; Preciado et al., 2004). CT imaging is used to evaluate bony pathology of the temporal bone that may explain hearing loss, including bony abnormalities, traumatic injury, and otosclerosis, whereas magnetic resonance (MR) imaging is better for evaluation of the membranous labyrinth and central auditory structures (Mafong, Shin, & Lalwani, 2002). CT imaging is highly recommended in the workup of the pediatric patient with hearing loss (Antonelli, Varela, & Mancuso, 1999; Mafong, Shin, & Lalwani, 2002; Preciado et al., 2004); the need for MR imaging may be less compelling, given its lower rate of abnormality detection in hearing loss (Preciado et al., 2004). The most common radiologic abnormality found in association with sensorineural hearing loss in children is large vestibular aqueduct (LVA), as seen in Fig. 5–3 (Antonelli, Varela, & Mancuso, 1999; Schroeder & Kuhn, 2000), followed by cochlear dysplasias and modiolar deficiencies. The vestibular aqueduct is a bony channel which contains the endolymphatic duct, a membranous structure that emerges from the vestibule and terminates in the en-

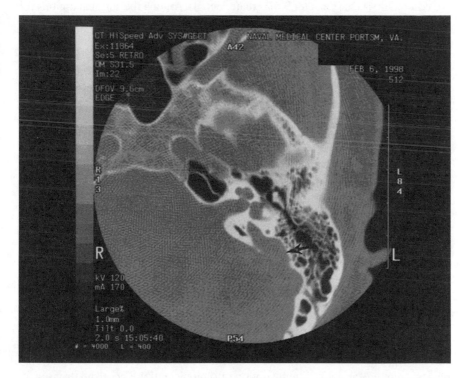

FIGURE 5–3. High-resolution axial CT showing enlarged left vestibular aqueduct, 5 mm in diameter (*arrow*). From Schroeder, A. A., & Kuhn, J. (2000). Imaging case of the month. Large vestibular aqueduct syndrome. *The American Journal of Otology, 21*, 433–434.

dolymphatic sac. In an important early study, Valvasorri and Clemins defined large vestibular aqueduct radiologically as having an anteroposterior diameter greater than 1.5 mm (Valvasorri & Clemins, 1978). The presence of LVA is clinically significant in that it may be found in association with Pendred syndrome, X-linked stapes gusher syndrome, or other ear malformations (Mafong, Shin, & Lalwani, 2002). Patients with LVA may be at increased risk for sensorineural hearing loss following minor head trauma (Walsh, Ayshford, Chavda, & Proops, 1999; Callison & Horn, 1998; Okumura, Takahashi, Honjo, Takagi, & Mitamura, 1995).

MANAGEMENT

Management options for the pediatric patient with hearing impairment will vary, depending on the etiology of hearing loss. Medical management may play a role in selected cases of pediatric hearing loss. Auditory amplification and/or surgical treatment are more commonly used management options. Types of auditory amplification include air conduction hearing aids, bone conduction hearing aids, and frequency-modulated (FM) systems (Gabbard & Schryer, 2003; Gregg, Wiorek, & Arvedson, 2004) (see Chapter 9 for greater detail). Among the surgical options for hearing loss are treatment for otitis media with effusion (OME) via myringotomy, tympanostomy tubes, and adenotonsillectomy, surgical correction of anatomic ear abnormalities or lesions, and cochlear implantation (Doyle & Ray, 2003; Kenna, 2004). For patients with conductive hearing loss, medical or surgical correction of the hearing loss is often considered initially; auditory amplification is recommended for poor surgical candidates or hearing loss refractory to correction. The bone-anchored hearing aid (BAHA) has emerged as an excellent tool for the treatment of both conductive hearing loss or complete unilateral sensorineural hearing loss (see Fig. 5–4). Auditory amplification can also help patients with sensorineural hearing loss. For those patients with bilateral severe to profound SNHL in whom auditory amplification provides little benefit, cochlear implantation (reviewed in greater detail in Chapter 7) may be a possible management option (Kenna, 2004).

Medical Management

In children with bacterial meningitis caused by *H. influenzae* type B, adjunctive treatment with dexamethasone may reduce the risk of meningitis-associated sensorineural hearing loss (McIntyre et al., 1997). A conductive hearing loss may result from swelling and occlusion of the external auditory canal (EAC) due to otitis externa. Appropriate treatment of otitis externa with EAC debridement, occasional placement of an ear wick, administration of ototopic antibiotic/steroid drops, and, if necessary, oral antibiotics will lead to resolution of the conductive hearing loss.

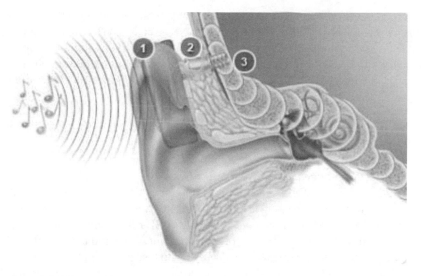

Figure 5–4. Diagram of bone-anchored hearind aid (BAHA), consisting of (1) a sound processor, (2) an external abutment, and (3) a bone-anchored titanium implant.Figure courtesy of
Cochler Ltd.

Conductive hearing loss due to the presence of cerumen or a foreign body is reme-
died by removal of the offending object from the EAC (Isaacson & Vora, 2003).

Auditory Amplification

Auditory amplification is designed to make speech and environmental sounds
audible without the use of high-intensity sounds that could risk further hearing
loss (Brookhouser, Beauchaine, & Osberger, 1999). The majority of children
with hearing aids have air conduction hearing aids, in which amplified sounds
are delivered directly into the external auditory canal. Children with a conductive component to their hearing loss may require amplification with a bone-
conduction hearing aid, in which amplified sound is transmitted to the cochlea
via a bone-conduction vibrator held tightly against the skull (Brookhouser,
Beauchaine, & Osberger, 1999; Gabbard & Schryer, 2003). The BAHA can be
used as an alternative for children who require permanent bone-conduction amplification, as is the case in patients with anatomic external and middle-ear
anomalies that have been refractory to conventional surgical therapy, as is often the case in patients with external canal atresia or absent ossicles (Tjellstrom,
Hakansson, & Granstrom, 2001; Gabbard & Schryer, 2003; Kenna, 2004). More
recently, the BAHA has been used in cases of unilateral sensorineural hearing
loss, as a form of surgical contralateral-routing-of-signal (CROS) aid; in this
method, placement of a BAHA on the side of a dysfunctional ear allows transmission of sound from the poor side via bone conduction to the functional cochlea, pro-

viding increased ability for sound reception and significantly decreasing the head-shadow effect (Niparko, Cox, & Lustig, 2003; Wazen et al., 2003; Hol, Bosman, Snik, Mylanus, & Cremers, 2004). In FM systems, another form of auditory amplification, the child wears a receiver in the ear, which receives amplified sounds from a microphone located at the sound source (e.g., school teacher) (Brookhouser, Beauchine, & Osberger, 1999).

Surgical Treatment

Surgical Management of Conductive Hearing Loss.   The primary surgical treatment option for OME is the insertion of tympanostomy tubes, which leads to an average 6- to 12-dB hearing level improvement. Adenoidectomy plus myringotomy is recommended for patients who have OME relapse after tympanostomy tube extrusion, because the need for future operations is reduced by 50%. The following categories of patients with OME should be considered for surgical treatment: children with OME for 4 months or longer with persistent hearing impairment; children at risk for developmental delay who have persistent or recurrent OME; and children who have OME and tympanic membrane or middle ear damage (American Academy of Family Physicians, American Academy of Otolaryngology—Head and Neck Surgery, American Academy of Pediatrics Subcommittee on Otitis Media with Effusion, 2004).

For patients with conductive hearing loss due to cholesteatoma, a locally destructive abnormal accumulation of squamous epithelium in the middle ear, temporal bone, or mastoid (Isaacson & Vora, 2003), complete surgical resection is necessary to halt the progression of the disease and to prevent hearing loss from worsening. The surgical procedures commonly used for cholesteatoma resection in pediatric patients are exploratory transcanal tympanotomy with removal of cholesteatoma and tympanoplasty, canal wall-up (CWU) tympanomastoidectomy, and canal wall-down (CWD) tympanomastoidectomy. Resection through a tympanotomy can be performed when disease is limited to the middle ear, but transcanal tympanotomy does not allow for adequate access to the epitympanum or mastoid (Shohet & de Jong, 2002). The CWU tympanomastoidectomy preserves the posterior EAC wall but limits exposure to the epitympanum and sinus tympani compared with the CWD tympanomastoidectomy. The CWD procedure is thought to be associated with less recidivism of disease, but also poorer hearing results secondary to alteration of the normal anatomic contour (Kazahaya & Potsic, 2004; Shohet & de Jong, 2002).

Conductive hearing loss due to congenital middle-ear anomalies can be addressed surgically as well. An exploratory tympanotomy should be performed to assess the integrity of the ossicular chain. Independent palpation of each ossicle is recommended to verify mobility. The ossicular chain should be reconstructed to create a stable means of sound conduction, with use of the appropriate prosthesis for optimal hearing results (Raz & Lustig, 2002).

Cochlear Implantation.   Cochlear implantation is a surgical option for the management of severe to profound sensorineural hearing loss in children. The cochlear implant is an electronic device consisting of an electrode array placed surgically within the cochlea, close to the auditory nerve, and an external unit through which sound is transduced into digital signals and transmitted to the internal electrode array. Delivery of digital signals to the electrode array leads to stimulation of the auditory pathway, ultimately leading to the perception of sound (Gates & Miyamoto, 2003). Cochlear implantation was approved for use in children in 1990 by the Food and Drug Administration (FDA). In 2000, the FDA approved the use of the Nucleus 24 device (Cochlear Corporation) in children as young as 1 year of age (Francis & Niparko, 2003). More detailed discussion of cochlear implantation is presented in the following chapter.

SURVEILLANCE

Comprehensive management of the pediatric hearing loss patient includes ongoing audiologic and medical surveillance. Successive audiometric assessments are needed to determine whether a child's hearing loss is stable, fluctuating, or progressive; this information may prove useful in identifying the etiology of hearing loss as well as optimizing medical or surgical management. In cases of fluctuating or progressive hearing loss, such as enlarged vestibular aqueduct syndrome, monthly reevaluations of hearing status should be performed until the pattern of hearing loss becomes apparent. Follow-up examinations are also important in evaluating the efficacy of the chosen intervention in managing the patient's hearing loss. For those children with hearing aids, for example, follow-up evaluations are recommended at the following intervals: every 3 months until age 2 years, every 6 months from ages 2 to 6 years, and annually from age 6 onward. At these intervals, hearing aids can be adjusted as needed, to accommodate functional changes in the child's audiologic status and growth-related changes in the child's external auditory canal shape with respect to earmold fit. Shorter intervals of monitoring are recommended at younger ages because obtaining feedback about hearing aid function is more difficult to obtain in younger children, and they tend to require growth-related earmold changes more frequently (Brookhouser, Beauchaine, & Osberger, 1999). For children with cochlear implants, postimplantation follow-up is necessary to optimize cochlear implant programming and to monitor for appropriate functioning (Balkany, Hodges, Miyamoto, Gibbin, & Odabasi, 2001).

CONCLUSION

Hearing impairment in children is a relatively common clinical condition that should not go undetected or untreated. Early diagnosis and intervention are key to the future success of the hearing-impaired child. Optimal care of the pediatric hearing loss patient requires a keen understanding of the etiologic factors involved in hearing loss and the management options for the given clinical situation. Conductive hearing loss can sometimes be reversed to normal or near-normal hearing with medical or surgical treatment, but sensorineural hearing loss presents a more difficult treatment challenge. Currently, sensorineural hearing loss is essentially irreversible, thus highlighting the need to recognize and avoid preventable causes of hearing loss. Fortunately, auditory rehabilitation in the form of hearing aids, auditory amplification, and cochlear implantation can provide tremendous help to the hearing-impaired child. Undoubtedly, future scientific and technological advances will lead to even better diagnostic and therapeutic options for patients.

REFERENCES

American Academy of Family Physicians, American Academy of Otolaryngology—Head and Neck Surgery, American Academy of Pediatrics Subcommittee on Otitis Media with Effusion (2004). Otitis Media with effusion. *Pediatrics, 113*, 1412–1429.

Antonelli, P. J., Varela, A. E., & Mancuso, A. A. (1999). Diagnostic yield of high-resolution computed tomography for pediatric sensorineural hearing loss. *Laryngoscope, 109*, 1642–1647.

Balkany, T. J., Hodges, A., Miyamoto, R. T., Gibbin, K., & Odabasi, O. (2001). Cochlear implants in children. *Otolaryngologic Clinics of North America, 34*, 455–467.

Bitner-Glindzicz, M. (2002). Hereditary deafness and phenotyping in humans. *British Medical Bulletin, 63*, 73–94.

Brookhouser, P. E., Beauchaine, K. L., & Osberger, M. J. (1999). Management of the child with sensorineural hearing loss. Medical, surgical, hearing aids, cochlear implants. *Pediatric Clinics of North America, 46*, 121–141.

Callison, D. M., & Horn, K. L. (1998). Large vestibular aqueduct syndrome: An overlooked etiology for progressive childhood hearing loss. *Journal of the American Academy of Audiology, 9*, 285–291.

Chiang, C. E. (2004). Congenital and acquired long QT syndrome. Current concepts and management. *Cardiology Reviews, 12*, 222–234.

Church, M. W., & Gerkin, K. P. (1988). Hearing disorders in children with fetal alcohol syndrome: Findings from case reports. *Pediatrics, 82*, 147–154.

Cone-Wesson, B., Vohr, B. R., Sininger, Y. S., Widen, J. E., Folsom, R. C., Gorga, M. P., & Norton S. J. (2000). Identification of neonatal hearing impairment: infants with hearing loss. *Ear and Hearing, 21*, 488–507.

Connolly, J. L., Carron, J. D., & Roark, S. D. (2005). Universal newborn hearing screening: Are we achieving the Joint Committee on Infant Hearing (JCIH) objectives? *Laryngoscope, 115*, 232–236.

de Kok, Y. J., van der Maarel, S. M., Bitner-Glindzicz, M., Huber, I., Monaco, A. P., Malcolm, S., Pembrey, M. E., Ropers, A. H., & Cremers, F. P. (1995). Association between X-linked mixed deafness and mutations in the POU domain gene POU3F4. *Science, 267*, 685–688.

Dennery, P. A., Seidman, D. S., & Stevenson, D. K. (2001). Neonatal hyperbilirubinemia. *New England Journal of Medicine, 344*, 581–590.

Doyle, K. J., & Ray, R. M. (2003). The otolaryngologist's role in management of hearing loss in infancy and childhood. *Mental Retardation and Developmental Disabilities: Research Reviews, 9*, 94–102.

Duggal, P., Vesely, M. R., Wattanasirichaigoon, D., Villafane, J., Kaushik, V., & Beggs, A. H. (1998). Mutation of the gene for IsK associated with both Jervell and Lange-Nielsen and Romano-Ward forms of Long-QT syndrome. *Circulation, 97,* 142–146.

Dyer, J. J., Strasnick, B., & Jacobson, J. T. (1998). Teratogenic hearing loss: A clinical perspective. *American Journal of Otology, 19,* 671–678.

Early identification of hearing impairment in infants and young children (1993). *National Institutes of Health Consensus Statement, 11,* 1–24. (No authors listed)

Everett, L. A., Glaser, B., Beck, J. C., Idol, J. R., Buchs, A., Heyman, M., Adawi, F., Hazani, E., Nassir, E., Baxevanis, A. A., Sheffield, V. C., & Green, E. D. (1997). Pendred syndrome is caused by mutations in a putative sulphate transporter gene (PDS). *Nature Genetics, 17,* 411–422.

Finsterer, J., & Fellinger, J. (2005). Nuclear and mitochondrial genes mutated in nonsyndromic impaired hearing. *International Journal of Pediatric Otorhinolaryngology, 69,* 621–647.

Fischel-Ghodsian, N. (2003). Mitochondrial deafness. *Ear and Hearing, 24,* 303–313.

Fortnum, H., & Davis, A. (1997). Epidemiology of permanent childhood hearing impairment in Trent Region, 1985–1993. *British Journal of Audiology, 31,* 409–446.

Francis, H. W., & Niparko, J. K. (2003). Cochlear implantation update. *Pediatric Clinics of North America, 50,* 341–61, viii.

Francis, H. W., Pulsifer, M. B., Chinnici, J., Nutt, R., Venick, H. S., Yeagle, J. D., Niparko, J. K. (2004). Effects of central nervous system residua on cochlear implant results in children deafened by meningitis. *Archive of Otolaryngology—Head and Neck Surgery, 130,* 604–611.

Francomano, C. A., Liberfarb, R. M., Hirose, T., Maumenee, I. H., Streeten, E. A., Meyers, D. A., & Pyeritz, R. E. (1987). The Stickler syndrome: Evidence for close linkage to the structural gene for type II collagen. *Genomics, 1,* 293–296.

Fraser, F. C., Sproule, J. R., & Halal, F. (1980). Frequency of the branchio-oto-renal (BOR) syndrome in children with profound hearing loss. *American Journal of Medical Genetics, 7,* 341–349.

Fraser, G. R. (1974). Epidemiology of profound childhood deafness. *Audiology, 13,* 335–341.

Friedman, T. B., Schultz, J. M., Ben Yosef, T., Pryor, S. P., Lagziel, A., Fisher, R. A., Wilcox, E. R., Riazuddin, S., Ahmed, Z. M., Belyantseva, I. A., & Griffith, A. J. (2003). Recent advances in the understanding of syndromic forms of hearing loss. *Ear and Hearing, 24,* 289–302.

Gabbard, S. A., & Schryer, J. (2003). Early amplification options. *Mental Retardation and Developmental Disabilities Research Review, 9,* 236–242.

Gates, G. A., & Miyamoto, R. T. (2003). Cochlear implants. *New England Journal of Medicine, 349,* 421–423.

Gregg, R. B., Wiorek, L. S., & Arvedson, J. C. (2004). Pediatric audiology: A review. *Pediatrics Reviews, 25,* 224–234.

Guillausseau, P. J., Massin, P., Dubois-LaForgue, D., Timsit, J., Virally, M., Gin, H., Bertin, E., Blickle, J. F., Bouhanick, B., Cohen, J., Caillet-Zucman, S., Charpentier, g., Chedin, P., Derrien, C., Ducluzeau, P. H., Grimaldi, A., Guerci, B., Kaloustian, E., Murat, A., Olivier, F., Paques, M., Paquis-Flucklinger, V., Porokhov, B., Samuel-Lajennesse, J., & Vialettes, B. (2001). Maternally inherited diabetes and deafness: A multicenter study. *Annals of Internal Medicine, 134,* 721–728.

Gurtler, N., & Lalwani, A. K. (2002). Etiology of syndromic and nonsyndromic sensorineural hearing loss. *Otolaryngology Clinics of North America, 35,* 891–908.

Hayes, D. (2003). Screening methods: Current status. *Otolaryngology Clinics of North America., 9,* 65–72.

Heath, P. T., Nik Yusoff, N. K., & Baker, C. J. (2003). Neonatal meningitis. *Archives of Disease in Childhood—Fetal and Neonatal Edition, 88,* F173–F178.

Hol, M. K., Bosman, A. J., Snik, A. F., Mylanus, E. A., & Cremers, C. W. (2004). Bone-anchored hearing aid in unilateral inner ear deafness: A study of 20 patients. *Audiology and Neurology, 9,* 274–281.

Hone, S. W., & Smith, R. J. (2001). Genetics of hearing impairment. *Seminars in Neonatology, 6,* 531–541.

Hone, S. W., & Smith, R. J. (2002). Medical evaluation of pediatric hearing loss. Laboratory, radiographic, and genetic testing. *Otolaryngology Clinics of North America, 35,* 751–764.

Hudson, B. G., Tryggvason, K., Sundaramoorthy, M., & Neilson, E. G. (2003). Alport's syndrome, Goodpasture's syndrome, and type IV collagen. *New England Journal of Medicine, 348,* 2543–2556.

Isaacson, J. E., & Vora, N. M. (2003). Differential diagnosis and treatment of hearing loss. *American Family Physician, 68,* 1125–1132.

Jerger, J. (1970). Clinical experience with impedance audiometry. *Archives of Otolaryngology, 92,* 311–324.

Jervell, A., & Lange-Nielsen, F. (1957). Congenital deaf-mutism, functional heart disease with prolongation of the Q-T interval and sudden death. *American Heart Journal, 54,* 59–68.

Johnson, K. C. (2002). Audiologic assessment of children with suspected hearing loss. *Otolaryngology Clinics of North America, 35,* 711–732.

Joint Committee on Infant Hearing, American Academy of Audiology, American Academy of Pediatrics, American Speech-Language-Hearing Association, and Directors of Speech and Hearing Programs in State Health and Welfare Agencies. (2000). Year 2000 position statement: Principles and guidelines for early hearing detection and intervention programs. *Pediatrics, 106,* 798–817.

Kazahaya, K., & Potsic, W. P. (2004). Congenital cholesteatoma. *Current Opinion in Otolaryngology Head and Neck Surgery, 12,* 398–403.

Keats, B. J., & Corey, D. P. (1999). The usher syndromes. *American Journal of Medical Genetics, 89,* 158–166.

Keats, B. J., & Savas, S. (2004). Genetic heterogeneity in Usher syndrome. *Americal Journal of Medical Genetics A, 130,* 13–16.

Kenna, M. A. (2004). Medical management of childhood hearing loss. *Pediatric Annals, 33,* 822–832.

Kim, S. Y., Bothwell, N. E., & Backous, D. D. (2002). The expanding role of the otolaryngologist in managing infants and children with hearing loss. *Otolaryngology Clinics of North America, 35,* 699–710.

Kopp, P. (2000). Pendred's syndrome and genetic defects in thyroid hormone synthesis. *Reviews in Endocrine and Metabolic Disorders, 1,* 109–121.

Kornblum, C., Broicher, R., Walther, E., Herberhold, S., Klockgether, T., Herberhold, C., & Schroder, R. (2005). Sensorineural hearing loss in patients with chronic progressive external ophthalmoplegia or Kearns-Sayre syndrome. *Journal of Neurology.*

Lee, M. P., Ravenel, J. D., Hu, R. J., Lustig, L. R., Tomaselli, G., Berger, R. D., Brandenburg, S. A., Litzi, T. J., Bunton, T. E., Limb, C., Francis, H., Gorelikow, M., Gu, H., Washington, K., Argani, P., Goldenring, J. R., Coffey, R. J., & Feinberg, A. P. (2000). Targeted disruption of the Kvlqt1 gene causes deafness and gastric hyperplasia in mice. *Journal of Clinical Investigation, 106,* 1447–1455.

Li, X. C., & Friedman, R. A. (2002). Nonsyndromic hereditary hearing loss. *Otolaryngology Clinics of North America, 35,* 275–285.

Liden, G. (1975). Application of tympanometry and acoustic reflex measurements. *Acta Otorhinolaryngologica Belgica, 29,* 802–813.

Liu, X. Z., Newton, V. E., & Read, A. P. (1995). Waardenburg syndrome type II: Phenotypic findings and diagnostic criteria. *American Journal of Medical Genetics, 55,* 95–100.

Lous, J., Burton, M. J., Felding, J. U., Ovesen, T., Rovers, M. M., & Williamson, I. (2005). Grommets (ventilation tubes) for hearing loss associated with otitis media with effusion in children. *Cochrane Database of Systematic Reviews,* CD001801.

Mafong, D. D., Shin, E. J., & Lalwani, A. K. (2002). Use of laboratory evaluation and radiologic imaging in the diagnostic evaluation of children with sensorineural hearing loss. *Laryngoscope, 112,* 1–7.

Maki-Torkko, E. M., Lindholm, P. K., Vayrynen, M. R., Leisti, J. T., & Sorri, M. J. (1998). Epidemiology of moderate to profound childhood hearing impairments in northern Finland. Any changes in ten years? *Scandinavian Audiology, 27,* 95–103.

Marsh, K. L., Dixon, J., & Dixon, M. J. (1998). Mutations in the Treacher Collins syndrome gene lead to mislocalization of the nucleolar protein treacle. *Human Molecular Genetic, 7,* 1795–1800.

Marszalek, B., Wojcicki, P., Kobus, K., & Trzeciak, W. H. (2002). Clinical features, treatment and genetic background of Treacher Collins syndrome. *Journal of Applied Genetic, 43,* 223–233.

McIntyre, P. B., Berkey, C. S., King, S. M., Schaad, U. B., Kilpi, T., Kanra, G. Y., & Perez, C. M. (1997). Dexamethasone as adjunctive therapy in bacterial meningitis. A meta-analysis of randomized clinical trials since 1988. *Journal of the American Medical Association, 278,* 925–931.

Melnick, M., Hodes, M. E., Nance, W. E., Yune, H., & Sweeney, A. (1978). Branchio-oto-renal dysplasia and branchio-oto dysplasia: Two distinct autosomal dominant disorders. *Clinical Genetics, 13,* 425–442.

Merchant, S. N., Burgess, B. J., Adams, J. C., Kashtan, C. E., Gregory, M. C., Santi, P. A., Colvin, R., Collins, B., & Nadof, J. B., Jr. (2004). Temporal bone histopathology in alport syndrome. *Laryngoscope, 114,* 1609–1618.

Mohri, I., Taniike, M., Fujimura, H., Matsuoka, T., Inui, K., Nagai, T., & Okada, S. (1998). A case of Kearns-Sayre syndrome showing a constant proportion of deleted mitochondrial DNA in blood cells during 6 years of follow-up. *Journal of the Neurologic Sciences, 158,* 106–109.

Nance, W. E. (2003). The genetics of deafness. *Mental Retardation and Developmental Disabilities Research Reviews, 9,* 109–119.

Nayak, C. S., & Isaacson, G. (2003). Worldwide distribution of Waardenburg syndrome. *Annals of Otology, Rhinology, and Laryngology, 112,* 817–820.

Newman, T. B., & Klebanoff, M. A. (1993). Neonatal hyperbilirubinemia and long-term outcome: Another look at the Collaborative Perinatal Project. *Pediatrics, 92,* 651–657.

Newton, V. (2001). Adverse perinatal conditions and the inner ear. *Seminars in Neonatology, 6,* 543–551.

Newton, V. E. (2002). Clinical features of the Waardenburg syndromes. *Advances in Otorhinolaryngology, 61,* 201–208.

Neyroud, N., Richard, P., Vignier, N., Donger, C., Denjoy, I., Demay, L., Shkolmikova, M., Pesce, R., Chevalier, P., Hainque, B., Coumel, P., Schwartz, K., & Guicheney, P. (1999). Genomic organization of the KCNQ1 K+ channel gene and identification of C-terminal mutations in the long-QT syndrome. *Circulation Research, 84,* 290–297.

Niparko, J. K., Cox, K. M., & Lustig, L. R. (2003). Comparison of the bone anchored hearing aid implantable hearing device with contralateral routing of offside signal amplification in the rehabilitation of unilateral deafness. *Otology and Neurotology, 24,* 73–78.

Nowak, C. B. (1998). Genetics and hearing loss: A review of Stickler syndrome. *Journal of Communication Disorders, 31,* 437–453.

Ocal, B., Imamoglu, A., Atalay, S., & Ercan, T. H. (1997). Prevalence of idiopathic long QT syndrome in children with congenital deafness. *Pediatric Cardiology, 18,* 401–405.

Ohlms, L. A., Chen, A. Y., Stewart, M. G., & Franklin, D. J. (1999). Establishing the etiology of childhood hearing loss. *Otolaryngology—Head and Neck Surgery, 120,* 159–163.

Okumura, T., Takahashi, H., Honjo, I., Takagi, A., & Mitamura, K. (1995). Sensorineural hearing loss in patients with large vestibular aqueduct. *Laryngoscope, 105,* 289–293.

Otitis media with effusion. (2004). *Pediatrics, 113,* 1412–1429.

Oysu, C., Oysu, A., Aslan, I., & Tinaz, M. (2001). Temporal bone imaging findings in Waardenburg's syndrome. *International Journal of Pediatric Otorhinolaryngology, 58,* 215–221.

Park, H. J., Shaukat, S., Liu, X. Z., Hahn, S. H., Naz, S., Ghosh, M., Kim, A. N., Moon, S. K., Abe, S., Tukamoto, K., Riazuddin, S., Kabra, M., Erdenetungalag, R., Radnaabazar, J., Khan, S., Pandya, A., Usami, S. I., Nance, W. E., Wilcox, E. R., Riazuddin, S., & Griffith, A. J. (2003). Origins and frequencies of SLC26A4 (PDS) mutations in east and south Asians: Global implications for the epidemiology of deafness. *Journal of Medical Genetics, 40,* 242–248.

Petit, C. (2001). Usher syndrome: from genetics to pathogenesis. *Annual Review of Genomics and Human Genetics, 2,* 271–297.

Phelps, P. D., Coffey, R. A., Trembath, R. C., Luxon, L. M., Grossman, A. B., Britton, K. E., et al. (1998). Radiological malformations of the ear in Pendred syndrome. *Clinical Radiology, 53,* 268–273.

Pletcher, S. D., & Cheung, S. W. (2003). Syphilis and otolaryngology. *Otolaryngology Clinics of North America, 36,* 595–605, vi.

Preciado, D. A., Lim, L. H., Cohen, A. P., Madden, C., Myer, D., Ngo, C., Bradshaw, J. K., Lawson, L., Choo, D. I., & Greinwald, J. H., Jr. (2004). A diagnostic paradigm for childhood idiopathic sensorineural hearing loss. *Otolaryngology Head and Neck Surgery, 131,* 804–809.

Raz, Y., & Lustig, L. (2002). Surgical management of conductive hearing loss in children. *Otolaryngologic Clinics of North America, 35,* 853–875.

Reardon, W., O'Mahoney, C. F., Trembath, R., Jan, H., & Phelps, P. D. (2000). Enlarged vestibular aqueduct: a radiological marker of pendred syndrome, and mutation of the PDS gene. *Quarterly Journal of Medicine, 93,* 99–104.

Rivas, A., & Francis, H. W. (2005). Inner ear abnormalities in a Kcnq1 (Kvlqt1) knockout mouse: A model of Jervell and Lange-Nielsen syndrome. *Otology Neurotology, 26,* 415–424.

Rivera, L. B., Boppana, S. B., Fowler, K. B., Britt, W. J., Stagno, S., & Pass, R. F. (2002). Predictors of hearing loss in children with symptomatic congenital cytomegalovirus infection. *Pediatrics, 110,* 762–767.

Rizk, D., & Chapman, A. B. (2003). Cystic and inherited kidney diseases. *American Journal of Kidney Disease, 42,* 1305–1317.

Roberts, J., Hunter, L., Gravel, J., Rosenfeld, R., Berman, S., Haggard, M., Hall, J., Lannon, C., Moore, D., Vernon-Feagaus, L., & Wallace, I. (2004). Otitis media, hearing loss, and language learning: controversies and current research. *Journal of Developmental and Behavioral Pediatrics, 25,* 110–122.

Roberts, J. E., Rosenfeld, R. M., & Zeisel, S. A. (2004). Otitis media and speech and language: A meta-analysis of prospective studies. *Pediatrics, 113,* e238–e248.

Robles, L., & Ruggero, M. A. (2001). Mechanics of the mammalian cochlea. *Physiological Reviews, 81,* 1305–1352.

Rodriguez, S. J. (2003). Branchio-oto-renal syndrome. *Journal of Nephrology, 16,* 603–605.

Roizen, N. J. (2003). Nongenetic causes of hearing loss. *Mental Retardation and Developmental Disabilities Research Review, 9,* 120–127.

Rosenfeld, R. M., & Kay, D. (2003). Natural history of untreated otitis media. *Laryngoscope, 113,* 1645–1657.

Schrijver, I. (2004). Hereditary non-syndromic sensorineural hearing loss: transforming silence to sound. *Journal of Molecular Diagnostics, 6,* 275–284.

Schroeder, A. A., & Kuhn, J. (2000). Imaging case of the month. Large vestibular aqueduct syndrome. *The American Journal of Otology, 21,* 433–434.

Shohet, J. A., & de Jong, A. L. (2002). The management of pediatric cholesteatoma. *Otolaryngologic Clinics of North America, 35,* 841–851.

Sininger, Y. S. (2003). Audiologic assessment in infants. *Current Opinion in Otolaryngology Head and Neck Surgery, 11,* 378–382.

Smith, R. J. (2004). Clinical application of genetic testing for deafness. *Americal Journal of Medical Genetics A, 130,* 8–12.

Smith, R. J., Bale, J. F., Jr., & White, K. R. (2005). Sensorineural hearing loss in children. *Lancet, 365,* 879–890.

Smith, R. J., & Schwartz, C. (1998). Branchio-oto-renal syndrome. *Journal of Communication Disorders, 31,* 411–420.

Stein, L. K. (1999). Factors influencing the efficacy of universal newborn hearing screening. *Pediatric Clinics of North America, 46,* 95–105.

Stickler, G. B., Hughes, W., & Houchin, P. (2001). Clinical features of hereditary progressive arthro-ophthalmopathy (Stickler syndrome): A survey. *Genetics in Medicine, 3,* 192–196.

Szymko-Bennett, Y. M., Mastroianni, M. A., Shotland, L. I., Davis, J., Ondrey, F. G., Balog, J. Z., et al. (2001). Auditory dysfunction in Stickler syndrome. *Archives of Otolaryngology Head and Neck Surgery, 127,* 1061–1068.

Tekin, M., Arnos, K. S., & Pandya, A. (2001). Advances in hereditary deafness. *Lancet, 358,* 1082–1090.

Tharpe, A. M., & Bess, F. H. (1999). Minimal, progressive, and fluctuating hearing losses in children. Characteristics, identification, and management. *Pediatric Clinics of North America, 46,* 65–78.

Thompson, D. C., McPhillips, H., Davis, R. L., Lieu, T. L., Homer, C. J., & Helfand, M. (2001). Universal newborn hearing screening: summary of evidence. *Journal of the American Medical Association, 286,* 2000–2010.

Tjellstrom, A., Hakansson, B., & Granstrom, G. (2001). Bone-anchored hearing aids: Current status in adults and children. *Otolaryngologic Clinics of North America, 34,* 337–364.

Tomaski, S. M., & Grundfast, K. M. (1999). A stepwise approach to the diagnosis and treatment of hereditary hearing loss. *Pediatrics Clinics of North America, 46,* 35–48.

Towbin, J. A., & Vatta, M. (2001). Molecular biology and the prolonged QT syndromes. *American Journal of Medicine, 110,* 385–398.

Tranebjaerg, L., Bathen, J., Tyson, J., & Bitner-Glindzicz, M. (1999). Jervell and Lange-Nielsen syndrome: A Norwegian perspective. *American Journal of Medical Genetics, 89,* 137–146.

Tunkel, A. R., & Scheld, W. M. (1993). Pathogenesis and pathophysiology of bacterial meningitis. *Clinical Microbiology Reviews, 6,* 118–136.

Valvasorri, G. E., & Clemins, J. D. (1978). The large vestibular aqueduct syndrome. *Laryngoscope, 88,* 723–728.

van Camp, G., & Smith, R. J. (2000). Maternally inherited hearing impairment. *Clinical Genetics, 57,* 409–414.

van de Bor, M., Ens-Dokkum, M., Schreuder, A. M., Veen, S., Brand, R., & Verloove-Vanhorick, S. P. (1992). Hyperbilirubinemia in low birth weight infants and outcome at 5 years of age. *Pediatrics, 89,* 359–364.

Van Naarden, K., Decoufle, P., & Caldwell, K. (1999). Prevalence and characteristics of children with serious hearing impairment in metropolitan Atlanta, 1991–1993. *Pediatrics, 103,* 570–575.

Vernon, M. (1969). Usher's syndrome—deafness and progressive blindness. Clinical cases, prevention, theory and literature survey. *Journal of Chronic Disease, 22,* 133–151.

Waardenburg, P. J. (1951). A new syndrome combining developmental anomalies of the eyelids, eyebrows and nose root with pigmentary defects of the iris and head hair and with congenital deafness. *Americal Journal of Human Genetics, 3,* 195–253.

Wallace, D. C. (1992). Diseases of the mitochondrial DNA. *Annual Review of Biochemistry, 61,* 1175–1212.

Walsh, R. M., Ayshford, C. A., Chavda, S. V., & Proops, D. W. (1999). Large vestibular aqueduct syndrome. *ORL Journal for Otorhinolaryngology and its Related Specialties, 61,* 41–44.

Wazen, J. J., Spitzer, J. B., Ghossaini, S. N., Fayad, J. N., Niparko, J. K., Cox, K., Brackmann, D. E., & Sofi, S. (2003). Transcranial contralateral cochlear stimulation in unilateral deafness. *Otolaryngology Head and Neck Surgery, 129,* 248–254.

Weingeist, T. A., Hermsen, V., Hanson, J. W., Bumsted, R. M., Weinstein, S. L., & Olin, W. H. (1982). Ocular and systemic manifestations of Stickler's syndrome: A preliminary report. *Birth Defects Original Article Series, 18,* 539–560.

Woods, C. R. (2005). Syphilis in children congenital and acquired. *Seminars in Pediatric Infectious Diseases, 16,* 245–257.

Year 2000 position statement: principles and guidelines for early hearing detection and intervention programs. Joint Committee on Infant Hearing American Academy of Audiology, American Academy of Pediatrics, American Speech-Language-Hearing Association, and Directors of Speech and Hearing Programs in State Health and Welfare Agencies (2000). *Pediatrics, 106,* 798–817. (No authors listed)

CHAPTER 6

Ototoxicity

Kathleen C. M. Campbell
Southern Illinois University School of Medicine

A number of compounds have been identified as ototoxic in the literature. The audiologist should be aware that simply because a drug is listed as ototoxic in the *Physician's Desk Reference* or in other materials, this does not necessarily mean that audiologic monitoring for ototoxicity is required. The degree or incidence of ototoxicity can vary widely across agents, and occasionally an agent may be listed as possibly ototoxic if there is only a suspicion of ototoxicity. Even among agents that are known to be ototoxic, the incidence of ototoxic hearing loss may be so low that formal ototoxicity monitoring may not be advised. In those cases the audiologist still needs to be aware that the drug may be ototoxic, so they can recognize it if a patient presents in the clinic after taking that particular medication.

CHEMOTHERAPEUTIC AGENTS

Chemotherapeutic agents constitute a major class of ototoxic medications. Unfortunately, the use of chemotherapy is typically restricted to situations of clinical exigency—usually malignant neoplastic disease—in which no other viable alternative exists. Chemotherapy, together with surgery and radiation therapy, is the primary method of almost all forms of cancer therapy.

The most ototoxic chemotherapeutic agent in common clinical use is cisplatin. Cisplatin was first approved by the Food and Drug Administration (FDA) in December 1978. Even though it has a relatively high incidence of permanent dose-related and cumulative cochlear toxicity, it continues to be used because it has excellent tumor kill properties for certain types of cancers and is sometimes the most effective option available. Other side effects include peripheral sensory and autonomic neuropathy and nephrotoxicity. Patients may also experience severe nausea and vomiting, although concomitant anti-emetic medications may help reduce this side effect. Cisplatin is used for a wide variety of cancers, including testicular, ovarian, head and neck, cervical, bladder, and lung tumors. The degree and incidence of ototoxicity vary according to the cumulative dose of cisplatin. Therefore, cancers that are generally discovered early and receive lower cumulative-dose cisplatin chemotherapy (e.g., testicular cancers) have a lower risk of ototoxicity, whereas cancers that are frequently discovered at relatively later stages (e.g., ovarian cancer) often require high-dose cisplatin chemotherapy, with a subsequently increased risk of ototoxicity.

Another platinum-based ototoxic chemotherapeutic drug is carboplatin. This drug is a second-generation platinum compound that was approved by the FDA in March 1989. Initially, carboplatin was thought to have little or no ototoxicity; however, because carboplatin is given at higher doses than cisplatin to reach therapeutic efficacy, ototoxicity can be seen in patients receiving carboplatin, particularly children. Depending on the dosing protocol, carboplatin-induced ototoxicity may occur, but with lower incidence and sometimes with a lesser degree of hearing loss than with cisplatin.

As for most ototoxic medications, hearing loss secondary to cisplatin and carboplatin treatment generally starts in the very high frequency range. If testing is conducted above 8,000 Hz, changes will first be observed in that region (Jacobson et al., 1969; Fausti et al., 1984a, 1984b; reviews by Campbell, 2004; Fausti et al., 2006). With continued use, the hearing loss will progress to lower frequencies until the hearing loss affects the frequencies from 250 Hz to 8,000 Hz, thus interfering with speech understanding. Tinnitus associated with cisplatin ototoxicity can be transient or permanent and is unpredictable. Tinnitus may precede or accompany the hearing loss. During the early stages of cisplatin-induced ototoxicity, the patient may only notice some difficulty in background noise or experience mild tinnitus and may ascribe these symptoms to the malaise accompanying chemotherapy or to the difficulties of dealing with a life-threatening illness. In cases of significant hearing loss, quality of life is further impaired during this challenging treatment period by the impaired ability to communicate.

In terms of cochlear histology, cisplatin-induced otoxicity first affects the outer hair cells in the basal turn, as consistent with clinical patterns of hearing loss. The damage then progresses into the middle or even apical turns with further drug administration (Schweitzer et al., 1984). In addition, the stria vascularis can be markedly affected (Meech et al., 1998; Campbell et al., 1999). Thus, with the combination of both strial and outer hair cell damage, hearing losses can range from mild to profound in degree. Similarly, carboplatin generally first affects the outer hair cells of the basal turn. The damage then progresses to the more apical turns. Selective inner hair cell loss has been found to occur in chinchilla models of ototoxicity (Wake et al., 1993), although these findings have not been found to extend to other animal models (Saito et al., 1989).

Cisplatin- and carboplatin-induced hearing loss is generally irreversible. It is very rare for a patient to recover hearing if hearing was lost secondary to either cisplatin or carboplatin treatment. Also, head- and neck-based tumors frequently require adjuvant radiation therapy, which can affect Eustachian tube function, thereby predisposing patients to the development of acute otitis media, which further compromises their ability to hear. Marked hearing loss can occur after the very first cycle of cisplatin treatment. Even if no threshold shift occurs after the first cycle of treatment, the patient may develop even profound hearing loss with continued platinum-based chemotherapy administration. Hearing loss is usually bilateral, and may be asymmetric at the high frequencies; in some cases, particularly for low dose regimens, hearing loss may be unilateral. Pediatric patients tend to be highly vulnerable to ototoxic threshold shift (Helson et al., 1978; Li et al., 2004).

It should be noted that although carboplatin- and cisplatin-induced hearing losses are related to cumulative dose, the relationship is not consistent. Intersubject variability is very high, and therefore prospective audiologic monitoring is essential. It is not unusual for two patients receiving the exact same dosing protocol to have widely different results on their hearing tests as treatment progresses. One patient receiving high-dose cisplatin chemotherapy may have no shift in hearing for the entire duration of therapy, while another patient on the exact same dosing protocol may have severe to profound hearing loss before the chemotherapy is completed. Much work remains to be done to determine the underlying causes of this intersubject variability. For patients receiving high-dose chemotherapy the incidence of permanent hearing loss affecting speech frequencies can exceed 50%, and hearing loss may continue to progress after the treatment is discontinued.

Cisplatin-induced hearing loss may be exacerbated by noise exposure or drug interactions, particularly with aminoglycoside antibiotics, or prior irradiation, particularly radiation to the head involving the cochlea. In some animal studies, loop diuretics exacerbated cisplatin-induced hearing loss, but we do not know yet whether that actually occurs at human therapeutic levels. Another factor is noise exposure. Most patients on ototoxic medications should avoid any noise exposure. All of these patients should be carefully counseled by the audiologist about protecting their hearing and wearing hearing protectors when they are around noise, not only during their treatment but for several months thereafter.

Other chemotherapeutic agents that can cause hearing loss include nitrogen mustard, difluoromethylornithine (DFMO), and vinca alkaloids (e.g., vincristine and vinblastine sulfate). Although nitrogen mustard is rarely used today in the United States, it is clearly associated with cochlear toxicity (Cummings, 1968). DFMO is a relatively new antineoplastic and antiparasitic drug. It is used primarily to treat colon cancer, although its areas of use are expanding (Ajani, 1990; Horn et al., 1987; O'Shaughnessy et al., 1999). It is also used to treat malignant melanomas, particularly metastatic recurrent malignant melanomas and metastatic liver disease, and as an adjuvant agent for brain cancers (Croghan et al., 1991; Levin et al., 2003). It is also used to treat African trypanosomiasis (sleeping sickness) and *Pneumocystis carinii* pneumonia in AIDS patients (Sjoerdsma et al., 1984; Legros et al., 2002; Sahai and Berry, 1989; see review by McAnn and Pegg, 1992). DFMO can cause transient or permanent dose-related ototoxicity. In many cases, DFMO patients are not referred prospectively for audiologic monitoring but are only referred once hearing loss has occurred. Therefore the audiologist may not have baseline information, which can render interpretation difficult. Because the hearing loss is frequently reversible, it is important that the audiologist recognize DFMO ototoxicity as soon as possible, because early identification may lead to treatment cessation or selection of another agent, with potential return of hearing. DFMO ototoxicity usually does not occur until the patient has had at least four weeks of treatment (Jansen et al., 1989; Lipton et al., 1989; Meyskens et al., 1994; Pasic et al., 1997). The hearing loss may progress from high to low frequencies (Horn et al., 1987; Creaven et al., 1993; Abeloff et al., 1986; Lipton et al., 1989), but flat hearing losses (Meyskens et al., 1986) and low-frequency hearing losses (Croghan et al., 1991; Pasic et al., 1997) have also been reported. If the drug is discontinued, hearing often recovers within about four to six weeks. (Meyskens et al., 1986; Croghan et al., 1988, 1991).

The vinca alkaloids are not strongly associated with hearing loss. Vincristine and vinblastine sulfate are chemotherapeutic agents frequently used in conjunction with other chemotherapeutic agents rather than as a single agent. Vinblastine can destroy hair cells in the organ of Corti, while leaving the spiral ganglion cells intact. There is only one reported case of ototoxicity, which was in 1999, which resulted in only mild high-frequency sensorineural hearing loss, although the patient had been reporting tinnitus after each treatment cycle (Moss et al., 1997). Unlike vinblastine, vincristine can affect not only the organ of Corti, but also the spiral ganglion cells. Reports of ototoxicity are also rare for vincristine, although the reports are more common than for vinblastine sulfate. The reports of ototoxicity secondary to vincristine are not typical for ototoxic hearing loss. Audiometric configuration ranges from relatively flat, moderate, bilateral sensorineural hearing loss with full recovery to sudden sensorineural hearing loss with only partial recovery. However, in prospective monitoring of larger groups of patients, ototoxicity generally has not been found to occur. Consequently, audiologic monitoring of these patients is usually not part of their care.

For a more thorough understanding of the ototoxicity of chemotherapeutic agents the reader is referred to "Cancer and Ototoxicity of Chemotherapeutics" by Rybak, Huang, and Campbell (2006).

AMINOGLYCOSIDES

Although aminoglycoside antibiotics have been recognized as ototoxic for decades, they remain very useful agents for the treatment of gram-negative bacterial infections. In the United States, close monitoring of peak and trough serum levels of aminoglycoside antibiotics has led to a decrease in both the degree and incidence of ototoxicity. Nevertheless, a recent study by Fausti et al. (1999) found that approximately one-third of patients in the Veterans Administration who received aminoglycoside antibiotics reached the ASHA 1994 criteria for significant ototoxic effects.

Aminoglycoside antibiotics cause hearing loss that generally starts in the high frequencies, especially those frequencies above 8000 Hz. Hearing loss progresses into the lower frequencies with continued drug administration. In some cases, aminoglycoside-associated ototoxicity is reversible. Additionally, aminoglycosides can be retained in the cochlea for several months after drug discontinuation. As a result, there may be a delayed onset of hearing loss or a progression in the hearing loss that has already occurred, requiring careful monitoring of these patients even after cessation of aminoglycoside therapy. Aminoglycoside ototoxicity can be exacerbated by noise exposure, concomitant administration of loop diuretics, and systemic illness, particularly when associated with renal failure, which leads to reduced clearance of the drug.

Several aminoglycosides are in clinical use in the United States. Each agent has an ototoxicity profile that is slightly different from the others. *Kanamycin* is one of the most ototoxic aminoglycosides, and it can cause complete deafness; however, it is rarely used systemically for any period of time, and is usually reserved for life-threatening infections or for very short-term application. *Amikacin* and *tobramycin* are also ototoxic and can cause hearing loss, but to a lesser degree than kanamycin. These agents exhibit greater cochleotoxicity rather than vestibulotoxicity. *Gentamicin* is more commonly vestibulotoxic than cochleotoxic, although it can affect both auditory and vestibular hair cells, as can most aminoglycosides. Gentamicin has recently come into clinical usage precisely because of its relatively selective vestibulotoxicity, as an intratympanic treatment agent applied to the round window, with the goal of destroying vestibular hair cells in patients with intractable vertigo from an otologic cause (such as Ménière's disease). *Netilmycin* is another aminoglycoside that is less commonly used in clinical practice, although it is also among the least ototoxic of the aminoglycoside antibiotics. *Neomycin* is another aminoglycoside antibiotic that is rarely used systemically because it is so highly ototoxic. Neomycin is used, however, in some ear drop formulations and could potentially cause hearing loss if the tympanic membrane is perforated and the neomycin ear drop reaches the round window. However, other non-ototoxic ear drop formulations, such as fluoroquinolone-based agents, are now becoming more commonly used.

The risk factors for aminoglycoside ototoxicity include the length of treatment, which can be quite long, since patients with serious infections, such as osteomyelitis, may stay on this medication for a period of several weeks. Other risk factors are concomitant use of other drugs, particularly loop diuretics, and possibly advanced age. One risk factor that is frequently difficult to ascertain is the use of previous aminoglycosides, which can predispose the patient to ototoxic hearing loss when more aminoglycosides are used at a subsequent date. As with other ototoxins, patients receiving aminoglycosides should avoid any noise exposure during, and for several months after, treatment.

As is the case for cisplatin, outer hair cells in the basal turn are first affected, with progression of hair cell loss toward the apical end of the cochlea with continued treatment. Inner hair cell loss can occur later. In severe cases, spiral ganglion cell loss can occur following inner hair cell loss, possibly due to a lack of synaptic transmission. Damage to the stria vascularis can also occur (see Schacht, 2007).

Two other non-aminoglycoside antibiotics may possibly cause hearing loss, but with a very low incidence. Erythromycin is not an aminoglycoside antibiotic, but rather a macrolide antibiotic. Erythromycin is a commonly used antibiotic and only very rarely causes hearing loss. Erythromycin-induced hearing loss may be sudden and severe in onset. Fortunately, if the cause of the hearing loss is recognized and the erythromycin is discontinued, hearing may recover in some cases. Vancomycin is a glycopeptide antibiotic, not an aminoglycoside antibiotic. It is sometimes used for severe or life-threatening infections. Its ototoxicity is debatable. Vancomycin is frequently used after the patient has received aminoglycoside antibiotics, which may be retained in the cochlea even while the vancomycin is later delivered. Consequently, if hearing loss occurs it is sometimes unclear whether the hearing loss is secondary to the aminoglycoside, the vancomycin, or the combination of the two drugs being present in the cochlea simultaneously. The incidence of vancomycin ototoxicity in isolation appears to be under 1% (Campbell et al., 2003).

LOOP DIURETICS

Loop diuretics, so named because of their effect on the glomerular loop of Henle of the kidney, induce a loss of free water, and are often used in cases of systemic fluid retention, such as in cases of congestive heart failure with subsequent pulmonary edema. These agents are not typically used as first-line diuretics for control of high blood pressure, even though they have antihypertensive properties as a result of their diuretic effects. The three most commonly used loop diuretics are furosemide (trade name Lasix), bumetanide (Bumex), and ethacrynic acid, which is seen less frequently in the United States.

In the adult patient population, loop diuretic-induced hearing loss is generally but not always reversible. Therefore, if the hearing loss is recognized as being secondary to the loop diuretic and the patient can be switched to a different diuretic, or temporarily stop treatment, the hearing may recover. The hearing loss secondary to loop diuretics can be more pronounced in either the middle or high frequencies, unlike cisplatin and aminoglycoside ototoxicity. Neonates may be at greater risk of permanent hearing loss from loop diuretics than adults. Bumetanide is a very potent diuretic, reported to be 40–60 times as great as furosemide. Because the diuresis of the bumetanide is so powerful, it is almost never used in neonates or young children. However, Fausti et al (1978) found no effect on 8,000- to 20,000-Hz thresholds for low-dose bumetanide treatment. As previously mentioned, the use of loop diuretics can greatly enhance the ototoxicity of aminoglycoside and possibly cisplatin if given concomitantly.

Both the stria vascularis and the outer hair cells can be affected by loop diuretics. In many animal studies, edema of the stria vascularis has been noted, with consequential changes in the endocochlear potential. The fact that loop diuretics primarily affect the stria vascularis may account for the variability in the audiometric configurations associated with this ototoxic agent (see review by Rybak, 2006).

Quinine is a drug that is rarely used in high doses in the United States. It has a history of causing severe ringing in the ears, vestibular disturbance, and hearing loss in patients using it as an antimalarial drug. However, in the United States, low-dose quinine dosing is sometimes used for leg cramps despite anecdotal reports of hearing loss, generally reversible, with low-dose quinine administration.

AUDIOLOGIC MONITORING

Audiologic monitoring for ototoxicity is an essential but sometimes challenging area of audiologic practice. Over the last few decades, the methodologies available to audiologists have greatly expanded (Campbell & Durrant, 1993; Campbell, 2004). Advances in high-frequency audiologic testing, otoacoustic emission detection, and auditory brainstem response testing have made ototoxicity monitoring possible in almost every patient. There are many difficulties inherent in monitoring for ototoxicity. Even experienced audiologists may require extra time for these patients, and yet rapid data collection is often required because of the poor medical condition of these patients, who may in addition be inattentive or difficult to transport physically. Bedside testing (e.g., in the intensive care unit) may be difficult because of acoustic and electrical noise, both of which complicate data interpretation. Baseline data, which are normally critical for accurate interpretation, are not always available. Both infectious disease patients and chemotherapy patients may be prone to otitis media, which can mask ototoxicity-induced sensorineural hearing loss. For these reasons, interpretation is not always initially straightforward.

In cases of patients exposed to ototoxic drugs, the audiologist may be able to make a critical difference for the patient and his or her family. This goal may be achieved in a number of ways. With prospective audiologic monitoring, the audiologist can work with the patient's physician and notify the physician when the patient may be showing early changes indicative of ototoxic hearing loss. In that case, the physician has the option of looking at possible alternative drug regimens for that particular patient, thus possibly preserving hearing function. In other cases, the audiologist may be told in advance that the drug regimen for this particular patient may not be changed for medical reasons; in these difficult cases, the audiologist may also be of great help to the patient and their family by monitoring the hearing loss as it develops, counseling the patient and family about how to alter the environment, such as reducing background noise as hearing loss develops and in providing amplification if needed or other communication strategies to maintain communication. It should be kept in mind that communication is largely dependent upon the ability to hear, and that the ability to communicate is extremely important during the last days of a terminal illness, for both the patient and family, many who may only have access to the patient through telephone. Monitoring for ototoxicity therefore has a potentially critical impact on a patient's quality of life.

Audiologists also need to become skilled collaborators on clinical trials for new drugs being developed through the FDA. In some cases ototoxicity monitoring is essential to determine if a new agent being developed is ototoxic. Audiologists can play a role in working with the drug companies in ensuring that the procedure is used and these clinical trials are appropriate and accurate for the study drug, whether that includes cochleotoxicity monitoring or vestibulotoxicity monitoring or both. Second, as new otoprotective agents are developed, the ototoxicity monitoring is critical in assessing whether the new drug significantly protects hearing or whether the changes observed in patient populations could be attributed to random variability. Therefore, audiologists must competently partner in these clinical trials. Even if the audiologist is clinically based and not research based, he or she will hopefully be able to collaborate with these research teams to ensure that the correct methods are selected and carried out appropriately.

Even audiologists that do not foresee prospective ototoxicity monitoring as a part of their usual clinical practice because they are not in a hospital setting, are not seeing patients on ototoxic medications, or are not involved in clinical trials of new medications of any sort, need to be aware of ototoxic medications. Virtually all audiologists at some point in time will see a patient that has had an ototoxic change in their hearing at some point, whether they recognize it or not. The audiologist may see the patient even many years after thy have had an ototoxic change in their hearing and the audiologist will need to know the implications of that drug regimen on their hearing, or they may see a patient that has had aminoglycoside many months ago and is now experiencing a change. Both the audiologist and the patient need to be aware that the change currently occurring may be related to prior drug therapy. Another reason that audiologists need to be fully aware of ototoxicity monitoring and ototoxic drugs is that many patients self administer medications and even over the counter drugs, such as aspirin, can be ototoxic at high does or in certain persons. Again, intersubject variability is very high for most ototoxic drugs. Therefore, if an audiologist sees a patient that has had a change in hearing, it is important to ask the patient about which medications, both prescription and over-the-counter, they are taking.

Monitoring Schedules for Ototoxicity

For prospective audiologic monitoring, one of the first decisions the audiologist must make is what monitoring schedule for ototoxicity will be followed. The audiologist should not simply rely on a physician referral for each visit, even if the insurance or other third-party payer does require a physician referral in each case. Rather, the audiologist should actively work with the physician and the nurse in prospectively setting up a schedule in conjunction with the patient.

The ototoxicity monitoring schedule will vary with the type of drug used. For cisplatin or carboplatin, usually audiologic testing will take place at baseline and then just before the next round of these two agents, whether given singly, in combination, or alternately. Usually these drugs are given once every three to four weeks. It is best to schedule the patient before they are even connected to the IV for drug delivery, as it makes examination more convenient and patients typically feel better at this stage of treatment. Other antineoplastic drugs, such as nitrogen mustard, vincristine, and vinblastine, are not generally prospectively monitored. For some other antineoplastic drugs there is actually some question as to whether or not they are actually ototoxic or whether the occasional hearing loss observed in those patients may be related to other factors.

Aminoglycoside antibiotics are generally only monitored when the patient is going to be on them for an extended period of time, such as the several week-long regimen required for the treatment of osteomyelitis. Testing is not generally performed if patients are only given an aminoglycoside antibiotic prophylactically for 24 hours to prevent a post-surgical complication or post-surgical infection. Drugs such as amikacin, gentamicin, and tobramycin are usually monitored once or twice per week. There is no clear relationship between the dosing level of the aminoglycoside and the degree of ototoxicity. Consequently there is not a truly safe level for these patients and it is difficult to modify the ototoxicity monitoring schedule according to dosing. The audiologist may need to work with the physicians to advise them that even when dosing is within the recommended peak and trough levels for the aminoglycoside antibiotic that ototoxicity can still occur and ototoxicity monitoring is still essential. Prospective audiologic monitoring for aminoglycoside ototoxicity will generally be scheduled to monitor amikacin, tobramycin, and gentamicin administration. Neomycin is almost never given systemically, and therefore does not need to be included in most ototoxicity monitoring protocols. Kanamycin is rarely given systemically, but when it is, severe ototoxicity can result. Patients will generally have a life threatening illness before kanamycin is used; consequently ototoxicity monitoring may be difficult to schedule. Other antibiotics, such as the macrolide erythromycin and the glycopeptide vancomycin, cause hearing loss so rarely relative to the number of patients taking it that prospective monitoring is not recommended.

Follow-up testing should be scheduled for patients on aminoglycoside antibiotics and the antineoplastic drugs cisplatin and carboplatin because late onset or progression of ototoxic hearing loss may occur. For both aminoglycoside antibiotics and the antineoplastic drugs cisplatin/carboplatin, the patient should always be advised at the time of each monitoring appointment to avoid noise exposure, and to wear earplugs when around noise when it is unavoidable. Hearing protection and noise reduction is critical for these patients, not only during treatment, but for several months thereafter.

For other classes of agents, such as loop diuretics, ototoxicity monitoring is generally not scheduled. The audiologist merely needs to be aware that if a patient on a loop diuretic does experience a hearing loss that the loop diuretic may be a factor. Hopefully the patient is not taking loop diuretics in combination with aminoglycoside drugs or in conjunction with platinum based chemotherapeutic drugs, because a synergistic reaction causing ototoxicity may occur. However, sometimes these combinations are unavoidable in the case of a life-threatening illness.

Patients taking salicylates generally take a low dose. Therefore, salicylates will not typically cause hearing loss unless the patient is self-administering a very high dose, or in the rare case in which a physician will recommend a very high dose as an anti-inflammatory agent. However prospective hearing monitoring will probably not be scheduled for those patients and usually, as with loop diuretics, if hearing loss occurs and the drug is discontinued, hearing will probably return to normal levels.

In the United States, audiologists will not commonly see patients treated with anti-malarial dosages of quinine. However, they may see patients from other countries showing the later effects of this treatment. It is possible that low-dose quinine generally used to treat leg cramps may cause ototoxic hearing loss, which may be reversible. However, monitoring is not typically scheduled in these cases.

Although there are no formal procedures for monitoring tinnitus in patients receiving ototoxic medications, the audiologist should ask the patient at each visit whether or not tinnitus has developed. There is some evidence that tinnitus sometime occurs before hearing threshold shift changes in cases of ototoxicity. Further, it will be an issue in patient management, because tinnitus can become very troublesome for these patients. However, formal assessment techniques for the tinnitus may or may not prove helpful to these patients, and frequently these patients are so ill that extended test protocols, such tinnitus matching, are difficult for them.

Currently, there are no broadly accepted guidelines for formally monitoring vestibular ototoxicity, and therefore there is also no recommended schedule for vestibulotoxicity monitoring, but the audiologist should certainly question patients about changes in balance when they see them for ototoxicity monitoring. Vestibulotoxicity appears to be very rare in cases of cisplatin or carboplatin, but may be more frequent with some of the aminoglycoside agents such as gentamicin.

Patients' families should be included in discussions of ototoxicity and monitoring whenever possible. Many times, when early ototoxic hearing loss begins, the patient may not recognize it as ototoxic hearing loss or a change in hearing, or their family may need to better understand the implications of high-frequency hearing loss. Without prospective audiologic monitoring, the onset of high frequency hearing loss, typical of ototoxic change, is often misinterpreted by the patient and their family as the patient simply being very distracted, not feeling well, being unable to concentrate, or other factors. In these seriously ill patients, these issues are often relevant factors, but hearing loss can greatly exacerbate the difficulties they present. Patients' families may feel ignored because the patients do not respond to them as they formerly had. In fact, the onset of a high-frequency hearing loss may underlie all of these difficulties in communication or certainly exacerbate them. Family members need to understand how to alter their communication patterns and the communication environment to help the patient experiencing ototoxic hearing loss along with the high stress of a serious medical condition. These issues can only be addressed if the family members are frequently present. For patients that are otherwise healthy, they may or may not be able to take information from the audiologist and carry it home to their family. In patients that are already seriously ill and perhaps overwhelmed with the life events they are currently dealing with, it may not be possible for them to retain information on communication strategies, assistive devices, amplification or other factors. Therefore, scheduling the patient's family in for some of these counseling sessions, particularly if hearing loss does occur, may greatly improve the patient's care.

As previously mentioned, baseline hearing testing is essential for proper ototoxicity monitoring. Given that hearing loss is common in our society as a whole, trying to determine if a hearing loss seen after a week with a treatment with an ototoxic drug is secondary to the drug or to a preexistent hearing loss is frequently impossible. Consequently, audiologists need to prospectively work with physicians to ensure that patients scheduled to receive the major ototoxic drugs are sent for baseline evaluations. In platinum based chemotherapy, a base line assessment should always be possible, as chemotherapy treatment typically begins well after the date of diagnosis. In the case of life-threatening infections, aminoglycoside antibiotics may be initiated immediately after the patient has been admitted to the hospital; prompt evaluation of hearing within a few days of treatment should allow for the acquisition of a reasonable baseline hearing test. The baseline evaluation may be more comprehensive than the follow up monitoring evaluations, simply so that a thorough profile of audiologic information is available for later comparison if an ototoxic change is noted. For example, the basic battery at baseline should include pure tone air conduction testing for the conventional frequency range of 250 Hz through 8,000 Hz. High-frequency audiometry up through 16,000 to 20,000 Hz is highly recommended if the patient has sufficient hearing to be monitored in those frequencies. High frequency audiometry may not be necessary if the audiologist knows in advance if that even if ototoxic change occurs, the medication protocol cannot be safely altered. In those cases, high frequency audiometry, which provides an early warning of ototoxic changes, may not alter the drug protocol and the patient management. In those cases the audiologist and the patient need to carefully consider whether an early warning will help the patient prepare for the eventual onset of hearing loss or whether it will only serve to increase the difficulties faced by the patient at that point. A baseline evaluation should also include bone conduction testing unless hearing is perfectly normal, because a conductive component, if present, could be addressed prior to treatment, and both the audiologist and patient should be aware that it may cause later fluctuation of hearing unrelated to ototoxic medication. It may also be helpful to know if there is a middle ear disorder or conductive hearing loss that could be addressed medically and perhaps resolved to improve the patient's hearing prior to treatment. Speech reception thresholds and word recognition are also essential at the baseline evaluation so if changes occur later, the patient and audiologist have a reference for where the patient was at the start, and how much of a change has occurred, not only in pure tone thresholds but in the patient's word recognition ability, as a result of the medication. Otoacoustic emissions may also prove valuable, particularly for pediatric patients.

For word recognition measures, the fifty word list should be employed and interpreted according to Thornton and Raffin (1977). Because these patients are often ill, audiologists may be tempted to use the 25-word list; however, this renders later interpretation of any significant change problematic and should be avoided. After the baseline evaluation, the follow-up assessment will generally consist of pure tone air conduction threshold testing, including high frequency audiometry. Otoacoustic emissions may also be useful in follow-up, as part of a test battery.

Over the years a number of significant change criteria have been suggested for determining ototoxic change. The most commonly used and the most widely validated criteria to determine ototoxic threshold shift were established in 1994 by the American Speech-Language Hearing Association. The criteria employed state that significant ototoxic change must meet one of the follow three criteria: 1) a threshold shift of 20 dB or greater at any one test frequency 2) threshold shifts of 10 dB or greater at any two adjacent frequencies or 3) loss of response at three consecutive frequencies where responses were previously obtained. The third criteria will usually be met only when at baseline thresholds were close to the limits of the audiometric test equipment. Changes are always interpreted relative to baseline measures, not just to the previous ototoxicity monitoring appointment of that patient. Also, if a change occurs, threshold measures must be reconfirmed within 24 hours to ensure it is an actual change and not simply random variability, particularly in the case of a very ill patient. It has been demonstrated in many studies that these criteria are quite sensitive to ototoxic change, and yet do not over identify patients (Frank, 2001; Fausti et al., 1999; Campbell et al., 2003a). Occasionally audiologists can be too aggressive in either identifying the number of agents to be prospectively monitored or in reporting ototoxic change or minimal threshold shifts, which will ultimately decrease the compliance of patients and physicians with ototoxicity monitoring protocols, because it will result in too many false positives. It should be noted that these criteria, as established by Campbell et al. (2003a), also work very well for determining ototoxic change for high frequency audiometry.

HIGH-FREQUENCY AUDIOMETRY:

High-frequency audiometry, sometimes called ultra-high-frequency audiometry, comprises air conduction two-tone threshold testing for the frequencies above 8,000 Hz. Special testing in this extended high frequency range occurs between 10,000 Hz and 20,000 Hz. Because most aminoglycoside- or cisplatin-induced hearing loss starts at the ultra high frequency range (Fee, 1980; Wright and Schaeffer, 1982; Schuknecht, 1993) this procedure allows early detection of ototoxic change (Jacobson et al., 1969; Fausti et al., 1984a, 1984b, 1992c; Rappaport et al., 1985; Tange et al., 1985; Kopelman et al., 1988). High-frequency audiometry was first studied several decades ago (Fletcher, 1929, 1965; Rosen et al., 1964; Zilis and Fletcher, 1966). However, initial problems with equipment and calibration limited its application. High-frequency audiometry has now been well documented as an effective test method over the last three decades and now should be standard procedure for most ototoxicity monitoring, particularly in adults, although it can be used with older children. Most patients that can cooperate with pure tone air conduction testing in the conventional frequency range can also cooperate with high frequency thresholds if they can tolerate the longer test period required for the additional frequencies. Some patients may not be eligible for high-frequency audiometry, simply because they do not have adequate hearing in the frequency range above 10,000 Hz. This deficit may be particularly common in older patients (Stelmachowizc et al., 1989; Wiley et al., 1998).

In early years, high-frequency audiometry was limited in its applications because of clinical equipment availability. However, now commercially available equipment is readily available and is also available on many standard audiometers as long as the additional high frequency earphones are also obtained. Calibration procedures have also now been standardized and are available for clinical use. In the early versions of high frequency transducers, small changes in placement techniques could yield significant changes in thresholds. But numerous investigators worked to largely resolve these issues (Fausti et al., 1979; Stelmachowizc et al., 1982; Tonndorf and Kurman, 1984; Northern and Ratkiewicz, 1985; Valente et al., 1992b). However, the new standardized clinical procedures and commercially variable equipment have significantly reduced that concern and the replicability of high frequency thresholds above 10,000 Hz are very similar to those below 8,000 Hz using the commercially available equipment.

Initially, concerns were expressed that high intersubject variability precluded the ability to establish an HL reference (Northern and Ratkiewicz, 1985). Even among patients with normal hearing thresholds in the 250–8,000 Hz range, hearing thresholds above 10,000 Hz may vary widely from subject to subject. This intersubject variability is not a problem for monitoring ototoxicity in these patients, because the audiologist uses the patient as his or her own reference over time using a serial monitoring protocol. With current commercially available equipment and standardized clinical procedures, intrasubject variability over time for high frequency audiometry is no greater than for testing in the conventional frequency range (Fausti et al., 1985; Dreschler et al., 1985; Feghali and Bernstein, 1991; Frank and Dreisbach, 1991; Frank, 1990, 2001; Campbell et al., 2003a). High-frequency audiometry can be conducted in a quiet hospital room (Valente et al. 1992a) although testing in the sound booth is recommended, whenever possible. Because some patients on ototoxic medications are so ill that they have trouble attending for a long period of time, some investigators have been developing abbreviated high frequency monitoring protocols using a restricted frequency range (Dreschler et al. 1989, Fausti et al. 1992 a, b, 1999). Another approach has been to use high-frequency auditory brainstem response thresholds to monitor ototoxicity (Fausti et al., 1992a,b, 2003), but these procedures are not in widespread clinical use.

OTOACOUSTIC EMISSIONS

Although not routinely used for ototoxicity monitoring in most clinics, otoacoustic emissions can certainly play a role in monitoring ototoxic changes, particularly in children. Otoacoustic emissions can quickly provide individualized ear information for pediatric test populations for outer hair cell function, which is usually a target of most ototoxic medications. For ototoxicity monitoring, otoacoustic emissions of interest are generally transient otoacoustic emissions and distortion product otoacoustic emissions. Spontaneous otoacoustic emissions and sustained frequency otoacoustic emissions are generally not used. Distortion product otoacoustic emissions are preferable because they provide greater frequency specificity across a wider frequency range. In addition, they are more sensitive to changes in the high frequency regions that are usually targeted by most ototoxic medications than transient otoacoustic emissions. Another advantage of distortion product otoacoustic emissions is that they can be present, depending on the stimulation protocol, even for patients with moderate hearing loss (Wier et al., 1988; Norton, 1992; Probst et al., 1991), while transient otoacoustic emissions generally are not present if the hearing threshold at a given frequency exceeds 30 dB HL. Nonetheless, both transient otoacoustic emissions (Plinkert and Kröber, 1991; Beck et al., 1992; Zorowka et al., 1993; Stavroulaki et al., 1999), and distortion product otoacoustic emissions (Muhleran and Degg, 1997; Ress et al., 1999; Lonsbury-Martin and Martin, 2001) are affected prior to hearing threshold changes in patients receiving most ototoxic medications. Distortion product otoacoustic emissions do appear to provide an earlier indication of injury than transient otoacoustic emissions (Lonsbury-Martin and Martin, 2001), but further research is needed.

The two greatest disadvantages of otoacoustic emission testing for ototoxicity monitoring are: 1) that there is no widely accepted standard for determining significant change while maintaining both sensitivity and specificity of the measures and 2) that OAEs can not be recorded in the presence of otitis media (Allen et al., 1998). As for all otoacoustic emission testing, patients with otitis media may not yield reliable results for the otoacoustic emissions measure or may yield no results (Owens et al., 1992). Nonetheless, otoacoustic emissions can be a valuable tool particularly for the pediatric patient or other patient that cannot cooperate with or complete behavioral test measures. Distortion product otoacoustic commissions can also provide an indication of the degree and configuration of hearing loss in those patients (Lonsbury-Martin and Martin, 1990; Martin et al., 1990). Hopefully, criteria for evaluation of otoacoustic omissions in ototoxicity monitoring will be firmly established in the future. Several criteria have been defined and proposed (Katbamna et al., 1999; Lonsbury-Martin and Martin, 2001), but these proposals require validation on larger patient populations.

PEDIATRIC TESTING

Increasingly, children are being referred for ototoxic monitoring. Audiologists can play an important role in evaluating the impact of hearing loss in children, which is critical not only for maintaining day to day communication but also for the proper development of vocabulary and language skills. Children that cannot communicate with their parents during a life-threatening illness may feel particularly isolated, and may not be able to articulate the extent of their hearing impairment to the parent or physician. As audiologists well know, children with hearing loss tend to have more behavioral problems that, coupled with a malignant brain tumor and the malaise accompanying chemotherapy, may seriously reduce the quality of life for that child and family. Therefore, it is the responsibility of each audiologist to communicate with their pediatric oncologist about the need for monitoring in these children.

A wide variety of test regimens are needed to evaluate children in this setting. Speed may be crucial in testing children because their attention span can be very limited. It is critical to obtain a relatively comprehensive baseline evaluation. For example, the audiologist may wish to always include otoacoustic emissions in the base line evaluation of children, even if the patient (at the time of initial evaluation) can cooperate with pure tone audiometry. If the child later becomes too ill or uncooperative, then otoacoustic emissions may be the only method available for monitoring that child's cochlear function. In addition, children are very prone to otitis media, and having the behavioral data available both in the conventional frequency range and in the high frequency range for pure tone air conduction thresholds may be critical because otoacoustic emissions may not obtainable in the future, if otitis media is present. Auditory brainstem response testing of children has been used and, as previously mentioned, high frequency auditory brainstem response testing is being investigated. However, because auditory brainstem response testing is relatively time consuming and may require sedation, using the ABR as a primary means of ototoxicity monitoring is probably not advisable for most patients. Given the frequently unpredictable behavior of children, flexible scheduling is a necessary accommodation for children with possible ototoxicity due to medication.

OTOTOXICITY TESTING FOR NEW DRUGS AND DEVELOPMENT

New drugs are constantly being developed. It is incumbent on us as a profession to develop guidelines for determination of ototoxicity in clinical trials and to actively collaborate in clinical trials when possible. By doing so, the audiologist may play a role in the development of new otoprotective agents or rescue agents to prevent permanent hearing loss from aminoglycoside otoxicity, chemotherapy based ototoxicity or noise induced hearing loss. At this time the FDA has not developed specific clinical practice guidelines specifically for monitoring ototoxicity during clinical trials. However, in my experience with a number of clinical trials, there are certain procedures that generally seem to be acceptable for FDA conducted trials. For example, Campbell et al. (2003a) reported a Phase I clinical trial for Dalbavancin, which is a glycopeptide antibiotic that was monitored both for possible cochleotoxicity and vestibulotoxicity throughout the phase I clinical trials. All audiologic methods were submitted to the FDA in advance of the clinical trials, as were the methods of data collection and analysis. The methods used in that study included air conduction testing in both the conventional (250–8,000 Hz) ranges as well as the high frequency ranges above 8,000 Hz. Bone conduction testing was included if the hearing was other than normal as indicated by air conduction thresholds for the conventional frequency range. Tympanometry and 50 word list/word recognition measures were also performed at baseline in case a subsequent ototoxic change was noted. Therefore all these measures would be later available for a comparison. We also designed patient inclusion and exclusion criteria and replicability criteria that were very stringent to avoid false positive and false negative findings. For vestibular assessment, prospective patient evaluation and formal balance testing was not employed; instead, the dizziness handicap inventory was used to monitor for possible vestibulotoxicity (other agents may require formal vestibular testing for evaluation of vestibulotoxicity). These methods then formed the basis of ototoxicity monitoring throughout Phase I for this particular agent. Such studies may serve as a model to assist others in developing clinical trial guidelines for ototoxicity evaluation.

ENVIRONMENTAL CHEMICALS

Although prospective ototoxicity monitoring will generally only occur for the patient receiving medications that are known to be ototoxic, audiologists should be aware that certain environmental chemicals can either enhance noise induced hearing loss or be ototoxic even in the absence of noise exposure. Exposure can occur in industrial environments, by deliberate exposure (e.g., glue sniffing) or by home improvement projects where adequate ventilation is not used in the presence of solvents or chemicals. A wide variety of chemicals can cause hearing loss, including organic solvents, asphyxiants, gases and heavy metals. These chemicals can affect both the auditory and vestibular system (Rybak, 1992; Morioka et al., 1999; Sulkowski et al., 2002). In some cases, workers may be monitored for noise exposure through the industrial Hearing Screening Programs, but the supervising audiologist should also inform the employer of the possibility of a synergistic relationship with chemicals in the environment. Sudden hearing loss may develop after exposure to chemicals, such as paint thinner; certain chemicals (eg. toluene) can be absorbed directly through the skin.

FUTURE DIRECTIONS

One of the most promising areas in ototoxicity research is the development of new otoprotective agents. In animal studies, a variety of new drugs have been developed that can prevent or significantly reduce cisplatin-induced, carboplatin-induced, aminoglycoside-induced, and noise-induced hearing loss. Some of these agents can even be delivered shortly after the ototoxic event and still provide protection from permanent hearing loss. Some drugs are currently in clinical trials and others should be in clinical trials within a few years. It is hoped that, within the next 5 to 10 years, there will be several FDA-approved drugs available to prevent or treat ototoxic and noise induced hearing loss. For example, one of the drugs that I have been researching in my lab for over 10 years, D-methionine can protect against cisplatin-induced, carboplatin-induced, aminoglycoside-induced, and noise-induced hearing loss, at least in animal studies (Campbell et al., 1996, 1999; Kopke et al., 1997; Sha and Schacht, 2000; Kopke et al., 2002; Campbell et al., 2003b). It is not yet known whether these drugs will be safe enough to routinely administer on a prophylactic basis, or whether they will only be used once hearing loss is manifest. It is sincerely hoped that through the development of new drugs and new methods for ototoxicity monitoring, the incidence of ototoxic hearing loss can be greatly reduced within the next decade.

REFERENCES

Abeloff, M. D., Rosen, S. T., Luk, G. D., Baylin, S. B., Zeltzman, M., & Sjoerdsma, Al. (1986). Phase II trials of alpha-diflumethylornithine, an inhibitor of polyamine synthesis in advanced small cell lung cancer. *Cancer Treatment Reports 70,* 843–845.

Ajani, J. A., Ota, D. M., Grossie, V. B., Jr., Abbruzzese, J. L., Faintuch, J. S., Patt, Y. Z., Jackson D. E., Levin, B., & Nishioka, K. (1990). Evaluation of continuous-infusion alpha-difluoromethylornithine therapy for colorectal carcinoma. *Cancer Chemother. Pharmacol., 26*(3), 223–226.

Allen, G. C., Tiu, C., Koike, K., Ritchy, A. K., Kurs-Lasky, M., & Wax, M. K. (1998). Transient-evoked otoacoustic emissions in children after cisplatin chemotherapy. *Otolaryngol. Head Neck Surg., 118*(5), 584–588.

American Speech-Language-Hearing Association. (1994). Guidelines for the audiologic management of individuals receiving cochleotoxic drug therapy. *ASHA, 36*(Suppl. 12), 11–19.

Beck, A., Maurer, J., Welkoborsky, H. J., & Mann, W. (1992). Changes in transitory evoked otoacoustic emissions in chemotherapy and with cisplatin and 5FU. *HNO, 40*(4), 123–127.

Campbell, K. C. M. (2004). Audiologic monitoring for ototoxicity. In P. Roland & J. Rutka (Eds.), *Ototoxicity* (pp. 153–160). Lewiston, NY: BC Decker.

Campbell, K. C. M., & Durrant, J. D. (1993). Audiologic monitoring for ototoxicity. *Otolaryngologic Clinics of North America, 26,* 903–914.

Campbell, K. C. M., Kelly, E., Targovnik, N., Hughes, L. F., Van Saders, C., Gottleib, A. B., et al. (2003a). Audiologic monitoring for potential ototoxicity in a phase I clinical trial of a new glycopeptide antibiotic. *Journal of the American Academy of Audiology: Special Edition on Ototoxicity, 14*(3), 157–169.

Campbell, K. C. M., Meech, R. P., Rybak, L. P., & Hughes, L. F. (2003b). The effect of D-methionine on cochlear oxidative state with and without cisplatin administration: Mechanisms of otoprotection. *Journal of the American Academy of Audiology: Special Edition on Ototoxicity, 14*(3), 144–156.

Campbell, K. C. M., Meech, R. P., Rybak, L. P., & Hughes, L. P. (1999). D-Methionine protects against cisplatin damage to the stria vascularis. *Hearing Research, 138,* 13–28.

Campbell, K. C., & Rybak, L. P. (2007). Otoprotective agents. In K. Campbell (Ed.), *Pharmacology and ototoxicity for audiologists* (pp. 287–296). Clifton Park, NY: Thomson Delmar Learning.

Campbell, K. C. M., Rybak, L. P., Meech, R. P., & Hughes, L. (1996). D-Methionine provides excellent protection from cisplatin ototoxicity in the rat. *Hearing Research, 102,* 90–98.

Creaven, P. J., Pendyala, L., and Petrelli, N. J. (1993). Evalution of alpha-difluoromethylornithine as a potential chemopreventive agent: Tolerance to daily oral administration in humans. *Cancer Epidemiology Biomarkers & Prevention, 2,* 243–247.

Croghan, M. K., Aickin, M. G., & Meyskens, F. L. (1991). Dose-related alpha-difluoromethylornithine ototoxicity. *Am. J. Clin. Oncol. (CCT), 14,* 331–335.

Croghan, M. K., Booth, A., & Meyskens, F. L., Jr. (1988). A phase I trial recombinant interferon-alpha and alpha-difluoromethylornithine in metastatic melanoma. *J. Boil Response Mod., 7*(4), 409–415.

Cummings, C. W. (1968). Experimental observations on the ototoxicity of nitrogen mustard. *Laryngoscope, 78*(4), 530–538.

Dreschler, W. A., van der Hulst, R. J., Tange, R. A., and Urbanus, N. A. (1985). The role of high frequency audiometry in early detection of ototoxicity. *Audiology, 24*(6), 387–395.

Dreschler, W. A., van der Hulst, R. J., Tange, R. A., and Urbanus, N. A. (1989). Role of high frequency audiometry in the early detection of ototoxicity. II. Clinical aspects. *Audiology, 28*(4), 211–220.

Fausti, S. A., Flick, C. L., Bobal, A. M., Ellingson, R. M., Henry, J. A., & Mitchell, C. R. (2003). Comparison of ABR stimuli for the early detection of ototoxicity: Conventional clicks compared with high frequency clicks and single frequency tonebursts. *Journal of the American Academy of Audiology, 14*(5), 239–250.

Fausti, S. A., Frey, R. H., Erickson, D. A., Rappaport, B. Z., & Cleary, E. J. (1979). A system for evaluating auditory function from 8000–20,000 Hz. *J. Acoust. Soc. of Am., 66*, 1713–1718.

Fausti, S. A., Frey, R. H., Henry, J. A., Olson, D. J., & Schaffer, H. I. (1992a). Early detection of ototoxicity using high frequency, tone-burst evoked auditory brainstem responses. *J. Am. Acad. Audiol., 3,* 397–404.

Fausti, S. A., Frey, R. H., Henry, J. A., Robertson, P. G., & Hertert, R. S. (1992b). Portable stimulus generator for obtaining high-frequency (8–14 kHz) auditory brainstem response responses. *J. Am. Acad. Audiol., 3,* 166–175.

Fausti, S. A., Frey, R. H., Rappaport, B. Z., & Erickson, D. A. (1978). And investigation of the effect of bumetanide on high frequency (8–20 kHz) hearing in humans. *J. Aud. Res., 18*(4), 243–250.

Fausti, S. A., Frey, R. H., Rappaport, B. Z., & Schechter, M. A. (1985). High frequency audiometry with an earphone transducer. *Seminars in Hearing, 6*(4), 347–357.

Fausti, S. A., Helt, W. J., Gordon, J. S., Reavis, K. M., Phillips, D. S., & Konrad-Martin, D. L. (2007). Audiologic monitoring for ototoxicity and patient management. In K. C. M. Campbell (Ed.), *Pharmacology and ototoxicity for audiologists* (pp. 230–248). New York: Thomson Delmar Learning.

Fausti, S. A., Henry, J. A., Helt, W. J., Phillips, D. S., Frey, R. H., Noffsinger, D., Larson, V. D., & Fowler, C. G. (1999). An individualized, sensitive frequency range for early detection of ototoxicity. *Ear Hear., 20*(6), 497–505.

Fausti, S. A., Henry, J. A., & Shaffer, H. I. (1992c). High-frequency audiometric monitoring for early detection of aminoglycoside ototoxicity. *The Journal of Infectious Diseases, 165,* 1026–1032.

Fausti, S. A., Rappaport, B. Z., Schechter, M. A., Frey, R. H., Ward, T. T., & Brummettt, R. E. (1984a). Detection of aminoglycoside ototoxicity by high frequency auditory evaluation: Selected case studies. *American Journal of Otolaryngology, 5,* 177–182.

Fausti, S. A., Schechter, M. A., Rappaport, B. Z., Frey, R. H., & Mass, R. E. (1984b). Early detection cisplatin ototoxicity: Selected case reports. *Cancer, 53,* 224–231.

Fee, W. E. (1980). Aminoglycoside ototoxicity in the human. *Laryngoscope, 90*(10 pt 2, Suppl. 24), 1–19.

Feghali, J. G., & Bernstein, R. S. (1991). A new approach to serial monitoring of ultra-high frequency hearing. *Laryngoscope, 101*(8), 825–829.

Fletcher, H. (1929). *Speech and hearing.* New York: Van Nostrand.

Fletcher, J. L. (1965). Reliability of high frequency thresholds. *J. Auditory Res., 5,* 133–137.

Frank, T. (1990). High-frequency hearing thresholds in young adults using a commercially available audiometer. *Ear & Hearing, 11,* 450–454.

Frank, T. (2001). High frequency (8 to 16 kHz) reference thresholds and intrasubject threshold variability relative to ototoxicity criteria using a Sennheiser HAD 200 earphone. *Ear & Hearing, 22*(2), 161–168.

Frank, T., & Dreisbach, L. E. (1991). Repeatability of high frequency thresholds. *Ear & Hearing, 12*(4), 294–295.

Helson, L., Okonkwo, E., Anton, L., & Cvitkovic, E. (1988). Cis-Platinum ototoxicity. *Clin Toxicol., 13,* 469–478.

Horn, Y., Schechter, P. J., & Marton, L. J. (1987). Phase I–II clinical trials with alpha-difluoromethylornithine—An inhibitor of polyamine biosynthesis. *Cancer Clin. Oncol., 23,* 1103–1107.

Jacobson, E. J., Downs, M. P., & Fletcher, J. L. (1969). Clinical findings in high frequency thresholds during known ototoxic drug usage. *J. Auditory Res., 9,* 379–385.

Jansen, C., Mattox, D. E., Miller, K. D., & Brownell, W. E. (1989). An animal model of hearing loss from alpha-difluoromethylornithine. *Arch. Otolaryngol. Head Neck Surg.*, *115*, 1234–1237.

Katbamna, B., Homnick, D. N., & Marks, J. H. (1999). Effects of chronic tobramycin treatment on distortion product otoacoustic emissions. *Ear Hear.*, *20*(5), 393–402.

Kopelman, J., Budnick, A. S., Kramer, M. B., Sessions, R. B., & Wong, G. Y. (1988). Ototoxicity of high-dose cisplatin by bolus administration in patients with advanced cancers and normal hearing. *Laryngoscope*, *98*(8 Pt 1), 858–864.

Kopke, R. D., Coleman, J. K. M., Liu, J., Campbell, K. C. M., & Riffenburgh, R. H. (2002). Enhancing intrinsic cochlear stress defenses to reduce noise-induced hearing loss. *The Laryngoscope, 112*, 1515–1532.

Kopke, R., Liu, W., Gabaizedeh, R., Jacano, A., Feghali, J., Spray, D., et al., (1997). Use of organotypic cultures of Corti's organ to study the protective effects of antioxidant molecules on cisplatin-induced damage of auditory hair cells. *The American Journal of Otology, 18*, 559–571.

Legros, D., Ollivier, G., Gastellu-Etchaegorry, M., Paquet, C., Burri, C., & Jannin, J. (2002). Treatment of human African trypanosomiasis—Present situation and need for research and development. *Lancet Infect. Dis., 2*, 437–440.

Levin, V. A., Hess, K. R., Choucair, A., Flynn, P. J., Jaeckle, K. A., Kyritsis, A. P., Garcia, P., Steinman, H., Malgrange, B., Ruben, R. J., Rybak, L., and Van de Water, T. R. (2003). Phase III randomized study of postradiotherapy chemotherapy with combination alpha-difluoromethylornithine-PCV versus PCV for anaplastic gliomas. *Clinical Cancer Research, 9*, 981–990.

Li, Y., Womer, R. B., & Silber, J.H. (2004). Predicting cisplatin ototoxicity in children: The influence of age and the cumulative dose. *Eur. J. Cancer, 40*, 2445–2451.

Lipton, A., Harvey, H. A., Glenn, J., Weidner, W., Strauss, M., Miller, S. E., Garcia, P., Steinman, H., Malgrange, B., Ruber, R. J., Rybak, L., Van de Water, T. R. (1989). A phase I study of hepatic arterial infusion using difluoromethylornithine. *Cancer, 63*, 433–437.

Lonsbury-Martin, B. L., & Martin, G. K. (1990). The clinical utility of distortion-product otoacoustic emissions. *Ear Hear.*, 11, 144–154.

Lonsbury-Martin, B. L., & Martin, G. K. (2001). Evoked otoacoustic emissions as objective screeners for ototoxicity. *Sem. Hearing, 22*(4), 377–391.

Martin, G. K., Ohlms, L. A., Franklin, D. J., & Lonsbury-Martin, B. L. (1990). Distortion product emissions in humans. III. Influence of sensorineural hearing loss. *Ann. Otol. Rhinol. Laryngol. (Suppl.), 147*, 30–42.

McCann, P. P., and Pegg, A. E. (1992). Ornithine decarboxylase as an enzyme target for therapy. *Pharmacol Ther, 54*(2), 195–215. Review. PMID: 1438532.

Meech, R., Campbell, K. C. M., Hughes, L. F., & Rybak, L. P. (1998). A semiquantitative analysis of the effects of CDDP on the rat stria vascularis. *Hear. Res., 124*, 44–59.

Meyskens, F. L., Kingsley, E. M., Glattke, T., Loescher, L., & Booth, A. (1986). A phase II study of alpha-difluoromethylornithine (DMFO) for the treatment of metastatic melanoma. *Invest New Drugs, 4*(3), 527–562.

Morioka, I., Kuroda, M., Miyashita, K., & Takeda, S. (1999). Evaluation of organic solvent ototoxicity by the upper limit of hearing. *Arch. Environ. Health, 54*(5), 341–346.

Moss, P. E., Hickman, S., & Harrison, B. R. (1997). Ototoxicity associated with vinblastine. *Ann. Pharmacother., 33*, 423–425.

Mulheran, M., & Degg, C. (1997) Comparison of distortion product OAE generation between a group requiring frequent gentamicin therapy and control subjects. *Br. J. Audiol., 31*, 5–9.

Northern, J. L., & Ratkiewicz, B. (1985). The quest for high-frequency normative data. *Seminars in Hearing, 6*(4), 331–339.

Norton, S. J. (1992). Cochlear function and otoacoustic emissions. *Semin. Hear., 13*, 1–14.

O'Shaughnessy, J. A., Demers, L. M., Jones, S. E., Arseneau, J., & Khandelwal, P. G. (1999). Alpha-difluomethylornithine as treatment for metastatic breast cancer patients. *Clinical Cancer Research, 5*, 3438–3444.

Owens, J. J., McCoy, M. J., Lonsbury-Martin, B. L., & Martin, G. K. (1992). Influence of otitis media on evoked otoacoustic emissions in children. *Semin. Hear., 13,* 53–66.

Pasic, T. R., Heisey, D., & Love, R. R. (1997). Alpha-difluoromethlylornithine ototoxicity. *Arch. Otolaryngol. Head Neck Surg., 123,* 1281–1286.

Plinkert, P. K., & Krober, S. (1991). Fruherkennung einer Cisplatin-Ototoxizitat durch evosierte otoakustische Emissionen. *Laryngorhinootologie, 70,* 457–462.

Probst, R., Lonsbury-Martin, B. L., & Martin, G. K. (1991). A review of otoacoustic emissions. *J. Acoust. Soc. Am., 20,* 2021–2027.

Rappaport, B. Z., Fausti, S. A., Schechter, M. A., Frey, R. H. N., & Hartigan, P. (1985). Detection of ototoxicity by high-frequency auditory evaluation. *Seminars in Hearing, 6*(4), 369–377.

Ress, B. D., Sridhar, K. S., Balkany, T. J., Waxman, G. M., Stagner, B. B., & Lonsbury-Martin, B. L. (1999). Effects of cis-platinum chemotherapy on otoacoustic emissions: The development of an objective screening protocol *Otolaryngology-Head and Neck Surgery, 121*(6), 693–701.

Rosen, S., Plester, D., El-Mofty, A., & Rosen, H. (1964). High frequency audiometry in presbycusis. *Arch. Otolaryngol., 79,* 18–32.

Rybak, L. P. (1992). Hearing: The effects of chemicals. *Otolaryngol. Head Neck Surg., 106*(6), 677–686.

Rybak, L. P. (2007). Renal function and ototoxicity of loop diuretics. In K. Campbell (Ed.), *Pharmacology and ototoxicity for audiologists* (pp. 177–183). Clifton Park, NY: Thomson Delmar Learning.

Rybak, L. P., Huang, X., & Campbell, K. C. (2007). Cancer and ototoxicity of chemotherapeutics. In K. Campbell (Ed.), *Pharmacology and ototoxicity for audiologists* (pp. 138–155). Clifton Park, NY: Thomson Delmar Learning.

Sahai, J., and Berry A.J. (1989). Eflornithine for the treatment of *Pneumocystis carinii* pneumonia in patients with the acquired immunodeficiency sydrome: A preliminary review. *Pharmacotherapy, 9,* 29–33.

Saito, T., Saito H., Saito K., Wakui, S., Manabe, Y., & Tsuda G. (1989). Ototoxicity of carboplatin in guinea pigs. *Auris Nasus Larynx, 16*(1), 13–21.

Schacht, J. (2007). Aminoglycoside ototoxicity. In K. Campbell (Ed.), *Pharmacology and ototoxicity for audiologists* (pp. 163–172). Clifton Park, NY: Thomson Delmar Learning.

Schuknecht, H. F. (1993). Disorders of intoxication. In *Pathology of the ear* (pp. 255–277). Philadelphia: Lea & Febiger.

Schweitzer, V. G., Hawkins, J. E., Lilly, D. J., Litterst, C. J., Abrams, G., & Davis, J. A. (1984). Ototoxic and nephrotoxic effects of combined treatment with cis-di-amminedichloroplatinum and kanamycin in the guinea pig. *Otolaryngol. Head Neck Surg., 92,* 38–49.

Sha, S., and Schacht, J. (2000). Antioxidants attenuate gentamicin-induced free radical formation in vitro and ototoxicity in vivo: D-methionine is a potential protectant. *Hear. Res., 142,* 34–40.

Sjoerdsma, A., Golden, J. A., Schechter, P. J., Barlow, J. L., and Santi, D. V. (1984). Successful treatment of lethal protozoal infections with the ornithine decarboxylase inhibitors, alpha-difluoromethylornithine. *Trans. Assoc. Am. Physicians, 97,* 70–79.

Stavroulaki, P., Apostolopoulos, N., Dinopoulo, D., Vossinakis, I., Tsakanikos, M., & Douniadakis, D. (1999). Otoacoustic emissions—An approach for monitoring aminoglycoside induced ototoxicity in children. *International Journal of Pediatric Otorhinolaryngology, 50,* 177–184.

Stelmachowicz, P. G., Beauchaine, K. A., Kalberer, A., and Jesteadt, W. (1989). Normative thresholds in the 8–20 kHz range as a function of age. *J. Acoust. Soc. Am., 86*(4), 1384–1391.

Stelmachowicz, P. G., Gorga, M. P., & Cullen, J. K. (1982). A calibration procedure for the assessment of thresholds above 8000 Hz. *J. Speech Hear. Res., 25,* 618–623.

Sulkowski, W. J., Kowalska, S., Matja, W., Guzek, W., Wesolowski, W., Szymczak, W., & Kostrezewski, P. (2002). Effects of occupational exposure to a mixture of solvents on the inner ear: A field study. *Int. J. Occup. Med. Environ. Health, 15*(3), 247–256.

Tange, R. A., Dreschler, W. A., & van der Hulst, R. J. (1985). The importance of high-tone monitoring for ototoxicity. *Arch. Otorhinolaryngol., 242*(1), 77–81.

Thornton, A., & Raffin, M. J. M. (1977). Speech discrimination scores modeled as a binomial variable. *J. Speech Hear. Res., 21*, 507–518.

Tonndorf, J., & Kurman, B. (1984). High frequency audiometry. *Ann. Otol. Rhinol. Laryngol., 93*(6 Pt 1), 576–582.

Valente, M., Potts, L.G., Valente, M., French-St. George, M., & Goebel, J. (1992a). High frequency thresholds: Sound suite versus hospital room. *J. Am. Acad. Audiol., 3*, 287–294.

Valente, M., Valente, M., & Goeble, J. (1992b). High-frequency thresholds: Circumaural versus insert earphone. *J. Am. Acad. Audiol., 3*, 410–418.

Wake, M., Takeno, S., Ibrahim, D., Harrison, R., & Mount, R. (1993). Carboplatin ototoxicity: An animal model. *J. Laryngol. Otol., 107*, 585–589.

Wier, C. C., Pasanen, E. G.., & McFadden, D. (1988). Partial dissociation of spontaneous otoacoustic emissions and distortion products during aspirin use in humans. *J. Acoust. Soc. Am., 84*, 230–237.

Wiley, T. L., Cruikshanks, K. J., Nondahl, D. M., Tweed, T. S., Klein, R., & Klein, B. E. K. (1998). Aging and high frequency hearing sensitivity. *JSHLR, 41*, 1061–1072.

Wright, C. G., & Schaefer, S. D. (1982). Inner ear histopathology in patients treated with cisplatin. *Laryngoscope, 92*, 1408–1413.

Zilis, T., & Fletcher, J. L. (1966). Relation of high frequency thresholds to age and sex. *J. Auditory Res., 6*, 189–198.

Zorowka, P. G., Schmitt, H. J., & Gutjahr, P. (1993). Evoked otoacoustic emissions and pure tone threshold audiometry in patients receiving cisplatinum therapy. *International Journal of Pediatric Otorhinolaryngology, 25*, 73–80.

CHAPTER 7

Auditory Electrophysiological Assessment

John A. Ferraro
University of Kansas Medical Center

Robert Folsom and Lisa R. Mancl
University of Washington

Annette Hurley and Robin Moorhouse
Louisiana State University Health Sciences Center

Auditory electrophysiology assessment provides an indirect, objective method of determining hearing sensitivity as well as identifying sensory and nervous system pathology. The units of this chapter cover electrocochleography testing, auditory brainstem response assessment of infants and children, and middle latency response assessment. Each unit covers test procedures, target populations, and summary test interpretations.

ELECTROCOCHLEOGRAPHY RECORDING TECHNIQUES

Recording Approach

There are two general approaches for recording electrocochleography (ECochG): Transtympanic (TT) and Extratympanic (ET). TT ECochG is an invasive procedure that involves passing a needle electrode through the tympanic membrane (TM) to rest on the cochlear promontory. This approach is still used in Europe and Australia and even by some physicians in the U.S. ET recordings are performed with an electrode resting against the skin of the ear canal or surface of the TM. For the latter recording site, the procedure can be referred to as "Tympanic (or TM) ECochG" (Ferraro & Ferguson, 1989), even though this approach is still considered to be ET. Pioneering work in ET recordings was performed by Sohmer and Feinmesser (1967), Coats and Dickey (1970), and Cullen et al. (1972), among others. Although ET ECochG can be performed using a needle electrode in the skin of the ear canal, this option is rarely, if ever, chosen. Thus, virtually all ET recordings are non-invasive, and therefore have been better accepted in the U.S. than TT techniques. Adult ECochG recordings are usually measured from the TM using an electrode patterned from that first described by Stypulkowski and Staller (1987). This device as well as other examples of ET electrodes is shown in Figure 7–1.

Although ET recordings require more signal averaging and tend to yield smaller component magnitudes than TT measurements, they are non-invasive (thus obviating the need for a medial setting and physician supervision) and within the scope of practice of audiologists (ASHA, 1990). These features have contributed to the popularity of ECochG not only among audiologists, but also physicians who offer auditory evoked potential (AEP) testing in their practices and utilize audiologists to perform these tests. In addition, we have found that the TM offers a good and practical compromise between ear canal and TT placements with respect to component magnitudes and, consequently, signal averaging time (Ferraro, Blackwell, Mediavilla, & Thedinger, 1994; Ferraro, Thedinger, Mediavilla, & Blackwell, 1994; Ruth & Lambert, 1989; Schoonhoven, Fabius, & Grote, 1995). Perhaps most importantly for clinical purposes, the response patterns nec-

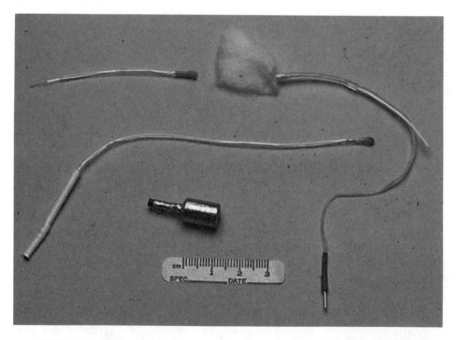

FIGURE 7–1.   Photographs of extratympanic ECochG electrodes. Tymptrode (modified version of electrode described by Stypulkoswski and Staller ((1987)) (top left), Lilly wick electrode (top right), and Bio-Logic ECochGtrode (middle) are placed on the surface of the tympanic membrane. Gold-foil TIPtrode (bottom) rests in the ear canal. From Ferraro (2000), page 429.

essary for interpreting the electrocochleogram are preserved in the ET approach when compared to TT recordings (Ferraro, Thedinger et al., 1994).

When performed correctly, TM ECochG should cause minimal-to-no discomfort to the patient. However, the technique of placing an electrode on the highly sensitive TM can sometimes result in more patient discomfort than is customary for other, non-invasive ET approaches (but certainly not as much as is usually associated with TT ECochG). Such discomfort may occur when the electrode is resting against the annular ligament instead of the TM itself (a situation that also will result in poor recordings).

Given the advantages and disadvantages of both approaches, the selection of ECochG recording approaches (i.e., TT or ET) depends on the traditional practices, personnel and attitudes of the clinic. Obviously, TT recordings are dependent on the availability of a physician who has the time and interest to perform the examination. While a physician is not needed for ET ECochG, placing an electrode on the TM is certainly a more delicate maneuver than attaching surface electrodes to the scalp or resting them in the ear canal. Unfortunately, one factor that is virtually overlooked in the decision to perform TT or ET ECochG is the attitude/preference of the patient. Given the choice with an understanding of the benefits and limitations of each approach, which one would you choose if you were in need of testing?

Recording Parameters

Since ECochG components generally occur within a latency epoch of 5 milliseconds (ms) following stimulus onset, they can be considered to be in the family of "early- or "short-latency" AEPs (Picton, Hillyard, Krausz, & Galambos, 1974). Thus, as relatives, ECochG responses and the auditory brainstem response (ABR) can be measured using similar recording parameters. There are some notable exceptions, however. Namely, when the Summating Potential (SP) is of interest, the filter band-pass must be wide enough to accommodate both a quasi-steady-state direct current (DC) component (the SP), and the alternating current (AC) component with a fundamental frequency of approximately 1 kHz which is the action potential (AP) of the auditory nerve. Other differences between ECochG and ABR recording parameters mainly involve the choice of electrode arrays and use of the TM electrode itself. The overall parameters for recording the SP and AP together, which are the components of interest when ECochG is used in the diagnosis of Meniere's disease/endolymphatic hydrops (MD/ELH), are described below.

Electrode Array

An electrode array that displays the AP as a downward (negative) deflection is generally preferred. For such a display, the primary electrode (i.e., the electrode connected to the +/non-inverting input of the differential preamplifier) should rest on the TM. Sites for the secondary (−/inverting) electrode include the vertex of the scalp, high forehead or contralateral earlobe or mastoid process. The earlobe or mastoid are preferred secondary (−)sites simply because electrodes tend to be easier to attach and secure to these areas. Choices for "ground" or "common" sites include the nasion and ipsilateral earlobe or mastoid. If one prefers to view the AP as an upward deflection (as it is seen as Wave I in conventional ABR tracings), reversing the + and − inputs to the preamplifier will accomplish this task.

Timebase (Averaging Window)

As indicated above, ECochG components represent the earliest voltage changes to occur in the ear in response to sound. For click stimuli, a timebase or averaging window of 10 ms allows for visualization of both ECochG components and subsequent ABR peaks. For longer duration stimuli (such as tonebursts) the timebase should extend beyond the duration of the stimulus envelope so that the entire response is observable within the averaging window (recalling that both the SP and CM persist for the duration of the stimulus). For example, we use a 20 msec. timebase for responses recorded to a 1000 Hz toneburst with a 2-cycle rise/fall time, and a 10 cycle plateau (i.e., a 14 ms envelope).

Amplification Factor

Amplification factor is selected to maximize the signal-to-noise ratio for a given recording condition. The amount of amplification needed for suitable recordings of the SP and/or AP for ET measurements generally ranges between 20,000 to 100,000 times greater than the input signal amplitude. In part, selection of this parameter is based on the level of the electrical noise floor, which incorporates several elements (i.e., myogenic and electroencephalographic activity, electrical artifact from the equipment and/or testing environment). The sensitivity setting of the signal averager's analog-to-digital converter also must be taken into account. Thus, amplification/sensitivity settings may vary from laboratory to laboratory and also among evoked potential units from different manufacturers. However, the manipulation of these variables to provide settings appropriate to recording conditions is easily accomplished in most commercial instruments.

Filter Settings

Adaptation notwithstanding, the SP, as fundamentally a DC potential, could last as long as the stimulus of any duration. Ideally, then, a DC recording amplifier is needed, but these devices are notoriously unstable for electrophsyiological recordings. Fortunately, the SP, as evoked for practical/clinical purposes using transient stimuli, is only quasi-steady-state, permitting the use of AC-coupled amplifiers (typically found in commercially manufactured systems for the measurement of the ABR and other AEPs). The high-pass cut-off, in turn, must allow for the amplification of the AP-N1, which has a fundamental frequency of approximately 1000 Hz. A filter bandpass for ECochG of 5 Hz–3000 Hz allows recording of the SP-AP complex without significant distortion of either component (Durrant & Ferraro, 1991). As a word of caution, however, and especially when recording the SP to tonal stimuli using modern AEP test systems, it is always best to be conservative re: filtering during the recording (i.e., over-filter is ill-advised), and to take advantage of post-hoc digital filtering to "clean up" the recording afterwards.

Repetitions

The number of stimulus repetitions needed to extract a well-defined electrocochleogram from the background noise will vary with recording conditions, and also the subject's degree of hearing loss. Regarding the former, and as described earlier, ET recordings require considerably more repetitions than TT approaches. For subjects with hearing loss in the 1000–4000 Hz range, more repetitions may be necessary than are usually needed for normally hearing subjects or those with low frequency losses. In general we have found a maximum of 1,000 repetitions to be sufficient for most ECochG applications. Under good recording conditions (from the TM) and especially for subjects with relatively normal hearing, a well-defined electrocochleogram should be apparent after 500–750 repetitions.

It should be noted that when sensorineural hearing loss in the mid-to-high frequencies exceeds 50–60 dB HL the use of ET ECochG is questionable. Losses of this magnitude generally involve (i.e., reduce the output of) the population of outer hair cells contributing to ECochG components, often rendering them absent or poorly defined. On the other hand, hearing loss of similar or greater magnitude often precludes the identification of wave I in the presence of wave V in the conventionally recorded ABR. An ECochG approach can be used in such conditions to record Wave I and thus measure the I-V interwave interval (Ferraro and Ferguson, 1989).

Stimulus Features

Choice of Stimuli

The broadband click continues to be the most popular stimulus for short-latency AEPs because it excites synchronous discharges from a large population of neurons to produce well-defined component peaks. In addition, 100 microseconds is a popular choice for the duration of the rectangular pulse that drives the transducer diaphragm because the first spectral null for a click of this duration occurs at 10,000 Hz. (i.e., 1/100 microseconds). Theoretically then, the acoustic signal contains equal energy at all frequencies below this value. In reality, the frequency range of the transducer does not extend this high and the outer and middle ears contribute additional filtering. Thus, the spectrum of the acoustic signal reaching the cochlea is not flat, nor as wide as 10,000 Hz.

Since the duration of both the CM and SP are stimulus-dependent, the brevity of the click makes it a less than ideal stimulus for studying these potentials. Despite this limitation, however, the use of clicks has proven to be very effective in evoking the SP-AP complex for certain ECochG applications, even though the duration of the SP is abbreviated under these conditions (Durrant & Ferraro, 1991).

Although the click continues to remain popular, toneburst stimuli also are used for many ECochG applications (Ferraro, Blackwell et al., 1994; Ferraro, Thedinger et al., 1994; Koyuncu, Mason, & Shinkwin, 1994; Levine, Margolis, Fournier, & Winzenburg, 1992; Margolis, Rieks, Fournier, & Levine, 1995; Orchik, She, & Ge, 1993). Since tonebursts provide a higher degree of response frequency-specificity than clicks (depending upon stimulus envelope and duration), they tend to be useful for monitoring cochlear status in progressive disorders (such as MD/ELH) where hearing is usually not affected at all frequencies during the initial stages. In addition, the use of extended-duration stimuli allows for better visualization of the SP and CM than can be achieved with clicks (Durrant & Ferraro, 1991).

A problem related to the use of toneburst stimuli for ECochG (and other AEPs) is the lack of standardization regarding stimulus parameters. Most studies employ tonebursts of only one or two frequencies, stimulus envelopes are different and there is no standardized approach to defining stimulus intensity. These inconsistencies make it difficult to compare data across laboratories/clinics. In our clinic we use tonebursts with linear rise-fall times of 2 ms and a 10 ms plateau.. Shorter plateaus (e.g., 5 ms) can sometimes be used to avoid (but generally do not eliminate) interference by ABR components (Levine et al., 1992).

Stimulus Polarity

Stimulus polarity is an important factor for ECochG. Presenting clicks or tonebursts in alternating polarity inhibits the presence of stimulus artifact and CM (which are phase-locked to the signal). The former can sometimes be large enough to obscure early ECochG components, and the latter generally overshadows both the SP and AP when these components are of interest. On the other hand, recording separate responses to condensation and rarefaction clicks may provide useful clinical information. In particular, certain subjects with MD/ELH display abnormal latency differences between AP-N1 latencies to condensation versus rarefaction clicks (Levine et al., 1992; Margolis & Lilly, 1989; Margolis, Fournier, Hunter, Smith, & Lilly, 1992; Margolis et al., 1995; Orchik, Ge, & Shea, 1997; Sass, Densert, & Arlinger, 1998). In deference to these studies, we measure separate responses to condensation and rarefaction clicks to assess the N1 latency difference, then add these waveforms off-line to derive the SP magnitude and SP/AP magnitude ratio. In addition, we also measure the SP and AP areas in our assessment of patients suspected of having MD/ELH. This procedure is accomplished with specialized software that allows us to set cursor points on the waveform and measure the "area under the curve" defined by these settings (Deviah et al., 2003; Ferraro and Tibbils, 1997).

Stimulus Rate

For ECochG, as with most signal-averaged AEPs, it is important that the cochlear/neural response to one stimulus be complete before the next stimulus is presented. For ECochG, however, increasing this rate beyond 10–30/second may cause unacceptable adaptation of the AP (Suzuki & Yamane, 1982). Indeed, rates on the order of 100/second have been used to cause extensive adaptation of the AP while leaving the SP relatively unaffected (Coats, 1981; Gibson et al., 1977). This approach has not proven to be very successful in the clinic, in part because the AP contribution is not completely eliminated, the SP may also be reduced under such conditions (Durrant, 1986; Harris & Dallos, 1989), and rapid clicks presented at loud levels tend to be obnoxious for patients.

Stimulus Level

When ECochG is performed to help diagnose Meniere's Disease/endolymphatic hydrops (MD/ELH), the stimulus should be intense enough to evoke a well-defined SP-AP complex. Thus, for this application we begin at a level near the maximum output of the stimulus generator (e.g., 95 dB nHL). As with all AEPs, the lack of standardization for stimuli regarding signal calibration and decibel (dB) reference presents problems for ECochG as well. Common references include dB Hearing Level (HL, or Hearing Threshold Level—HTL), dB normal Hearing Level (nHL), dB Sensation Level (SL), and dB peak equivalent Sound Pressure Level (peSPL). Thus, the selection of the "dial setting" to begin ECochG testing may differ among laboratories/clinics and the particular AEP unit being used. If this level is calibrated in nHL (i.e., based on the average threshold of a group of normal listeners) it is important to remember that 0 dB nHL for clicks corresponds to approximately 30 dB peSPL (Stapells et al., 1982). Thus, presenting clicks at 95 dB nHL corresponds to a peSPL level of approximately 125 dB. Masking of the contralateral ear is not a concern for conventional ECochG since the magnitude of any electrophysiological response from the non-test ear is very small (especially when tubal insert earphones are used) and ECochG components are generated prior to crossover of the auditory pathway.

Stimulus Artifact

A final note regarding stimuli relates to stimulus artifact, which can be quite large for ECochG. The nature of ET (especially TM) electrodes is that they tend to have high impedance and are vulnerable to radiation from the transducer and other electrical sources in the environment. To help avoid such contamination of the waveform, we:

- use a tubal insert transducer;
- separate the transducer from the electrode cables as much as possible;
- braid the electrode cables;
- test subjects in a shielded sound booth with the examiner and AEP unit located outside of the booth;
- plug the AEP unit into an isolated socket equipped with a true-earth ground;

- use a grounded cable for the primary electrode (such cables are commercially available);
- turn off the lights in the testing room and unplug unnecessary electronic equipment (it also may be necessary to turn off the lights in the examiner room).

Under certain conditions when the noise is particularly troublesome, encasing the transducer in grounded Mu metal shielding may also be necessary to achieve good recordings.

Subject/Patient Considerations

Most patients are unfamiliar with ECochG and therefore confused and often fearful as to what it is, why they need it, and how it will be performed. The complex term, "electrocochleography," adds to this confusion. Therefore, it is important to provide instructions to the patient with an assurance that the examination is non-invasive and painless, that the test will take approximately 1 hour, and they can sleep through it if they wish. The patient also is informed as to why their physician has requested this examination (e.g., to help determine if there is too much fluid in the inner ear). Engaging patients in conversation at this point and watching them walk also provides some insight about the status of their hearing and balance. Once in the sound booth, the patient rests comfortably in a reclining examination chair, which can be adjusted to maximize comfort of the head, neck and upper back. Remove eyeglasses and/or earrings, and food/chewing gum/candy/etc. must be swallowed or discarded. When the patient is comfortable and attentive, explain the testing procedures beginning with a description of the electrodes and how they will be attached to the scalp. Also, alert the patient that the TM electrode might feel strange and maybe a little uncomfortable, but that it should not be particularly painful. However, they are instructed to inform the clinician if the latter condition should occur at any time. Describe the procedures for preparing the skin and placing the surface electrodes (commercially-available, pre-gelled and disposable with an adhesive backing) while performing these tasks. Surface electrode application for ECochG is identical to that used for ABR testing. Skin preparation merely involves cleaning site and rubbing it with a mild abrasive solution. The abrasive substance should be removed before attaching the electrode as it can impede current flow. After the surface electrodes are attached (or beforehand, for that matter) otoscopy is performed to assess the patency of the ear canal and normalcy of the TM. Cerumen removal may be necessary to visualize the TM and clear a pathway along the ear canal large enough for the electrode. Once the surface electrodes have been positioned and otoscopy performed, the TM electrode can be placed. If either the ear canal or TM appears abnormal or damaged, ECochG should not be performed at all, or at least not without first consulting the patient's physician.

As a final note regarding subject considerations, both ears should be tested, even if unilateral disease is suspected. Comparison between affected and unaffected sides can provide important diagnostic information. Our practice is to test the affected side first in case the patient becomes restless as the examination progresses.

Construction and Placement of the TM Electrode (Tymptrode)

The photograph of ET electrodes in Figure 1 include the tymptrode (originally described by Stypulkowski and Staller, 1987, and modified by Ferraro and Ferguson, 1989), the Lilly wick electrode (Lilly & Black, 1989), and the TM-ECochGtrode manufactured by Bio-Logic. The latter two electrodes are commercially available. The tymptrode can be fabricated using commercially available materials that include: medical grade silicon (Silastic) tubing (0.058", inner diameter, 0.077" outer diameter); Teflon-insulated sliver wire (0.008" bare diameter, 0.011" insulated diameter); a wad of cotton; standard electrode gel (not paste or cream); fine, needle-nosed forceps; 1 cc disposable tuberculin syringe with needle; and a copper microalligator clip soldered to the end of an electrode cable (Ferraro, 1997).

Briefly, the procedure for constructing the tymptrode involves cutting the wire and tubing into segments a few centimeters (cm) longer than the ear canal, with the wire approximately 2 cm longer than the tubing. The fine forceps are used to scrape the insulation off both ends of the wire (a crucial step), which is then threaded through the tubing. One end of the wire protruding from the tubing remains bare, while the other end is hooked to the end of a small plug (approximately 2 mm × 3 mm) of cotton. Once again using the fine forceps, that portion of the cotton plug hooked to the wire is tucked into the end of the tubing to leave only a small portion of the cotton extending beyond the tubing. A drawing of the fabricated tymptrode and its components is shown in Figure 7–2. Tymptrodes, at

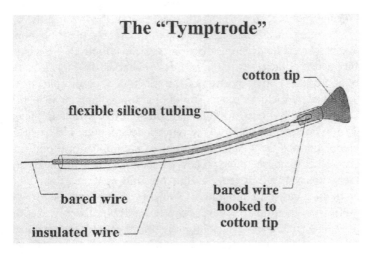

FIGURE 7–2.   Components of the "tymptrode" electrode used for surface recordings from the tympanic membrane. From Ferraro and Durrent (2006, p. 55).

this stage, can be made and stockpiled for indefinite periods of time. Immediately prior to use, the cotton tip of the tymptrode must be impregnated with electrode gel. This step is accomplished by filling the tuberculin syringe with gel and injecting the entire piece of cotton until it is thoroughly saturated (including that portion of the foam/cotton within the tubing attached to the wire). Attach the microalligator clip of the electrode cable to the other (bare) end of the wire, and the tymptrode is ready to use.

Inserting the Tymptrode

To gain the assistance of gravity when placing the tymptrode, the patient is instructed to gently roll over onto his/her side so that the test ear is facing up. The tymptrode is then inserted into the entrance of the ear canal and gently advanced (by hand or using the fine forceps) until the tip makes contact with the TM. The latter is confirmed via otoscopy and electrophysiological monitoring. It also helps to ask the patient when they feel the electrode touching the TM. Even with an otoscope, it is difficult to actually see the point of contact between the tymptrode tip and TM. However, monitoring the electrophysiological noise floor during electrode placement helps to achieve proper contact with the TM. As the electrode is being advanced into the ear canal, the raw EEG/noise floor is displayed on-screen. Large, spurious and cyclic or peak-clipped voltages (i.e., an open-line situation) characterize this electrical activity. When proper contact of the tymptrode tip with the TM is achieved, the noise floor drops dramatically and becomes more stable and less cyclic. Using both visual and electrophysiological monitoring provides the best opportunity for achieving proper contact with the TM on the "first try."

Once the tymptrode is in place, the foam tip of the sound delivery tube is compressed and inserted into the ear canal alongside the tymptrode tubing. Care must be taken during this stage to not push the electrode further against the TM when inserting the earplug, as this can cause some discomfort to the patient and a conductive loss. However, the materials that comprise the tymptrode are relatively soft and flexible, which allows the tip to compress or bend at the TM rather than penetrate the membrane. Only a portion of the transducer earplug needs to be inserted into the canal to achieve proper stimulation for evoking the ECochGm. Figure 7–3 is a drawing of the tymptrode and sound delivery tube in the ear canal (modified from Ferraro, 1992). With the tymptrode and other electrodes attached to the preamplifier and the sound tube in place, and the patient comfortable, relaxed and still, the signal averaging process can begin. Even with the most delicate contact, the tymptrode tends to leave a slight blushing spot (i.e., light red in color) on the TM in most cases. In hundreds of subjects and patients that I have tested over the years, this condition has never proven to be an untoward reaction, clears up within minutes, and is even a useful indicator of exactly where the electrode was situated (should this be difficult to visualize upon placement or the electrode moved).

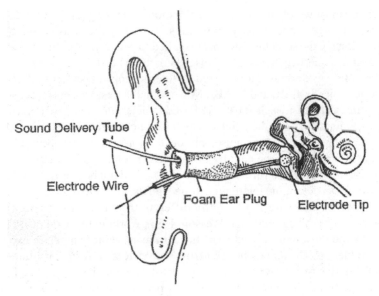

FIGURE 7–3.   Schematic illustration of the tymptrode in place. Modified from Ferraro (1992), page 28.

AUDITORY BRAINSTSTEM TECHNIQUES FOR INFANTS AND YOUNG CHILDREN: THE APPROACH AT THE UNIVERSITY OF WASHINGTON'S CENTER ON HUMAN DEVELOPMENT AND DISABILITY

The use of short-latency auditory-evoked potentials, such as the auditory brainstem response, has had a great impact on pediatric audiology. With the advent of universal newborn hearing screening and diagnosis of hearing loss at increasingly younger ages, the ABR is the essential tool in diagnosing the degree, type, and configuration of hearing loss in the very young pediatric population. The use of these scalp-recorded potentials, in conjunction with existing behavioral information, has improved the ability to estimate hearing levels in children early in life and has thus made a major contribution to early intervention and, it follows, the management of hearing disorders. Further, for some children, behavioral testing is not successful due to behavior or intellectual disability at ages well into early childhood. The ABR is a crucial test in determining hearing levels in these patients, as well.

Definition and Basic Measurement of the ABR

Multiple auditory-evoked potentials are available anytime electrodes are attached to the scalp; the ABR being one of these. This section will focus on ABRs because they are the most widely used for the estimation of hearing levels in infants and children. However, other evoked potentials, primarily those from longer time epochs following the stimulus, have been applied to pediatric populations for hearing assessment and will be discussed elsewhere in this text.

The ABR waveform is characterized by three prominent peaks usually labeled Roman numerically I, III, and V. ABR Wave V, the largest and most robust wave across stimulus intensities, is most often used to determine the ABR threshold or visual detection threshold (the point at which a replicated response can be visually differentiated from background noise), although in early infancy, depending on filter settings, wave III can be equally prominent (Klein, 1984; Stuart and Yang, 1994; Weber, 1982). The term "ABR threshold" should not be confused with hearing threshold as determined with pure-tone signals, since ABRs and the stimuli used to generate them are substantially different from behavioral responses to sound (Sininger, Abdala, and Cone-Wesson, 1997; Worthington and Peters, 1980). Latency is the most widely used ABR measurement value. There are two basic latency values which can be obtained from the ABR waveform: absolute latencies and relative or interwave latencies. Absolute latencies are defined as the elapsed time from stimulus onset to the ABR peak of interest. Interwave latency is the difference between the absolute latency of two wave peaks (e.g., waves I and V) and implies that it is the elapsed time between one generator site and another. Although not entirely accurate, this is often referred to as "central transmission time" or "neural conduction time" (Don, Ponton, Eggermont, and Kwong, 1998). Absolute latencies of the ABR have an inverse relationship with stimulus level, in that as intensity is decreased, latencies increase (Hecox and Galambos, 1974). This latency change is roughly equivalent for all waves of the response, suggesting that peripheral changes (such as stimulus level or peripheral hearing loss), will first affect the latency of wave I with subsequent waves shifting accordingly.

In general, the interwave latencies are not substantially affected by peripheral hearing loss (Fowler and Noffsinger, 1983). Prolongation of the wave I to V interval suggests a disorder that involves the retrocochlear portion of the auditory pathway, rather than the peripheral portion as with a conductive or sensory hearing loss (Eggermont, Don, & Brackmann, 1980; Musiek & Lee, 1995). If all waves within the ABR are available for latency measurement, a disorder affecting the peripheral portion of the pathway can usually be differentiated from a disorder involving the central portion (Musiek, Josey, and Glasscock, 1986). This is of great advantage in infant hearing assessment, for example, when attempting to differentiate between those with significant hearing loss and those with neurological disorder or immaturity (Hecox, Cone, & Blaw, 1981). It should be noted that wave I is not always easily resolved in the ABR, particularly in patients who have substantial high-frequency hearing loss (Bauch, Rose, & Harner, 1982).

Getting Ready: Recording Considerations and Set-up

Electrodes and electrode array: The use of disposable electrodes, usually silver/silver chloride impregnated adhesive Mylar, are typically the standard of care in infant electrophysiologic recordings. We have had good experience with this type of electrode and find it superior to other electrode types with regard to infection control. Cleaning the skin at each electrode site with water and, typically, a commercial electrode paste, increases the likelihood of low (< 5kΩ) electrode/skin impedance. Unless otherwise indicated, we use a single-channel recording approach, placing electrodes at Fz (just below the anterior fontanelle) and at each mastoid (A1, A2). Balanced impedance across electrode sites is preferable, putatively resulting in improved common mode rejection and, it follows, increased response amplitude above the background physiologic noise.

Amplifier filters: Improving the relationship between the response and background physiologic noise is fundamental to recording short-latency potentials and filtering unwanted noise is an important part of the process. For adult recordings, when using clicks or high-frequency tonal stimuli, typical band pass settings are 100–3000 Hz. For low-frequency stimuli, it is common use a high pass setting of 30 or 40 Hz which allows for the recording of the resultant broader, lower-frequency ABR waveform. We routinely use a 30 Hz high-pass setting in our clinical band pass settings (3000 Hz low-pass) when assessing infants, regardless of stimulus frequency (Stuart & Yang, 1994). This added low frequency activity in the ABR adds to the amplitude of ABR wave V as well as the negative trough following wave V. The resulting increased amplitude aids in the identification of the wave V complex to lower-frequency spectral content in the infant ABR waveform, particularly using low-frequency stimuli. It is possible, of course, that in ABRs recorded with a reduced high-pass setting the increased wave V amplitude is due to the inclusion of additional noise rather than an actual increase the ABR amplitude. Therefore, this increased amplitude is not necessarily all beneficial, and care must be taken when using a 30 to 40 Hz high-pass setting that additional noise is not introduced into the response. A reduced high-pass setting should be reserved for when the infant is sleeping quietly.

Analysis window: To guard against truncating the later components of the ABR in infant patients, we use a 15 ms analysis window for all of our recordings. This is sufficient under most conditions, including allowance for the time delay imparted by the insert transducer. By keeping a constant time window, the visual display is uniform from one waveform to the next and across frequencies. Occasionally, using a 500 Hz tone burst at low intensity levels, a time window of 20 ms is required.

Signal averaging: Our experience has shown that a maximum of 2,000 stimulus repetitions (and subsequent trigger pulses) are sufficient to resolve the ABR in most infants. When the recording conditions are less than optimal (e.g., increased physiologic noise) or in the presence of high-frequency hearing loss, additional repetitions may be necessary. However, since the signal to noise ratio improves by the √ of the number of repetitions, improvement of the signal to noise ratio by 2 requires that the typical 2000 sweeps be multiplied by the square of that number (4), resulting in 8000 repetitions. We find an economy of time by keeping the number of sweeps fixed at 2000 and repeating the recordings two or three times to judge the extent to which the repeated waveforms replicate the initial averaged waveform.

Transducers: Insert earphones are the transducer of choice in infant/pediatric assessment. Insert transducers provide a more consistent and comfortable delivery of the stimulus in the ear canal (compared to a supra-aural earphone) and guard against low-frequency acoustic leakage (Johnson & Nelson, 1991). Importantly, insert earphones eliminate any possibility of ear canal collapse, a common problem with supra-aural phones, and the subsequent false-positive findings. For frequency specific applications, the ~0.9 ms delay between the electrical event at the transducer and delivery of the stimulus to the ear canal afforded by insert earphones is essential for separation of the stimulus artifact from early portions of the response. Clearly, an adjustment in absolute latency (i.e., the subtraction of the 0.9 ms delay) is essential for accurate comparison to norms derived using standard earphones.

Bone conduction: Bone conduction ABR has become an indispensable tool in pediatric assessment using the ABR (Campbell, Harris, Hendricks, & Sirimanna, 2004). We use standard bone oscillators in our recordings; in our experience the Radioear B-71 delivers the least artifact. We achieve a 50–55 dBnHL stimulus level using the stimulus output of the ABR system. As with air-conducted stimuli, age-matched latency norms are required although the ABR visual detection threshold is the typical measurement used in our clinic. For adequate stimulus levels in infant testing, placement of the oscillator on the mastoid is mandatory (Stuart, Yang, & Stenstrom, 1990) since incompletely ossified skull sutures result in substantial attenuation of bone conduction stimuli delivered to the forehead. One of the challenges in bone conduction ABR testing with infants is obtaining a good placement of the bone vibrator and transmission of the stimulus on the mastoid of the child. To ensure good transmission, adequate tension must be applied to the oscillator. On our pediatric patients, either a pediatric headset or a commercially available Velcro headband is used; neither are ideal, both can provide satisfactory placement and consistent pressure.

Repetition rate: We have found that a moderate repetition rate of 33.3/sec results in a high-quality waveform. This rate is slow enough to be free from the adaptation effects of higher stimulus repetition rates and yet rapid enough to acquire sufficient data to estimate hearing levels in each ear in a reasonable amount of time. It would seem that the fastest rate of presentation would be the most efficient since the identification of ABR wave V is the primary goal of these recordings, however there is a trade-off between overall response clarity and repetition rate. Further, there is a complex relationship between repetition rate and high intensities revealed in the ABRs of infants that can be avoided by keeping the rate below 30 or 40/sec. If no response or poor waveform morphology is noted to tone burst stimuli, then we typically use a slow-rate click (13.3/sec) at a high intensity level (90 dBnHL) to maximize the generation of the response.

Stimulus Considerations

Stimulus frequency: Whenever possible, it is our practice to use tone burst stimuli to generate ABR waveforms for estimating hearing levels in infants. The use of these stimuli, usually between 500 and 4000 Hz, is the most straightforward approach for estimating frequency-specific hearing levels and obtaining some semblance of hearing loss configuration. With this approach, we can typically obtain hearing level estimates at 3 or 4 frequencies in each ear in one recording session. These data provide sufficient resolution of estimated hearing levels across frequency to initiate hearing aid fitting and develop a family habilitation plan. Under circumstances where no response can be generated using high frequency tone bursts, we will turn to broadband clicks as our most abrupt stimulus and attempt to obtain high frequency hearing information. However, the putative high-frequency specificity of clicks can change in the presence of high frequency hearing loss leaving doubt regarding the frequencies tested.

We use digitally generated tone bursts that have a 3-cycle rise/fall with no plateau gated using a Blackman window (Gorga, Kaminski, Beauchaine, & Jesteadt, 1988; Gorga & Thornton, 1989; Orlando & Folsom, 1995). This creates a stimulus that is sufficiently abrupt to provide the necessary neural synchrony to generate a response as well as a satisfactorily narrow spectrum, with reduced side lobes, for greatest possible frequency specificity. In particular, the reduced spectral side lobes obtained with a Blackman window are an advantage when differentiating hearing levels across frequency in a steeply sloping (or rarely, rising) hearing loss configuration.

We maintain a constant 30 or 40 Hz high-pass filter setting infant recordings and this works well for our frequency specific recordings as well (Sininger, 1995). As described above, the ~1 ms delay introduced by separation between the electrical event at the transducer and the delivery of the stimulus in the ear canal is usually adequate to avoid substantial stimulus artifact, in particular any interference in observing a clear wave V. To avoid any latency shift and subsequent response cancellation, we do not alternate the polarity of the stimulus. As described below, we use a sequence of 2000 and 500 Hz in each ear and then fill in 4000 Hz and 1000 Hz as time allows.

Stimulus intensity: As is true for most clinical laboratories, we establish hearing levels (re 0 dBnHL) for our stimuli by averaging the behavioral hearing thresholds for the stimulus using a jury of young, normal hearing listeners. For our click stimuli (generated using a 100 μsec electric pulse to the insert transducer in a 2 cc coupler) 0 dBnHL corresponds to 36 dBpSPL which is typical of other clinical labs using a 33.3/second repetition rate (Stapells, Picton, and Smith, 1982). For frequency specific stimuli, the underlying dBpSPL is dependent on such a high number of factors (e.g., windowing, duration) that any description of stimulus SPL would be idiosyncratic and ineffective as guidance for the clinician. The output limit of our clinical system is 90 to 110 dBnHL across frequency. Our sequence of intensity presentations is described below.

Age-matched norms: Published data are available for normative values across age for latency and thresholds to click and frequency-specific stimuli (e.g., Gorga, Kaminski, Beauchaine, Jesteadt, & Neely, 1989; Gorga, Reiland, Beauchaine, Worthington, & Jesteadt, 1987). Clinics can rely on published values until adequate clinic normative data have been gathered.

Measuring the ABR

Sleep: Due to the limited number of clinics available to do sedated ABR testing, and the risks inherent in administering sedatives, many clinics opt to perform ABR testing without sedation. At the UW Pediatric Audiology Clinic, ABR tests are routinely and successfully performed on children under the age of 12 months during natural sleep. To maximize the length of the child's sleep session, parents are given specific information by phone and by letter instructing them to bring the child to the clinic tired and ready to take a nap, with no significant sleep within 2 hours prior to the appointment. After the electrodes have been applied to the child, the parent is seated in a comfortable lounge chair in a darkened room and given time to soothe the child to sleep in the parent's arms.

Test session protocol: The goal of a diagnostic ABR is to determine the degree of hearing loss in each ear, the nature of the loss, and the configuration of the loss. Ideally, frequency specific thresholds will be obtained for stimuli from 500 to 4000 Hz in each ear, in addition to bone-conduction testing. However, audiologists cannot presume to obtain all of this information in one test session due to the possibility of a child awakening and the testing being terminated at any point. In our clinic, we establish a clinic plan for the session that delineates the starting ear, level, and frequency order, given what is known about the patient. Other tests in the battery that can be completed prior to the ABR session will be helpful in guiding testing sequence. Immittance testing provides crucial information about the status of the outer and middle ear systems prior to the ABR test. Results of OAE testing are not crucial prior to the ABR, but are often available in patients who have failed OAE screenings. However, OAE results are a critical piece of the test battery in patients with absent ABRs in distinguishing between profound hearing loss and auditory dysynchrony/neuropathy.

Plan for testing: Beginning the session with frequency specific stimuli ensures that if limited threshold information is obtained, clinical decisions can be made regarding hearing aids and intervention. Some audiologists prefer to start with a broadband click stimulus. However, the click is an ideal stimulus for screening purposes and neurological assessment, but is not ideal for determining frequency-specific ABR thresholds and the hearing loss configuration. Recording ABR thresholds to 4 frequencies per ear is ideal, but it is unlikely that all frequencies can be completed in both ears in one test session.

Frequency: ABR thresholds at 2000 Hz and 500 Hz are recommended as minimum frequencies for establishing estimates of audiometric configuration. If time allows, additional thresholds at 1000, and 4000 Hz should be established in each ear. In our clinic, we use a frequency order that alternates between high and low frequency stimuli (2000, 500, 4000, 1000 Hz), so that if the session is terminated suddenly, we have thresholds at both ends of the audiometric frequency range. If ABR responses are absent at maximum output levels or if the waveform morphology is poor, then we move to a slow rate (13.3) click stimulus to maximize recording the ABR in patients whose neurological integrity is compromised.

Which ear first? If previous hearing screening information indicates abnormal results only in one ear, than testing should begin with "the ear of concern," ensuring that if testing is halted, information is at least obtained about this ear. However, it also crucial to establish hearing levels in both ears, even if previous screening results showed concerns about only one ear. We typically obtain thresholds for 2000 and 500 Hz in the first ear, and then adjust the child's position in the parent's arms, insert the earphone in the second ear and obtain thresholds for 2000 and 500 Hz. Alternating frequently between ears increases the risk of disturbing and waking the child.

Starting level: Ideally, ABR recordings should begin approximately 20 dB above ABR threshold, allowing for a clear identification of wave V prior to searching for threshold. For a child who has failed previous otoacoustic emission testing, a 50 dB starting level is recommended. If the starting level is too high, the audiologist will spend an inordinate amount of time decreasing the level to find threshold, with the added potential of awakening a child with a high level stimulus. If the starting level is too low, the audiologist will be starting data collection at a level where the ABR is not observed. For a child who has had a previous ABR screening at specific levels, then starting level should be increased accordingly. For example, for a child who has failed a screening ABR with no responses at a 70 dBnHL screening level, we would recommend starting testing at 90 dBnHL.

Step size: A down 20, up 10 dB step size is recommended to efficiently establish hearing levels. However, for the purposes of precise setting of hearing aids based on ABR thresholds, a 5 dB step size is worthwhile.

Bone conduction: ABR bone conduction testing is a crucial piece of information in diagnosing hearing loss in determining if an air-bone gap exists and in quantifying the degree of the conductive component. Because of bone oscillator output limitations and stimulus artifact from the oscillator, maximum output levels are typically 50–55 dBnHL. Bone conduction testing should be instituted early enough in the session before the child awakes, typically after both 2000 and 500 Hz air conduction thresholds have been established in each ear.

Masking: During air conduction testing, using insert earphones, the interaural attenuation of the stimulus is typically 70 dB (Van Campen, Sammeth, & Peek, 1990) in infants and children. Therefore, if the difference between air conduction thresholds across ears is greater than 70 dB at any test frequency, narrow band noise masking must be presented to the non-test ear to prevent crossover. During bone conduction testing, infants typically show interaural attention of 25 dB (Yang, Rupert, & Mousegian, 1987).

Maximizing accuracy of the session:

Trouble-shooting: As the clinician moves quickly during the recording session, we find that errors can arise in the transducer choice, electrode array and the clinician may unknowingly be presenting stimuli to the wrong ear, wrong transducer, or recording from the contralateral ear. After making any changes in electrodes or transducer, we do a crosscheck of the patient's set-up prior to resuming data collection. Likewise, if at any point in the session the ABR is absent or poorly formed, we pause data collection and complete a crosscheck. This crosscheck involves checking the placement of the earphone, the configuration of the electrodes, and the impedance of the electrodes. It may be necessary to re-position electrodes or apply new electrodes if impedance has increased. The quality of the ABR recording is always maximized by minimizing the contribution of physiologic noise produced by movement of the child. The clinician monitors the ongoing EEG activity and pauses data collection when the child is moving.

Interpreting results: We are typically conservative in interpreting the presence of an ABR response. If there is doubt about the agreement between two averaged responses, we obtain an additional replication to "break the tie" and determine if the response is absent or present. If a response is present, the audiologist can quickly estimate and record the latency of wave V and a more careful determination of latency can be made after the end of the data collection session. Tracking the latency of wave V across dB level is helpful in determining which peak to choose as the wave V response. Referring to age-matched norms is also a crucial tool in assisting the audiologist in interpreting the ABR. For example, wave V thresholds may be elevated and wave V latencies prolonged compared to normative values in a child with conductive hearing loss.

Making recommendations based on ABR results: At the completion of an ABR test session, the audiologist is often in the position of diagnosing hearing loss for the first time in an infant or young child. If inadequate information has been obtained such that the audiologist cannot make conclusions about degree and type of hearing loss in each ear, the audiologist may need to have the child return to complete data collection. However, typically we are able to complete an ABR test session using the protocol described and counsel the parents of the child regarding the degree of hearing loss for low and high frequency stimuli in both ears, the nature of the loss (conductive vs. sensorineural). In addition, the audiologist is able to use data from immittance and otoacoustic emission testing to complete the final diagnosis.

MIDDLE LATENCY RESPONSE

The middle latency response (MLR) was first reported by Geisler, Frishkopt, and Rosenblith in 1958. The MLR occurs in the epoch following the auditory brainstem response (ABR) but before the late latency response (LLR) covering the range of 12–70 milliseconds (msec). Although the MLR was once considered to be an "early" response, after much interest in the ABR, it was re-named the "middle" response.

There has been considerable controversy and some misunderstanding surrounding this recording which may have limited its clinical use. The MLR time epoch has been defined as 10–80 ms (Kraus, Kileny, & McGee, 1994), 10–50 ms (Polich & Starr, 1983) and 12–50 msec (Davis, 1976). Clearly, the post-stimulus analysis window for these responses is not rigid. The MLR is characterized by negative and positive waves listed alphabetically, Na, Pa, Nb, and Pb. Normally, the positive peaks are more useful diagnostically. In terms of identification, wave Pa occurs around 25 msec and wave Pb occurs approximately at 50 msec. Often there is a small positive waveform before Pa labeled Po. A normal MLR recording is depicted in Figure 7–4.

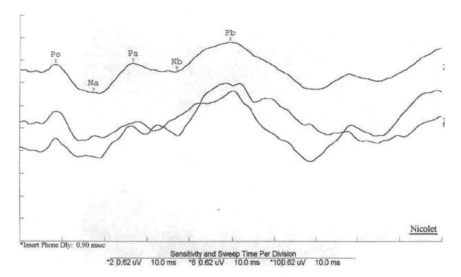

FIGURE 7–4.   This figure shows a "normal" MLR from a seven year old male. The top tracing is a summed response of the two lower individual recordings.

Originally, Geisler et al. (1958) reported that these potentials were neurogenic in nature, but this was later disputed by Bickford, Jacobson, & Cody (1964) who attributed these potentials to myogenic artifact from the neck and head muscles. Although at high intensities, myogenic activity can interfere with these recordings, investigators have shown that at low or moderate stimulus levels, neurogenic activity is responsible for these potentials (Harker, Hosick, Voots, & Mendel, 1977). It is important for the clinician to recognize when myogenic activity is present as it can be mistaken for neurogenic responses (Cody, 1976; Picton, Hillyard, Kraus, & Galambos, 1974). The use of earlobes, rather than the mastoids as reference electrode sites, may reduce the post-auricular muscle artifact.

Each wave in the MLR is the result of the activation of multiple generator sites. The underlying auditory generators of the MLR include the thalamocortical pathway (Kileny, Paccioretti, & Wilson, 1987; Kraus, Ozdamar, Hier, & Stein, 1982; Ozdamar & Kraus, 1983), the reticular formation (Kraus, Kileny, & McGee, 1994), and the inferior colliculus (McGee, Kraus, Comperatore, & Nicol, 1991). Specifically, the early middle latency components (waves Na, and Pa) might arise from the medial geniculate and thalamus, while the association areas of the cortex might be responsible for waves Nb and Pb (Geisler et al., 1958).

Recording Considerations

Much of the debate about the utility of the MLR has stemmed from the recording parameters. The average peak-to-peak amplitude of wave Pa is about 1 μvolt in normal adult subjects. MLR amplitude will increase and there will be a slight de-

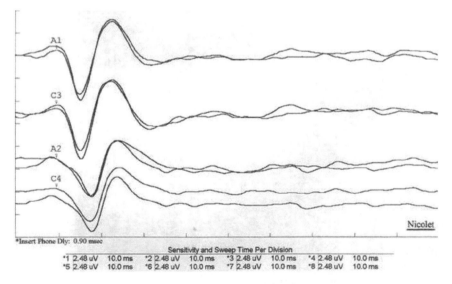

FIGURE 7–5.   Post-auricular muscle (PAM) artifact is evident in all electrode channels of this recording. This muscle artifact which occludes wave Pa is approximately 7μVolts in amplitude.

crcasc in latency with increasing stimulus intensity to moderate levels, around 50–60 dBnHL (Ozdamar & Kraus, 1983). Approximately 500 stimulus presentations are required for one averaged response. Usually clinicians collect several averages and later sum the individual averaged responses. Stimulus onset or rise time in the frequency specific tone pips may also affect the amplitude of the MLR response (Lane, Kupperman, & Goldstein, 1971).

Recordings are made from the scalp. Most often, the electrode placement follows the 10–20 system of the International Federation (Jasper, 1958). Recordings are made from vertex to earlobes (A1 or A2) or mastoids (M1 or M2) as the reference. Although one or two channel recordings are routinely performed for most evaluations, a four channel recording using additional electrode recording sites is recommended when completing an auditory processing disorder (APD) evaluation.

The MLR is affected by various stimulus parameters. MLR recordings are made to either auditory clicks or tonal stimuli. Tonal stimuli may be useful if frequency specific thresholds are desired. The latency of wave Pa is slightly earlier in response to click stimuli rather than tonal stimuli.

Much of the spectral energy of the MLR recording in a 100 msec window is bctwccn 3–3000 Hz (McGee, Kraus, & Manfredi, 1988), but some investigators may change the low pass filter to 3000 Hz and simultaneously record the ABR and MLR (Ozdamar and Kraus, 1983). However, in order to accomplish this, a sophisticated averaging computer that will allow recording or offline data analysis in dual time windows is necessary. The choice of filter bands (narrow vs. wide) will also affcct the morphology of the waveform, with the narrower bandwidth sometimes causing either ringing or distortions of the waveform.

Stimulus presentation rates of less than 5/sec are recommended for optimal amplitude. Higher stimulus rates produce some amplitude decline and make detection of wave Pa difficult in infants (Jerger, Chmiel, Glaze, & Frost, 1987). Even though the MLR recording occurs between 10 and 70 msec, the time window for the MLR recording should be at least 100 msec.

Subject Age

Although the MLR is primarily used with adults, it can be recorded in infants. However, there are significant differences in these populations. Suzuki, Hirabayahi, and Kobayashi (1983) reported prolonged MLR latencies and poorer morphology in infants as well as greater intra-subject variability. Wolf and Goldstein (1980) reported that only the recording that is ipsilateral to the ear that is stimulated is present in neonatal recordings; the contralateral is not. In normal adults, both ipsilataeral and contralateral recordings are present, regardless of the ear that is stimulated.

The detectability of wave Pa increases with age. In general, the MLR recording in children does not reach adult like maturity until 8–10 years of age. Perhaps this is one factor that discouraged clinicians from utilizing this recording. However, these recordings are proving to be valuable in assessing maturation of the central auditory nervous system. Researchers have reported an increase in Pa amplitude with age (Kelly-Ballweber & Dobie, 1984; Chambers & Griffiths, 1991) but have also found that amplitude is affected by peripheral hearing sensitivity. The latency of wave Pa remains stable with increasing age (Erwin & Buchwald, 1986) after reaching mature values.

Endogenous Factors

The MLR is not affected by attention to the stimulus. It may be obtained while the subject is ignoring the stimulus, reading a book, watching a video, or quietly playing a hand-held game.

However, investigators have reported that sleep state can interfere with the detectability of the MLR (Kileny, 1983; Krause, Smith, Reed, Stein, & Cartee, 1985; Suzuki et al., 1983) and that during stage 4 of sleep, the MLR is usually absent (Kraus, McGee, & Comperatore, 1989). There have been conflicting reports on the effect of sleep on wave Pa in adults. Osterhamel, Shallop, & Terkildsen (1985) reported a decrease in amplitude as a function of sleep stage. The MLR can be recorded in stage 1 and 2 of sleep, sometimes in stage 3 but is not detectable in stage 4 sleep. Similarly, general anesthesia eliminates the response of the MLR (Goff, Allison, & Lyons, et al., 1977).

Threshold Assessment

There is little doubt that the ABR is the test of choice for high frequency electrophysiological threshold measures. However, without using a carefully structured toneburst, high frequency energy can limit their value for low frequency threshold measures. The MLR is less dependent upon neural synchrony and may be used in assessing low frequency thresholds (Kraus & McGee, 1990; Xu, De Vel, Vink, & Van Cauwenberge, 1995). This may be very in assessing thresholds in patients suffering from brainstem lesions which affect neural synchrony. However, because of the effect of sleep on the MLR and its variability in infants, the MLR is limited in its usefulness for threshold assessment. Several investigations have reported similar thresholds for both the ABR and MLR for low frequency thresholds (Kavanagh, Harker, & Tyler, 1984; Mackersie, Down, & Stappells, 1993; Oates & Stapells, 1997; Wu and Stapells, 1994).

40 Hz Response

Often the 40 Hz recording has been used in assessing hearing thresholds. This recording was first described by Galambos, Makeig, & Talmachoff, 1981. This recording is elicited by presenting an acoustic stimulus at a rate of 40 per second. The response mimics the stimulating sinusoid so that there is a positive waveform at the period of the 40 Hz stimulation rate or every 25 msec. Results of the 40 Hz recordings are similar to audiometric thresholds. Again, though, this response is not reliable in young children and is affected by sleep, sedation, and anesthesia (Plourde & Picton, 1990; Stappels, Galambos, Costello, & Makeig, 1988). A 40

Hz response can also be elicited by visual and somatosensory stimuli (Galambos et al., 1981). It is important to note that the underlying generators for this response are not completely understood.

Assessment for Cochlear Implant Function

Investigators have reported that MLR may be useful in cochlear implant evaluation (Gardi, 1985; Miyamoto, 1986; Kileny & Kermink, 1987; Kileny, Kermink, & Miller, 1989). Electrically generated MLRs (EMLRs) are very similar in morphology to those generated acoustically. However latencies in the EMLR are shorter. The EMLR has been used as an objective assessment of neural integrity in pre-operative cochlear implant evaluations and as an objective measurement of comfortable listening level in post-operative cochlear implant mapping sessions.

Auditory Processing Disorder Assessment

The MLR recording can be a valuable tool in assessing maturity of the central auditory pathway. Inter-subject variability of the MLR is great in the pediatric population, so there are no normative latency and amplitude data available for very young children. Again, it is important to note that the MLR does not reach adult maturity until around age 8–10 years. However, it is significant if the MLR is absent (Chermak & Musiek, 1997). The MLR recording is also proving its usefulness in assessing the efficacy of some APD therapy programs.

Generally, waves Na and Pa are the only waves that are used diagnostically in APD evaluations (Chermak & Musiek, 1997) providing amplitude and latency measures for interpretation. However, amplitude may be a more sensitive measure than latency (Kraus et al., 1982; Scherg & von Cramon, 1986).

A four channel recording is recommended for APD evaluations. The amplitude of wave Pa is compared when measured from vertex to earlobes or mastoids and from coronal electrode sites (C3 and C4) to earlobes or mastoids. Amplitude measures that are less than 50 percent in comparison to other electrode sites are diagnostically significant. If there is a lesioned area, the amplitude from the electrode closest to the lesioned area will be compromised. This reduced amplitude is referred to as an electrode effect (Musiek, Baran, & Pinheiro, 1994). An example of an electrode effect for C3 is shown in Figure 7–6. This effect was evident regardless of the ear that was stimulated, i.e. an ipsilateral or a contralateral response.

Other investigators have also reported "Ear Effects," a reduction of the amplitude of one ear, regardless of which ear is stimulated (Chermak & Musiek, 1997). However, the "ear-effect" is not as diagnostically significant as the electrode effect (Kelly, Lee, Charette, & Musiek, 1996; Shehata-Dieler, Shimizu, Soliman, & Tusa, 1991).

MLR recordings have also been useful in documenting plasticity of the central auditory nervous system Previous investigators have reported increased amplitude of the MLR after the patient has completed an intensive auditory training program (Morlet, Berlin, Norman, & Ray, 2003). Other investigators have re-

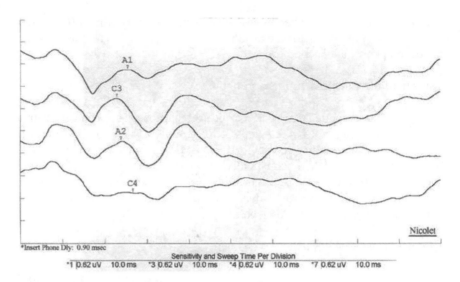

FIGURE 7–6.   These four tracings are summed responses for electrodes A1, C3, A2, and C4 for right auditory stimulation. An electrode effect is evident for tracing C4 as wave Pa is not evident in this tracing.

ported the appearance of wave Pb after intensive auditory training (Morlet et al., 2003). Greater amplitude of wave Pa is depicted in Figure 7–7 for one patient showing both the right and left ears post Fast ForWord. Although post testing showed improvement in behavioral tests, the MLR offers objective evidence of changes in the auditory nervous system.

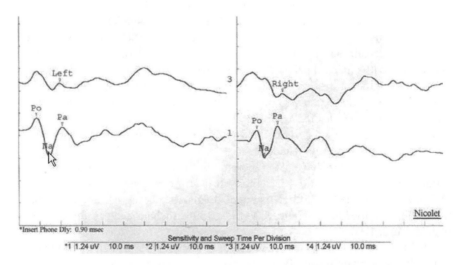

FIGURE 7–7.   Improved MLRs as displayed in tracings 1 and 2 are evident for both left and right auditory stimulation after Fast ForWord™ training. Waves 3 and 4 are pre-test recordings for the left and right ears, respectively. All tracings are summed responses of 2 individual averages.

Learning Disorders

Investigators have reported conflicting results in the MLR recordings in children with learning disorders. Arehole, Augustine, & Simhadri (1995) reported prolonged Pa latency in 5 of 11 subjects with learning disorders. Other researchers have reported similar findings, i.e., abnormal MLRs in a group of children with learning disabilities (Jerger, Martin & Jerger, 1987; Kileny et al., 1987). However, Kraus, et al. (1985) reported no difference in the MLR recording in children with learning disorders and a normal group. Differences in these findings may be in part related to the wide heterogeneity of the group and selection criterion into each group.

Clinical Populations

Although most clinicians have used only waves Na and Pa for clinical interpretation, investigators have reported interesting neurological findings associated with wave Pb. Wave Pb has been reported to be abnormal in patients with Alzheimer's disease (Buchwald, Erwin, Read, Van Lancker, & Cummings 1989). These investigators reported a decrease in Pb amplitude in comparison to normal subjects. They attributed this decrease to a dysfunction in the cholinergic cells found in the midbrain, that are responsible for wave Pb. It must be noted that this finding has not been used as a diagnostic marker for Alzheimer's disease.

Abnormal wave Pbs (absent, or delayed) have also been reported in patients with Parkinson's disease (Pekkonen et al., 1998). However after a surgical procedure (posterior ansapallidotomy), wave Pb returned to normal (Mohammed et al., 1996).

The MLR has also been studied in patients with multiple sclerosis (Celebisoy, 1996; Robinson & Rudge, 1977; Versino Bergamaschi, Romani, Banfi, et al., 1992), many of whom may also have had cortial lesions. Often these patients have absent waves Na and Pa. Robinson and Ruge (1977) reported normal ABR recordings and abnormal MLR recordings in 12% of their patients. Analyses of serial MLR recordings could distinguish between active and quiescent disease state. This supports the contention that the MLR may be valuable in assessing patients with neurologic diseases.

Of interest in interpreting wave Pb is the finding that left-handed patients show a longer Pb latency than right handed adults (Hood, Martin, & Berlin, 1990). This finding was later supported by Stewart, Jerger, and Lew (1993) who reported prolonged Pa and Pb latencies in left handed individuals. Therefore, it is important to note the handedness of patients and subjects.

Central Lesions

Abnormal MLR recordings have been reported in patients with central and temporal lesions (Woods, Knight, & Neville, 1984) and absent temporal lobes (Hood, Berlin, & Allen, 19—) Often, however, in these types of cases, the MLR may be normal (Kraus et al., 1982; Kileny et al., 1987). Investigators must compare the amplitude of the response from various recording sites to determine if there is an

TABLE 7–1
MLR

Stimulus	100 μsec clicks
Rate	3.3/second
Stimulus Level	75 dB nHL
Filter	10Hz -1500Hz
Electrode Montage	Cz-A1, Cz-A2
	C3-A1, C4-A2
Time Window	100 msec

ear or electrode effect. Often the amplitude of the MLR will be reduced over the lesioned area.

Clinical Use

The MLR is routinely recorded as part of the APD test battery. Stimulus parameters are listed in Table 7–1.

First, the latency of waves Na and Pa are noted. Next, amplitude comparisons across the electrode sites are analyzed to determine if there is an ear effect or electrode effect. The presence of wave Pb is also reported for each recording. Recordings can be made while the patient watches a video, or quietly plays a handheld game.

REFERENCES

Arehole, S., Augustine, L. E., & Simhadri, R. (1995). Middle latency response in children with learning disabilities: Preliminary findings. *Journal of Communication Disorders, 28,* 21–38.

ASHA. (1990) *Competencies in auditory evoked potential measurement and clinical applications.* Working Group on Auditory Evoked Potential Measurements of the Committee on Audiologic Evaluation (Suppl 2).

Bauch, C. D., Rose, D. E., & Harner, S. G. (1982). Auditory brainstem response results from 255 patients with suspected retrocochlear involvement. *Ear Hear, 3,* 83–86.

Bickford, R. G., Jacobson, J. L., & Cody, T. R. (1964). Nature of average evoked potentials to sound and other stimuli in man. *Annals of the New York Academy of Sciences, 112,* 204–223.

Buchwald, J. S., Erwin, R. J., Read, S., Van Lancker, D., & Cummings, J. L. (1989). Mid-latency auditory evoked responses: Differential abnormality of P1 in Alzheimer's disease. *Electroencephalography Clinical Neurophysiology, 74,* 378–384.

Campbell, P. E., Harris, C. M., Hendricks, S., & Sirimanna, T. (2004). Bone conduction auditory brainstem responses in infants. *Journal of Laryngol Otology, 118,* 117–122.

Celebisoy, N., Aydogdu, I., Ekmekci, O., & Akurekli, O. (1996). Middle latency auditory evoked potentials (MLAEPs) in MS. *Acta Neurologica Scandinavica, 93,* 318–321.

Chambers, R. D., & Griffiths, S. K. (1991). Effects of age on the adult auditory middle latency response. *Hearing Research 51,* 1–10.

Chermak, G. D., & Musiek, F. E. (1997). Central Auditory Processing Disorders New Perspectives. San Diego, CA: Singular.

Coats, A. C., & Dickey, J. R. (1970). Non-surgical recording of human auditory nerve action potentials and cochlear microphonics. *Annals of Otology, Rhinology and Larygology; 29,* 844–851.

Coats, A. C. (1981). The summating potential and Meniere's disease. *Arch Otolaryngol 104,* 199–208.

Cody, D. T. R. (1976). Averaged responses evoked by acoustic stimuli. In C. A. Smith & J. A. Vernon (Eds.), Handbook of auditory and vestibular research methods (pp. 246–279). Springfield, IL: Charles C. Thomas.

Cullen, J. K., Ellis, M. S., Berlin, C. I., & Lousteau, R. J. (1972). Human acoustic nerve action potential recordings from the tympanic membrane without anesthesia. *Acta Otolaryngologica 74,* 15–22.

Davis, H. (1976). Principles of electric response audiometry. *Annals of Otology, Rhinology and Laryngology, 85,* 1–96.

Devaiah, A. K., Dawson. K. L., Ferraro, J. A., & Ator, G. (2003). Utility of area curve ratio: Electrocochleography in early Meniere's Disease. *Arch Otolaryngol Head Neck Surg, 129,* 547–551.

Don, M., Ponton, C.W., Eggermont, J.J., & Kwong, B. (1998). The effects of sensory hearing loss on cochlear filter times estimated from auditory brainstem latencies. *J Acoust Soc Amer, 104,* 2,280–2,289.

Durrant, J. D., & Ferraro, J. A. (1991). Analog model of human click-elicited SP and effects of high-pass filtering. *Ear and Hearing 12,* 144–148.

Durrant, J. D. (1986). Combined ECochG-ABR versus conventional ABR recordings. *Seminars in Hearing 7,* 289–305.

Erwin, R., & Burchwald, J. S. (1986). Middle latency auditory evoked responses: Differential effects of sleep in the human. *Electroencephalography and Clinical Neurophysiology, 65,* 383–392.

Ferraro, J. A., Blackwell, W., Mediavilla, S. J., & Thedinger, B. (1994). Normal summating potential to tonebursts recorded from the tympanic membrane in humans. *J Am Acad Aud 5,* 17–23.

Ferraro, J. A. (2000). Electrocochleography. In R. Roesser, M. Valente & H. Hosford-Dunn (Eds.), *Audiology: diagnoses* (pp. 425–450). New York: Thieme.

Ferraro, J. A., & Durrant, J. D. (2006). Electrocochleography in the evaluation of Meniere's disease/endolymphatic hydrops. *J. Am. Acad. Aud. 17,* 45–68

Ferraro, J. A., & Ferguson, R. (1989). Tympanic ECochG and conventional ABR: A combined approach for the identification of wave I and the I-V interwave interval. *Ear and Hearing 3,* 161–166.

Ferraro, J. A., Thedinger, B., Mediavilla, S. J., & Blackwell, W. (1994). Human summating potential to tonebursts: Observations on TM versus promontory recordings in the same patient. *J Am Acad Aud 6,* 217–224.

Ferraro, J. A., & Tibbils, R. (1999). SP/AP area ratio in the diagnosis of Meniere's disease. *Am J Aud 8,* 21–28.

Ferraro, J. A. (1992). Electrocochleography: How, Part I. *Audiology Today 4,* 26–28.

Ferraro J. A. (1997). *Laboratory exercises in auditory evoked potentials.* San Diego, CA: Singular Publishing Group, Inc.

Galambos, R., Makeig, S., & Talmachoff, P. J. (1981). A 40-Hz auditory potential recorded from the human scalp. *Proc Natl Acad Sci USA 78,* 2643–2647.

Gardi, J. N. (1985). Human brain stem and middle latency responses to electrical stimulation: A Preliminary observation. In R. Schindler & M. Merzenich (Eds.), *Cochlear implants* (pp. 351–363). New York: Raven Press.

Geisler, C. D., Frishkopf, L. S., & Rosenblith, W. A. (1958). Extracranial responses to acoustic clicks in man. *Science, 128,* 1210–1211.

Gibson, W. P. R., Moffat, D. A., & Ramsden, R. T. (1977). Clinical electrocochleography in the diagnosis and management of Meniere's disorder. *Audiology 16,* 389–401.

Goff, W. R, Allison, T., & Lyons, W. (1977). The functional neuroanatomy of eventrelated potentials. In E. Callaway, P. Tueting, and S. H. Koslow (Eds), *Event related brain potentials in man.* New York: Academic Press.

Gorga, M. P., & Thornton, A. R. (1989). The choice of stimuli for ABR measurements. *Ear Hear, 10,* 217–230.

Gorga, P. M., Kaminski, J. R., Beauchaine, K. A., & Jesteadt, W. (1988). Auditory brainstem responses to tone bursts in normally hearing subjects. *J Speech Hear Res, 31,* 87–97.

Gorga, P. M., Kaminski, J. R., Beauchaine, K. A., Jesteadt, W., & Neely, S. T. (1989). Auditory brainstem responses from children three months to three years of age: II. Normal patterns of response. *J Speech Hear Res, 32,* 281–288.

Gorga, P. M., Reiland, J. K., Beauchaine, K. A., Worthington, D. A., & Jesteadt, W. (1987). Auditory brainstem responses from graduates of an intensive care nursery: Normal patterns of response. *J Speech Hear Res, 30,* 311–318.

Harker, L. A., Hosick, E., Voots, R. J., & Mendel, M. I. (1977). Influence of succinylcholine on middle component auditory evoked potentials. *Archives of Otolaryngology, 103,* 133–37.

Harris, D., & Dallos, P. (1979). Forward masking of auditory nerve fiber responses. *J Neurophysiol 42,* 1083–1107.

Hecox, K., & Galambos, R. (1974). Brain stem auditory evoked responses in human infants and adults. *Arch Otolaryngol, 99,* 30–33.

Hood, L. J., Martin, D. A., & Berlin, C. I. (1990). Auditory evoked potentials differ at 50 miliseconds in right-and left handed listeners. *Hearing Research 45,* 115–122.

Jasper, H. H. (1958). The ten-twenty electrode system of the international federation. *Electroencephalography and Clinical Neurophysiology, 10:* 371–375.

Jerger, J., Chmiel, R., Glaze, D., & Frost, J. D. (1987). Rate and filter dependence of the middle latency responses in infants. *Audiology, 26,* 269–283.

Jerger, J., Martin, R. C., & Jerger, J. (1987). Specific auditory perceptual dysfunction in a learning disabled child. *Ear Hearing, 8,* 78–86.

Johnson, S. E., & Nelson, P. B. (1991). Real ear measures of auditory brain stem response click spectra in infants and adults. *Ear Hear, 12,* 180–183.

Kavanagh, K. T., Harker, L. A., & Tyler, R. S. (1984). Auditory brainstem and middle latency responses I. Effects of response filtering and waveform identification. II. Threshold responses to a 500 Hz tone pip. *Acta Otolaryngol; 108,* 1–12.

Kelly, T., Lee., W., Charette, L., & Musiek, F. (1996). *Middle latency evoked response sensitivity and specificity.* Paper presented at the Annual Meeting of the American Auditory Society, Salt Lake City, UT.

Kelly-Ballweber, D., & Dobie, R. A. (1994). Binaural interaction measured behaviorally and electrophysiologically in young and old adults. *Audiology, 23,* 181–194.

Kileny, P. (1983). Auditory evoked middle latency responses: Current issues. *Seminars in Hearing, 4,* 403–412.

Kileny, P. R., & Kermink, J. L. (1987). Electrically evoked middle-latency auditory potential s in cochlear implant candidates. *Archives of Otolaryngology-Head and Neck Surgery, 113,* 1072–1077.

Kileny, P. R., Paccioretti, D., & Wilson, A. F. (1987) Effects or cortical lesions on middle-latency auditory evoked responses (MLR). *Electroencephalography Clinical Neurophysiology, 66,* 108–120.

Koyuncu, M., Mason, S. M., & Shinkwin, C. (1994) Effect of hearing loss in electrocochleographic investigation of endolymphatic hydrops using tone-pip and click stimuli. *J Laryngol Otol 108,* 125–130.

Kraus, N., Kileny, P., & McGee, T. (1994). Middle latency auditory evoked potentials. In J. Katz (Ed.), Handbook of clinical audiology, 4th ed. (pp. 387–405). Baltimore, MD: Williams & Wilkins..

Kraus, N., & McGee, T. (1990). Clinical application s of the middle latency response. *Journal of the American Academy of Audiology, 1,* 130–133.

Kraus, N., McGee, T., & Comperatore, C. (1989). MLRs in children are consistently present during wakefulness stage I and REM sleep. *Ear Hear, 10,* 339–345.

Kraus, N., Ozdamar, O, Hier, D., & Stein, L, (1982). Auditory middle latency response (MLRs) in patients with cortical lesions. *Electroencephalogr Clin Neurophysiolo, 54,* 275–287.

Kraus, N., Smith, D., Reed, N., Stein, L., & Cartee, C. (1985). Auditory middle latency responses in children; effects of age and diagnostic category. *Electroencephalogr Clin Neurophysiol, 62,* 343–351.

Lane, R. H., Kupperman, G. L., & Goldstein, R. (1971). Early components of the averaged electroencephalic response in relation to rise-decay time and duration of pure tones. *Journal of Speech and Hearing Research, 14,* 408–415.

Levine, S. M., Margolis, R. H., Fournier, E. M., & Winzenburg, S. M. (1992). Tympanic electrocochleography for evaluation of endolymphatic hydrops. *Laryngoscope 102,* 614–622.

Lilly, D. J., & Black, F. O. (1989). Electrocochleography in the diagnosis of Meniere's disease. In J. B. Nadol (Ed.), Meniere's disease (pp. 369–373). Berkeley, CA: Kugler and Ghedini.

Mackersie, C., Down, K. E., & Stapells, D. R. (1993). Pure-tone masking profiles for human auditory brainstem and middle latency responses. *Hear Research, 65,* 61–68.

Margolis, R. H., Levine, S. M., Fournier, M. A., Hunter, L. L., Smith, L. L., & Lilly, D. J. (1992). Tympanic electrocochleography: Normal and abnormal patterns of response. *Audiology 31,* 18–24.

Margolis, R. H., & Lilly, D. J. (1989). Extratympanic electrocochleography: Stimulus considerations. *Asha 31,* 183(A).

Margolis, R. H., Rieks, D., Fournier, M., & Levine, S. M. (1995). Tympanic electrocochleography for diagnosis of Meniere's disease. *Arch Otolaryngol Head & Neck Surg 121,* 44–55.

McGee, T., Kraus, N., & Manfredi, C. (1988). Toward a strategy for analyzing the auditory middle latency response waveform. *Audiology, 27,* 119–130.

McGee, T., Kraus, N., Comperatore, C., & Nicole, T. (1991). Subcortical and cortical components of the MLR generating system. *Brain Research, 54,* 211 220.

Mohammed, A. S., Iacono, R. P., & Yamada, S. (1996). Normalization of middle latency auditory P1 potential following posterior ansa-pallidootomy in idiopathic Parkinson's disease. *Neurol Res, 18,* 516–520.

Morlet, T., Berlin, C. I., Norman, M., & Ray, M. (2003). Fast ForWord™: Its scientific basis and treatment effects on the human efferent auditory system. In C. I. Berlin & T. G. Weyand (Eds), The brain and sensory plasticity: Language acquisition and hearing (pp 129–148). New York: Delmar Learning.

Musiek, F. E., Josey, A. F., & Glasscock, M. E. (1986). Auditory brain stem response—Interwave measurements in acoustic neuromas. *Ear Hear, 7,* 100–105.

Musiek, F. E., & Lee, W. W. (1995). The auditory brain stem response in patients with brain stem of cochlear pathology. *Ear Hear, 16,* 631–636.

Musiek, F. E., Baran, J. A., & Pinheiro, M. L. (1994). *Neuroaudiology case studies.* San Diego: Singular Publishing Group.

Oates, P., & Stapells, D. (1997). Frequency specificity of the human auditory brainstem and middle latency responses to brief tones I. *High Pass Noise Masking J. Acoust Soc Amer, 102:* 3597–3608.

Orchik, J. G., Ge, X., & Shea, J. J. (1997). Action potential latency shift by rarefaction and condensation clicks in Meniere's disease. *Am J Otol 14,* 290–294.

Orlando, M. S., & Folsom, R. C. (1995). The effects of reversing the polarity of frequency-limited single-cycle stimuli on the human auditory brain stem response. *Ear Hear, 16,* 311–320.

Osterhammel, P. A., Shallop, J. K., & Terkildsen, K. (1985). The effect of sleep on the auditory brainstem response (ABR) and the middle latency response (MLR). *Scandinavian Audiology, 14,* 47–50.

Ozdamar, O., & Kraus, N. (1983). Auditory middle latency responses in humans. *Audiology, 22,* 34–49.

Pekkonen, E., Ahveninen, J., Virtanan, J., & Teravainen, H. (1998). Parkinson's disease selectively impairs preattentive auditory processing: An MEG study. *NeuroReport, 9,* 2949–2952.

Picton T. W., Hillyard, S. H., Frauz, H. J., & Galambos, R. (1974). Human auditory evoked potentials. *Electroenceph Clin Neurophysiol 36,* 191–200.

Picton, T. W., Hillyard, S. A., Kraus, H. I., & Galambos, R. (1974). Human auditory evoked potentials, I. Evaluation of components. *Electroencephalography & Clinical Neurophysiology 36,* 179–190.

Plourde, G., & Picton, T. W. (1990). Human auditory steady-state response during general anesthesia. *Anesth Analg 71,* 460–468.

Polich, J. M., & Starr, A. (1983). Middle-late- and long-latency auditory evoked potentials. In E. J. Moore (Ed.), Bases of auditory brain stem evoked responses (pp. 345–361). New York: Grune & Stratton.

Robinson, K., & Rudge, P. (1978). The stability of the auditory evoked potentials in normal man and patients with multiple sclerosis. *J. Neurol. Science, 36,* 147–156.

Ruth, R. A., & Lambert, P. R. (1989). Comparison of tympanic membrane to promontory electrode recordings of electrocochleographic responses in Meniere's patients. *Otolaryngol Head Neck Surg 100,* 546–552.

Sass, K., & Densert, B., Arlinger, S. (1997). Recording techniques for transtympanic electrocochleography in clinical practice. *Acta Otolaryngol (Stockh) 118,* 17–25.

Scherg, M., & von Cramon, D. (1986). Evoked dipole source potentials of the human auditory cortex. *Electroencephalogr Clin Neurophysiol, 65,* 344–360.

Schoonhoven, R., Fabius, M. A. W., & Grote, J. J. (1995). Input/output curves to tonebursts and clicks in extratympanic and transtympanic electrocochleography. *Ear & Hearing 16,* 619–630.

Shehata-Dieler, W., Shimizu, H., Soliman, S. M., & Tusa, R. J. (1991). Middle latency auditory evoked potentials in temporal lobe disorder. *Ear Hear, 12,* 377–388.

Sininger, Y. S. (1995). Filtering and spectral characteristics of averaged auditory brainstem response and background noise in infants. *J Acoust Soc Amer, 98,* 2048–2055.

Sininger, Y. S., Abdala, C., & Cone-Wesson, B. (1997). Auditory threshold sensitivity of the human neonate as measured by the auditory brainstem response. *Hear Res, 104,* 27–38.

Sohmer, H., & Feinmesser, M. (1967). Cochlear action potentials recorded from the external canal in man. *Ann Otol Rhinol Otolaryngol 76,* 427–435.

Stapells, D., Picton, T. W., & Smith, A. D. (1982). Normal hearing thresholds for clicks. *J Acoust Soc Am 72,* 74–79.

Stappels, D. R.,Galambos, R., Costello, J., & Makeig, S. (1988). Inconsistency of auditory middle latency and steady-state responses in infants. *Electroencephalography and Clinical Neurophysiology, 71,* 289–295.

Stewart, M. G., Jerger, J., & Lew, H. L. (1993). Effect of handedness on the middle latency auditory evoked potential. *American Journal of Otology, 14,* 595–600.

Stuart, A., & Yang, E. Y. (1994). Effects of high-pass filtering on the neonatal auditory brainstem response to air- and bone-conduction clicks. *J Speech Hear Res, 37,* 475–479.

Stuart, A., Yang, E. Y., & Stenstrom, R. (1990). Effect of temporal are bone vibrator placement on auditory brainstem response in newborn infants. *Ear Hear, 11,* 363–369.

Stypulkowski, P. H., & Staller, S. J. (1987). Clinical evaluation of a new ECoG recording electrode. *Ear and Hearing 8,* 304–310.

Suzuki, J. L., & Yamane, H. (1982) The choice of stimulus in the auditory brainstem response test for neurological and audiological examinations. *Ann New York Acad Sci 388,* 731–736.

Suzuki, T., Hirabayashi, M., & Kobayashi, K. (1983). Auditory midlle latency responses in young children. *British Journal of Audiology, 17,* 5–7.

Van Campen, L. E., Sammeth, C. A., Hall, J. W., & Peek, B. F. (1992). Comparison of Etymotic insert and TDH supra-aural earphones in auditory brainstem response measurement. *J Am Acad Audiol, 3,* 315–323.

Van Campen, L. E., Sammeth, C. A., & Peek, B. F. (1990). Interaural attenuation using Etymotic ER-3A insert earphones in auditory brainstem response testing. *Ear Hear, 11,* 66–69.

Versino, M., Bergamaschi, R., Romani, A., Banfi, P., Callieco, R., Citterio, A., Gerosa, E., & Cosi, V. (1992). Middle latency auditory evoked potentials improve detection of abnormalities along auditory pathways in multiple sclerosis patients. *Electroencephalogr Clin Neurophysiolo, 84,* 296–299.

Wolf, K. E., & Goldstein, R. (1980). Middle component AERs from neonates to low-level tonal stimuli. *J Speech Hearing Res, 23,* 185–201.

Wu, C., & Stapells, D. R. (1994). Pure-tone masking profiles for human auditory brainstem and middle latency responses to 500-Hz tones. *Hear Research, 78,* 169–174.

Xu, Z. M., De Vel, E., Vink, B., & Van Cauwenber, P. (1995). Application of cross-correlation function in the evaluation of objective MLR thresholds in the low and middle frequencies. *Scandinavian Audiology, 24,* 231–236.

Yang, E. Y., Rupert, A. L., & Mousegian, G. (1987). A developmental study of bone conduction auditory brainstem responses in infants. *Ear Hear, 8,* 244–251.

CHAPTER 8

Cochlear Implants: A Brief Overview

Brian Dunham
Johns Hopkins Hospital

Charles J. Limb
National Institutes of Health and Johns Hopkins Hospital

A cochlear implant (CI) is a sophisticated electronic device designed to enable sound detection and improve speech understanding in individuals with severe-to-profound sensorineural hearing loss who receive little benefit from hearing aids. Implants differ from other forms of auditory rehabilitation in that implants interact directly with the nervous system. They receive, process, and convert acoustic signals into electrical impulses that stimulate the auditory nerve. CIs are the first manufactured prostheses to successfully integrate a sensory modality (Gantz & Turner, 2003).

In the intact human auditory pathway, the cochlea is populated by approximately 15,000 hair cells, which are divided into two populations. *Inner hair cells* stimulate afferent fibers of the auditory nerve and act as the primary transducer of acoustic information to the central auditory pathway. The *outer hair cells* receive both afferent and efferent innervation and possess a rapid electromotile response, which is thought to account for the cochlea's active mechanical properties. It is the outer hair cells' contraction and elongation, which are hypothesized to amplify the vibration of the organ of Corti and enable the exquisite sensitivity and frequency selectivity of the ear (Oghalai, 2004). Most often, sensorineural hearing loss occurs because of malfunction or loss of cochlear hair cells. Yet, despite the loss of hair cell function and the resultant decrease in synaptic activity, many fibers of the auditory nerve retain their viability and excitability. It is these fibers that CIs electrically stimulate, effectively bypassing the failing hair cell transduction system. Although implants maintain the flow of acoustic energy into neural impulses, they do not instantly restore normal hearing; typically, the signals delivered to

171

the brain can only be interpreted as meaningful sounds after considerable training and rehabilitation.

HISTORICAL BACKGROUND AND DEVELOPMENT

The history of electrical auditory stimulation dates back at least 200 years. Alessandro Volta is often credited with the first observation of electrical stimulation of hearing in the late 18th century. He connected a group of batteries to two metal rods inserted in his auditory canals. After completing the circuit, he experienced a rather unpleasant "secousse dans la tête" (a blow in the head) followed by a sound that he associated with thick, boiling soup (Volta, 1800).

The first direct neural stimulation occurred over a century and a half later. On February 25, 1957 (at a time when there was considerable apprehension about the safety of inserting prosthetic material into the inner ear), Djourno and Eyriès positioned a monopolar electrode onto the eighth nerve of a patient with bilateral profound sensorineural hearing loss (Djourno & Eyries, 1957). Their report is commonly cited as a major catalyst for the development of cochlear implants. The patient had undergone both left and right temporal bone resections for large cholesteatomas. These operations had bilaterally ablated his labyrinths, cochleae, and facial nerves, leaving him with profound deafness and complete facial paralysis. The consequent bony defect on his right allowed the apposition of an electrode directly onto the stump of his auditory nerve at the level of the lateral internal auditory canal. Stimulation three days postoperatively produced auditory percepts that the patient compared to the sounds of crickets and whistles. While speech remained unintelligible to him, he was on occasion able to discern simple words such as: "allo," "maman," and "papa" (Djourno & Eyries, 1957; Djourno, Eyries, & Vallancien, 1957; Djourno, Eyries, & Vallancien, 1957; Eisen, 2003).

By 1957, an important evolution in temporal bone surgery had taken place, with the development of the transmastoid facial recess approach, which provided good access to the round window. Via the facial recess, which is a space in between the facial nerve and chorda tympani nerves, insertion of an electrode into the cochlea could be acomplished (Sheehy, 1959). During that same year, a patient brought Djourno and Eyriès' work to the attention of Dr. William F. House. Drs. F. Blair Simmons, Robin Michelson, and William House, all leading separate investigational teams, propelled the early development of cochlear implants.

In the 1960s and early 1970s, House, Michelson, and Simmons all began to electrically stimulate the human cochlear nerve (Doyle, Jr., Doyle, Turnbull, Abbey, & House, 1963; Michelson, 1971a, 1971b; Simmons, Mongeon, Lewis, & Huntington, 1964). The first step was to record the electrical activity of the eighth nerve and observe the effects of electrical stimulation. In collaboration with a neurosurgeon and an engineer, House placed electrodes directly on the eighth nerve in patients undergoing vestibular nerve sectioning for treatment of Meniere's disease (Doyle, Jr., Doyle, Turnbull, Abbey, & House, 1963; Doyle, Doyle, & Turnbull, 1964). He also placed electrodes onto the promontory or directly through the open oval window into the perilymph of patients undergoing stapes surgery. Patients reported a greater sense of loudness when the voltage amplitude of the electrical stimulation was increased. Similarly, an increase in frequency resulted in an increase in pitch. Of importance was the finding that direct stimulation in the perilymph did not seem to cause discomfort, dizziness, or clinically observable facial nerve activity with signals above 30 Hz. However, with stimulation frequencies of 20 Hz or less, patients experienced dizziness (House, 1976).

In 1961, studies indicated that biphasic currents minimized chances of damage to cochlear tissue, and in that same year, House introduced a single gold wire electrode and subsequently a five-wire system in the scala tympani of a deaf patient (House, 1976). His subject reported pleasant auditory sensations from electrical stimulation. Unfortunately, the insulating material used on the electrodes was a major problem; it allowed fluids to penetrate into the electrodes, leading to their eventual failure. In 1964, Simmons placed a bipolar electrode directly onto the modiolar portion of the cochlea (Simmons, Mongeon, Lewis, & Huntington, 1964).

In the 1970s, CIs began to receive considerable public attention. However, it would be another decade before implants were commercially available. In 1972, House implanted the first single wire induction coil system, which was developed in conjunction with the engineer, Jack Urban (House & Urban, 1973). In that same year, the House 3M single-electrode implant became commercially available and was the first implant to receive U.S. Food and Drug Administration (FDA) approval in 1984. Professor Graeme Clark and his colleagues at the University of Melbourne, Australia, developed the first multichannel device for clinical trial in 1982; this device received FDA approval in 1985.

In the 1990s, advances in sound processing led to substantial improvements in speech recognition. Blake Wilson developed the continuous interleaved sampling (CIS) strategy for multielectrode CIs and compared it to the standard compressed analog (CA). The latter presents analog waveforms simultaneously to all electrodes, whereas the CIS strategy presents brief pulses to each electrode in a non-overlapping sequence. Seven experienced implant users, selected for their excellent performance with the CA processor, participated as subjects. The new strategy produced large improvements in the scores of speech reception tests for all subjects (Wilson et al., 1991). In 1995, Hugh McDermott reported the use of a novel speech processing strategy (SPEAK) in a study with 24 postlinguistically deafened adults. The results showed improved performance with the SPEAK coding strategy. By far the greatest improvement observed was for sentence recognition in noise, with the mean score across subjects for the SPEAK strategy twice that obtained with the previously used strategy (Whitford et al., 1995). In 2004, Lan reported on a novel speech-processing strategy incorporating tonal information for CI patients who use tonal languages such as Chinese (Lan, Nie, Gao, & Zeng, 2004).

In the modern cochlear implant, the external components have become progressively smaller and now routinely offer more than one sound processing strategy. Recent years have also seen a trend towards perimodiolar electrode designs.

These electrodes are designed to place stimulating contacts close to the spiral ganglion cells, to reduce power consumption and refine stimulation selectively (Balkany, Eshraghi, & Yang, 2002; Eshraghi, Yang, & Balkany, 2003).

DEVICE MANUFACTURERS

As of 2007, over 100,000 people worldwide have received CIs. Currently, there are three manufacturers with FDA approved devices on the market. The **Cochlear Corporation** is the offspring of Professor Graeme Clark's work. The parent company is based in Australia with American headquarters in Englewood, Colorado. Over 60,000 people across 120 countries have received their devices. Cochlear Corporation produces the Nucleus Freedom that has a 22-channel, self-curling electrode array. Its receiver-stimulator is encased in a soft polymer enabling greater conformation to the shape of the skull and has a removable magnet to allow for magnetic resonance imaging (MRI) up to 1.5 Tesla. **Advanced Bionics Corporation** is based in California. This company first received FDA approval in 1996 for its Clarion device, and they now produce the Clarion Hi-Res 90K device. This device also has a soft silicone housing and removable magnet, with 16 electrode contacts that are designed to focus stimulation toward the nerve fibers. The **Med El** Corporation is headquartered in Innsbruck, Austria. It launched the PulsarCI^{100} device in 2004. Its implant is housed in a hard ceramic case. The company offers a variety of electrode arrays, which carry a total of 12 electrodes. The standard electrode array is approximately 31-mm long and is designed for deep insertion. The medium array has moderate contact spacing for cases where deep insertion is not desired or is not possible due to anatomic restrictions. The compressed array similarly has 12 pairs of electrode contacts spaced over 12.1 mm for insertion into partially ossified cochlear lumens. The split array is designed for severely ossified or malformed cochlear lumens. It has two separate electrode branches, one with five and one with seven pairs of electrode contacts, all of which are spaced in compressed fashion. These electrodes branches are designed for insertion into two separate cochleostomies, one at the basal turn and another placed into the cochlea in front of the oval window. The PulsarCI^{100} is currently the only FDA approved for MRI use (0.2 Tesla) without removal of the magnet.

COCHLEAR IMPLANT DESIGN

Overview

All cochlear implants today have both external and internal components. The surgically implanted portion carries a radio frequency receiving coil, a stimulator, and an electrode array. The external portion consists of a microphone, a speech processor, a radio frequency transmitting coil, and a power source.

The external and internal mechanisms are not in direct contact with each other, but communicate via radio frequency signals. The internal receiver/stimu-

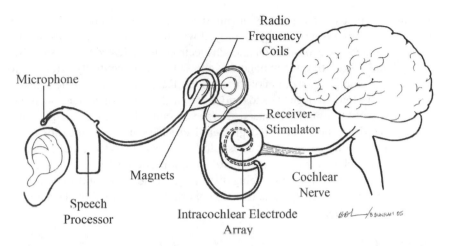

FIGURE 8–1.   Cochlear Implant Components. This illustration shows both the external and internal components. The implanted portion carries a radio frequency receiving coil, a stimulator, and an electrode array. The external portion consists of a microphone, a speech processor, a radio frequency transmitting coil, and a power source. The internal receiver/stimulator houses a hermetically-sealed magnet that aligns the external radio frequency coil, enabling transcutaneous signaling.

lator houses a hermetically-sealed magnet that aligns the external radio frequency coil, enabling transcutaneous signaling. The external components are placed and the device is activated two to four weeks after implantation. This delay allows for healing of the tissues, and abatement of postoperative edema. As the wound heals, a fibrotic capsule tightly envelopes the receiver-stimulator, which helps to secure it in position.

The microphone detects the acoustic energy of both speech and environmental sound, and relays it to the speech processor, which is essentially a miniaturized computer. The speech processor acts like a transducer, converting the acoustic energy into a signal that is then transmitted by radio frequency. The analog signals are digitized and separated into frequency bandwidths, which are assigned to specific electrodes. The digitized and filtered signals are then transmitted via radiofrequency to the implanted device, which translate the radiofrequency signals into electrical discharges at the respective assigned electrodes. The processors faces the challenge of taking a wideband signal with a dynamic range greater than 100 dB and converting it into a set of parallel narrowband signals each with a maximum "data transfer" rate of a few thousand spikes per second, which is the upper limit of auditory nerve phase-locking with electrical stimulation, and a restricted dynamic range of approximately 2 dB, which is the typical dynamic range for electrical stimulation of an auditory nerve (Rubinstein, 2004). Upon receiving the radio frequency signal, the stimulator converts the information into an electrical signal that is distributed to the electrodes, which directly stimulate surviving spiral ganglion cells. The distribution pattern and timing of the electrical stimulation is partly determined by the number of available electrodes and partly by the speech processing strategy employed which will filter, extract from, amplify, or compress the acoustic signal. Each electrode is dedicated to a specific frequency band. These frequency band assignments are sequentially arranged to match the tonotopic organization of the cochlea. The processed acoustic signal is divided into discrete frequency bands and sent to its frequency-matched electrode. The intensity of the stimulus is encoded in the amount of electrical energy delivered, with louder sounds receiving a greater electrical stimulus. At the time of activation, the audiologist measures threshold levels as well as the loudness comfort levels at each electrode. They create an amplitude mapping to render the electrical signals audible without being disturbingly loud. Most of the other parameters are set by the manufacturer and are not ordinarily adjusted by the audiologist (Shannon, 2002).

MICROPHONES

Contemporary microphones are diminutive in size, usually directional, and are typically housed within the speech processor. Current CIs can provide high levels of speech performance in quiet environments. However, performance deteriorates rapidly with increasing levels of background noise (Fu, Shannon, & Wang, 1998). Strategies that enhance microphone efficiency and minimize distortion are evolving. Bilateral two-microphone noise reduction techniques have demonstrated increased speech intelligibility (van Hoesel & Clark, 1995). Similarly, a monaural two-microphone noise reduction system can lead to improved signal-to-noise ratio (Wouters & Vanden Berghe, 2001).

SPEECH PROCESSORS

The external battery-powered speech processor accepts signals from the microphone and encodes the information for transmission to the implanted receiver-stimulator. Initially, the processors were sizeable, bulky devices worn on the body, normally on a belt or clip. The evolution of microchip technology has enabled a substantial reduction in the size of the speech processor. All three manufacturers now offer processors that sit behind the ear, similar to conventional behind-the-ear hearing aids. Improved battery technology now routinely allows 1–5 days of use from a battery pack, depending on hours of daily usage. At the time of implant activation, an audiologist begins programming the signal processing strategies, storing them in the memory of the processor. Multiple strategies can be encoded to deal with a variety of listening situations.

Additionally, externally fitted or built-in telecoils now provide access to systems equiped with assistive listening devices (ALDs), including induction loops and infrared or FM systems. The telecoils allow CI recipients to use phones including cell phones, CD players, and MP3 players, while also enhancing their experiences in venues such as galleries, movie theaters, and concert halls outfitted with ALDs.

PROCESSING STRATEGIES

There have been steady improvements in speech recognition with CIs over the past two decades. Our ability to improve upon the design and function of CIs is directly dependent on our understanding of the relative roles played by the cochlea and central nervous system in speech recognition. Currently far more is understood about cochlear function than about central neural processing of sound. Speech is an extremely complex auditory signal, which requires a large amount of neural processing. Which acoustic cues are most important for speech recognition? Recent research on amplitude, temporal, and spectral cues in speech show that speech recognition is only mildly distorted by alterations in the amplitude and temporal domains, but is highly sensitive to manipulations in the frequency spectrum (Shannon, 2002).

Speech recognition is relatively resistant to amplitude deterioration. Experiments which manipulate amplitude have shown only modest performance impairment in the recognition of phonemes (Drullman, 1995; Fu & Shannon, 1998; Loizou, Dorman, Poroy, & Spahr, 2000). Amplitude mapping is therefore important to the extent that the acoustic signal be audible to the listener. Once the stimulation is audible, the exact mapping of amplitude is relatively less important to speech recognition (Shannon, 2002). Similarly, distortions in temporal cues do not appear to greatly affect intelligibility. Temporal cues in speech can transmit information on envelope (< 50 Hz), periodicity (50–500 Hz), and spectral fine structure (> 500 Hz). Removal or distortion of all temporal information above 20 Hz has a negligible effect on speech recognition (Fu & Galvin, 2001; Saberi & Perrott, 1999; Shannon, 2002; Vandali, Whitford, Plant, & Clark, 2000). Saberi and Perrott provided a dramatic demonstration of the corrective capacity of the human speech encoding system. They highly distorted temporal cues by subdividing a digitized sentence into equal segments and played each segment backwards in time. For reversed segments below 100 ms, intelligibility remained high (Saberi & Perrott, 1999). The effective temporal "window" for speech appears to be about 50 ms. Speech with complete spectral cues is more resistant to temporal distortion than speech with reduced spectral resolution (Shannon, 2002).

In contrast to amplitude and temporal cues, both the quantity and quality of spectral cues are essential to speech recognition (Shannon, 2002). Four spectral channels are needed for speech recognition in quiet (Dorman, Loizou, & Rainey, 1997; Fu, Shannon, & Wang, 1998; Shannon, Zeng, Kamath, Wygonski, & Ekelid, 1995). Speech recognition in noise is more challenging for CI recipients and requires more than four channels (Fu, Shannon, & Wang, 1998). Music recognition calls for the greatest number of channels, requiring at least 16 channels (Kong, Cruz, Jones, & Zeng, 2004; Smith, Delgutte, & Oxenham, 2002). For unknown reasons, CI listeners' speech recognition reaches maximal performance near 8 spectral channels, whereas normal-hearing listeners experience continued improvement in speech recognition up to at least 20 spectral channels (Fishman, Shannon, & Slattery, 1997; Friesen, Shannon, Baskent, & Wang, 2001; Lawson, Wilson, & Finley, 1993; Shannon, 2002).

In an experiment to examine the deleterious effect of spectral gaps on speech recognition, Shannon used a 20-band processor in CI listeners, and a 20-band noise processor in normal-hearing listeners. Eliminating electrodes or noise carrier bands in the basal, middle, or apical regions of the cochlea created 1.5 to 6mm "holes" in the tonotopic representation of sound along the cochlea. Both groups of listeners could tolerate a large deficit in the basal or middle regions, provided that the rest of the spectrum was intact. Deficits in the apical low-frequency region, however, were severely damaging to speech recognition for both normal-hearing and CI listeners (Shannon, Galvin, & Baskent, 2002).

Speech recognition requires that spectral information be delivered to the "normal" cochlear tonotopic region (Shannon, 2002; Shannon, Zeng, & Wygonski, 1998). If the spectral stimulus is shifted by more than 3 mm, speech recognition is appreciably degraded (Dorman, Loizou, & Rainey, 1997; Shannon, 2002). Tonotopic patterns of information for speech appear to be stored and retrieved in the brain in terms of absolute cochlear location—distortions or shifts in the frequency-to-place mapping can result in substantial decreases in performance (Dorman, Loizou, & Rainey, 1997; Shannon, 2002).

Speech processing strategies have evolved considerably in the past couple of decades. Their evolution has resulted in important improvements in speech intelligibility. A major advance occurred with development of continuous interleaved sampling (CIS), which was proposed as an alternative to standard compressed analog (CA) processing (Wilson et al., 1991). The CA method uses an analog filter

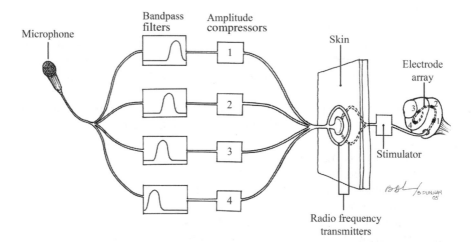

FIGURE 8–2A.   Compressed Analogue Strategy. This figure illustrates a multichannel analog processor. Sound is sampled by a microphone. Bandpass filters separate incoming sound into different frequencies. The amplitude compressors then decrease the dynamic range within each channel to match the constricted dynamic range of electrical hearing. The radio frequency coils communicate the signals transcutaneously from the processor to the receiver-stimulator. The stimulator then simultaneously delivers the electrical signals to the respective intracochlear electrodes.

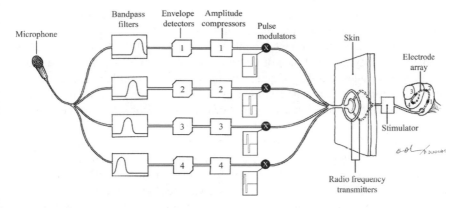

FIGURE 8–2B. Continuous Interleaved Sampling Strategy. This figure illustrates a multi-channel pulsatile processor. In contrast to the compressed analogue strategy, the intracochlear electrical pulses are non-simultaneous, eliminating a principal component of electrode inter-actions due to summation of electrical fields.

bank strategy in which microphone signals varying over a wide dynamic range are compressed to the narrow dynamic range of electrically evoked hearing. Using an automatic gain control, the output is filtered into four contiguous frequency bands for presentation to each of four electrodes. Sinusoidal currents are distributed simultaneously to the electrodes.

Speech information is contained in the relative stimulus amplitude delivered through the four electrodes and in the temporal structure of the waveforms for each channel. With CA processing, most patients experience limited access to the presented acoustic information. For example, they have difficulty perceiving frequency changes in stimulus waveforms above a "pitch saturation limit" around 400 Hz. As a result, many temporal details are inaccessible to the typical user. Furthermore, the simultaneous presentation of stimuli is likely to produce substantial channel interaction from the summation of electrical fields generated by closely arranged electrodes. The electrical overlap is thought to degrade the salience of channel-related cues (Wilson et al., 1991).

CIS processing circumvents channel interaction by the use of interleaved non-simultaneous stimulation. Using a series of digital filters, CIS pre-processes and digitizes the sound input. Trains of balanced biphasic pulses are directed to each electrode with temporal offsets, eliminating any overlap across channels. In contrast to the four-channel CA strategy, between four and twelve bandpass filters and stimulation channels are typically used. The amplitude of each stimulus pulse is determined by mathematical transformation of the corresponding channel's envelope signal at that time, compressing the signal into the appropriate dynamic range (Skinner, Arndt, & Staller, 2002; Wilson et al., 1991). A key feature of CIS is its high rate of channel stimulation. It uses brief pulses and minimal delays, allowing rapid variations in speech to be tracked by pulse amplitude variations. The channel stimulation rate is flexible and usually exceeds 800 pulses per second; it remains constant during both voiced and unvoiced intervals. Thus, CIS reduces channel interaction and retains most if not all of the temporal information that can be perceived by the implant patient (Wilson et al., 1991). CIS offers considerable flexibility in the choice of stimulated sites from all the available intracochlear electrodes, number of active channels, rate of stimulation, and order in which electrodes are stimulated within a cycle. The default setting stimulates in an apical to basal direction, but a staggered or basal to apical mode can be selected (Skinner et al., 2002).

Unlike the CIS strategy, the spectral peak strategy (SPEAK) focuses on spectral cues rather than temporal cues. SPEAK was described by Seligman and McDermott, and Skinner et al. in the mid 1990s (Seligman & McDermott, 1995; Skinner et al., 1994). Like CIS, it operates on a filter bank stratagem. Frequency bands of incoming sound are assigned to a maximum of 20 channels that span the range from 116 to 8000 Hz. Frequency bands are assigned in a tonotopic fashion, with the lowest frequency band assigned to the most apical electrode. The amplitude outputs of the channel filters are examined; the processor then selects between six and nine that have the highest amplitude or "maxima," for stimulation during each cycle. The selected channels within a cycle are stimulated in a basal to apical order. The frame repetition rate is 250 Hz, resulting in delivery of a new frame of electrical pulses every 4 milliseconds (Skinner, Arndt, & Staller, 2002; Skinner et al., 2002).

The CIS strategy differs in that it divides the frequency spectrum into a smaller number of channels (between four and twelve) than does SPEAK. In CIS each of these channels is sequentially stimulated with every new frame. The CIS frame repetition, typically between 720 and 2400 Hz, is higher than with SPEAK (Skinner et al., 2002). Its high frame repetition, combined the stimulation of all its selected electrodes, gives CIS more detailed temporal information than SPEAK does.(Loizou, 1999) On the other hand, SPEAK offers greater spectral detail than CIS because more channels are stimulated (Skinner et al., 2002).

The advanced combination encoder (ACE) speech coding strategy combines the advantages of SPEAK's spectral representation and CIS' temporal representation. Much like SPEAK, ACE processing divides the frequency into as many as 22 bands, each of which is assigned to an electrode. Like SPEAK, there is a dynamic selection of the frequency bands with the highest amplitude. The number of bands chosen is constant and is determined by a value programmed into the speech coding software; this number is usually between eight and twelve. The frame repetition rate in ACE, much like the CIS strategy, is relatively high; the rates usually chosen range between 500 and 2400 Hz. Similar to the SPEAK processing strategy, electrode stimulation in ACE follows a basal to apical order.

ELECTRODE ARRAYS

Signals are transcutaneously conveyed via radio frequency from the processor to the receiver/stimulator, which generates electrical impulses; these impulses then travel via a connecting lead to an array of electrodes surgically positioned within the scala tympani of the cochlea. The electrodes deliver electrical currents, depolarizing surviving auditory afferent neurons seated in the modiolus. Since two contacts are prerequisite to establishing a current, each active electrode must be paired to a ground electrode. Monopolar electrode designs use a single extracochlear ground electrode, which is typically placed under the temporalis muscle, to service one or multiple active intracochlear electrodes. Bipolar electrode configurations closely pair both active and ground electrodes within the cochlea. While monopolar electrodes deliver a broader electrical stimulus, bipolar electrodes provide a more discrete electrical impulse. Bipolar electrodes however have to overcome greater resistance; they, consequently, minimize channel interaction but have greater power requirements and deplete batteries more rapidly (Niparko, Francis, Tucci, Dawsey, & Chinnici, 2003).

In observance of the tonotopic arrangement of the cochlea, the electrodes of a multichannel array are longitudinally positioned. Deep placement, therefore, theoretically enables a greater spectral range; current electrode carriers are typically inserted up to 30 mm. While the ideal depth of electrode insertion remains unknown, placement beyond the first portion of the cochlea's basal turn seems intuitively necessary to reach lower frequency neurons (Niparko, Francis, Tucci, Dawsey, & Chinnici, 2003). Recent perimodiolar electrode designs have targeted closer apposition of the electrode to the target neurons within the modiolus, in an effort to reduce power consumption, increase stimulation selectivity, and decrease channel interaction (Eshraghi, Yang, & Balkany, 2003; Fayad, Luxford, & Linthicum, 2000). These designs use either a Silastic positioning shim or an increased curvature of flexible arrays. In 2002, a spike in the incidence of meningitis in the cochlear implant population and documented consequent intracochlear damage with the use the Silastic positioners raised suspicion; an association found between the incidence of meningitis and the use of shims led to their discontinued use (Cohen, Roland, & Marrinan, 2004; Nadol & Eddington, 2004; O'Donoghue et al., 2002; Richter et al., 2002). The investigation into the rise of meningitis incidence has led to an increased focus on preoperative vaccination as well as the judicious sealing of the cochleostomy with soft tissue (Cohen, Roland, & Marrinan, 2004; Dahm et al., 1994). The flexible, contoured arrays have not been implicated in the increase in meningitis and their use continues today.

In 1990, Abbas reported the first successful recording of Evoked Compound Action Potentials (ECAP) in human cochlear implant users (Brown, Abbas, & Gantz, 1990). An ECAP is the synchronized reaction from peripheral auditory nerves to an electrical stimulus delivered by an intracochlear electrode and measured by a neighboring electrode, amplified, and encoded for transmission via radio frequency back to the speech processor (Dillier et al., 2002). Telemetry systems have evolved to allow the measurement of the impedance of individual electrodes within the implant, to monitor whether the implant delivers the specified stimulation current, as well as the physiologic response of the auditory nerve. This bi-directional neural telemetry offers a non-invasive recording of the ECAPs of the peripheral auditory nerves in-situ, without the need for sedation. Patients can be sitting up without affecting the quality of the recordings. Since muscle activity is less of a problem than with electrically evoked auditory brain stem response recording, relatively long recording sessions are possible (Abbas et al., 1999). Measurements can be taken with relative ease and speed in younger children, who would otherwise be more difficult to assess (Abbas et al., 1999; Kaplan-Neeman et al., 2004; Seyle & Brown, 2002). Bi-directional telemetry offers an alternative method to behavior-based programming of the cochlear implant. It can map the electrical stimulation parameters since it can help determine both which electrodes to include or exclude in the patient's program and threshold and comfort levels at each electrode site. Additionally, telemetry information can be used to monitor both the integrity of the implant as well as the neural responses over time. This technology is expected to promote the evolution of carefully tailored programming most appropriate for the individual user (Abbas et al., 1999).

IMPLANT CANDIDACY EVALUATION:

The Food and Drug Administration regulates cochlear implants, which are considered medical devices. During periods of investigation, exacting criteria of patient inclusion and exclusion govern study patient selection. Post-investigational patient selection is based on those criteria. The original selection criteria have relaxed substantially over the years as cochlear implants have shown evidence of very few serious complications and patients' speech reception scores steadily improved. For example, children were once excluded and now patients 12 months old are routinely receiving implants. On special indications such as labyrinthitis ossificans due to meningitis, even younger patients are receiving implants (Cohen, 2004; James & Papsin, 2004; Rizer & Burkey, 1999; van den Broek et al., 1995). Not surprisingly, selection criteria continue to evolve as cochlear implant performance and the underlying technology improve. The selection process is rarely simple and requires a fairly large multidisciplinary team that is specifically trained for cochlear implant management. The team is comprised of an administrative and coordinating staff, psychologists, speech and language therapists, otologic surgeons, nurses, and audiologists. Patient and family education plays an important role in setting appropriate expectations. The post-operative rehabilitation can be challenging and may require several therapeutic approaches, which again underscores the importance of a well-organized multidisciplinary team.

AUDIOLOGIC CRITERIA

The audiologic evaluation is a key component of cochlear implant candidacy assessment and includes both aided and unaided audiograms as well as a minimal speech battery in adults. The detailed device-dependent criteria, which are usually set by the manufacturers, are specified in the product labeling or in training manuals. The original criteria requiring profound bilateral sensorineural hearing loss have been relaxed to now include adults patients with bilateral severe-to-profound hearing loss. Therefore, patients 18 years old or older should have an unaided three frequency pure-tone average (PTA) (measured at 500, 1000, and 2000

Hz) of 70 dB or greater in their better hearing ear. In addition to documented sensorineural hearing loss, a demonstrated lack of benefit from appropriately fitted hearing aids is essential. In general and under best-aided conditions, appropriate adult candidates will have a score of 40–50 percent or less (device dependent) in the ear to be implanted and 60 percent or less (device dependent) in the non-implant ear on open-set hearing in noise sentence testing (HINT). Medicare coverage sets more stringent demands requiring scores of 30 percent or less on sentence recognition test for postlingually deafened adults under best-aided conditions.

The audiologic criteria for children are similar. The most liberal criteria found in the product labeling allow for bilateral severe-to-profound sensorineural hearing loss from the ages of 25 months on, and bilateral profound sensorineural hearing loss from the ages of 12 to 24 months. As a rule, a trial period of three to six months of appropriate amplification is mandated (device dependent) and is beneficial in preparing young patients to wear the external behind-the-ear components of a cochlear implant. In younger children less than two years old, little or no benefit from amplification is defined by a lack of progress in the development of simple auditory milestones such as spontaneously responding to name in quiet or to environmental sounds. In older children, 2 years old and up, lack of aided benefit is characterized by a score of 20–30 percent or less (device dependent) on simple open-set word recognition tests, such as the Lexical Neighborhood Test (LNT) or the Multisyllabic Lexical Neighborhood Test (MLNT).

Medical and Otologic Evaluation

Every potential candidate should undergo a complete history and physical with a focus on general medical as well as otologic issues. Successful cochlear implantation mandates a patent cochlea, an absence of retrocochlear pathology that would prevent the neural transmission of signals to the central auditory pathway, as well as sufficient general health to withstand the surgical procedure and postoperative rehabilitation. Appropriate laboratory studies are routinely obtained to rule out any medical contraindications to implantation. Since implantation requires the ability to tolerate general anesthesia, the patient should be healthy enough to withstand the physiologic rigors of a general anesthetic. Since the operation is typically not a lengthy procedure, rare is the patient whose health is so poor that they cannot undergo implantation. In those patients who present unacceptably high anesthetic risks, implantation under local anesthesia has been reported (Toner, John, & McNaboe, 1998). This approach, however, significantly limits the extent of retrosigmoid bony and soft tissue dissection, and has little to offer outside the truly exceptional case (Niparko, Francis, Tucci, Dawsey, & Chinnici, 2003).

The otologic portion of the history should detail the onset, pattern of progression, and duration of hearing impairment, and if possible, its etiology. The cause of hearing loss is rarely a contraindication to implantation but can prove useful in developing an appropriate treatment strategy. Meningitis offers a critical example of the potential importance of knowing the etiology; the accompanying inflammation can lead to a progressive obstructive ossification of the cochlea that can limit and sometimes prevent intracochlear insertion. Its presence can call for an accelerated timeline to implantation. The history should also elicit all attempts at aural rehabilitation including hearing amplification and education. Previous otologic operations should be reviewed. The details of the operation should be known whenever possible, since the patient's anatomy may have been significantly altered, affecting the surgical approach. The presence of a canal-wall-down mastoidectomy does not preclude implantation (Karatzanis, Chimona, Prokopakis, Kyrmizakis, & Velegrakis, 2003; Pasanisi et al., 2002). The otologic exam notes the function of the facial nerve since this is one of the most important structures at risk of injury during the operation. Otoscopic or microtoscopic examination verifies the health of external auditory canal and tympanic membrane. Any active infection or significant tympanic perforation should be addressed prior to implantation.

There has been considerable concern about the safety of cochlear implantation in the pediatric population since implantation occurs during the age with the highest prevalence of otitis media (OM). The fear is that the infection could potentially extend along the electrode array into the cochlea or, even further, into the central nervous system. Recently released information about an increased incidence of post-implantation meningitis by the FDA has heightened this concern ("FDA Public Health Web Notification: Cochlear implant recipients may be at greater risk for meningitis (Updated September 25, 2003)," July 24, 2002). So far, however, research has not confirmed this fear (Fayad, Tabaee, Micheletto, & Parisier, 2003; Kempf, Stover, & Lenarz, 2000; Luntz, Teszler, & Shpak, 2004; Luntz, Teszler, Shpak, Feiglin, & Farah-Sima'an, 2001). Several studies have shown that the incidence of OM does not increase after implantation, and that when OM does occur after implantation, there are relatively few severe complications (Balkany, Hodges, Miyamoto, Gibbin, & Odabasi, 2001; House, Luxford, & Courtney, 1985; Luntz, Hodges, Balkany, Dolan-Ash, & Schloffman, 1996). In a study of 366 children (ages 1 to 14) undergoing implantation, 5.6 percent of the patients suffered from acute otitis media (AOM) post surgically over a follow-up period of up to 8 years (Kempf, Stover, & Lenarz, 2000). Of the 20 infected ears this represented, 9 were on the non-implanted side. No cases of meningitis were reported. In a prospective study of 60 pediatric implant patients, divided into OM-prone (n = 34) and non-OM-prone (n = 26) groups, 38 percent of the OM-prone and 7.6 percent of the non-prone group develop an episode of AOM. The incidence of OM decreased in the OM-prone group after implantation (Kempf, Stover, & Lenarz, 2000). The drop in OM after implantation may be explained by meticulous pre-operative OM management, the natural decline of OM incidence with age, and also possibly by the therapeutic benefit of mastoidectomy (House, Luxford, & Courtney, 1985; Luntz, Teszler, & Shpak, 2004). Most importantly, authors agree that a history of OM should not delay implantation (Fayad, Tabaee, Micheletto, & Parisier, 2003; Luntz, Teszler, & Shpak, 2004; Luntz, Teszler, Shpak, Feiglin, & Farah-Sima'an, 2001). Placement of a ventilation tube should be considered either before or at the time of implantation in an OM prone patient. Some authors advocated the continuous use of a ventilating tube in OM-prone implantees until they outgrow their susceptibility to OM (Luntz, Teszler, & Shpak, 2004). Subsequent episodes of OM should be treated diligently with conventional therapy, namely orally and otically administered antibiotics.

RADIOLOGIC EVALUATION

Radiologic imaging is necessary to determine whether or not implantation will be feasible since the cochlea has to be patent in order to accommodate the electrode array. Computed tomography (CT) and magnetic resonance imaging (MRI) play complimentary roles in the evaluation of an implant candidate. Most cochlear implant centers today rely on high-resolution CT as their primary imaging modality. CT nicely details bony anatomy while MRI is more adept at the description of soft tissues, such as neural structures. Some authors support the use of CT scans primarily, reserving MRI studies for adjunctive evaluations, (Nair, Abou-Elhamd, & Hawthorne, 2000) while others advocate MRI alone and in particular the fast spin echo (FSE) MRI technique (Ellul, Shelton, Davidson, & Harnsberger, 2000; Tien, Felsberg, & Macfall, 1992). High-resolution CT scans using a bone algorithm are useful in guiding surgical planning: these scans can reveal detailed bony anatomy of the mastoid, detect anomalies in the course of the facial nerve, and confirm the presence of the cochlea and its patency. Their predominant limitation is in the description of the cochlear patency. Fibrous obliteration of the cochlea is visible only on gradient-echo T2-weighted (MRI) images and not on CT images; CT, however, is needed to confirm the presence of calcifications which cannot be distinguished from fibrous obliteration on MRI (Casselman, 2002). In cases of meningitis or in cases where high-resolution CT scans reveal abnormally narrow internal auditory canals (Cho, Na, Jung, & Hong, 2000), MRI serves an important role in evaluating for both cochlear patency and the presence of the cochlear nerve. The presence of cochlear ossification or fibrous obstruction does not preclude implantation, whereas severe cochlear malformation and agenesis will. A history of meningitis should alert the surgeon to consider using specially designed shorter arrays. An implant may yield less satisfactory results in a cochlea whose patency is compromised.

PSYCHOLOGIC EVALUATION

The psychologic hardship of auditory rehabilitation is considerable. The presence of a robust social support network considerably facilitates this rehabilitation. The patient's (or the patient's parents') expectations should be clearly discussed; their motivations should be understood. All candidates (and/or their families) should understand that cochlear implants do not restore "normal" hearing and that they require considerable rehabilitation post-operatively. At first, implant recipients often describe the sound as being "synthetic"; this artificial sound gradually dissipates after several weeks of use. There is unfortunately no means to always accurately predict who will be able to understand language well. Counseling should be provided to individuals and families with unrealistic expectations of the benefits of cochlear implants. A cochlear implant can and usually does involve a lifetime commitment to its use, as well as understanding of its susceptibilities. Patient may have to face certain lifestyle changes including an awareness of static electricity, which can temporarily or permanently damage a cochlear implant, a dependency on batteries to be able to hear, and an understanding that their implant will interact with the electronic environment. The latter is due to the fact that implants can set off security systems, be affected by cellular phones, and can interact with computers and magnetic fields unpredictably. Furthermore, the external components are vulnerable to damage by water. Physical trauma to the head can damage the implant, even from a low velocity impact sustained during a fall. Therefore, a formal psychological evaluation is helpful in screening for any psychopathology that may limit the patient's ability to take care of their device and derive benefit from it.

SURGERY

The operative side is determined preoperatively; this is a decision that is usually guided by differences in hearing, in the length of hearing impairment, and in the patency of the cochleae. At our institution, the worst hearing ear is typically chosen if both cochleae are patent (Francis, Yeagle, Brightwell, & Venick, 2004; Friedland, Venick, & Niparko, 2003). There are, however, other institutions which preferentially implant the better hearing ear (Gomaa, Rubinstein, Lowder, Tyler, & Gantz, 2003; Rubinstein, Parkinson, Tyler, & Gantz, 1999). If the cochlear dimensions are similar and hearing loss is symmetric but of unequal duration, it is preferable to implant the ear with the shortest period of impairment. If there is no difference in either the quality of the cochlear lumens, the ability to hear, or the length of hearing impairment, it is preferable to place the implant on the patient's dominant hand side to facilitate manipulation of the external components.

Barring any medical conditions or complications requiring hospitalization, cochlear implantation is usually done on an outpatient basis. The patient is typically discharged to home after a brief stay of a few hours in the post-anesthesia care unit. Depending on the patient's anatomy, the operation takes about 2 to 3 hours to complete in the hands of an experienced team.

The patient is placed on the operating table in the supine position. After general anesthesia is established, the patient is intubated and ventilated. The endotracheal tube, which rests between the true vocal cords, can cause a mild sore throat 12 to 36 hours post-operatively. Subcutaneously placed electrodes monitor the electrical activity of the orbicularis oris and obicularis oculi muscles, which are innervated by the facial nerve. This allows the surgeon to monitor the activity and integrity of the facial nerve during the operation; it is, however, an assistive device and does not substitute for a thorough understanding of facial nerve anatomy.

The head is turned slightly to the non-operative side. The postauricular hair is shaved and the operative site is infiltrated with a local anesthetic agent with epinephrine, a vasonconstrictive agent that reduces bleeding. The area is then sterily prepared and drapped. There are a variety of available incisions that can be used.

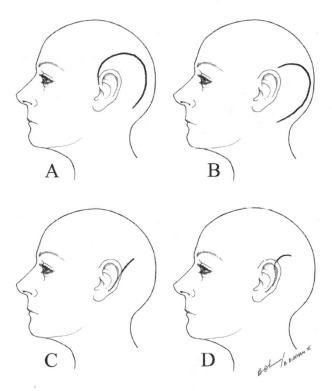

FIGURE 8-3.   Incisions. As shown in the illustration, a variety of incisions are possible during cochlear implantation. The larger incisions, shown in figures A and B, have slowly been abandoned for the shorter ones in figures C and D. The latter have been accompanied with less soft tissue manipulation and improved postoperative pain. Regardless of the incision used, it is important to not position the incision directly over the internal receiver/stimulator as a wound dehiscence could directly expose the implant.

The best approach is the one that offers good access to the tissues while minimizing tissue handling. After the incision, soft tissue elevation allows exposure of the mastoid cortical bone. The transmastoid, transfacial recess approach of cochlear implantation is a modification of long-standing techniques used for chronic mastoid and middle ear infections. A drill removes the cortical bone of the mastoid and bony air cells found within its cavity. A bony well is positioned posterosuperior to the mastoid to seat the receiver-stimulator, with adequate allowance for the positioning of a behind-the-ear speech processor.

Key surgical landmarks, including the tegmen mastoideum, fossa incudis, short process of the incus, and lateral semicircular canal, guide the subtractive process of bony removal within the mastoid cavity. Their presence greatly facilitates the identification of the facial recess and facial nerve whose vertical segment rests within the mastoid cavity, in close proximity to the bony external canal wall. It is imperative for the surgeon to thoroughly understand the normal as well as abnormal courses of the facial nerve to avoid injury to the nerve.

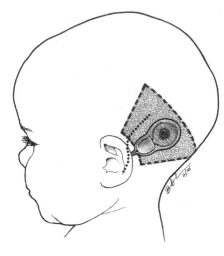

FIGURE 8–4. Position of the Receiver-Stimulator. The surgeon creates a post-auricular bony well behind the mastoidectomy to seat the receiver-stimulator, allowing enough room for a behind-the-ear speech processor to be worn comfortably without overlapping the receiver- stimulator. The incision, shown as a line, is ideally placed at least one centimeter away from the body of the receiver-stimulator. The receiver-stimulator itself can be positioned at a variety of angles, as shown by the shaded area. This is a decision which is partly dictated by the size and shape of the skull as well as the surgeon's preference.

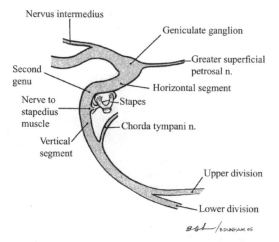

FIGURE 8–5.   Facial Nerve Anatomy. The facial nerve emerges from the brain stem and travels with the cochlear nerve and both the inferior and superior vestibular nerves through the approximately 1-cm long bony internal auditory canal. As it exits the internal auditory canal, the facial nerve travels anteriorly between the vestibule of the inner ear and the ampullated end of the superior semicircular canal. Immediately beyond, the bulbous swelling of the geniculate ganglion appears, which leads to the first genu of the facial nerve. At this genu, the nerve bends posteriorly and passes through through the middle ear. This continuation distal to the geniculate ganglion is known as the horizontal segment. The nerve then curves inferiorly forming the second genu, and passes just anteroinferiorly to the prominence of the lateral semicircular canal. As it travels inferiorly it is known as the vertical or mastoid segment of the facial nerve; it is this segment that is most vulnerable to injury during cochlear implantation. As it courses through the mastoid, the facial nerve gives off two branches, the nerve to the stapedius muscle and farther inferiorly the chorda tympani, which provides taste sensation to the ipsilateral anterior two thirds of the tongue. The chorda tympani and the vertical segment form the anterior and posterior boundaries of the facial recess, a space which when opened allows access to the promontory of the middle ear to drill the cochleostomy.

The tegmen, or roof of the mastoid cavity that separates it from the overlying temporal lobe of the brain, is identified and followed anteriorly to the antrum, a large mastoid air cell that communicates with the middle ear cavity. The horizontal semicircular canal is identified; its hard smooth bone distinguishes it from the surrounding air cells. The vertical segment of the facial nerve runs inferiorly to this important landmark; the nerve can be visualized through bone by its vascular pattern and a salmon-colored blush, if the surrounding bone is sufficiently thin. The posterior external auditory canal is carefully delineated and thinned to a point

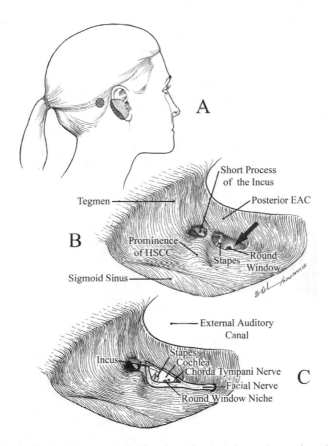

FIGURE 8–6.   Surgical Approach. A. The triangular shaded area shows where the mastoidectomy occurs. The shaded circular area shows approximately where the well for the receiver-stimulator is placed. B. View of the completed mastoidectomy and facial recess. The short process of the incus is visible through the mastoid antrum. The posterior external auditory canal (EAC) is thinned to near translucency. The prominence of the horizontal semicircular canal (SCC) serves as a major landmark during bony removal, as does the tegemen. The arrow points through the facial recess, which is bounded anteriorly by the chorda tympani and posteriorly by the facial nerve, to where the cochleostomy is placed, anterior and inferior to the round window niche. This placement allows the electrode array to be inserted into the scala tympani. C. View of the completed mastoidectomy. This illustration more clearly delineates the relationship of the facial nerve to the facial recess.

of near translucency; this is critical to avoid injury to the facial nerve and to optimize the view into the middle ear. The short process of the incus, lying within the fossa incudis, is identified; it and its overlying bony buttress are used to guide the drilling of the facial recess, which is performed under binocular microscopy. The facial recess is a triangular aerated bony tract that is bounded by the facial nerve posteriorly, by the fossa incudis superiorly, and by the chorda tympani nerve anteriorly, which provides taste sensation to the ipsilateral anterior two thirds of the tongue. The recess provides access to the middle ear from the mastoid cavity and offers a view of the incudostapedial joint and round window. If the facial recess is too small to permit insertion of an electrode, the chorda tympani can be sacrificed. With the cochlear promontory in sight through the facial recess, the cochleostomy is typically placed anteroinferiorly to the round window niche to permit electrode insertion into the scala tympani.

Careful assessment of the cochlear surface anatomy is critical in patients with anomalous cochlear anatomy. A helpful guide is the fact that the round window niche is invariably about 2mm away from the inferior margin of the oval window. During the drilling of the cochleostomy, careful avoidance of the basilar membrane minimizes physical acoustic trauma. The electrode is then delicately advanced into position to minimize damage to the delicate soft tissues of the cochlea. A full insertion will place the tip of the electrode array approximately 25 to 30mm within the cochlear lumen. The internal receiver-stimulator can be seated in its bed either before or after the insertion of the electrode array. The cochleostomy site is then sealed with either a piece of fascia or temporalis muscle. The wound is carefully closed and a pressure dressing is applied. The external device is not fitted until two to four weeks later at which time the device is typically activated.

COMPLICATIONS

The risks of cochlear implantation are similar to the risks of chronic ear surgery: bleeding, infection, facial nerve paresis or paralysis, taste disturbance, further loss of natural hearing, cerebrospinal fluid (CSF) leak, meningitis, and auricular numbness. In addition, cochlear implantation carries a risk of device failure as well as device extrusion or exposure. Also the presence of an implant may preclude medical treatment that includes neurostimulation, the use of monopolar electrocautery near the implant site, electroconvulsive therapy, and ionic radiation therapy. The presence of an implant may also limit the patient's access to MRI imaging. Today, most MRI scanners have a magnet strength between 1.5 and 4 Telsa. High strength MRI scans (1.5 Tesla and above) cannot be done in a routine manner with the implant's magnet in position (Hochmair, Teissl, Kremser, & Hochmair-Desoyer, 2000; Sonnenburg et al., 2002).

Currently the Med El device has FDA approval for 0.2 Tesla imaging without removal of the magnet. Both Advanced Bionics' HiRes 90K and Cochlear's Nucleus Freedom implants have a removable magnet and are MRI safe up to 1.5 Tesla. Implantation in children is not felt to carry a greater risk of complication (Parisier, Chute, Popp, & Hanson, 1997; Waltzman & Cohen, 1998). The largest postnatal changes in the temporal bone are thought to occur in the mastoid. Expansions in length, width, and depth of the mastoid have been described from birth until at least the teenage years. The facial recess enlarges throughout fetal life with the development of the facial canal and the tympanic annulus; however, it probably reaches adult size by birth, allowing surgical access for cochlear implantation in very young children (Eby, 1996).

One of the most feared complications of implantation is damage to the facial nerve. Its vertical course through the mastoid in close proximity to the surgical site puts it at risk. Facial nerve injury can lead to either a temporary or permanent weakness or paralysis. A dense paralysis of the nerve results in the inability to contract the muscles of facial expression and an inability to close the ipsilateral eye. The latter carries a substantial risk of developing an exposure keratitis, which can result in considerable visual loss. As we are considerably dependent on facial expression for communication, facial paralysis can be psychologically traumatic. Fortunately, facial nerve injury is relatively rare with a reported incidence between 0.27 percent and 3 percent of cases (Cohen & Hoffman, 1991; Fayad, Wanna, Micheletto, & Parisier, 2003; Kempf, Tempel, Johann, & Lenarz, 1999; Makhdoum, Snik, & van den Broek, 1997; Webb et al., 1991). Another associated risk to the facial nerve is stimulation from electrodes. The chorda tympani is a small nerve that branches from the facial nerve and travels through the middle ear space. Because it forms the anterior border of the facial recess during dissection, a narrow facial recess can mandate its transection to accommodate the insertion of the electrode. Disruption of the chorda tympani's continuity will lead to a taste disturbance on the anterior two thirds of the ipsilateral tongue. Patients often describe a metallic taste. This typically spontaneously resolves within a few months.

A CSF leak is rare. It occurs typically from a defect in the bony tegmen that separates the mastoid cavity from the cranial middle fossa. It also arises in the setting of a CSF gusher where, upon entering the cochlea, CSF rushes out of the cochleostomy. The latter is due to a bony defect in the inner ear and is treated by insertion of the array into its normal position with sealing of the cochleostomy. Wound infection can lead to other complications, such as flap necrosis with extrusion of the device, as well as meningitis. Fortunately, the majority of infections can be treated without further sequelae or adverse effect on device performance, provided that infections are diagnosed early and treated aggressively (Bhatia, Gibbin, Nikolopoulos, & O'Donoghue, 2004). Meningitis, as previously mentioned, has received much attention recently. As of May 2003, the FDA was aware of 118 cases of cochlear implant recipients worldwide who developed bacterial meningitis, 55 of which occurred in the United States. The patients ranged in age from 13 months to 81 years, with the vast majority of the U.S. cases occurring in children no older than five. In the non-U.S. cases, the incidence was equally distributed among children and adults. The FDA and Centers for Disease Control (CDC) reviewed the medical records of 4,264 children under the age of six; of these, 26 developed meningitis. The number of cases, however, was too small to clearly identify the etiology of the meningitis. The FDA/CDC study did show that cochlear implants with positioners led to a greater risk of meningitis. In July 2002, Advanced Bionics withdrew its positioner from the market.("FDA Public Health Web Notification: Cochlear implant recipients may be at greater risk for meningitis (Updated September 25, 2003)," July 24, 2002) Interestingly, a recent study of cochlear implantations performed in England did not find an association between bacterial meningitis and implantation with a positioner, as was found in the United States and Europe in 2002 (Summerfield et al., 2004).

RESULTS:

A detailed discussion of CI outcomes is beyond the scope of this chapter. Both adult and pediatric groups have derived significant benefit from implantation, and there are numerous data to quantify this benefit. Most impressive has been the ability of children to acquire language, and the subsequent effect of CI on language development. Svirsky et al. showed that the rate of language development in children after CI paralleled those of their normal-hearing counterparts, and that any lag in language development was attributable to the duration of deafness prior to implantation (Svirsky, Robbins, Kirk, Pisoni, & Miyamoto, 2000). This finding has been borne out in school placement, with increasing rates of participation of implanted children in mainstream schooling systems. In adults, detailed quality of life analyses and cost analyses have supported the merits of CI, including the elderly population (Wyatt, Niparko, Rothman, & deLissovoy, 1996). Duration of deafness and preoperative scores on test of sentence recognition are both significant predictors of word recognition with a cochlear implant and account for 80 percent of the variance in word recognition achieved with a cochlear implant (Niparko, Mertes, & Limb, 2005).

FUTURE:

The past two decades have seen remarkable improvement in the performance of cochlear implants. As stated earlier, most of that progress is attributable to advances in processing strategies (Skinner et al., 1994; Wilson et al., 1991). Cochlear implants are arguably the most successful prosthetic interface with the human nervous system, but much work remains. Patients continue to fare far better in quiet conditions than in noisy ones, especially in the face of competing speech. Music and tonal language appreciation offer ample room for improvement. Current efforts to further improve implant benefit include bilateral cochlear implantation, combining conventional acoustic amplification with cochlear implantation for patients with significant residual low-frequency hearing, and increasing levels of neural control with implants.

BILATERAL IMPLANTS

The benefits of bilateral cochlear implantation is an active area of investigation (Gantz et al., 2002; Muller, Schon, & Helms, 2002; Schon, Muller, & Helms,

2002; Tyler et al., 2002; Van Hoesel, Ramsden, & Odriscoll, 2002). Speech perception in noise is important during everyday communication since much of our communication takes place in noisy environments (Gantz et al., 2002). Possible advantages of bilateral implantation include restoration of sound localization abilities and the signal-to-noise advantages that accompany those abilities (Wilson, Lawson, Muller, Tyler, & Kiefer, 2003). Bilateral implants may also lend a "head shadow" benefit for listening in noisy environments. The "head shadow" effect is a purely physical phenomenon: the head creates an acoustic barrier preventing noise from reaching the ear on the opposite side, which preferentially attenuates high frequency sounds (Gantz et al., 2002; Wilson, Lawson, Muller, Tyler, & Kiefer, 2003).

Another potential advantage of binaural hearing lies in the central processing from two independent sources. Listeners with normal hearing use bilateral input, and interaural timing, amplitude, and spectral differences to separate sounds into different "streams." In other words, they separate one acoustic source from other competing acoustic sources. When speech and noise come from different locations, the brain may be able to differentiate them by using their distinct localization cues and therefore improve their intelligibility. This is known as "binaural squelch" (Gantz et al., 2002; Middlebrooks & Green, 1991; Wilson, Lawson, Muller, Tyler, & Kiefer, 2003).

The data collected on bilateral cochlear implants so far is encouraging. The majority of the studied subjects have shown a complete or nearly complete "head shadow" benefit and a significantly better ability to localize sound with both implants, compared to patients with unilateral implants. Additionally, some subjects have shown binaural squelch effects. So far, there has been no evidence of a decrement in speech reception or sound localization for any of the studied subjects. Lastly, subjects have expressed a strong preference for bilateral over unilateral implantation (Wilson, Lawson, Muller, Tyler, & Kiefer, 2003).

COMBINING ACOUSTIC AND ELECTRICAL HEARING IN THE SAME EAR

The most common form of adult hearing loss is a high-frequency sensorineural deficit due to hair cell damage in the basal turn of the cochlea. In these individuals the apical hair cells still function normally, accurately perceiving low-frequency sounds. The primary difficulty is the inability to distinguish the higher-frequency sounds of speech, such as consonants, that are crucial for human communication (Gantz & Turner, 2003). Traditional hearing aids are often ineffective in transmitting these sounds in people with severe high-frequency hearing loss (Ching, Dillon, & Byrne, 1998).

Gantz reported the results of combining acoustic and electrical stimulation in post-lingual adults with severe high-frequency loss (Gantz & Turner, 2004; Gantz & Turner, 2003; Turner, Gantz, Vidal, Behrens, & Henry, 2004). The cochlear implant used had a unique 6-channel electrode array that was based the Nucleus 24 multichannel implant. The electrode array was short, being 6 or 10mm long. Low-frequency hearing was preserved in all patients. Patients who had received the 10mm array were able to understand 83–90 percent of monosyllabic words using the implant and binaural hearing aids, which represented a doubling of the preoperative scores using hearing aids alone. The improvement in speech recognition was primarily due to the increased perception of high-frequency consonant speech cues; this improvement required several months to be apparent (Gantz & Turner, 2004). This preliminary research shows that the human ear has the capacity to integrate both acoustic and high-frequency electrically stimulated speech information. The authors concluded that a device combining electrical and acoustic speech processing has the potential to improve speech recognition in the large number of people whose hearing losses are not severe enough in the low frequencies to justify implantation with the current generation of long-electrode cochlear implants.

TOTALLY IMPLANTABLE COCHLEAR IMPLANT

The presence of the external components in modern cochlear implants does present some limitations. For example, patients cannot hear without the aid of the external device nor they cannot swim with the external device in place. A completely implantable device is therefore very attractive. Its development is currently in a relative infancy. It is unlikely to need a magnet, making it truly MRI compatible. A totally implantable cochlear implant will require a rechargeable power supply as well as an implantable microphone. The latter will be challenging since it will have to be placed where it is capable of great sensitivity, yet not exposed to interference or the risk of extrusion (Cohen, 2004). Also, because the amount of energy a power source can produce is often size limited, a totally implantable system would benefit from a significant reduction of power consumption. Norman has reported the development of a penetrating electrode that will potentially be able to reduce the power consumption of an implant (Hillman, Badi, Normann, Kertesz, & Shelton, 2003; Jones, Campbell, & Normann, 1992; Maynard, Nordhausen, & Normann, 1997). It consists of an array of 1-mm long silicon-based electrode needles that project out from a common 0.2-mm thick silicon base. The electrodes penetrate into neural tissue creating direct electrode-neuron contact. Whereas current devices have a power consumption of approximately 37 μW per electrode, a penetrating electrode could reduce the power requirement to 20 μW per electrode. If and when the totally implantable cochlear implant becomes a reality, it is likely to require modification of current surgical techniques and possibly coupling a microphone mechanism to the ossicular chain (Cohen, 2004; Maniglia, Murray, Arnold, & Ko, 2001; Zenner et al., 2000; Zenner et al., 2004).

AUDITORY BRAINSTEM IMPLANTS

An offshoot of cochlear implant technology is the auditory brainstem implant, which received FDA approval in 2000. Over 141 have been implanted at the House Ear Institute and 300 worldwide (Otto, Brackmann, Hitselberger, Shannon, &

Syms, 2005; Schwartz, Otto, Brackmann, Hitselberger, & Shannon, 2003). With an electrode placement over the cochlear nucleus complex, its main utility has been in the treatment of patients with neurofibromatosis II who develop bilateral vestibular schawnnomas. The complete resection of these tumors often results in permanent disruption of the auditory nerve and, therefore, deafness (Kuchta, Otto, Shannon, Hitselberger, & Brackmann, 2004; Otto, Brackmann, & Hitselberger, 2004; Otto, Brackmann, Hitselberger, Shannon, & Kuchta, 2002; Otto, House, Brackmann, Hitselberger, & Nelson, 1990; Otto et al., 1998; Schwartz, Otto, Brackmann, Hitselberger, & Shannon, 2003).

Similar to cochlear implants, there is an external device housing a microphone and speech processor that communicates to an internal receiver/stimulator via a radio frequency coil. Its electrode design is significantly different however. The array does not linearly arrange its electrodes but rather has a footplate of 2.5 × 8mm with 21 electrodes contacting the neural tissue. Implantation requires a neurosurgical and not an otologic operation. Compared to cochlear implants, the performance benefits of auditory brainstem implants require a longer rehabilitation. While auditory brainstem implant performance is poorer than that of a cochlear implant, there are individuals who benefit significantly and display cochlear implant-like speech recognition. New penetrating microelectrodes and new speech processing strategies hold the promise of improved performance and will soon be tested in humans (Kuchta, Otto, Shannon, Hitselberger, & Brackmann, 2004; Otto, Brackmann, Hitselberger, Shannon, & Syms, 2005; Schwartz, Otto, Brackmann, Hitselberger, & Shannon, 2003).

REFERENCES

Abbas, P. J., Brown, C. J., Shallop, J. K., Firszt, J. B., Hughes, M. L., Hong, S. H., et al. (1999). Summary of results using the nucleus CI24M implant to record the electrically evoked compound action potential. *Ear Hear, 20*(1), 45–59.

Balkany, T. J., Eshraghi, A. A., & Yang, N. (2002). Modiolar proximity of three perimodiolar cochlear implant electrodes. *Acta Otolaryngol, 122*(4), 363–369.

Balkany, T. J., Hodges, A., Miyamoto, R. T., Gibbin, K., & Odabasi, O. (2001). Cochlear implants in children. *Otolaryngol Clin North Am, 34*(2), 455–467.

Bhatia, K., Gibbin, K. P., Nikolopoulos, T. P., & O'Donoghue, G. M. (2004). Surgical complications and their management in a series of 300 consecutive pediatric cochlear implantations. *Otol Neurotol, 25*(5), 730–739.

Brown, C. J., Abbas, P. J., & Gantz, B. (1990). Electrically evoked whole-nerve action potentials: data from human cochlear implant users. *J Acoust Soc Am, 88*(3), 1385–1391.

Casselman, J. W. (2002). Diagnostic imaging in clinical neuro-otology. *Curr Opin Neurol, 15*(1), 23–30.

Ching, T. Y., Dillon, H., & Byrne, D. (1998). Speech recognition of hearing-impaired listeners: predictions from audibility and the limited role of high-frequency amplification. *J Acoust Soc Am, 103*(2), 1128–1140.

Cho, Y. S., Na, D. G., Jung, J. Y., & Hong, S. H. (2000). Narrow internal auditory canal syndrome: Parasaggital reconstruction. *J Laryngol Otol, 114*(5), 392–394.

Cohen, N. L. (2004). Cochlear implant candidacy and surgical considerations. *Audiol Neurootol, 9*(4), 197–202.

Cohen, N. L., & Hoffman, R. A. (1991). Complications of cochlear implant surgery in adults and children. *Ann Otol Rhinol Laryngol, 100*(9, Pt. 1), 708–711.

Cohen, N. L., Roland, J. T., Jr., & Marrinan, M. (2004). Meningitis in cochlear implant recipients: The North American experience. *Otol Neurotol, 25*(3), 275–281.

Dahm, M. C., Clark, G. M., Franz, B. K., Shepherd, R. K., Burton, M. J., & Robins-Browne, R. (1994). Cochlear implantation in children: Labyrinthitis following pneumococcal otitis media in unimplanted and implanted cat cochleas. *Acta Otolaryngol, 114*(6), 620–625.

Dillier, N., Lai, W. K., Almqvist, B., Frohne, C., Muller-Deile, J., Stecker, M., et al. (2002). Measurement of the electrically evoked compound action potential via a neural response telemetry system. *Ann Otol Rhinol Laryngol, 111*(5, Pt. 1), 407–414.

Djourno, A., & Eyries, C. (1957). [Auditory prosthesis by means of a distant electrical stimulation of the sensory nerve with the use of an indwelt coiling.]. *Presse Med, 65*(63), 1417.

Djourno, A., Eyries, C., & Vallancien, B. (1957). [Electric excitation of the cochlear nerve in man by induction at a distance with the aid of micro-coil included in the fixture.]. *C R Seances Soc Biol Fil, 151*(3), 423–425.

Djourno, A., Eyries, C., & Vallancien, P. (1957). [Preliminary attempts of electrical excitation of the auditory nerve in man, by permanently inserted micro-apparatus.]. *Bull Acad Natl Med, 141*(21–23), 481–483.

Dorman, M. F., Loizou, P. C., & Rainey, D. (1997). Speech intelligibility as a function of the number of channels of stimulation for signal processors using sine-wave and noise-band outputs. *J Acoust Soc Am, 102*(4), 2403–2411.

Doyle, J. B., Jr., Doyle, J. H., Turnbull, F. M., Abbey, J., & House, L. (1963). Electrical Stimulation In Eighth Nerve Deafness. A Preliminary Report. *Bull Los Angel Neuro Soc, 28*, 148–150.

Doyle, J. H., Doyle, J. B., Jr., & Turnbull, F. M., Jr. (1964). Electrical Stimulation Of Eighth Cranial Nerve. *Arch Otolaryngol, 80*, 388–391.

Drullman, R. (1995). Temporal envelope and fine structure cues for speech intelligibility. *J Acoust Soc Am, 97*(1), 585–592.

Eby, T. L. (1996). Development of the facial recess: Implications for cochlear implantation. *Laryngoscope, 106*(5, Pt. 2, Suppl. 80), 1–7.

Eisen, M. D. (2003). Djourno, Eyries, and the first implanted electrical neural stimulator to restore hearing. *Otol Neurotol, 24*(3), 500–506.

Ellul, S., Shelton, C., Davidson, H. C., & Harnsberger, H. R. (2000). Preoperative cochlear implant imaging: Is magnetic resonance imaging enough? *Am J Otol, 21*(4), 528–533.

Eshraghi, A. A., Yang, N. W., & Balkany, T. J. (2003). Comparative study of cochlear damage with three perimodiolar electrode designs. *Laryngoscope, 113*(3), 415–419.

Fayad, J. N., Luxford, W., & Linthicum, F. H. (2000). The Clarion electrode positioner: Temporal bone studies. *Am J Otol, 21*(2), 226–229.

Fayad, J. N., Tabaee, A., Micheletto, J. N., & Parisier, S. C. (2003). Cochlear implantation in children with otitis media. *Laryngoscope, 113*(7), 1224–1227.

Fayad, J. N., Wanna, G. B., Micheletto, J. N., & Parisier, S. C. (2003). Facial nerve paralysis following cochlear implant surgery. *Laryngoscope, 113*(8), 1344–1346.

FDA Public Health Web Notification: Cochlear implant recipients may be at greater risk for meningitis (Updated September 25, 2003). (July 24, 2002). from www.fda.gov/cdrh/safety/cochlear/html

Fishman, K. E., Shannon, R. V., & Slattery, W. H. (1997). Speech recognition as a function of the number of electrodes used in the SPEAK cochlear implant speech processor. *J Speech Lang Hear Res, 40*(5), 1201–1215.

Francis, H. W., Yeagle, J. D., Brightwell, T., & Venick, H. (2004). Central effects of residual hearing: Implications for choice of ear for cochlear implantation. *Laryngoscope, 114*(10), 1747–1752.

Friedland, D. R., Venick, H. S., & Niparko, J. K. (2003). Choice of ear for cochlear implantation: The effect of history and residual hearing on predicted postoperative performance. *Otol Neurotol, 24*(4), 582–589.

Friesen, L. M., Shannon, R. V., Baskent, D., & Wang, X. (2001). Speech recognition in noise as a function of the number of spectral channels: comparison of acoustic hearing and cochlear implants. *J Acoust Soc Am, 110*(2), 1150–1163.

Fu, Q. J., & Galvin, J. J., III. (2001). Recognition of spectrally asynchronous speech by normal-hearing listeners and Nucleus—22 cochlear implant users. *J Acoust Soc Am, 109*(3), 1166–1172.

Fu, Q. J., & Shannon, R. V. (1998). Effects of amplitude nonlinearity on phoneme recognition by cochlear implant users and normal-hearing listeners. *J Acoust Soc Am, 104*(5), 2570–2577.

Fu, Q. J., Shannon, R. V., & Wang, X. (1998). Effects of noise and spectral resolution on vowel and consonant recognition: acoustic and electric hearing. *J Acoust Soc Am, 104*(6), 3586–3596.

Gantz, B. J., & Turner, C. (2004). Combining acoustic and electrical speech processing: Iowa/Nucleus hybrid implant. *Acta Otolaryngol, 124*(4), 344–347.

Gantz, B. J., & Turner, C. W. (2003). Combining acoustic and electrical hearing. *Laryngoscope, 113*(10), 1726–1730.

Gantz, B. J., Tyler, R. S., Rubinstein, J. T., Wolaver, A., Lowder, M., Abbas, P., et al. (2002). Binaural cochlear implants placed during the same operation. *Otol Neurotol, 23*(2), 169–180.

Gomaa, N. A., Rubinstein, J. T., Lowder, M. W., Tyler, R. S., & Gantz, B. J. (2003). Residual speech perception and cochlear implant performance in postlingually deafened adults. *Ear Hear, 24*(6), 539–544.

Hillman, T., Badi, A. N., Normann, R. A., Kertesz, T., & Shelton, C. (2003). Cochlear nerve stimulation with a 3-dimensional penetrating electrode array. *Otol Neurotol, 24*(5), 764–768.

Hochmair, E. S., Teissl, C., Kremser, C., & Hochmair-Desoyer, I. (2000). Magnetic resonance imaging safety of the Combi 40/Combi 40+ cochlear implants. *Adv Otorhinolaryngol, 57*, 39–41.

House, W. F. (1976). Cochlear implants. *Ann Otol Rhinol Laryngol, 85 suppl 27*(3Pt2), 1–93.

House, W. F., Luxford, W. M., & Courtney, B. (1985). Otitis media in children following the cochlear implant. *Ear Hear, 6*(3 Suppl.), 24S–26S.

House, W. F., & Urban, J. (1973). Long term results of electrode implantation and electronic stimulation of the cochlea in man. *Ann Otol Rhinol Laryngol, 82*(4), 504–517.

James, A. L., & Papsin, B. C. (2004). Cochlear implant surgery at 12 months of age or younger. *Laryngoscope, 114*(12), 2191–2195.

Jones, K. E., Campbell, P. K., & Normann, R. A. (1992). A glass/silicon composite intracortical electrode array. *Ann Biomed Eng, 20*(4), 423–437.

Kaplan-Neeman, R., Henkin, Y., Yakir, Z., Bloch, F., Berlin, M., Kronenberg, J., et al. (2004). NRT-based versus behavioral-based MAP: a comparison of parameters and speech perception in young children. *J Basic Clin Physiol Pharmacol, 15*(1–2), 57–69.

Karatzanis, A. D., Chimona, T. S., Prokopakis, E. P., Kyrmizakis, D. E., & Velegrakis, G. A. (2003). Cochlear implantation after radical mastoidectomy: management of a challenging case. *ORL J Otorhinolaryngol Relat Spec, 65*(6), 375–378.

Kempf, H. G., Stover, T., & Lenarz, T. (2000). Mastoiditis and acute otitis media in children with cochlear implants: Recommendations for medical management. *Ann Otol Rhinol Laryngol Suppl, 185*, 25–27.

Kempf, H. G., Tempel, S., Johann, K., & Lenarz, T. (1999). [Complications of cochlear implant surgery in children and adults]. *Laryngorhinootologie, 78*(10), 529–537.

Kong, Y. Y., Cruz, R., Jones, J. A., & Zeng, F. G. (2004). Music perception with temporal cues in acoustic and electric hearing. *Ear Hear, 25*(2), 173–185.

Kuchta, J., Otto, S. R., Shannon, R. V., Hitselberger, W. E., & Brackmann, D. E. (2004). The multichannel auditory brainstem implant: how many electrodes make sense? *J Neurosurg, 100*(1), 16–23.

Lan, N., Nie, K. B., Gao, S. K., & Zeng, F. G. (2004). A novel speech-processing strategy incorporating tonal information for cochlear implants. *IEEE Trans Biomed Eng, 51*(5), 752–760.

Lawson, D. T., Wilson, B. S., & Finley, C. C. (1993). New processing strategies for multichannel cochlear prostheses. *Prog Brain Res, 97*, 313–321.

Loizou, P. C. (1999). Introduction to cochlear implants. *IEEE Eng Med Biol Mag, 18*(1), 32–42.

Loizou, P. C., Dorman, M., Poroy, O., & Spahr, T. (2000). Speech recognition by normal-hearing and cochlear implant listeners as a function of intensity resolution. *J Acoust Soc Am, 108*(5 Pt 1), 2377–2387.

Luntz, M., Hodges, A. V., Balkany, T., Dolan-Ash, S., & Schloffman, J. (1996). Otitis media in children with cochlear implants. *Laryngoscope, 106*(11), 1403–1405.

Luntz, M., Teszler, C. B., & Shpak, T. (2004). Cochlear implantation in children with otitis media: Second stage of a long-term prospective study. *Int J Pediatr Otorhinolaryngol, 68*(3), 273–280.

Luntz, M., Teszler, C. B., Shpak, T., Feiglin, H., & Farah-Sima'an, A. (2001). Cochlear implantation in healthy and otitis-prone children: A prospective study. *Laryngoscope, 111*(9), 1614–1618.

Makhdoum, M. J., Snik, A. F., & van den Broek, P. (1997). Cochlear implantation: a review of the literature and the Nijmegen results. *J Laryngol Otol, 111*(11), 1008–1017.

Maniglia, A. J., Murray, G., Arnold, J. E., & Ko, W. H. (2001). Bioelectronic options for a totally implantable hearing device for partial and total hearing loss. *Otolaryngol Clin North Am, 34*(2), 469–483.

Maynard, E. M., Nordhausen, C. T., & Normann, R. A. (1997). The Utah intracortical Electrode Array: A recording structure for potential brain-computer interfaces. *Electroencephalogr Clin Neurophysiol, 102*(3), 228–239.

Michelson, R. P. (1971a). Electrical stimulation of the human cochlea. A preliminary report. *Arch Otolaryngol, 93*(3), 317–323.

Michelson, R. P. (1971b). The results of electrical stimulation of the cochlea in human sensory deafness. *Ann Otol Rhinol Laryngol, 80*(6), 914–919.

Middlebrooks, J. C., & Green, D. M. (1991). Sound localization by human listeners. *Annu Rev Psychol, 42*, 135–159.

Muller, J., Schon, F., & Helms, J. (2002). Speech understanding in quiet and noise in bilateral users of the MED-EL COMBI 40/40+ cochlear implant system. *Ear Hear, 23*(3), 198–206.

Nadol, J. B., Jr., & Eddington, D. K. (2004). Histologic evaluation of the tissue seal and biologic response around cochlear implant electrodes in the human. *Otol Neurotol, 25*(3), 257–262.

Nair, S. B., Abou-Elhamd, K. A., & Hawthorne, M. (2000). A retrospective analysis of high resolution computed tomography in the assessment of cochlear implant patients. *Clin Otolaryngol, 25*(1), 55–61.

Niparko, J. K., Francis, H. W., Tucci, D. L., Dawsey, D., & Chinnici, J. (2003). Auditory rehabilitation: Cochlear implants. In L. Lustig, & J. K. Niparko (Eds.), *Clinical neurotology: Diagnosing and managing disorders of hearing, balance and the facial nerve* (1st ed., pp. 291–331). London: Martin Dunitz Ltd.

Niparko, J. K., Mertes, J. L., & Limb, C. J. (2005). Cochlear implants: results, outcomes, and rehabilitation. In C. W. Cummings, P. W. Flint, L. A. Harker, B. H. Haughey, M. A. Richardson, K. T. Robbins, D. E. Schuller, & J. R. Thomas (Eds.), *Otolaryngology head & neck surgery* (4th ed., Vol. 4, pp. 3650–3671). Philadelphia, PA: Elsevier Mosby.

O'Donoghue, G., Balkany, T., Cohen, N., Lenarz, T., Lustig, L., & Niparko, J. (2002). Meningitis and cochlear implantation. *Otol Neurotol, 23*(6), 823–824.

Oghalai, J. S. (2004). The cochlear amplifier: Augmentation of the traveling wave within the inner ear. *Curr Opin Otolaryngol Head Neck Surg, 12*(5), 431–438.

Otto, S. R., Brackmann, D. E., & Hitselberger, W. (2004). Auditory brainstem implantation in 12- to 18-year-olds. *Arch Otolaryngol Head Neck Surg, 130*(5), 656–659.

Otto, S. R., Brackmann, D. E., Hitselberger, W. E., Shannon, R. V., & Kuchta, J. (2002). Multichannel auditory brainstem implant: Update on performance in 61 patients. *J Neurosurg, 96*(6), 1063–1071.

Otto, S. R., Brackmann, D. E., Hitselberger, W. E., Shannon, R. V., & Syms, M. J. (2005). Auditory brainstem implant. In R. K. Jackler & D. E. Brackmann (Eds.), *Neurotology* (2nd ed., pp. 1323–1330). Philadelphia, PA: C. V. Mosby.

Otto, S. R., House, W. F., Brackmann, D. E., Hitselberger, W. E., & Nelson, R. A. (1990). Auditory brain stem implant: effect of tumor size and preoperative hearing level on function. *Ann Otol Rhinol Laryngol, 99*(10, Pt. 1), 789–790.

Otto, S. R., Shannon, R. V., Brackmann, D. E., Hitselberger, W. E., Staller, S., & Menapace, C. (1998). The multichannel auditory brain stem implant: Performance in twenty patients. *Otolaryngol Head Neck Surg, 118*(3, Pt. 1), 291–303.

Parisier, S. C., Chute, P. M., Popp, A. L., & Hanson, M. B. (1997). Surgical techniques for cochlear implantation in the very young child. *Otolaryngol Head Neck Surg, 117*(3, Pt. 1), 248–254.

Pasanisi, E., Vincenti, V., Bacciu, A., Guida, M., Berghenti, T., Barbot, A., et al. (2002). Multichannel cochlear implantation in radical mastoidectomy cavities. *Otolaryngol Head Neck Surg, 127*(5), 432–436.

Richter, B., Aschendorff, A., Lohnstein, P., Husstedt, H., Nagursky, H., & Laszig, R. (2002). Clarion 1.2 standard electrode array with partial space-filling positioner: radiological and histological evaluation in human temporal bones. *J Laryngol Otol, 116*(7), 507–513.

Rizer, F. M., & Burkey, J. M. (1999). Cochlear implantation in the very young child. *Otolaryngol Clin North Am, 32*(6), 1117–1125.

Rubinstein, J. T. (2004). How cochlear implants encode speech. *Curr Opin Otolaryngol Head Neck Surg, 12*(5), 444–448.

Rubinstein, J. T., Parkinson, W. S., Tyler, R. S., & Gantz, B. J. (1999). Residual speech recognition and cochlear implant performance: Effects of implantation criteria. *Am J Otol, 20*(4), 445–452.

Saberi, K., & Perrott, D. R. (1999). Cognitive restoration of reversed speech. *Nature, 398*(6730), 760.

Schon, F., Muller, J., & Helms, J. (2002). Speech reception thresholds obtained in a symmetrical four-loudspeaker arrangement from bilateral users of MED-El. cochlear implants. *Otol Neurotol, 23*(5), 710–714.

Schwartz, M. S., Otto, S. R., Brackmann, D. E., Hitselberger, W. F., & Shannon, R. V. (2003). Use of a multichannel auditory brainstem implant for neurofibromatosis type 2. *Stereotact Funct Neurosurg, 81*(1–4), 110–114.

Seligman, P., & McDermott, H. (1995). Architecture of the Spectra 22 speech processor. *Ann Otol Rhinol Laryngol Suppl, 166*, 139–141.

Seyle, K., & Brown, C. J. (2002). Speech perception using maps based on neural response telemetry measures. *Ear Hear, 23*(1 Suppl.), 72S—79S.

Shannon, R. V. (2002). The relative importance of amplitude, temporal, and spectral cues for cochlear implant processor design. *Am J Audiol, 11*(2), 124–127.

Shannon, R. V., Galvin, J. J., III, & Baskent, D. (2002). Holes in hearing. *J Assoc Res Otolaryngol, 3*(2), 185–199.

Shannon, R. V., Zeng, F. G., Kamath, V., Wygonski, J., & Ekelid, M. (1995). Speech recognition with primarily temporal cues. *Science, 270*(5234), 303–304.

Shannon, R. V., Zeng, F. G., & Wygonski, J. (1998). Speech recognition with altered spectral distribution of envelope cues. *J Acoust Soc Am, 104*(4), 2467–2476.

Sheehy, J. L. (1959). A review of operations on the temporal bone. *Calif Med, 91*, 137–142.

Simmons, F. B., Mongeon, C. J., Lewis, W. R., & Huntington, D. A. (1964). Electrical Stimulation Of Acoustical Nerve And Inferior Colliculus. *Arch Otolaryngol, 79*, 559–568.

Skinner, M. W., Arndt, P. L., & Staller, S. J. (2002). Nucleus 24 advanced encoder conversion study: Performance versus preference. *Ear Hear, 23*(1 Suppl.), 2S–17S.

Skinner, M. W., Clark, G. M., Whitford, L. A., Seligman, P. M., Staller, S. J., Shipp, D. B., et al. (1994). Evaluation of a new spectral peak coding strategy for the Nucleus 22 Channel Cochlear Implant System. *Am J Otol, 15 Suppl 2*, 15–27.

Skinner, M. W., Holden, L. K., Whitford, L. A., Plant, K. L., Psarros, C., & Holden, T. A. (2002). Speech recognition with the nucleus 24 SPEAK, ACE, and CIS speech coding strategies in newly implanted adults. *Ear Hear, 23*(3), 207–223.

Smith, Z. M., Delgutte, B., & Oxenham, A. J. (2002). Chimaeric sounds reveal dichotomies in auditory perception. *Nature, 416*(6876), 87–90.

Sonnenburg, R. E., Wackym, P. A., Yoganandan, N., Firszt, J. B., Prost, R. W., & Pintar, F. A. (2002). Biophysics of cochlear implant/MRI interactions emphasizing bone biomechanical properties. *Laryngoscope, 112*(10), 1720–1725.

Summerfield, A. Q., Cirstea, S. E., Roberts, K. L., Barton, G. R., Graham, J. M., & O'Donoghue G. M. (2005). Incidence of meningitis and of death from all causes among users of cochlear implants in the United Kingdom. *J Public Health (Oxf), 27*(1), 55–61.

Svirsky, M. A., Robbins, A. M., Kirk, K. I., Pisoni, D. B., & Miyamoto, R. T. (2000). Language development in profoundly deaf children with cochlear implants. *Psychol Sci, 11*(2), 153–158.

Tien, R. D., Felsberg, G. J., & Macfall, J. (1992). Fast spin-echo high-resolution MR imaging of the inner ear. *AJR Am J Roentgenol, 159*(2), 395–398.

Toner, J. G., John, G., & McNaboe, E. J. (1998). Cochlear implantation under local anaesthesia, the Belfast experience. *J Laryngol Otol, 112*(6), 533–536.

Turner, C. W., Gantz, B. J., Vidal, C., Behrens, A., & Henry, B. A. (2004). Speech recognition in noise for cochlear implant listeners: Benefits of residual acoustic hearing. *J Acoust Soc Am, 115*(4), 1729–1735.

Tyler, R. S., Gantz, B. J., Rubinstein, J. T., Wilson, B. S., Parkinson, A. J., Wolaver, A., et al. (2002). Three-month results with bilateral cochlear implants. *Ear Hear, 23*(1 Suppl), 80S–89S.

van den Broek, P., Cohen, N., O'Donoghue, G., Fraysse, B., Laszig, R., & Offeciers, E. (1995). Cochlear implantation in children. *Int J Pediatr Otorhinolaryngol, 32 Suppl*, S217–223.

Van Hoesel, R., Ramsden, R., & Odriscoll, M. (2002). Sound-direction identification, interaural time delay discrimination, and speech intelligibility advantages in noise for a bilateral cochlear implant user. *Ear Hear, 23*(2), 137–149.

van Hoesel, R. J., & Clark, G. M. (1995). Evaluation of a portable two-microphone adaptive beamforming speech processor with cochlear implant patients. *J Acoust Soc Am, 97*(4), 2498–2503.

Vandali, A. E., Whitford, L. A., Plant, K. L., & Clark, G. M. (2000). Speech perception as a function of electrical stimulation rate: using the Nucleus 24 cochlear implant system. *Ear Hear, 21*(6), 608–624.

Volta, A. (1800). On the electricity excited by mere contact of conducting substances of different kinds. *R Soc Phil Trans, 90*(403–431).

Waltzman, S. B., & Cohen, N. L. (1998). Cochlear implantation in children younger than 2 years old. *Am J Otol, 19*(2), 158–162.

Webb, R. L., Lehnhardt, E., Clark, G. M., Laszig, R., Pyman, B. C., & Franz, B. K. (1991). Surgical complications with the cochlear multiple-channel intracochlear implant: Experience at Hannover and Melbourne. *Ann Otol Rhinol Laryngol, 100*(2), 131–136.

Whitford, L. A., Seligman, P. M., Everingham, C. E., Antognelli, T., Skok, M. C., Hollow, R. D., et al. (1995). Evaluation of the Nucleus Spectra 22 processor and new speech processing strategy (SPEAK) in postlinguistically deafened adults. *Acta Otolaryngol, 115*(5), 629–637.

Wilson, B. S., Finley, C. C., Lawson, D. T., Wolford, R. D., Eddington, D. K., & Rabinowitz, W. M. (1991). Better speech recognition with cochlear implants. *Nature, 352*(6332), 236–238.

Wilson, B. S., Lawson, D. T., Muller, J. M., Tyler, R. S., & Kiefer, J. (2003). Cochlear implants: some likely next steps. *Annu Rev Biomed Eng, 5*, 207–249.

Wouters, J., & Vanden Berghe, J. (2001). Speech recognition in noise for cochlear implantees with a two-microphone monaural adaptive noise reduction system. *Ear Hear, 22*(5), 420–430.

Wyatt, J. R., Niparko, J. K., Rothman, M., & deLissovoy, G. (1996). Cost utility of the multichannel cochlear implants in 258 profoundly deaf individuals. *Laryngoscope, 106*(7), 816–821.

Zenner, H. P., Leysieffer, H., Maassen, M., Lehner, R., Lenarz, T., Baumann, J., et al. (2000). Human studies of a piezoelectric transducer and a microphone for a totally implantable electronic hearing device. *Am J Otol, 21*(2), 196–204.

Zenner, H. P., Limberger, A., Baumann, J. W., Reischl, G., Zalaman, I. M., Mauz, P. S., et al. (2004). Phase III results with a totally implantable piezoelectric middle ear implant: Speech audiometry, spatial hearing and psychosocial adjustment. *Acta Otolaryngol, 124*(2), 155–164.

CHAPTER 9

Treatment of Vestibular Disorders

Benjamin L. Judson and H. Jeffrey Kim
Georgetown University Medical Center

Vestibular system disorders cause a spectrum of symptoms from acute debilitating vertigo to barely noticeable mild imbalance. The time course of injury to the vestibular system and a naturally occurring vestibular compensation process in the central nervous system (CNS) determines the clinical course experienced by these patients. Understanding the CNS compensation process and its dynamic relation with the pathophysiology of the disease affecting the vestibular system is important for managing patients with these disorders. Frequently symptoms resulting from vestibular system injury, such as vertigo, are self-limiting because of CNS compensation. However, several factors can delay or impair normal CNS compensation and in these cases medical, rehabilitative or surgical intervention may be helpful. This chapter reviews the mechanism of vestibular compensation and provides an overview of the pathophysiology of common vestibular disorders such as viral labyrinthitis, migraine headache, Ménière's disease, benign paroxysmal positional vertigo, and different types of labyrinthine fistula. The medical, rehabilitative and surgical treatments for these diseases are reviewed, including symptomatic and disease specific treatments.

CLASSIFICATION OF VESTIBULAR DISORDERS

Vestibular disorders are classified according to the time course of injury to the vestibular system. Disorders can cause a single acute injury, ongoing or chronic injury, or they may have a recurrent or relapsing course with periods of chronic or repeated acute injury. Some diseases have a bilateral effect while others result in unilateral injury. The time course of each disease is important for understanding its relationship to CNS vestibular compensation and the role of treatment. One common disease pattern is acute unilateral vestibulopathy which results in vertigo, nausea and vomiting that usually lasting several days (Table 9-1). These symptoms

TABLE 9–1
Common Patterns of Vestibular Disease

Acute unilateral vestibulopathy	Chronic bilateral vestibulopathy	Recurrent acute vestibulopathy
Viral neuronitis	Ototoxic injury	Benign paroxysmal positional vertigo
Labyrinthitis		Migraine's
Acute labyrinthitis		Vertibrobasilar insufficiency
Surgical/Iatrogenic		Ménière's disease
Temporal bone fracture		
Stroke		
Perilymphatic fistula		

disappear over days, weeks and even months as a result of the vestibular compensation process. Another common disease pattern is a chronic bilateral vestibulopathy which frequently occurs from a slow ongoing injury to the vestibular system. These patients frequently do not have acute symptoms because of ongoing vestibular compensation but may eventually experience a general imbalance or even oscillopsia, which is a perception that the environment is moving when the head is moved. For example, with oscillopsia walking generates a sensation that the environment is moving when there is head movement.

Recurrent acute vestibulopathies cause an acute vestibular dysfunction and symptoms (see Table 9–2). However, the dysfunction abates before compensation occurs and then re-occurs in the future. Examples of this pattern include the most common cause of vertigo, benign paroxysmal positional vertigo, as well as vertiginous migraine headaches, and vertibrobasilar insufficiency. A recurrent acute vestibulopathy that also has a progressive nature to its course is Ménière's disease. With this poorly understood disease there is vestibular dysfunction that resolves and recurs over time but there can be an overall progressive course of vestibular dysfunction. Vestibular compensation occurs, however there can be ongoing acute symptoms because of the ongoing change in vestibular function. The persistence of acute vestibular symptoms makes this disease debilitating.

TABLE 9–2
Symptoms from Unilateral Acute Vestibular Injury

Vertigo	Sensation that the environment or patient's body is moving when neither is occurring. Frequently described as a whirling or spinning sensation.
Nystagmus	Involuntary rhythmic eye movement away from the side of the vestibular injury. Spontaneous nystagmus is present initially. After recovery of spontaneous nystagmus, there may still be nystagmus induced by head movement or other stimuli.
Head and body tilt	Head and body tilt toward the side of the lesion.
Ataxia and imbalance	Difficulty coordinating ambulation with imbalance and tendency to turn or fall toward the side of the vestibular injury.
Nausea and emesis	Sensation of having to vomit or actually vomiting.

VESTIBULAR COMPENSATION

An acute unilateral vestibulopathy can cause vertigo, nystagmus, head and body tilt, nausea, diaphoresis, ataxia, and imbalance (see Table 9–2). Following vestibular injury a central nervous system (CNS) compensation process occurs. Vestibular compensation can be most easily demonstrated when it occurs in response to an acute unilateral vestibulopathy. However, it occurs with all vestibular injury. Vestibular compensation is a heterogeneous process. First, the symptoms of acute vestibular injury improve over different periods of time (see Table 9–3). Second, some symptoms resolve completely while others may persist indefinitely. Finally, the process is significantly dependent on the function of other peripheral and central systems. Therefore, young otherwise healthy patients may exhibit a remarkable recovery from significant vestibular injury while other patients with confounding medical conditions affecting their vision, musculoskeletal system, or peripheral or central nervous system may have limited recover from a much smaller injury.

Current theories explain vestibular compensation in terms of CNS plasticity (or flexibility) and substitution. At rest, sensory hair cells in the peripheral vestibular organs (semicircular canals, saccule and utricle) have a tonic rate of firing. When stimulated positively the rate of depolarization of the different cells increases and when stimulated negatively the rate decreases. Each sense organ has a corresponding contralateral sensory organ. For example the left anterior semicircular canal is in the same plane as the right posterior semicircular canal. Their configuration is such that head movement that stimulates one side positively, will stimulate the other side negatively. Therefore there is a "push-pull" balance between the two sides. When one side is injured, the imbalance of tone is perceived as movement and is responsible for acute symptoms of vestibular injury. There is no recovery of tone in neurons from the damaged vestibular sensory cells. However, the vestibular nucleus compensates by increasing the rate of firing on the injured side and decreasing the rate of firing on the un-injured side until an

TABLE 9–3
Stages of Compensation of Acute Unilateral Vestibular Injury

System Affected	Acute (hours to days)	Short-term (days to weeks)	Long-term (months to years)
Vestibulo-thalamo-cortical network	Severe vertigo	Mild or positional vertigo	Rare to absent
Vestibulo-autonomic pathways	Nausea Emesis Sweating pallor	Mild nausea	Rare to absent
Vestibulo-ocular reflexes	Spontaneous Nystagmus	Inducible nystagmus	Inducible nystagmus uncommon
Vestibulo-spinal reflexes	Severe ataxia Head and body tilt	Lessening of severity, disequilibrium	Symptomatic resolution (abnormalities detectable with testing)

equilibrium is again established. This compensation is responsible for the resolution of spontaneous nystagmus and is thought also to be responsible for the resolution of vertigo (Black, 2003). However, testing of the vestibulo-occular reflexes (VOR) reveals that even in asymptomatic individuals who clinically appear to have completely compensated, there is a reduction in the gain of the VOR. Therefore even in patients who are clinically completely compensated, testing can reveal underlying deficits in vestibular functioning.

SYMPTOMATIC MEDICAL TREATMENTS FOR VERTIGO

The treatment of acute vestibular symptoms is accomplished primarily with vestibular suppressants and anti-emetics. If vestibular symptoms are present for more than 30 minutes medical treatment may provide some relief. Medical therapies for specific vestibular pathologies will be discussed in the next section. Vestibular suppressants include anticholinergics, antihistamines, and benzodiazepines. The most commonly used vestibular suppressants are listed in Table 9–4. Vestibular suppressants have a significant side effect of general sedation.

Vestibular suppressants have been shown in animal models to retard vestibular compensation. This can be a beneficial or deleterious effect depending on the

TABLE 9-4
Commonly Used Vestibular Suppressants

Medication	Dose	Mechanism	Adverse effects
Anticholinergics			
scopolamine	0.5 mg patch every 3days	Anticholingergic	Topical allergy, Precaution with glaucoma and prostatic enlargement
Antihistamines			
meclizine	12.5–50 mg every 4–6 hours	Histamine (H1) antagonist Muscarine antagonist	Sedation Caution with prostatic enlargement
dimenhydrinate	50 mg every 4 hours	Histamine (H1) antagonist Muscarine antagonist	Sedation Caution with prostatic enlargement
Benzodiazepines			
clonazepam	0.5 mg twice a day	GABA agonist	Sedating Drug dependency
diazepam	2–10 mg every 4 hours	GABA agonist	Sedation Respiratory depressant Dependency Caution in glaucoma
lorazepam	0.5 mg twice a day	GABA agonist	Sedating Drug dependency

TABLE 9–5
Antiemetics Commonly Used in Patients with Vertigo

Medication	Dose	Mechanism	Adverse effects
Granisetron	1 mg orally or IV	Serotonin 5-HT3 antagonist	Headache
Meclizine	12.5–50 mg every 4–6 hours	Histamine (H1) antagonist Muscarine antagonist	Sedation Precaution with glaucoma and prostate enlargement
Metoclopramide	10 mg orally or IM TID	Dopamine antagonist stimulates upper gastrointestinal motility	Fatigue Sedation Restlessness Confusion
Ondansetron	4 mg orally or IV	Serotonin 5-HT3 antagonist	Headache Diarrhea Fever
Prochlorperazine (Compazine)	5–10 mg orally every 6–8 hours or 25 mg rectally every 12 hours	Muscarinic antagonist Dopamine (D2) antagonist	Sedating Extrapyramidal
Promethazine (Phenergan)	25 mg orally every 6–8 hours or 25 mg rectally every 12 hours	Histamine (H1) antagonist Muscarinic antagonist Dopamine (D2) antagonist	Sedating Extrapyramidal

etiology of the vestibular injury. For example, in patients with acute unilateral vestibular damage, such as after surgery for a vestibular schwanoma, this would be a detrimental effect. Vestibular compensation is the pathway to recovery in these patients. Therefore dampening their compensation with vestibular suppressants can impair their ultimate function. However in patients with Ménière's disease, where the amount of vestibular dysfunction varies over time and compensation to a "recovered" level of vestibular function can be symptomatic, this effect of vestibular suppressants may be beneficial in controlling bothersome symptoms.

VESTIBULAR REHABILITATION

The initial vestibular compensation following acute vestibular injury is enhanced by head movement and delayed by inactivity. Following acute vestibulopathy, sensory stimulus which results in the unpleasant experience of vertigo appears to be the stimulus for compensation. Also, the degree of compensation in the acute phase seems to have an impact on long term compensation. This is the theoretical basis for vestibular rehabilitation and intervention (Strupp, 2001). Vestibular rehabilitation has been shown to benefit patients with acute as well as chronic vestibulopathies. Therapists will identify the very movements or positions that provoke symptoms and then develop programs which reproduce these movements. The goal is to extinguish the symptoms through habituation or compensation. Other aspects of vestibular rehabilitation include postural control exercises for patients found to have postural control abnormalities, visual vestibular exercises for patients with bilateral vestibular deficits, and conditioning activities for patients who have adopted a sedentary lifestyle to avoid vertigo symptoms.

SPECIFIC PATHOLOGIES AND THEIR TREATMENTS

Ménière's Disease

Meniere's disease is a triad of vertigo, fluctuating hearing loss, and tinnitus. Frequently patients also experience aural fullness. Early hearing loss usually improves only to recur. Over time, Meniere's can cause persistent sensorineural hearing loss. Vestibular injury also follows an intermittent recurring course. Vertigo attacks typically are intense over a period of minutes and then subside over minutes to hours. They occur at irregular intervals and can have long periods of remission. Meniere's can progress to a "burned out" stage with severe sensorineural hearing loss, less vigorous vertigo, and decreased vestibular function. Up to one third of patients go on to develop bilateral sensorineural hearing loss. Diagnosis depends on documentation of fluctuating hearing loss, typically with greater loss at lower frequencies. The pathophysiology of Meniere's disease is poorly understood but is thought to be related to endolymphatic hyprops.

Treatment of Meniere's disease includes acute symptomatic vestibular suppression as described earlier. Also, medical measures aimed at reducing endolymphatic hydrops, such as diuretics and a low salt diet are effective for controlling vertigo in approximately 70 to 95 percent of patients. Patients who fail medical management are candidates for more aggressive medical and surgical treatments. Over the last decade, the use of transtympanic gentamicin has become increasingly popular. This aminoglycoside, known for its toxicity to the inner ear, is used to ablate vestibular function. The success rate for eliminating vertigo is over 80 percent with almost all patients experiencing some improvement. Thirty percent of patients have some hearing loss, although it is difficult to determine whether the

TABLE 7–6
Treatment of Meniere's Disease

Management of Meniere's Disease	
Acute phase	Short term use of vestibular suppressants and anti-emetics
Chronic phase	Low sodium diet
	Diuretics
Chronic phase if medical therapy fails	Transtympanic gentamicin injection
	Labyrinthectomy
	Vestibular nerve section
	Endolymphatic mastoid shunt

gentamicin or the Meniere's is responsible. There are several surgical interventions also used for patients who fail medical management. Labrinthectomy has a vertigo control rate of over 95 percent, although involves loss of hearing. Vestibular neurectomy, a hearing preserving procedure, also has a vertigo control rate over 95 percent, but involves a craniotomy. Endolymphatic mastoid shunt operations (EMS) is also a hearing preserving surgery although does not have as high a success rate. With either chemical or surgical vestibular ablation there is a risk of unsteadiness if the contralateral vestibular function is impaired or if there are other co-morbidities which impair vestibular compensation (Kaylie, 2005).

Benign Paroxysmal Positional Vertigo

The most common cause of vertigo is benign paroxysmal positional vertigo (BPPV). Patients with BPPV have abrupt attacks of vertigo precipitated by positional change. This classically occurs with turning over in bed, sitting up, or bending over and then straightening up. The vertigo lasts only seconds to a minute and then resolves even if the provocative position is maintained. Diagnosis is achieved with history as well as physical exam including a Dix Hallpike test. This is a positional test that when positive stimulates the vertigo attack and nystagmus. During the Dix-Hallpike procedure the nystagmus should have latency and fatigability (Fig. 9–1).

BPPV is thought to occur because of canalolithiasis or calcium carbonate crystals floating freely within a semicircular canal, most commonly the posterior semicircular canal. These crystals are thought to create a clot which then generates pressure with movement that stimulates the cupula. The stimulation results in the sensation of vertigo.

The primary treatment of BPPV is canolith repositioning maneuvers, most commonly the Epley maneuver (Fig. 9–2). This positional maneuver resolves the symptoms in 80–90 percent of patients. Some patients do recur and require repeat treatments. Because of the success of canolith reposition techniques and the short duration of the vertigo attacks, medical suppressants are usually not helpful in the management of BPPV. Although the classic presentation of BPPV is consistent with posterior canal canalolithiasis, there are atypical cases that point to the involvement of other semicircular canals.

Perilymphatic Fistula

Various causes of an abnormal opening into the labryrinth can cause a vestibulopathy. The fluid-filled membranous labyrinth and perilymphatic fluid compartments are normally encased in the dense bone of the otic capsule except around the oval and round windows. Disruption in the labyrinthine bone or in the membranes around the oval or round window can result in audiovestibular dysfunction. One cause of such a disruption is known as a perilymphatic fistula (PLF).

Perilymphatic fistulas are thought to be caused by blunt head trauma, barotruama, or by a complication of stapes surgery (Fitzgerald, 2001). A leak of perilymph occurs around the oval or round window and resulting in sensorineural

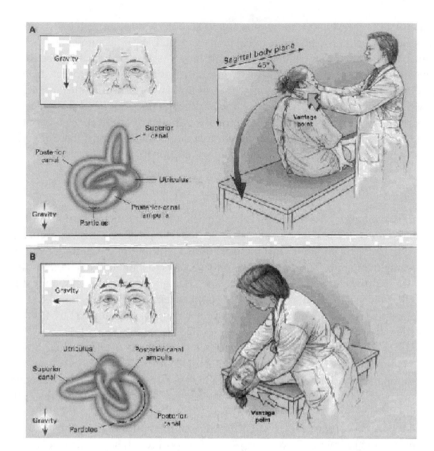

FIGURE 9–1.   The Dix-Hallpike Test of a Patient with Benign Paroxysmal Positional Vertigo Affecting the Right Ear. In Panel A, the examiner stands at the patient's right side and rotates the patient's head 45 degrees to the right to align the right posterior semicircular canal with the sagittal plane of the body. In Panel B, the examiner moves the patient, whose eyes are open, from the seated to the supine right-ear-down position and then extends the patient's neck slightly so that the chin is pointed slightly upward. The latency, duration, and direction of nystagmus, if present, and the latency and duration of vertigo, if present, should be noted. The red arrows in the inset depict the direction of nystagmus in patients with typical benign paroxysmal positional vertigo. The presumed location in the labyrinth of the free-floating debris thought to cause the disorder is also shown. Reprinted with permission from Furman JM. Cass SP. Benign paroxysmal positional vertigo. New England Journal of Medicine. 341(21):1590–6, 1999 Nov 18.

hearing loss, episodic vertigo or chronic imbalance. Except in rare spontaneous cases of PLF, the diagnosis is based on a clinical history of a precipitating event involving increased middle ear or intracranial pressure or trauma. Abnormal electrocochleography and positive fistula tests based on either videonystagmography (VNG) or pressure platform posturagraphy can be seen in the patients with PLF; however, the specificity and sensitivity of these tests for PLF are not well

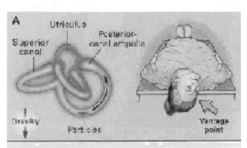

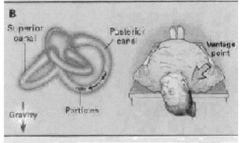

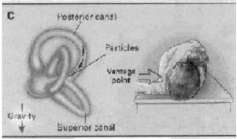

FIGURE 9–2.   Bedside Maneuver for the Treatment of a Patient with Benign Paroxysmal Positional Vertigo Affecting the Right Ear. The presumed position of the debris within the labyrinth during the maneuver is shown in each panel. The maneuver is a three-step procedure. First, a Dix-Hallpike test is performed with the patient's head rotated 45 degrees toward the right ear and the neck slightly extended with the chin pointed slightly upward. This position results in the patient's head hanging to the right (Panel A). Once the vertigo and nystagmus provoked by the Dix Hallpike test cease, the patient's head is rotated about the rostral-caudal body axis until the left ear is down (Panel B). Then the head and body are further rotated until the head is face down (Panel C). The vertex of the head is kept tilted downward throughout the rotation. The maneuver usually provokes brief vertigo. The patient should be kept in the final, face-down position for about 10 to 15 seconds. With the head kept turned toward the left shoulder, the patient is brought into the seated position (Panel D). Once the patient is upright, the head is tilted so that the chin is pointed slightly downward. Reprinted with permission from Furman JM. Cass SP. Benign paroxysmal positional vertigo. New England Journal of Medicine. 341(21):1590–6, 1999Nov 18.

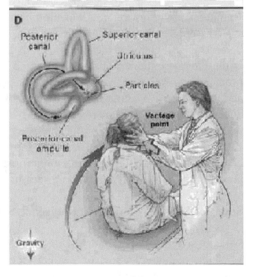

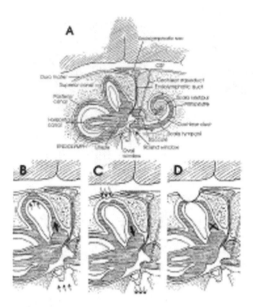

FIGURE 9–3. Mechanism of symptoms and signs with superior semicircular canal dehiscence syndrome. (A) Schematic drawing of inner ear. There are normally two windows in the bony capsule—the oval window (filled by the stapes foot plate) and the round window. A third window in the bony wall of the superior semicircular canal leads to vertigo and nystagmus with loud sounds or pressure changes in the middle ear or CSF (B and C). If the window is large enough, the superior semicircular canal can be blocked (D). See text for details. Reprinted with permission from Baloh RW. Superior semicircular canal dehiscence Syndrome; Leaks and squeaks can make you dizzy. Neurology. 2004; 62:684–685.

determined. When conservative medical therapy, including avoidance of elevated intracranial and middle ear pressure, does not resolve the clinical symptoms, surgical patching of the fistula around the oval and round windows can lead to stabilization of hearing and to resolution of vertigo.

Labyrinthine Fistula

Another cause of an abnormal opening into the labyrinth is when cholesteatoma, often associated with chronic otitis media, causes an erosion of the labyrinthine bone. The most common location of a bony labyrinthine fistula from cholestaomea is the lateral semicircular canal followed by the oval window region and the promonatory. Patients can experience sound and pressure induced attacks of vertigo and have a positive fistula sign manifested by transient horizontal nystagmus produced by applying pressure to the affected ear. In a majority of cases, the surgical treatment requires removal of the cholesteatoma matrix and inflammatory granulation tissue followed by closure of the labyrinthine fistula with a fascia graft. In all cases the underlying cholesteatoma must be surgically addressed in order to prevent further and potentially more serious complications.

Superior Semicircular Canal Dehisence Syndrome

Superior semicircular canal dehiscence syndrome (SCCDS) is a recently described vestibular pathology associated with absence of the bone covering over the superior semicircular canal (Minor, 2000). Because the bony dehiscence creates a "third" mobile window within the inner ear, loud sounds, increased outer and middle ear pressure, or increased intracranial pressure (e.g., by Valsalva maneuver) can result in vertigo, nystgmus, pulsatile tinnitus, and sometimes hearing loss. Positive pressure in the outer and middle ear causes inward motion of the stapes footplate. When there is a mobile "window" in the vestibular system there is flow within the semicircular canal resulting in vestibular excitation and the abnormal sensation of motion.

Migraine-related dizziness

Migraine headaches are diagnosed on the basis of criteria established by the International Headache Society (IHS). Most commonly they present as intermittent and recurrent headaches that are unilateral, disabling, throbbing, associated with nausea and sensitivity to sounds and light. It is not uncommon for patients with migraine headaches to have dizziness or vertigo with the incidence as high as 55 percent of migraine patients (Furman, 2003). One subtype of headache in the IHS classification, basilar artery migraine, has vertigo as a chief characteristic. Migraine patients have vestibular findings, including positional and spontaneous nystagmus and abnormal posturography. Abnormal vestibular function on caloric testing also occurs. Vertigo symptoms have a variable duration lasting from seconds to days. Although there have been recent advances in the understanding of the patolphysiology of migraines in general, the understanding of how migraines cause vertigo is limited. Some patients have non-localizing central vestibular findings suggesting a central affect. However, the prevalence of unilateral reduced caloric response may point to an inner ear or nerve effect. Theories include the release of vasoactive peptides by the eighth nerve and vasospasm induced vestibular ischemia. Finally, it is important to make sure there there is no other cause of vestibular symptoms in a migraine patient.

Patients who have migrainous vertigo usually have resolution of their vertigo symptoms with successful treatment of their migraines. Medical treatment includes abortive medications, taken at the first sign of a migraine, and preventive medications aimed at avoiding the next migraine. Abortive medications include nonsteroidal anti-inflammatory medications (NSAIDs), ergotamines, serotonin receptor agonists (such as triptans), and vasoconstrictors (such as isometheptene mucate and dichloralphenazone). Preventive medications include NSAIDs, tricyclic antidepressants, selective serotonin reuptake inhibitors (SSRI), other antidepressants (such as trazadone and buproprion), beta blockers, calcium channel blockers, and anti-convulsant medications. Neurological evaluation should be a part of the evaluation for all patients suspected to have vertiginous or basilar migraines.

Viral Neuronitis

The acute onset of vestibular symptoms including severe vertigo, nausea and emesis lasting for several days in the absence of auditory or neurologic symptoms is a classic presentation of acute viral neuronitis. More than 50 percent of these patients report an upper respiratory tract infection prior to symptom onset. The term viral labyrinthitis is sometimes used to describe this process. However pathologic examination reveals atrophy of one or more vestibular nerve trunks with sparing of the labyrinth. Attempts to isolate a virus responsible for the injury have largely been unsuccessful, although herpes zoster infections have been occasionally identified.

Viral neuronitis represents an acute vestibulapathy. Patients undergo classical vestibular compensation barring any co-morbidities or other impediments. Initial management with vestibular suppressants followed by mobilization to facilitate compensation is indicated for treatment.

Vertebrobasilar insufficiency

The vertebrobasilar circulation supplies the brainstem as well as the eighth nerve and labyrinth. Transient ischemic attacks (TIAs) in this system can cause abrupt onset vertigo, nausea, emesis and imbalance. Typically patients also experience visual blurring or deficits, diplopia, drop attacks, weakness or numbness of the extremities and headache. With TIAs in the vertebrobasilar system, the symptoms can occur at different times but the presence of brainstem symptoms even if initially not coincident with the vertigo, should raise suspicion for this process. A stroke in this system will cause some a similar constellation of symptoms although will not abate as with a TIA. Magnetic resonance imaging provides good assessment of the affected areas whether a TIA or stroke. Magnetic resonance angiography can identify vascular disease in the vessels in the neck or base of brain. Diagnosis and treatment of TIAs and stroke should involve a neurologist. Following a stroke, vestibular compensation will occur and treatment is aimed at palliating initial symptoms and then facilitating compensation through early mobilization of patients.

Conclusion

Vestibular compensation underlies the treatment of diverse and in some instances poorly understood vestibular pathology. The judicious use of vestibular suppressants is important for not impairing vestibular compensation. Vestibular rehabilitation seems to facilitate compensation. Finally, making the diagnosis of each underlying pathology allows the use of appropriate treatments for the primary disease process.

REFERENCES

Badke, M. B., Shea, T. A., Miedaner, J. A., & Grove, C. R. (2004). Outcomes after rehabilitation for adults with balance dysfunction. *Archives of Physical Medicine and Rehabilitation, 85,* 227–233.

Baloh, R. W. (1998). Vertigo. *The Lancet 352,* 1841–1846.

Baloh, R. W. (2004). Superior semicircular canal dehiscence Syndrome; Leaks and squeaks can make you dizzy. *Neurology, 62,* 684–685.

Black, F. O., & Pesznecker, S. C. (2003). Vestibular adaptation and rehabilitation. *Current Opinions in Otolaryngology, Head & Neck Surgery, 11,* 355–360.

Brandt, T. (2000). Managemtent of vestibular disorders. *Journal of Neurology. 247*, 491–499.

Carey, J. (2004). Intratympanic gentamicin for the treatment of Meniere's Disease and other forms of peripheral vertigo. *Otolaryngologic Clinics of North America. 37*, 1075–1090.

Crevits L., & Bosman, T., (2005). Migraine-related vertigo: towards a distinctive entity. *Clinical Neurology and Neurosurgery 107*, 82–87.

Darlington, C. L., & Smith, P. F. (2000). Molecular mechanisms of recovery from vestibular damage in mammals: recent advances. *Progress in Neurobiology, 62*, 313–325.

Enticott, J. C., et al. (2005). Effects of vestibulo-ocular reflex exercises on vestibular compensation after vestibular schwannoma surgery. *Otology & Neurotology, 26*, 265–269.

Furman, J. M., & Cass, S. P. (1999). Benign paroxysmal positional vertigo. *New England Journal of Medicine. 341*(21),1590–1596.

Furman, J. M., Marcus, D. A., & Baladan, C. D. (2003). Migranous vertigo: development of a pathogenetic model and structured diagnostic interview. *Current Opinions in Neurology 16*, 5–13.

Hain, T. C., & Uddin, M. (2003). Pharmocological treatment of vertigo. *CNS drugs 17*(2), 85–100.

Kaylie, D. M., Jackson, C. G., & Gardener, E. K. (2005). Surgical management of Meniere's disease in the era of gentimicin. *Otolaryngology Head and Neck Surgery 132*, 443–445

Lacour, M., & Sterkers, O. (2001). Histamine and Betahistine in the treatment of vertigo; Elucidation of mechanisms of action. *CNS drugs 15*(11), 853–870.

Strupp, M., Arbusow, V., & Brandt, T. (2001). Exercise and drug therapy alter recovery from labyrinth lesion in humans. *Annals of the New York Academy of Sciences, 942*, 79–94.

Topuz, O., Topuz, B., Ardic, F. N., Sarhus, M., Ogmen, G., & Ardic, F. (2004). Efficacy of vestibular rehabilitation on chronic unilateral vestibular dysfunction. *Clinical Rehabilitation, 18*, 76–83.

Whitney, S. L., Wrisley, D. M., Brown, K. E., & Furman, J. M. (2000). Physical therapy for migraine related vestibulopathy and vestibular dysfunction with history of migraine. *Larngoscope, 110*, 1528–1534.

Yardley, L., Donovan-Hall, M., Smith, H. E., Walsh, B. M., Mullec, M., & Bronstein, A. M., (2004). Effectiveness of primary care-based vestibular rehabilitation for chronic dizziness. *Annals of Internal Medicine, 141*, 598–605.

CHAPTER 10

Hearing Instrument Fitting
for Infants and Young Children

Jeffrey Simmons, Kathryn Laudin Beauchaine, and
Leisha R. Eiten

Boys Town National Research Hospital

First sounds. First words. Parents wait expectantly to hear their baby's voice and first words. Hearing loss can disrupt and delay the process of speech and language development. The rationale for fitting amplification as early in life as possible is to minimize the deleterious effects of hearing loss (Yoshinago-Itano et al., 1998). With earlier identification of hearing loss through universal newborn hearing screening, amplification can be provided soon after the hearing loss is identified, as young as 2–4 months of age. Guidelines for pediatric amplification fitting are now available that articulate the considerations that must be made when working with this population (American Academy of Audiology (AAA), 2003; Pediatric Working Group (PWG), 1996).

The overall goal of early amplification is to provide an acoustic signal that is audible and comfortable for a wide range of inputs. The attainment of this goal may be compromised by the degree and configuration of hearing loss and by limitations of current technologies. The expected outcomes from fitting amplification vary with the degree and configuration of the hearing loss. The expected outcomes may also be influenced by other factors, including cognitive, medical, socio-economic and parental involvement to name a few.

Early amplification has come to mean fitting amplification within the first month following the identification of hearing loss, with the identification of hearing loss occurring within the first 3 months of life. The Joint Committee on Infant Hearing (JCIH, 2000; under revision) recommends that hearing loss be identified and intervention begun by 6 months of age. As recently as 2003, data was reported suggesting that there was a national trend toward approaching this goal (Harrison, Roush, & Wallace, 2003). Thus, an increasing number of audiologists are faced with the need to provide amplification for younger hearing instrument users within the context of their family environment, their medical home, and in concert with early intervention services.

There are several identified roadblocks to the implementation of early amplification. The primary roadblocks include those related to securing third party payment or financial eligibility, illness including the presence of otitis media, recommendations for further audiological testing (Harrison & Roush, 1996; Sjoblad, Harrison, Roush & McWilliam, 2001), as well as delays due to the suspicion of auditory neuropathy (Harrison, Roush & Wallace, 2003).

PEDIATRIC LISTENING AND AMPLIFICATION NEEDS

Research supports that infants and children have different listening needs when compared to adults. The following studies highlight these differences. Children require increased intensity levels (Nozza, Rossman, & Bond, 1991) and greater signal-to-noise ratios (Allen & Wightman, 1994; Nozza, Rossman, Bond, & Miller, 1990; Stuart, 2005) in order to achieve adult-like performance. Infants and/or young children tend to have poorer temporal resolution (Werner et al., 1992), and they do not use contextual cues as effectively as older listeners (Nittrouer & Boothroyd, 1990; Stelmachowicz et al., 2000). Other studies demonstrate the importance of high-frequency information when children perform detection and/or discrimination tasks (Stelmachowicz et al., 2001, 2002; Stelmachowicz et al., 2004).

In addition to the differences in listening needs suggested by research, infants and young children present with an array of other factors that affect hearing instrument use. At very young ages, they are not able to independently or effectively change their position or location to optimize their listening environment. Infants and young child explore their environment and they have a tendency to pull out their hearing instruments and put them in their mouths. All of these factors are considered when fitting hearing instruments on this population. Some of these factors will be explored below.

One of the most obvious differences between an adult listener and a young listener is size. This becomes important for both practical and acoustical reasons. Additionally, small pinnae may not readily support behind-the-ear (BTE) hearing instruments, requiring adhesives or other supports to assist keeping the devices in place.

The young listener's hearing instruments require safety features, such as tamper resistant battery cases and programmed or mechanical volume-control locks. It has been reported that young children swallowing hearing instrument batteries account for the majority of accidental ingestion of button battery reports (Dire, 2005).

Kruger (1987) studied the acoustics of the infant ear canal and demonstrated how the changing dimensions of the ear alter the resonant frequency of the ear canal. This, in turn, may require subsequent changes in hearing instrument frequency-gain characteristics. Age-related changes in real-ear-to-coupler-differences (RECDs) are discussed in detail in the Verification Section.

There are audibility issues related to the infant and young child's inability to situate themselves to improve their listening environment. This, in combination with the literature that suggests that the very young listener needs a more salient signal, lends support to the use of FM systems for this population. It has been demonstrated that FM-use for infants and young children is feasible (Gabbard, 2005).

PROTOCOL DEVELOPMENT

Given the unique characteristics of infants and young children, it is clear that typical adult-driven protocols and prescriptive methods are not appropriate for the young listener. There are two published national guidelines specific to pediatric patients. The Pediatric Working Group (PWG, 1996) developed the first of these. More recently, the American Academy of Audiology (AAA) published a Pediatric Amplification Guideline (2003).

One component that the PWG and AAA documents both emphasize is the importance of an evidence-based prescriptive method to determine the gain and/or output required to ensure speech audibility. Both the Desired Sensation Level (DSL) (Cornelisse et al., 1995; Scollie et al., 2005; Seewald et al., 2005) and the NAL-NL1 (Dillon, 1999; Byrne et al., 2001) provide targets with the goal of speech audibility and provide real-ear saturation response (RESR) targets. The DSL method emphasizes *habilitative audibility* (Seewald et al., 2005); that is, children learn to use the audibility that is provided to them. In contrast, the NAL-NL1 emphasizes *effective audibility;* that is, audibility that has been found to be effective with post-lingually impaired listeners. In addition to these prescriptive methods, each hearing instrument manufacturer has proprietary algorithms developed for their respective hearing instruments, which are typically aimed at the adult user. Many hearing instrument manufacturers have incorporated DSL and NAL-NL1 targets into their fitting software.

The process of fitting amplification described here includes the following steps:

1. Pre-selection
2. Verification
3. Orientation
4. Validation
5. Planned follow-up

It is important to remember that this process occurs in the context of a family-centered, culturally sensitive remediation strategy. This is an active process whereby each step is revisited numerous times during the child's life as new information becomes available. The hearing instrument process is just one aspect of a comprehensive aural habilitation/educational program. The fitting process is only initiated after the family has been informed of the test findings that support the need for use of amplification, and the family is ready to move forward with amplification.

Step One: Pre-Selection

In the first step, Pre-selection, amplification options are reviewed with the family. The first two decisions that are made involve the style and type of earmolds and hearing instruments.

Amplification options are explored in order to provide audibility of speech in the maximum number of situations. Age and developmental factors, family needs and wants, and the degree and configuration of the hearing loss are considered. Pros and cons of various options are explored with the family so that they can make an informed choice in a timely manner. "Families have the right to information that is comprehensive, and based on research and tested practices." (Sass-Lehrer, 2004). There is an overriding goal that amplification use is initiated within one month following the identification of the hearing loss. This timeline of fitting within one month following the identification of hearing loss is in keeping with the recommendation from the Joint Committee on Infant Hearing (2000; under revision). If the decision for personal amplification is delayed for any reason, a short-term loan of hearing instruments is a possibility. Reasons for delays may include the need for additional test information, the need to locate funding sources, or other circumstances. The use of loaner hearing instruments is also useful for those inevitable times when the hearing instruments are sent for repair. While it is recognized that every clinic does not have the ability to provide loaner-hearing instruments, it is recommended that a clinic specializing in pediatric audiology have a loaner hearing instrument program or have access to such programs.

Pre-selection of Earmolds

The earmold style and material that are selected depend on the degree and configuration of the hearing loss. For infants and young children, the style that is generally selected is a full-shell earmold. Smaller ears do not adequately support or provide sufficient retention for smaller earmold styles, such as skeleton or canal locks.

Venting options are limited in small ears, but can be considered when the ear canal is large enough and as appropriate for the degree and configuration of hearing loss. It is important to consider the effects of venting on the frequency response. For example, a diagonal vent decreases high frequencies. For small ear canals, venting is not an option. In fact, for very small ears, it can be difficult to fit a standard #13 tube into the ear canal portion of the earmold, which can create a reverse horn effect.

Earmold material choices include vinyl (PVC), silicone and acrylic/hard lucite. There are increasing color choices in all materials. For young infants, vinyl is typically recommended. It is firmer than silicone, so it maintains its shape in a small ear canal. Vinyl also accepts glue or solvents, allowing the tubing to be bonded to the earmold; an important feature when children are at the age where they frequently remove hearing instruments by pulling on them, stressing the point where the tubing and the earmold connect. Vinyl has a tendency to shrink and discolor; however, that is not an issue for very young children where earmolds are replaced at regular intervals due to the child's growth. Although silicone is a soft material, it is difficult to modify. For children with very small ear canals, the canal portion of a silicone earmold might be so thin that is can collapse in the ear canal. To stabilize tubing in a silicone earmold, a tubing retention ring is attached to the tubing. This retention ring can create a slight bulge in the canal portion of the earmold, creating a possible source of discomfort. Although silicone material does not harden over time, it can tear more easily than vinyl. Lucite, due to its hardness, is not recommended for young ears.

Pre-selection of Hearing Instruments

A major challenge in the pre-selection phase is to balance technology options, listening needs and costs to determine which hearing instruments will best meet the patient's needs. The prescriptive targets largely determine the electroacoustic characteristics and the output/gain requirements for a given audiogram. For example, when working with infants and young children, DSL targets are used to ensure that speech is audible and that signals do not exceed predicted upper limits of comfort. Many hearing instrument manufacturers have the option of using DSL for pediatric hearing instrument fittings. It is important to note that the manufacturer's computer simulations of predicted real ear gain and output, require electroacoustic confirmation with either real-ear probe microphone measure or with coupler measures (Hawkins & Cook, 2003).

The following need to be considered in device selection:

- Electroacoustic appropriateness, including frequency response
- FM compatibility
- Tamper resistant features (battery compartment, volume control, program switches)
- Advanced features (e.g., directional microphones, multiple memories, and the ability to en/disable those not needed at the time of the fitting)
- Pediatric sized tone hooks
- Cost
- Durability
- Warranty
- Battery life
- Color options

The hearing instrument style of choice for infants and young children is behind-the-ear (BTE). With BTE hearing instruments the earmolds can be replaced as frequently as needed without requiring that the entire hearing instrument be sent in, as is necessary for custom products. These BTE instruments, for the most part, accept FM and the working parts are outside of the ear canal. The latter consideration is an important safety issue for active, young children.

As children mature, concerns about the appearance of BTEs may arise. Older children may request custom hearing instruments such as in-the-ear (ITE), in-the-canal (ITC) or completely in the canal (CIC) styles. There is no specific age when this style change should be considered. It is important to advise the child and family that a custom product will limit or prohibit FM access, in addition to the considerations mentioned above.

The use of binaural amplification for those with binaural hearing loss is considered a standard recommendation. Typically, monaural hearing instrument use is limited to those with nonfunctional word recognition in one ear, those with very large asymmetries in thresholds between ears, and those with other medical reasons that prohibit wearing a device in one ear (e.g., atresia, chronic ear drainage). For children with unilateral hearing loss, amplification use is considered on a case-by-case basis. Research results have shown that unilateral hearing loss is associated with academic concerns for as many as one-third of students (Bess et al., 1998). While there is little research supporting the use of CROS hearing instruments in children or a hearing instrument on the unilaterally impaired ear (Kentworthy et al., 1990; Updike, 1994), parents/caregivers should be informed of the various options that are available.

Digital hearing instrument choices continue to expand, and the features that are possible in these instruments must be evaluated before introducing special-feature use with very young children. While there is not a known and accepted "best" compression threshold for any given hearing loss, it is generally accepted that the compression threshold should be as low as possible to ensure that softer speech or softer speech components have the maximum likelihood of being audible (Dillon, 2001). Recent work by Marriage et al. (2005) suggests that WDRC circuits may be appropriate for children even when there is severe to profound hearing loss.

The necessary number of channels in the hearing instrument varies with the configuration of hearing loss. Pittman & Stelmachowicz (2003) showed that unusual audiometric configurations are more apt to be encountered in the pediatric population as compared to adults with later-onset hearing loss. Multiple channels allow for more flexibility in frequency shaping. However, it is important to remember that some frequency shaping can be accomplished by using filtered tone hooks, as shown in Figure 10–1.

Hearing instruments with multiple programs/memories are common. One practical application of a second program is to have an FM + environmental microphone (EM) program. The use of multiple programs for infants and young children should be approached with caution. If the program switch is active, the child could inadvertently change settings, and the parent/caregiver could be unaware of the program that the child is using. Thus, it is prudent to periodically check that the program selection is correct. Another option is a remote control used by parents/caregivers to switch programs as needed. Alternately, it is possible to disable memory/program capabilities until the child is old enough to make appropriate choices. Although older children can use multiple programs effectively (Jenstad et al., 1995), each family will have to assess their child's ability to change

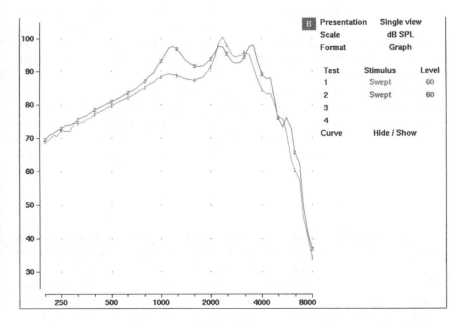

FIGURE 10–1. Example of the effect on the coupler measures for two tone hooks. The response with a 680 Hz filter (upper line) and a 1000 Hz filter (second curve from top) is shown.

programs in a thoughtful and communication-enhancing manner. The age at which this occurs requires further research (Marriage et al., 2005).

Feedback reduction methods are available on many hearing instruments. The way that this feature affects high frequency gain varies. The audiologist must be cognizant of how each feedback-control system works. Some systems simply reduce gain in the region of feedback, which may result in less audibility than intended, while others implement phase cancellation or notch filtering.

Many hearing instruments have features that allow reduction of interference from background noise. Noise reduction strategies, however, may reduce the audibility of important environmental sounds. For the very young listener, the presence and meaning of environmental sounds is important information.

Directional microphones are another feature that should be used cautiously with the young listener. Children learn language through incidental listening and learn about their environments by over-hearing speech and sounds around them. There is a concern that directional microphones could compromise this incidental listening. For example, directional microphones might make it difficult for the child to hear warning signals as the child toddles away. One hearing instrument option is an adaptive noise feature that automatically enables directional microphones with either an adaptive or fixed polar pattern. The use of adaptive directionality in infants and young children has not been studied.

In a laboratory study, Gravel et al. (1999) showed that children as young as 4 years had better word and sentence scores when listening in noise with a directional microphone. Importantly, recent research with adults has suggested that improved word or sentence scores observed in laboratory-based directional microphone studies do not always directly translate into real-world benefit (Cord et al., 2004). Ricketts & Tharpe (2005) have begun to study directional microphone benefit for children in classrooms.

In summary, during the pre-selection process, numerous decisions are made that have long-term implications for auditory communication skill development. With rapidly changing technology, the audiologist must stay current and implement amplification changes when supported by research. It is critical, however, to cautiously view technological changes when considering applying them to the pediatric population.

Step Two: Verification

The second step in the pediatric amplification process is verification of hearing instrument performance. The goal of amplification is to provide optimal access to the speech spectrum for soft, average and loud inputs to maximize the potential to develop oral speech and language. The focus is on achieving audibility of speech to the greatest degree possible given the patient's hearing loss and given the limits of hearing instrument performance characteristics. It is critically important that the audiologist assess the performance of the hearing instruments in a manner that provides information about how well this goal is being met. It is the audiologist's responsibility to verify hearing instrument performance in terms of gain and output across frequencies. As stated above, this step involves assessment beyond viewing the computer simulation of hearing instrument performance in Manufacturer Software Screens.

Experts in pediatric amplification stress that verification strategies be evidence-based (AAA, 2003; PWG, 1996). A systematic verification process, with a defined rationale that has been shown to provide benefit, should be used. This point might seem obvious, however, a survey published in 1996 (Hedley-Williams et al.) indicated that 50 percent of the respondents used a *personal* fitting strategy rather than a formal prescriptive method for pediatric amplification. A similar survey in 2001 (Tharp et al.) showed a positive change; however, 18 percent of audiologists who reported fitting amplification on children were still using an *informal personal method* for prescribing and verifying amplification characteristics.

How is hearing instrument performance verified? Traditionally, audiologists have used two methods to verify hearing instrument performance: behavioral and electroacoustic. Behavioral methods include amplified speech perception testing and amplified sound-field thresholds (ASFT) or functional gain measures. Electroacoustic methods are comprised of real-ear measurements or simulated real-ear measurements of hearing instrument gain and output. The effectiveness and usefulness of these methods and their respective benefits and limitations in verifying the performance of hearing instruments are explored below.

Behavioral Verification

Behavioral verification methods include amplified speech perception testing and amplified sound-field thresholds (ASFT). The former is not reliable with normally developing children under approximately 3 years of age, who are in the early stages of speech-language development. The latter is often used to determine functional gain, defined as the difference in dB between amplified and unamplified thresholds at a given frequency or for speech inputs. In the past, functional gain was the only available method to quantify the performance of amplification devices, and surveys indicate that a number of clinicians fitting amplification on pediatric patients continue to rely exclusively on it (Tharpe et al., 2001). Since the advent of probe-microphone technology, questions have been raised regarding the continued utility of ASFTs for hearing instrument performance verification in young children.

AAA (2003) stated that behavioral methods are not the recommended method for verifying amplification fittings in children. The primary reason is that behavioral tests of auditory responsiveness cannot be reliably completed with infants. JCIH (2000) instituted the goal of identification of hearing loss by 3 months of age and initial fitting of amplification by 6 months of age. With the implementation of universal newborn hearing screening across the United States, great strides have been made toward reaching these goals. Because of this, audiologists routinely see patients at a much younger age than was common in the past.

What are other reasons that ASFTs are not recommended when verifying amplification on children? First, it should be noted that ASFTs provide information about responses to sound pressure levels that may or may not be related to the conversational speech spectrum. Consequently, it is difficult to form conclusions regarding the audibility of speech for the listener. This is especially true when the hearing instrument is utilizing non-linear amplification. In these non-linear devices, the amount of gain varies with the level of the input signal. In other words, gain provided for sounds of lower intensity may be greater than the gain for typical speech inputs (Stelmachowicz & Lewis, 1988). This can lead to faulty estimations of the audibility of the amplified speech signal. In addition, ASFTs provide no reliable information regarding real ear saturation response (RESR). Thus, the audiologist is unable to determine if the RESR is set too low in a way that might reduce sensation levels of speech and limit optimal use of residual hearing. Likewise, it cannot be determined if the RESR is set so high that there is risk to residual hearing or loudness discomfort that could lead to device rejection.

Other limitations of behavioral methods of verification involve test-retest reliability and frequency resolution. Test-retest reliability in infants and young children can be compromised. With the limited time window for testing generally encountered in some infants and young children, it is common to obtain only a few reliable thresholds in a test session. Amplitude resolution is likewise limited, because behavioral measurements are typically conducted in increments no finer than 5 dB. Adjustments to the hearing instruments, on the other hand, can occur in steps of 1 dB. With a 5 dB behavioral test increment and typical test-retest variability of 5 dB, it is extremely difficult to demonstrate the effects of small adjustments made to the hearing instrument's gain. A study by Hawkins, et al (1987) indicated that two amplified sound-field thresholds, for adults, must differ by 15 dB or more in order to be considered significantly different (the volume control was not fixed between test sessions). ASFT test-retest variability in children (5–9 years and 10–14 years) was investigated by Stuart et al. (1990), and those test findings indicated that a 10 dB difference in ASFTs is a significant difference at the 95 percent confidence level *if the volume control setting is the same in each session.*

The above information begs the question: Should behavioral verification methods such as functional gain or ASFTs be eliminated? AAA (2003) recommends that ASFTs not be used as the *primary* means of verifying hearing instrument performance. However, there are situations in which functional gain measures can be of use in verification. Functional gain may be the only feasible method for verifying the performance of bone conduction hearing devices. In the overwhelming majority of clinics, equipment necessary for electroacoustic testing of bone conduction amplification, such as an artificial mastoid, is not available. Another device for which ASFTs are useful is the digital frequency compression hearing instrument. These devices compress or transpose high frequency stimuli to a lower frequency region where the listener has better hearing sensitivity. Current electroacoustic analysis equipment generally does not provide accurate, objective information about this specific function of the hearing instrument. Therefore, in order to assess the effectiveness of the frequency compression and audibility of select high-frequency inputs, a behavioral measure such as ASFT must be utilized. The limitations regarding behavioral verification discussed above apply to bone conduction and frequency compression devices as well.

The ASFTs plotted on an audiogram traditionally have been used to illustrate to parents and school personnel how a child is responding to amplification. As mentioned above, though, this information cannot reliably predict the audibility of speech, which is the primary signal of interest.

Another use for ASFTs is to help determine if responses obtained from a child during audiometric testing are auditory responses or vibrotactile responses. The adult listener can differentiate and report when a stimulus is perceived tactilely rather than through the auditory system. Adults can be instructed not to respond to the former. The very young listener may respond to both types of perception and may be unable to indicate if the stimulus perceived was vibrotactile or auditory. When functional gain is much less than that predicted by electroacoustic measures, it is possible that the child's responses are vibrotactile, and hearing instrument benefit will be limited.

Aside from the exceptions mentioned above, ASFTs should generally only be used as a supplement to objective electroacoustic verification measures, rather than the primary tool in this process. Aided speech perception tests, however, may be useful in demonstrating improvements in performance if the child is old enough to perform a picture-pointing or word-repetition task.

Electroacoustic verification

Probe microphone measurement of sound pressure levels in the child's ear canal with hearing instruments and earmolds in place is the most accurate means of verifying that amplification is performing as closely as possible to desired targets. However, the degree of cooperation required for accurate measurements is typically more than can be provided by a young child. When verifying hearing instrument performance with infants and young children, the audiologist often relies on coupler measurements. There is simply no choice in most instances, because of poor head control and an inability to provide the amount of cooperation needed for traditional probe microphone measures. However, the 2-cc coupler is intended to approximate the average adult ear. The infant ear canal is considerably smaller than the adult ear canal. When the same signal is introduced into two cavities of differing sizes, a greater sound pressure level is developed in the smaller cavity. Consequently, the output SPL of a hearing instrument will be greater in the young child's ear than in the 2-cc coupler. The audiologist needs to account for this difference in order to accurately determine audibility of the speech signal as well as to determine if maximum output of the hearing instrument is at an acceptable level.

There is a procedure that provides the audiologist with the means to use probe microphone measurements for patients who are very young. This procedure is known as the real-ear-to-coupler difference (RECD) (Moodie et al., 1994; Bagatto et al., 2005). The RECD is the difference, in decibels across frequency, between the SPL of a given signal measured in a 2-cc coupler and the same signal measured in the ear with an earmold in place. The RECD is a measurement of the acoustic properties for an individual ear. Therefore, it is applied to both the thresholds and to the hearing instrument coupler results. For threshold measurements, the RECD is added to the thresholds in dB HL and the reference equivalent threshold sound pressure level (RETSPL) to obtain the estimated threshold in SPL at the tympanic membrane. For the hearing instrument, it is added to coupler values to estimate real-ear responses.

The details of conducting the RECD procedure with a specific probe microphone system vary; however, there are four essential steps:

1. The sound pressure level in decibels (dB SPL) for a particular test signal is measured in a 2-cc coupler.
2. A probe microphone is placed in a patient's ear along with the earmold, and the same test signal is introduced into the ear canal.
3. The SPL of the test signal is then measured in the ear.
4. The difference between the SPL of the test signal in the coupler and the SPL of the same signal in the ear is determined, and applied to the coupler values as an estimate of real-ear responses.

A DVD illustrating the RECD procedure was produced by Phonak AG (2004). Although it shows how to perform the measurement with a particular real-ear system, the procedure can be generalized to other systems. Positive RECD values illustrate the degree to which levels measured in the ear canal exceed levels measured in the 2-cc coupler. The completed measurement accounts for the variable acoustic effects of the occluded ear canal. Figure 10–2 shows an example of a typical RECD.

It is important to note that not all RECDs will be similar in appearance to the one shown here. There may be instances when some of the RECD values are negative. That is, the SPL in the ear canal is less than the SPL in the 2-cc coupler. At low frequencies, this typically results from acoustic leakage due to a loose fitting earmold or a vent in the mold larger than 1 mm (Bagatto, 2001). The presence of the probe-microphone tube during the actual measurement of the RECD can cause a slit leak, reducing sound pressure level in the ear canal. Marked negative RECD values are also observed in the presence of a tympanic membrane perforation or a patent tympanostomy tube. These negative values result from a coupling with the middle ear space that effectively increases the volume of the occluded ear canal and lowers the SPL of the input signal. In these cases the negative RECD can be as great as −10 dB to −5 dB in the lower to mid frequencies and is most pronounced in the 750 to 1000 Hz region (Bagatto, 2001; Liu & Lin, 1999; Martin et al., 2001; Martin et al., 1997). In these cases, the configuration of the RECD also can show a characteristic dip in the 1000 Hz region. Application of RECD values will be discussed below. Figure 10–3 shows an example of an RECD in an ear with a patent tympanostomy tube.

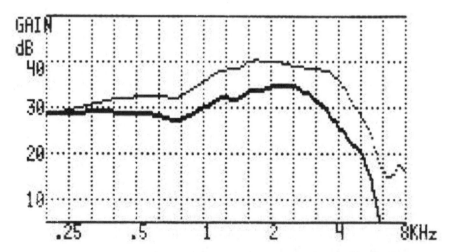

FIGURE 10–2.   An example of a typical RECD. The heavier black line represents the response from a 2-cc coupler, and the thin black line shows the response for the same input signal in the ear canal with a custom earmold in place.

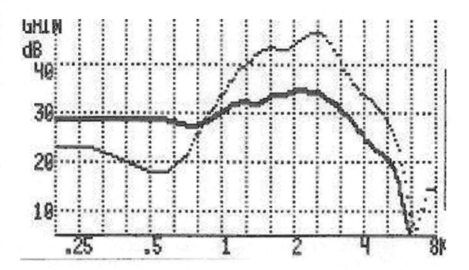

FIGURE 10–3.   An example of an RECD measurement obtained in an ear with a patent tympanostomy tube. Following the convention of Figure 2.

Tips to Assist in Measuring the Recd

1. Become highly familiar with the equipment and with the procedure prior to attempting the RECD measurement with a child.

2. Familiarize the parent(s) with the process and rationale before proceeding.

3. Use otoscopy to observe the ear canal. Determine its overall size and shape. Check for cerumen accumulation that may need to be avoided (or removed).

4. Mark the probe tube for an insertion depth of 15 to 25 mm, depending on the child's age and ear canal size. When the probe tube is placed in the ear, locate the marking at the intertragal notch. An alternative is to mark the tube in reference to the earmold so that it extends approximately 5 mm beyond the tip of the mold's canal. There are other options for achieving proper insertion, but these tend to be the most common. In any case, the goal is to place the probe-tube's tip within 5 to 6 mm of the tympanic membrane to avoid standing waves.

5. Apply a small amount of earmold lubricant to the side of the probe tube. This may help the tube adhere to the ear canal, and reduce friction that may move the tube when the earmold is inserted. Be cautious not to block the tip of the tube with the lubricant.

6. Check the placement of the tube with the otoscope after insertion to insure sufficient depth and avoidance of obstruction.

7. Adhesive can be used to stabilize the tube at the intertragal notch. This is another means of preventing the tube from moving during insertion of the earmold.

8. With toddlers, holding a mirror in a position that allows the child to view your actions may engage his/her attention enough to decrease movement of the head.
9. Record the RECD while the child and parent remain quiet.

Research has shown that the RECD measurement is reliable, with mean test-retest differences close to 0 dB in adults (Munro & Davis, 2003; Munro & Toal, 2005). Differences reported by Sinclair et al. (1996) were less than 2 dB, even for the infants in the study. Tharpe et al. (2001) examined the reliability of the RECD in a population of infants across their first 12 months of life. They noted somewhat poorer test-retest correlations and greater standard deviations than did the other studies. This was especially true for the highest (3 and 4 kHz) and lowest (.25 kHz) frequencies tested. It is of note that in the Tharpe et al. study, the infants were tested regardless of whether they were quiet, noisy or uncooperative. This may have introduced variables influencing the RECD that were not present in the other studies. Nevertheless, the authors concluded that the RECD measure was a reliable tool for use in hearing instrument fitting for young children.

When the RECD for a given individual is known, it can be added to coupler measures of gain or output to provide an accurate prediction of real ear SPL (Munro & Hatton, 2000; Seewald et al., 1999). This allows the audiologist to adjust any number of parameters (e.g., gain, frequency response, compression characteristics, maximum output, and tone hook filtering) on the device within the controlled environment of the hearing instrument test chamber without the need for the patient to be present.

Although age-related average RECD values exist, it is recommended that the measurement be completed for every child being fit with amplification. This is due to the fact that research studies have indicated high intersubject variations in RECD values (Feigin et al., 1989; Bagatto et al., 2002). An individual's RECD is influenced by factors such as residual ear canal volume, earmold characteristics (e.g., depth of insertion, amount of acoustic leakage, length of soundbore, earmold material), middle ear impedance and ear canal length. It is, therefore, difficult to predict RECD without error. Nevertheless, an effort has been made to establish age-related average values in cases where real-ear measurements cannot be reliably completed due to factors such as lack of cooperation from the child, or drainage or cerumen that repeatedly occlude the probe tube. Recently, Bagatto et al. (2002) reported a set of average RECD values in age increments of 1 month that can be used from birth through 10 years of age. The data from this study indicated that RECD values change with age, and that the greatest degree of change occurs over the first two years of life and for the higher frequencies. As the ear canal grows, the RECD becomes smaller and approaches average adult values by approximately 7 years of age (Feigin et al., 1989)

For a variety of reasons, it may be possible to obtain the RECD for only one ear. Should age related averages be used for the unmeasured ear, or can the results from one ear be used to reasonably predict the RECD for the other? Tharpe et al. (2001) reported that between-ear RECD values for their subjects were moderately correlated, and they concluded that it was generally reasonable to use the same RECD for both ears when measurement could be completed for only one. Exceptions included when only one ear had a tube or tympanic membrane perforation or other difference. Another study (Munro & Buttfield, 2004) compared between-ear RECDs for a group of adult subjects and reported that the difference was less than or equal to 3 dB in the 500 Hz to 4000 Hz range. Munro and Hatton (2000) reported on the difference between the actual real-ear aided response (REAR) and a derived REAR calculated by using 2-cc measures and the RECD from the opposite ear. The mean difference between the measured and derived values was within 3 dB at the main audiometric frequencies. It appears that predicting the RECD for one ear by using values from the opposite ear may carry less chance of error than using age related averages.

An effective format to illustrate speech audibility provided by a particular amplification device is the SPL-o-gram used in the Desired Sensation Level (DSL) prescriptive method (Cornelisse et al., 1995). In the SPL-o-gram, all relevant variables—the patient's audiometric characteristics, the unamplified long-term average speech spectrum (LTASS), predicted or measured maximum output, and acoustic characteristics of the amplification device—are expressed in terms of a common reference: dB SPL at the tympanic membrane. This provides a picture of how well the goal of speech audibility is being met. Without this type of approach, the audiologist is left to compare variables measured in different units at different reference points. An example of an SPL-o-gram is shown in Figure 10–4. Similar to a standard audiogram, amplitude is plotted as a function of frequency. However, the SPL-o-gram uses a scale of dB sound pressure level (SPL) rather than the dB hearing level (HL) utilized in the audiogram. Revit (1997) and Seewald and Scollie (1999) provide explanations of the process used to convert dB HL thresholds to dB SPL at the eardrum. Thresholds are plotted using circles for the right ear or x's for the left ear. The unamplified LTASS is the shaded area. XX Targets for REAR (+) and RESR (*) are shown.

Figure 10–5 shows the verification SPL-o-gram with the hearing instrument. The amplified LTASS for conversational level speech is within the auditory area, and maximum output of the device approximates the RESR targets without significantly exceeding them. The output of the hearing instrument is derived from measurements in the 2-cc coupler with the addition of RECD values and microphone location effects (Bentler & Pavlovic, 1989), when appropriate.

The clinician should also be aware of a situation in which use of the RECD + 2-cc coupler procedure can result in an underestimation of real-ear SPL. Specifically, when negative RECD values occur due to acoustic leakage or venting, sound also enters the ear canal along the same pathways. When this occurs at frequencies where there is minimal or no hearing loss, negative RECD values should not be applied to the coupler responses for targets or estimates of REAR/RESR. This situation occurs rarely, and in general, the method discussed provides an accurate prediction of amplified real-ear sound pressure level (Hoover et al., 2000).

Digital hearing instrument programming software allows clinicians to view hearing instrument settings and predicted performance on the computer screen.

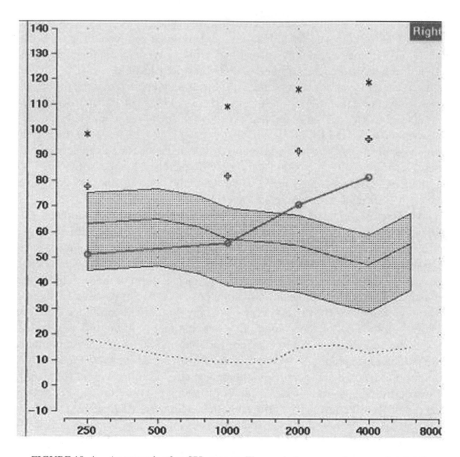

FIGURE 10–4.   An example of an SPL-o-gram. The graph shows sound pressure level at the tympanic membrane on the vertical axis and frequency on the horizontal axis. The circles (0) represent hearing sensitivity thresholds for the right ear. Plus (+) signs show the targets for the amplified long-term average speech spectrum, and asterisks (*) indicate targets for maximum output of the hearing instrument or real-ear saturation RESR. The unamplified speech long-term average speech spectrum is shown as a shaded area.

Many of the manufacturers also have automatic fit capabilities that can set the devices based on a selected prescriptive method. For some programs, patient's RECDs can also be entered and included in the process of determining suggested parameter settings. There is concern that, in some cases, clinicians may be relying on these representations of performance in place of actual verification measures. This is unacceptable when fitting amplification with the pediatric population. As Hawkins and Cook (2003) indicated, the representation of the hearing instrument generated by manufacturer programming software is a simulation only. It does not indicate the real-ear performance of the hearing instrument for a particular patient. Due to tolerances of the hearing instrument components, the simulation may even differ from 2-cc coupler measures. Figure 10–6 illustrates this

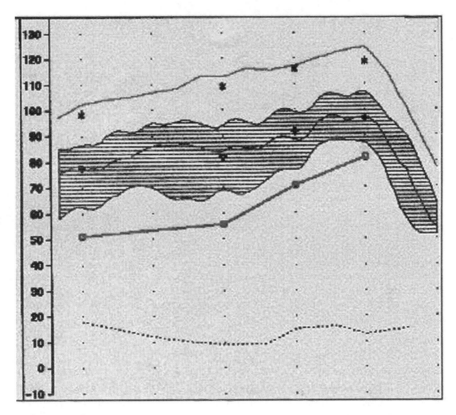

FIGURE 10–5   An example of an SPL-o-gram reflecting data obtained from electroacoustic measurement of a hearing instrument, following the convention of Figure 10–4. The portion of the amplified speech spectrum that is audible (above sensitivity threshold) can be visualized as the hatched area. The single thin line indicates the RESR.

point. The top panel shows the simulated or predicted response of a hearing instrument after selecting an automatic fit to match DSL-prescribed targets, which is also shown. The right panel displays the changes in the simulated response following adjustments made to meet DSL targets during electroacoustic verification. The automatically-generated settings would have resulted in the patient being inadequately amplified.

Using the manufacturer's fitting software as a shortcut without performing electroacoustic verification can easily result in inaccuracies, and an automatic fit should be used only as a starting point to be followed by the electroacoustic methods discussed in this chapter (Scollie, 2003).

The ideal signal to be used in verification is real speech, because it is most likely to show how the hearing instruments will process speech, the primary signal of interest. Hearing instrument clinical test equipment is capable of producing and analyzing calibrated speech signals. In equipment that does not include

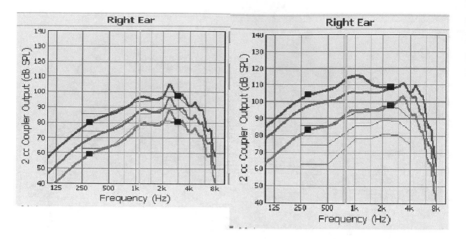

FIGURE 10–6.   Views from programming software showing a hearing instrument's predicted response after an automatic fit to match DSL targets (left panel) and following adjustments to meet actual DSL targets during electroacoustic verification measurements. In each panel the heavy lines indicate predicted hearing instrument responses for three input levels and the thin lines are the software-generated DSL targets. Note the discrepancy between the automatic fit and the actual match to DSL targets.

this capability; the signal used to test hearing instrument performance should represent the frequency, intensity and temporal characteristics of speech as closely as possible (American Academy of Audiology, 2003; Scollie, 2003; Stelmachowicz et al., 1996). The more a test signal deviates from real speech with regard to these parameters, the less likely the test results will accurately predict amplified speech. In addition, if a test signal other than speech is used with digital hearing instruments that utilize noise reduction, the possibility exists that the device will determine that the test signal is not speech, and gain may be adjusted accordingly. It is recommended that, if possible, the noise reduction feature be disabled when verifying the hearing instrument with a signal other than speech or a speech-like modulated signal (Scollie, 2003).

In 2002, Scollie and Seewald described their proposed characteristics of an adequate verification protocol. They indicated that verification should tell how the hearing instrument processes speech and at what levels output is limited. In addition, it should be efficient, reliable, and valid. Finally, it should be capable of being used with infants. A verification protocol utilizing electroacoustic measurements—either Real Ear Measures or Simulated Real Ear Measures—meets these criteria. With electroacoustic verification, measurements can be made of the hearing instrument response to speech or speech-like signals. This verification procedure can typically be performed in significantly less time than functional gain testing. The literature shows that the RECD measurement is reliable, regardless of the age of the patient. It has also been shown that electroacoustic measures of the hearing instrument in a 2-cc coupler with the addition of an RECD and established microphone location effects provides a valid representation of real ear sound pressure levels with a particular device. There are no age constraints on the use of the described electroacoustic verification procedure, because no response or active participation is required from the patient. Finally, viewing a SPL-o-gram that illustrates the relationship between the audiometric characteristics of the patient and the electroacoustic characteristics of the hearing instrument provides meaningful, direct information with regard to how well the goal of audibility of speech is being met.

Mention should also be made regarding use of real ear insertion gain (REIG) or real ear insertion response (REIR) as a means of verifying hearing instrument performance in infants and young children. Although REIG and REIR are electroacoustic measurements, they should not be used in the amplification verification process with this population because they do not provide direct information about audibility of the speech spectrum (American Academy of Audiology, 2003).

Step Three: Orientation

Although the orientation phase of a pediatric amplification fitting appears to be a straightforward to-do list, its quality can determine the success of establishing hearing instrument use. During this time, parents are still in the grieving process related to their child's diagnosis of hearing loss. Yet they are being asked to learn new, unexpected skills, which involve new vocabulary, new equipment and new challenges. Orientation may be better viewed as a process, rather than a one-time event. It serves the pediatric audiologist well to consciously review and plan what information needs to be shared with caregivers and when that information should be presented. Taking the time to discover the family's preferences and needs will make the process more effective. Depending on many factors, some topics covered in this section are more appropriately introduced early in the process and others should be presented or reviewed at later stages.

No matter how thorough the audiologist is in providing information, a fitting will not be successful until the child's parents are ready to proceed with amplification. An often over-looked purpose of the orientation process is to assist parents in dealing with their reactions to their child's hearing loss and to help focus on coping with that loss. In Elfenbein's (2000) review of counseling needs related to hearing instrument orientation, she states: "Audiologists must be as concerned with the emotional reactions to their message as they are with the communication of facts." If the audiologist is only focused on facts that must be reviewed, an excellent opportunity to begin a collaborative relationship with the parents may be lost. Forming a collaborative relationship can assist the family in moving from grief to empowerment. With this in mind and before beginning any formal orientation, the audiologist should discover what questions the family may have about the hearing loss diagnosis or about the hearing instrument fitting process. Knowing what the family wants to accomplish helps to focus the orientation time and will assist in planning for future appointments.

At the most basic level of orientation, the child's family, and ultimately the child need to learn how the hearing instruments function, how to put them on, and how to care for them. This translates into a long list of detailed information that covers the following basic areas:

- Daily use and care
- Listening checks
- Cleaning
- Moisture prevention
- Wearing schedule
- Insertion, removal, retention and storage of devices and earmolds
- Insertion, removal, storage and disposal of batteries
- Maintenance of devices
- Troubleshooting
- Use with telephone and assistive devices

Sample Orientation Checklist:

- Fit earmold, cut tubing and attach to the hearing instrument
- Demonstrate and review function of main components of the hearing instrument system:
    Earmold
    Microphone
    Battery compartment
    Volume/gain control
    Receiver
  Switches/remote controls
- Demonstrate and practice earmold insertion and hearing instrument placement
- Demonstrate and practice battery placement
- Demonstrate and practice daily listening checks, regular cleaning and maintenance, using appropriate literature for caregivers to follow along

Rather than simply showing caregivers and children how to use and maintain their hearing instruments, structured activity and practice is recommended. The emphasis needs to be on skill development. This sends the message that care and maintenance are important. Hands-on practice provides opportunities to acknowledge the parents' achievements. As they master skills, anxiety about hearing instrument use decreases. Tools to facilitate care, maintenance and troubleshooting should be provided to the family at the time of the orientation appointment in order to make the process as seamless as possible. Some hearing instrument manufacturers make care kits that have most or all of the tools noted below:

- Earmold blower
- Battery tester

- Extra batteries
- Listening tube or hearing instrument stethoscope
- Hearing instrument dehumidifier
- Brush and wax pick for earmolds
- Retention devices

Hearing Instrument Retention

The audiologist often takes responsibility for checking retention of the hearing instrument at the beginning of any fitting process, but over time caregivers will need instruction and practice in checking retention for their child. Regardless of who is responsible, the following information may be helpful in providing the best retention possible.

A well-fitted mold is essential to good retention, including fitting with an earmold that is tubed at the correct angle and cut to the correct length.

A step-by-step guide to achieve a good earmold fit follows:

- Measure with the BTE in place, with glasses on, if worn
- Put the earmold in
- Mark the length of tube needed by comparing it to the tonehook of the hearing instrument
- Remove the earmold and cut the tubing based on the marking
- Connect the earmold to the BTE and double check placement over the ear

The use of a correctly sized tonehood may improve retention. Many manufacturers have a choice of pediatric-sized tone hooks that can be interchanged.

In some cases, the weight of a hearing instrument on soft cartilage or a small ear causes it to flop off the pinna. The use of wig tape or water-soluble body adhesives (such as It Stays™) serves to fix the instrument in place against the head. Adhesives placed on the side of the BTE case may also be needed if a child has a tendency to pull on the instrument. Huggie™ or retention rings can be used to prevent the instrument from flopping off. However, the rings can sometimes cause the pinna to curl when the device is in place. Children who pull on their hearing instruments may find the ring to be a convenient removal handle! The use of eyeglasses can complicate hearing instrument retention, with all devices needing to fit closely behind the ear.

As infants and young children become more active, loss-prevention options need to be introduced and encouraged. Options include: clips that connect from the body of the BTE hearing instrument to the child's clothing or a thin fabric cap that covers the hearing instrument. The use of a cap can be used to deter removal of the devices; however, it may increase the chance of acoustic feedback. The cap must be evaluated to confirm that the material is acoustically transparent. This can be accomplished by comparing covered and uncovered electroacoustic responses either in a test chamber or on the child's ear using probe microphone measures.

As much as is possible, all topics reviewed and practiced during orientation should be supported with written information. Written material serves as a reference for information that might be forgotten. Most manufacturers provide thorough, model-specific brochures or booklets that review device function, basic care and maintenance and troubleshooting tables that are often available in multiple languages.

Warranty and Insurance

In general, new hearing instruments are dispensed with some type of manufacturer's warranty covering repair and/or device loss. The length of the manufacturer's warranty may vary, and extended warranties can be obtained through many manufacturers for an additional fee.

Near the end of the manufacturer's renewable warranty, the family should be informed about independent hearing instrument insurance plans. Infants and children generally experience more repairs, breakage and loss than a typical adult hearing instrument user. The cost of even one hearing instrument replacement justifies the cost of an annual insurance premium. Some homeowner's policies may also cover hearing instrument loss, less the individual's co-pay amount on a claim, but may not cover damage or repair charges for general wear and tear.

Step Four: Validation

Validation of amplified auditory function is a demonstration of the benefits and limitations of amplified hearing abilities, and begins immediately after amplification use is initiated. Validation is an ongoing process designed to ensure that the child is receiving optimal speech input from others and that his or her own speech is adequately perceived (PWG, 1996).

Hearing instruments may be recommended, instruments may be programmed, verified and fit, but are they providing the expected benefit? Validation measures tell the audiologist if a positive difference has been achieved. In recent years, the fields of health-care and education have moved to outcome-based assessment and the provision of amplification and hearing intervention crosses both disciplines. Validation cannot be an afterthought. It should be regarded as an important step in the provision of amplification services. Validation measures are either subjective or objective.

Subjective Validation

Subjective measures of validation typically involve use of functional assessment tools. These tools are often questionnaires, where parents, teachers and sometimes children are asked to judge attention and listening performance in a variety of real-world environments. Some of these functional assessment tools require detailed evaluation and may not be appropriate for use during a typical clinical audiology appointment. However, the pediatric audiologist may recommend or facilitate the use of such tools to assist in evaluating amplification benefit. A variety of people may be involved in the administration of subjective validation tools, including the audiologist, early interventionist, parent and teacher(s).

A list of some subjective validation tools, many suitable only for older children, follows:

- **CHILD** (Children's Home Inventory of Listening Difficulties), by Anderson and Smaldino (2000), is an inventory completed by parents for children 3–12 years of age. A child's format of the scale can be completed by children as young as 7–8 years of age. The illustration of an "Understand-O-Meter" is used to rate the ability to hear and understand in a variety of situations. The CHILD is available as a downloadable file from http://www. phonak.com/com_child_questionnaire_gb.pdf.

- **C-APHAP** (Child's Abbreviated Profile of Hearing Aid Performance) (Kopun & Stelmachowicz, 1998) is a self-report questionnaire for children 10–16 years of age, and is a modification of the APHAP (Cox & Alexander, 1995).

- **COW** (Children's Outcome Worksheet) is a children's version of the COSI (Client Oriented Scale of Improvement) (Dillon, et al, 1999). The COW is designed for use with children 4–12 years of age. Parents and children specify their goals for amplification, and indicate when those goals have been met. It can be downloaded from http://www.oticon.com/eprise/main/Oticon/US_en/SEC_Professionals/PowerSupport/Downloads/AudSupportAnd ProductMaterials/.

- **ELF** (Early Listening Function), by Anderson (2002), is appropriate for infants and toddlers. The ELF uses the illustration of the "sound bubble" to describe responses to sounds at different distances. The ELF is available as a downloadable file from http://www.phonak.com/com_elf_questionnaire_ gb.pdf.

- **FAPI** (Functional Auditory Performance Indicators), by Stredler-Brown and Johnson (2001, 2003, 2004) evaluates seven categories of auditory skills in a hierarchical order, from sound awareness through linguistic auditory processing. No age limits are stated for this tool, and many different skills can be evaluated over time. The FAPI is available as a downloadable file from http://www.csdb.org/chip/resources/docs/fapi6_23.pdf.

- **LIFE** (Listening Inventory for Education) by Anderson and Smaldino (1998) is a teacher and school-age student appraisal of listening difficulty in a variety of environments and situations. The teacher version can be used to compare performance before and after an amplification or assistive device change. Test forms are available in a downloadable format at http://www.hear2learn.com/.

- **MAIS / IT-MAIS** (Meaningful Auditory Integration Scale; Infant / Toddler version; Robbins, et al, 1991; Zimmerman-Phillips, et al, 1997) are parent report scales that allow the examiner to evaluate a child's auditory skills in meaningful, real-world situations. The scales are more appropriate for children who have severe-profound hearing loss. Unstructured probes are presented to the parent to elicit their description about the child's spontaneous listening in their home and family environments. Test administration and forms are available in a downloadable format for the MAIS at http://www.medicine.iu.edu/documents/otolaryngology/mais.pdf and for the IT-MAIS at http://www.bnionic-implants.org/printables/it-mais_ brochure.pdf

- **SIFTER (Anderson, 1989)/ Preschool SIFTER (Anderson & Matkin, 1996) / Adolescent SIFTER (Anderson, 2004)** (Screening Inventory for Targeting Educational Risk), by Anderson, were developed to screen children's performance in five areas: academics/pre-academics, attention, communication, class participation and social behavior, with specific forms for different ages. Administration forms are available as a downloadable file from http://www.hear2learn.com/.

Objective Validation

Objective validation measures often are completed in a controlled clinical environment, such as an audiological test booth. Most objective tools compare performance with and without hearing instruments, or before and after a hearing instrument modification. These tools typically evaluate how well the child can identify or understand environmental signals and/or speech. Language and vocabulary development of the child will determine which objective measures can be used. Many of the available measures are not applicable for children under 36 months language age.

Objective validation measures should include the use of age-appropriate speech recognition materials such as:

- **BKB-SIN Speech-in-Noise Test** (Bench, Koval, Bamford-Speech in Noise Sentences) (Bench, Koval & Bamford, 1979) is an open-set sentence repetition task in increasing levels of noise for use with children 5 years and older.
- **CASPA** (Computer Assisted Speech Perception Assessment) by Boothroyd (2004) is a word repetition task with no age parameters specified. The CASPA manual is available as a downloadable file from http://www -rohan.sdsu.edu/~aboothro/files/CASPA/caspa_manual.pdf
- **Early Speech Perception Task (ESP)** (Moog & Geers, 1990) is a closed-set picture or object pointing response to assess pattern and word recognition in children who have severe-to-profound hearing loss. It has standard and low-verbal versions.
- **Functional Listening Evaluation** (FLE) by Johnson and Von Almen (1997) and revised by Johnson (2001) is designed to simulate actual listening conditions and evaluate the effects of noise, distance and visual input for school age children using a word or sentence repetition response. The FLE is available as a downloadable file from http://www.cde.state.co.us/cdesped/ download/pdf/s4-FunListEval.pdf.

- **GASP** (Glendonald Auditory Screening Procedure) (Erber, 1982) is a word repetition task for 6–10 year olds.
- **PSI Test** (Pediatric Speech Intelligibility) (Jerger, et al, 1980) is intended for 3–10 year olds.
- **SAT** (Speech Awareness Threshold) amplified and unamplified measures for 6 months and older.
- **SRT** (Speech Reception Threshold) amplified and unamplified measures for picture-pointing or word-repetition using spondee words, for 3 years and older.

A comprehensive list of common speech recognition tests to use with children is detailed in the PWG (1996) document.

Step Five: Planned Follow-Up and Monitoring

A planned, regular schedule for follow-up testing and monitoring is important for the long-term success of a child with hearing loss. Rapid growth, increasing reliability of behavioral results, the possibility of fluctuation or progression in hearing loss and the needed changes in hearing instrument settings are some of the many reasons for regular evaluation and monitoring with infants and young children.

At a minimum, pediatric amplification guidelines recommend audiological follow-up every three months during the first 2 years of life, and every 6 months until 5–6 years of age. If a child exhibits fluctuation or progression in hearing thresholds, follow-up may be recommended more frequently. Behavioral audiometric evaluation and tympanometry is recommended at each of these visits, along with the following:

- Check the fit and condition of the child's earmolds, with earmold replacements as needed
- Repeat RECD measures with new earmolds or at least annually if earmolds are not replaced
- Test hearing instrument performance, including both electroacoustic evaluation and listening checks
- Adjust hearing instruments, as needed
- Complete measures of amplified auditory performance, as appropriate for the child's age and developmental level

Counseling and orientation should be considered an on-going process that is part of follow-up and monitoring. Once again, focusing only on a checklist of tests to complete may cause the audiologist to lose sight of important information that is available from the family. As a child develops, his or her listening needs change and parents often have new questions and concerns. The incorporation of technical features such as directional microphones and multiple listening programs must be considered and discussed. Parents also need information and support if they choose to incorporate the use of assistive devices such as FM systems at home. Eventually families have questions about when to upgrade their child's hearing instrument technology.

As relationships are established over time, parents may also bring up personal concerns with the audiologist. Issues such as dealing with temper tantrums or concerns about the child's self-esteem and social acceptance may be presented during follow-up visits. The audiologist must be mindful of when a referral to a psychologist or social worker is warranted. The pediatric audiologist is in a unique counseling position because of the long-term relationship that is established with families. Counseling coursework (English et al., 1999) as part of Audiology training programs has potential to improve patient-clinical communication. Further, several books and publications have been produced in recent years that provide audiologists with further information and assistance in developing their counseling skills (Clark & English, 2004; Clark & Martin, 1994; English, 2005).

As children's listening needs change, so too does their level of independence. The family and audiologist should work together over time to increase the child's independence in terms of self-care and self-advocacy. Taking the time to explain audiological test results and hearing instrument verification at the level of the child's understanding encourages the child to be part of the decision-making process. Experienced pediatric audiologists can likely share stories about children who mistakenly thought that they would outgrow their hearing loss when they became an adult, or who had little understanding about what audiological test results meant in relationship to everyday listening.

Appropriate assistive technology needs to be introduced along the way to increase independence in everyday activities such as talking on the telephone, waking up, and alerting and safety at home. Regular follow-up visits provide many opportunities to share information that helps the family's understanding about hearing loss and about the variety of assistive technology that is available. These visits also create bonds of trust between families and the audiologist.

SUMMARY

An evidence-based approach to providing audiological care to infants, children and their families is presented. Although the process is presented in a step-by-step manner, from Pre-selection to Planned follow-up, it is emphasized that these steps are interactive. Additionally, provision of amplification is just one component of care provided in the aural habilitation and rehabilitation of infants and children with hearing loss.

REFERENCES

Allen, P., & Wightman, F. (1994). Psychometric functions for children's detection of tones in noise. *Journal of Speech and Hearing Research, 37,* 205–215.

American Academy of Audiology Pediatric Amplification Protocol. (2003). http://www.
    audiology.org/NR/rdonlyres/53D267792-E321-41AF-850F-CC253310F90b/0/pedamp.
    pdf
Anderson, K. L. (1989). *Screening instrument for targeting educational risk (SIFTER)*.
    Tampa, FL: Educational Audiology Association. http://home.earthlink.net/~karen
    landerson/sifter.html
Anderson, K. L. (2002). *Early listening function (ELF)*. Tampa, FL: Educational Audiolgoy
    Association. http://home.earthlink.net/~karenlanderson/ELF.html
Anderson, K. L., & Matkin, N. D. (1996). *Screening instrument for targeting educational
    risk in preschool children (age 3-kindergarten) (Preschool SIFTER)*. Tampa, FL:
    Educational Audiology Association. http://home.earthlink.net/~karenlanderson/
    presifter.html
Anderson, K. L., & Smaldino, J. (2000). Children's home inventory of listening diffi-
    culties (CHILD). *Educational Audiology Review, 17*(3), Suppl. http://home.earthlink
    .net/~karenlanderson/child.html
Anderson, K. L., & Smaldino, J. (1998). *The listening inventory for education (LIFE)*.
    Tampa, FL: Educational Audiology Association.
Bagatto, M. P. (2001). Optimizing your RECD measurements. *Hearing Journal, 54*(32),
    34–36.
Bagatto, M., Moodie, S., Scollie, S., Seewald, R., Moodie, S., Pumford, J., & Liu, K. P.
    (2005). Clinical protocols for hearing instrument fitting in the desired sensation level
    method. *Trends in Amplfication, 9*(4) 199–226.
Bagatto, M. P., Scollie, S. D., Seewald R. C., Moodie, K. S., & Hoover, B. M. (2002). Real-
    ear-to-coupler difference predictions as a function of age for two coupling procedures.
    Journal of the American Academy of Audiology, 13, 407–415.
Bagatto, M. P., Seewald, R., Scollie, S., Liu, R., & Hyde, M. (2004). *Integrating frequency-
    specific ABR thresholds into the hearing instrument fitting process*. Poster presented at
    Sound Foundations Conference, November, Chicago, IL.
Bench, J., Koval, A., & Bamford, J. (1979). The BKB (Bamford-Koval-Bench) sentence
    lists for partially-hearing children. *British Journal of Audiology 13*, 108–112.
Bentler, R. A., & Pavlovic, C. V. (1989). Transfer functions and correction factors used in
    hearing aid evaluation and research. *Ear and Hearing, 10*, 58–63.
Bess, F. H., Dodd-Murphy, J., & Parker, R. A. (1998). Children with minimal sensorineural
    hearing loss: Prevalence, educational performance, and functional status. *Ear and
    Hearing, 19*(5), 339–354.
Boothroyd, A. (2004). *CASPA (Computer assisted speech perception assessment) 3.3a*.
    http://www-rohan.sdsu.edu/~aboothro/files/CASPA/caspa_manual.pdf
Byrne, D., Dillon, H., Ching, T., Katsch, R., & Keidser, G. (2001). NAL-NL1 procedure for
    fitting nonlinear hearing aids: Characteristics and comparisons with other procedures.
    Journal of American Academy of Audiology, 12(1), 37–51.
Clark, J. G., & English, K. (2004). *Counseling in audiologic practice: Helping patients and
    families adjust to hearing loss*. Boston: Allyn & Bacon.
Clark, J.G. and Martin, F.N. (1994). *Effective Counseling in Audiology: Perspectives and
    Practice*. Boston: Allyn & Bacon.
Cord, M. T., Surr, R. K., Walden, B. E., & Drylund, O. (2004). Relationship between lab-
    oratory measures of directional advantage and everyday success with directional mi-
    crophone hearing aids. *Journal of American Academy of Audiology, 15*(5), 353–364.
Cornelisse, L. E., Seewald, R. C., & Jamieson, D. G. (1995). The input/output formula: A
    theoretical approach to the fitting of personal amplification devices. *Journal of the
    Acoustical Society of America, 97*, 1854–1864.
Cox, R. M., & Alexander, G. C. (1995). The abbreviated profile of hearing aid benefit. *Ear
    and Hearing, 16*, 176–183.

Dillon, H. (2001). *Hearing Aids.* New York: Theime.

Dillon, H. (1999). NAL-NL1: A new prescriptive fitting procedure for non-linear hearing aids. *The Hearing Journal, 52*(4),10–16.

Dillon, H., Birtles, G., & Lovegrove, R. (1999). Measuring the outcomes of a national rehabilitation program: Normative data for the Client Oriented Scale of Improvement (COSI) and the Hearing Aid User's Questionnaire (HAUQ). *Journal of the American Academy of Audiology, 10*(2), 7–79.

Dire, D. (2005). *Disk battery ingestion.* http://www.emedicine.com/emerg/topic139.htm

Elfenbein, J. L. (2000) Batteries required: Instructing families on the use of hearing instruments. *A Sound Foundation Through Early Amplification,* 141–150.

Ellis, M. R., & Wynne, M. K. (1999). Measurements of loudness growth in ½-octave bands for children and adults with normal hearing. *American Journal of Audiology, 8,* 40–46.

English, K. (2005). Get ready for the next big thing in audiologic counseling. *The Hearing Journal, 58*(7), 10–15.

English, K., Lucks Mendel, L., Rojeski, T., & Hornak, J. (1999). Counseling in Audiology, or in learning to listen: Pre- and post-measures from an Audiology Counseling Course. *American Journal of Audiology, 8,* 34–39.

Erber, N. P. (1982). *Auditory training.* Washington, DC: Alexander Graham Bell Association for the Deaf.

Feigin, J. A., Kopun, J. G., Stelmachowicz, P. G., & Gorga, M. P. (1989). Probe microphone measures of ear-canal sound pressure levels in infants and children. *Ear and Hearing, 10,* 254–258.

Gabbard, S. (2005). The use of FM technology for infants and young children. In R. Seewald & J. Bamford (Eds.), A sound foundation through early amplification: Proceedings of the third international conference (pp.155–162). Stafa, Switzerland: Phonak AG.

Gravel, J. S., Fausel, M., Liskow, C., & Chobot, J. (1999). Children's speech recognition in noise using omni-directional and dual-directional microphone hearing aids technology. *Ear and Hearing, 20,* 1–11.

Harrison, M., & Roush, J. (1996). Age of suspicion, identification and intervention for infants and young children with hearing loss: A national study. *Ear and Hearing, 17,* 55–62.

Harrison, M., Roush, J., & Wallace, J. (2003). Trends in age of identification and intervention in infants with hearing loss. *Ear and Hearing, 24,* 89–95.

Hawkins, D. B., & Cook, J. A. (2003). Hearing aid software predictive gain values: How accurate are they? *Hearing Journal, 56*(7), 8–42.

Hawkins, D. B., Montgomery, A. A., Prosek, R. A., & Walden, B. E. (1987). Examination of two issues concerning functional gain measurements. *Journal of Speech and Hearing Disorders, 52,* 56–63.

Hedley-Williams, A., Tharpe, A. M., & Bess, F. H. (1996). Fitting hearing aids in the pediatric population: A survey of practice procedures. In F. H. Bess, J. S. Gravel, & A. M. Tharpe (Eds.), Amplification for children with auditory deficits (pp. 193–213). Nashville, TN: Bill Wilkerson Center Press.

Hoover, B. M., Stelmachowicz, P. G., & Lewis, D. E. (2000). Effect of earmold fit on predicted real ear SPL using a real ear to coupler difference procedure. *Ear & Hearing, 21,* 310–317.

Jerger, S., Lewis, S., Hawkins, J., & Jerger, J. (1980). Pediatric speech intelligibility test: I. Generation of test materials. *International Journal of Pediatric Otorhinolaryngology, 2,* 217–230.

Jenstad, L. M., Seewald, R. C., Cornelisse, L. E., & Shantz, J. (1999). Comparison of linear gain and wide dynamic range compression hearing aid circuits: Aided speech perception measures. *Ear and Hearing, 20,* 17–126.

Johnson, C. D., & Von Almen, P. (1993). The functional listening evaluation. In Johnson, Benson, & Seaton (Eds.), Educational audiology handbook (pp. 336–339). San Diego: Singular Publishing Group, Inc.

Johnson, C. D. (2001). *Revised functional listening evaluation.* http://www.cde. state.co.us/cdesped/download/pdf/s4-FunListEval.pdf

Joint Committee on Infant Hearing. (2000). Principles and guidelines for early hearing detection and intervention programs. *Audiology Today, Special Issue*, 2000.

Kentworthy, O. T., Klee, T., & Tharpe, A. M. (1990). Speech recognition ability of children with unilateral sensorineural hearing loss as a function of amplification, speech stimuli and listening condition. *Ear and Hearing, 11,* 264–270.

Kopun, J. G., & Stelmachowicz, P. G. (1998). Perceived communication difficulties of children with hearing loss. *American Journal of Audiology, 7,* 30–38.

Kruger, B. (1987). An update on the external ear resonance in infants and young children. *Ear and Hearing, 8*(6), 333–336.

Liu, T., & Lin, K. (1999). Real-ear to coupler difference in patients with ear drum perforation. *ORL Journal for Oto-Rhino-Laryngology and Its Related Specialties, 61,* 345–349.

Macpherson, B. J., Elfenbein, J. L., Schum, R. L., & Bentler, R. (1991). Thresholds of discomfort in young children. *Ear and Hearing, 12,* 401–408.

Marriage, J, Moore, B. C. J., Stone, M. A., & Baer, T. (2005). Effects of three amplification strategies on speech perception by children with severe and profound hearing loss. *Ear and Hearing, 26,* 35–41.

Martin, H. C., Munro K. J., & Lam, M. C. (2001). Perforation of the tympanic membrane and its effect on the real ear-to-coupler difference acoustic transform function. *British Journal of Audiology, 35,* 259–264.

Martin, H. C., Munro K. J., & Langer, D. H. (1997). Real-ear to coupler differences in children with grommets. *British Journal of Audiology, 31,* 63–69.

Moodie, K. S., Seewald, R. C., & Sinclair, S. T. (1994). Procedure for predicting real-ear hearing aid performance in young children. *American Journal of Audiology, 3,* 23–31.

Moog, J. S., & Geers, A. E. (1990). Early speech perception test. St. Louis, MO: CID.

Munro, K. (2004). Integrating the RECD into the hearing instrument fitting process. Phonak Focus 33. Stafa, Switzerland: Phonak AG

Munro, K. J., & Buttfield, L. (2004). RECD measurements: A comparison of right and left ear. Presentation at NHS 2004: The International Conference on Newborn hearing Screening, Diagnosis, and Intervention, Como, Italy.

Munro, K. J., & Davis, J. (2003). Deriving the real-ear SPL of audiometric data using the "coupler-to-dial difference" and the "real-ear-to-coupler difference". *Ear and Hearing, 24,* 100–110.

Munro, K. J., & Hatton, N. (2000). Customized acoustic transform functions and their accuracy at predicting real-ear hearing aid performance. *Ear and Hearing, 21,* 59–69.

Munro, K. J., & Toal, S. (2005). Measuring the real-ear to coupler difference transfer function with an insert earphone and a hearing instrument: Are they the same? *Ear and Hearing, 26,* 27–34.

Nittrouer, S., & Boothroyd, A. (1990). Context effects in phoneme and word recognition by young children and older adults. *Journal of the Acoustical Society of America, 87,* 2705–2715.

Nozza, R. J., Rossman, R. N. F., & Bond, L. C. (1991). Infant-adult differences in unmasked thresholds fro the discrimination of consonant-vowel syllable pairs. *Audiology, 30,* 102–112.

Nozza, R. J., Rossman, R. N. F., Bond, L. C., & Miller, S. L. (1990). Infant speech-sound discrimination in noise. *Journal of the Acoustical Society of America, 87,* 339–350.

Oticon for the Children's Outcome Worksheet. http://www.oticon.com/eprise/main/ Oticon/US_en/SEC_Professionals/PowerSupport/PowerSupportPDF/cow_form.PDF

Pediatric Working Group of the Conference on Amplification for Children with Auditory Deficits. (1996). Amplification for infants and children with hearing loss. *American Journal of Audiology, 5,* 77–88.

Phonak DVD. (2004). *Hearing care for infants: Strategies for a sound beginning.* http://www.phonak-us.com/com_professional_pediatrics_video_referenceguide.pdf

Pittman, A. L., & Stelmachowicz, P. G. (2003). Hearing loss in children and adults: Audiometric configuration, asymmetry, and progression. *Ear and Hearing, 24,* 198–205.

Revit, L. J. (1997). The circle of decibels: Relating the hearing test, to the hearing instrument, to the real ear response. *Hearing Review, 4,* 35–38.

Ricketts, T. A., & Tharpe, A. M. (2005). Potential for directivity-based benefit in actual classroom environments. In R. Seewald and J. Bamford (Eds.), A sound foundation through early amplification: Proceedings of the Third International Conference (pp. 143–153). Phonak AG: Stafa, Switzerland.

Robbins, A. M. (2002). Empowering parents to help their newly diagnosed child gain communication skills. *The Hearing Journal, 55*(11), 55–59.

Robbins, A. M., Renshaw, J. J., & Berry S. W. (1991). Evaluating meaningful auditory integration in profoundly hearing-impaired children. *Am J Otol. 12 Suppl,* 144–150.

Sass-Lehrer, M. (2004). Early detection of hearing loss: Maintaining a family-centered perspective. In J. P. Preece (Ed.), Issues in Family-Centered Pediatric Audiology. *Seminars in Hearing, 25*(4).

Scollie, S. D. (2003). Hearing aid test signals: What's new and what's good for kids. *Hearing Journal, 56*(9), 10–15.

Scollie, S., & Seewald, R. (2002). Electroacoustic verification measures with modern hearing instrument technology. In R. Seewald and J. Gravel (Eds.), A sound foundation through early amplification: Proceedings of the Second International Conference (pp. 121–137). Stafa, Switzerland: Phonak AG.

Scollie, S. D., Seewald, R. C., Cornelisse, L. E., & Jenstad, L. M. (1998). Validity and repeatability of level-independent HL to SPL transforms. *Ear and Hearing, 19,* 407–413.

Scollie, S., Seewald, R., Cornelisse, L., Moodie, S., Bagatto, M., Larunagaray, D., Beaulac, S., & Pumford, J. (2005). The Desired Sensation Level mulitstate input/output algorithm. *Trends in Apmlification, 9*(4).

Scollie, S. D., Seewald, R. C., Moodie, K. S., & Dekok, K. (2000). Preferred listening levels of children who use hearing aids: Comparison to prescriptive targets. *Journal of the American Academy of Audiology, 11,* 230–238.

Scollie, S., Seewald, R., Sinclair-Moodie, S., Cornelisse, L., Bagatto, M., & Beaulac, S. (2004). *The Desired Sensation Level (DSL) Method in 2004: DSL m[i/o] version 5.0.* Poster presented at Sound Foundations Conference, November, Chicago, IL.

Seewald, R. C. (1995). The desired sensation level (DSL) method for hearing aid fitting in infants and children. *Phonak Focus 20.* Stafa, Switzerland: Phonak, AG.

Seewald, R. C., Moodie, S., Scollie, S., & Bagatto, M. (2005). The DSL method for pediatric hearing instrument fitting: Historical perspective and current issues. *Trends in Amplification, 9*(4), 145–157.

Seewald, R. C., & Scollie, S. D. (1999). Infants are not average adults: Implications for audiometric testing. *Hearing Journal, 52*(10), 64–72.

Seewald, R. C., Moodie, K. S., Sinclair, S. T., & Cornelisse, L. E. (1996). Traditional and theoretical approaches to selecting amplification for infants and children. In F. H. Bess, J. A. Gravel, & A. M. Tharpe (Eds.). Amplification for children with auditory deficits. Nashville, TN: Vanderbilt Press.

Seewald, R. C., Moodie, K. S., Sinclair, S. T., & Scollie, S. D. (1999). Predictive validity of a procedure for pediatric hearing instrument fitting. *American Journal of Audiology, 8,* 143–152.

Seewald, R., & Scollie, S. (2003). An approach for ensuring accuracy in pediatric instrument fitting. *Trends in Amplification, 7*(1), 1–9.

Sinclair, S. T., Beauchaine, K. L., Moodie, K. S., Feigin, J. A., Seewald, R. C., & Stelmachowicz, P. G. (1996). Repeatability of a real-ear-to-coupler difference measurement as a function of age. *American Journal of Audiology, 5,* 52–56.

Sjoblad, S., Harrison, M., Rousch, J., & McWilliam, R. (2001). Parents' reactions and recommendations after diagnosis and hearing aid fitting. *American Journal of Audiology, 10*(1), 24–31.

Stelmachowicz, P. G., Kopun, J. K., Mace, A. L., & Lewis, D. E. (1996). Measures of hearing aid gain for real speech. *Ear & Hearing, 17,* 520–527.

Stelmachowicz, P. G., & Lewis, D. L. (1988). Some theoretical considerations regarding the relation between functional gain and insertion gain. *Journal of Speech and Hearing Research, 31,* 491–496.

Stelmachowicz, P. G., Hoover, B., Lewis, D. E., Kortekass, R. W. L., & Pittman, A. L. (2000). The relation between stimulus context, speech audibility, and perception for normal-hearing and hearing-impaired children. *Journal of Speech, Language, and Hearing Research, 43,* 902–914.

Stelmachowicz, P. G., Hoover, B., Lewis, D. E., & Brennan, M. (2002). Is functional gain really functional? *Hearing Journal, 55*(11), 38–42.

Stelmachowicz, P., Lewis, D., Kalberer, A., & Creutz, T. (1994). Situational Hearing-Aid Response Profile (SHARP, Version 2.0). User's Manual. Omaha, NE: BTNRH. http://www.boystownhospital.org/BasicClinic/clinic-behavioral/Situational_aid.asp

Stelmachowicz, P. G., Pittman, A. L., Hoover, B., & Lewis, D. E. (2001). Effect of stimulus bandwidth on the perception of /s/ in normal- and hearing-impaired children and adults. *Acoustical Society of American, 110*(4), 2183–2190.

Stelmachowicz, P. G., Pittman, A. L., Hoover, B., & Lewis, D. E. (2002). Aided perception of /s/ and /z/ by hearing-impaired children. *Ear and Hearing, 23,* 316–324.

Stelmachowicz, P. G., Pittman, A. L., Hoover, B., Lewis, D. E., & Moeller, M. P. (2004). The importance of high-frequency audibility in the speech and language development of children with hearing loss. *Archives of Otolaryngology Head and Neck Surgery, 130,* 556–562.

Stredler-Brown, A., & Johnson, C. D. (2001, 2003, 2004). Functional auditory performance indicators: An integrated approach to auditory skill development. Retrieved from http:www.cde.state.co.uscdesped/download/pdf/FAPI_3-1-04g.pdf

Stuart, A. (2005). Development of auditory temporal resolution in school-age children revealed by word recognition in continuous and interrupted noise. *Ear and Hearing, 26*(1), 78–88.

Stuart, A., Dureiux-Smith, A., & Stenstrom, R., (1990). Critical differences in aided sound field thresholds in children. *Journal of Speech and Hearing Reseach, 33,* 612–615.

Tharpe, A. M., Fino Szumski, M. S., & Bess, F. H. (2001). Survey of hearing aid fitting practices for children with multiple impairments. *American Journal of Audiology, 10,* 32–40.

Tharpe, A. M., Sladen, D., Huta, H. M., & McKinley Rothpletz, A. (2001). Practical considerations of real-ear-to-coupler difference measures in infants. *American Journal of Audiology, 10,* 1–9.

The Pediatric Working Group. (1996). *Amplification for infants and children with hearing loss.* Nashville, TN: Bill Wilkerson Press. http://www.phonak.com/com_028–0601– Xx_focus_23.pdf

Updike, C. D. (1994). Comparison of FM auditory trainers, CROS aids, and personal amplification in unilaterally hearing impaired children. *Journal of American Academy of Audiology, 5,* 204–209.

Werner, L. A., Marean, G. C., Halpin, C. F., Spetner, N. B., & Gillenwater, J. M. (1992). Infant auditory temporal acuity: Gap detection. *Child Development, 63*(2), 260–272.

Yoshinaga-Itano, C., Sedy, A. L., Coulter, D. K., & Mehl, A. L. (1998). Language of early- and later-identified children with hearing loss. *Peditatrics, 102*(5), 1161–1171.

Zimmerman, S., Osberger, M. J., & Robbins, A. M. (1998). Infant-Toddler: Meaningful Auditory Intergration Scale (IT-MAIS). In W. Estabrooks (Ed.), *Cochlear implants for kids.* Washington, DC: AG Bell Association for the Deaf.

CHAPTER 11

Adult Amplification

Stephen Boney
University of Nebraska

Current estimates indicate that there are 31.5 million people in the United States who have a hearing loss, which translates to approximately 10 percent of the population (Kochkin, 2005). Further, the prevalence of hearing loss increases with age, especially over the age of 40 (National Center for Health Statistics, 2004). With the projected increase in the number of adults aged 50+ over the next 15 years, we can expect to see a parallel increase in the number of patients with hearing loss (U.S. Bureau of the Census). The majority of these adults will have a sensorineural hearing loss which will not be medically treatable. Many of these individuals will seek aural rehabilitation in the form of hearing aids.

The sensory technology most often recommended to address sensorineural hearing loss is a hearing aid. More that 2 million hearing aids were sold in 2004, with a projected retail market value of $3.7 billion (Strom, 2005). Despite strong sales and a market increase of nearly 7.5 percent, the penetration rate for hearing aids remains at approximately 22 percent (Kochkin, 2001). This means that only 1 in 5 individuals who could benefit from hearing aid actually have purchased them. Numerous attempts by hearing aid manufacturers to increase the penetration rate have been met with limited success. Recent advances in hearing aid technology and expanded fitting capabilities may improve the number of hearing-impaired individuals seeking and benefiting from amplification.

Hearing aids are considered a medical device and therefore regulated by the Food and Drug Administration (FDA). The FDA classifies hearing aids as Class I devices which carry a low health risk and do not need premarket review. It would be beneficial to the reader to review the FDA requirements regarding labeling of devices and conditions for sale. These requirements can be accessed at www.fda.gov. It should be noted that these regulations were promulgated in 1977 and are in need of updating.

The information in this chapter will draw largely from clinical experience in dispensing hearing aids along with evidence-based practice (EBP). EBP should form the basis of what we do clinically, regardless of what audiological services we are providing. This requires that the audiologist integrate clinical expertise, current best evidence, and patient values to provide optimal clinical services on an individual basis (ASHA, 2005). With the field of amplification changing at a fast pace it is important that practicing dispensing audiologists maintain a current knowledge base to provide patients with optimal services.

This chapter will address the process of fitting adults with air-conduction hearing aids. A complete discussion of fitting other forms of amplification (e.g., implantable prosthetic devices or bone conduction hearing aids) is beyond the scope of this chapter. References will be made throughout the chapter to some of these devices as possible amplification alternatives. The chapter will begin with a discussion of how hearing aids operate and the various types of signal processing available in current hearing aids followed by a description of the basic styles of hearing aids and earmolds. The remainder of the chapter will focus on the hearing aid fitting process. The fitting process will be divided into the following sections: candidacy, device selection, fitting/orientation, verification and validation, and follow-up. The reader is reminded that the fitting of hearing aids is a dynamic process and that each of the above sections does not necessarily represent a mutually exclusive part of the hearing aid fitting process for adults.

SIGNAL PROCESSING

The purpose of a hearing aid is to amplify acoustic signals from a listeners environment so that these signals are audible and within a comfort range for the patient. A hearing aid accomplishes this in the following manner. Acoustic signals from the patient's environment are picked up by a *microphone* and converted to an electrical analog in the form of a voltage. Microphones are a class of electrical devices called a transducer which convert energy from one form to another. The electrical signal created at the microphone travels to an *amplifier circuit* which is designed to increase the amplitude of the signal. In reality, the electrical signal goes through several stages of amplification. Once the amplification process is completed, the signal is sent to a *receiver (loudspeaker)*, which is a transducer that changes the electrical signal back into an acoustic form, and is then channeled to the listener's ear. The hearing aid is powered by a small, pill shaped *zinc- air battery* which generates approximately 1.4 volts. The above represent the basic components of a hearing aid. Contemporary hearing aids often have other components. Table 11–1 provides a description of some of these components and their function along with signal processing technologies that are being incorporated in many of the hearing aids currently on the market.

Even though all hearing aids share basic components, the manner in which signals are processed may vary. Currently, there are three types of signal processing that are available in hearing aids: analog, digitally controlled analog (DCA), and digital. Figure 11–1 depicts block diagrams of these three types of signal processing.

Briefly, *analog* hearing aids process sound in a continuous manner. The electrical voltage in the hearing aid is analogous to the input SPL of the hearing aid. This type of signal processing has been used in hearing aids as far back as the

TABLE 11–1
Description of Various Components and Technologies Used in Current Hearing Aids

Technology	Description
Direct Audio Input (DAI)	Feature which allows direct electrical connection between ALD and hearing aid. Most often used for connection to FM receivers.
Directional Microphone	Microphones which are differentially sensitive to sound from varying directions. Used to improve SNR for the listener.
Feedback Systems (managers)	Electronic systems used to control (reduce or eliminate) feedback in hearing aids. Current active systems include use of gain reduction, notch filtering, and phase control.
Listening Programs	Sets of algorithms that are programmed and stored in the hearing aid to optimize communication in various listening situations (e.g. music, noise, telephone).
Noise reduction algorithms	Signal processing scheme that attempts to statistically analyze the input signal to the hearing aid into speech and noise components. Identified noise components are reduced using various algorithms.
Remote control	Devices which allow the hearing aid user to change various functions of the hearing aid.
Telecoil (T-coil)	Small coil of wire placed inside the hearing aid that picks up alternating magnetic fields. Used for telephones and ALDs.
Volume control	Feature used to increase or decrease the volume of the hearing aid. May be analog or digital.
Wide dyamic range compression (WDRC)	Non-linear form of amplification. Gain varies across a wide range of input signals to the hearing aid. Used to better match the wider range of environmental sounds to the limited dynamic range of the listener

1920s in vacuum tube hearing aids. The number of features and types of adjustments that can be made with these instruments are limited.

The addition of *DCA* instruments came about in the mid-1980s. These instruments added the dimension of programmability to analog circuitry. In these instruments the electroacoustic characteristics of the analog path in the hearing aid are controlled by digital circuits. How these digital circuits function is controlled by instructions that are programmed into the hearing instrument by an external programming device connected to the hearing aids via a set of cables. This type of arrangement allows the hearing aid dispenser to easily change how these circuits function by establishing and storing a new set of instructions. DCA instruments have the advantage of increased electroacoustic flexibility, but still the signal processing is essentially analog.

In the late 1990s hearing aids with digital signal processing (DSP) were introduced on the hearing aid market. DSP aids convert the analog signal coming into the hearing aid into a digital binary form via the use of an analog to digital converter (A/D). The signal is then stored and modified by a series of algorithms programmed and stored in the hearing aid. The modification of the signal does take time; however, the time delay from input to output is typically short enough so it does not affect the listener's perception. After being modified, the signal is then put back into an analog form using a digital to analog (D/A) converter before being delivered to the listener's ear as audible sound. Like DCA instruments,

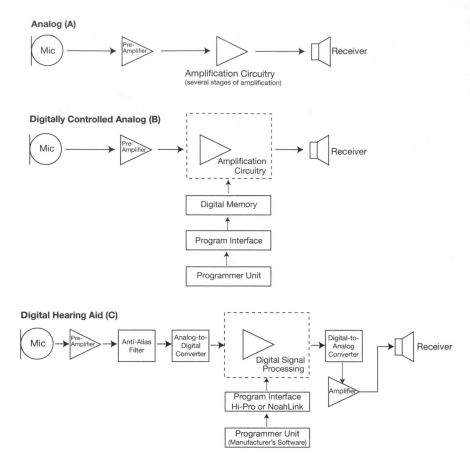

FIGURE 11–1.   Block diagram of three signal processing technologies currently available in hearing aids: (a) analog, (b) digitally controlled analog, and (c) digital.

instructions on how the hearing aid is to process signals are programmed into the hearing aid by an external device. More about this process will be provided in the section on fitting hearing aids. The advantages of DSP hearing aids include: miniaturization and fewer internal components, low internal noise, greater precision in signal reproduction, increased electroacoustic flexibility through programming, and reduced power consumption.

In 2004, 83 percent of the hearing aids dispensed were digital, 5 percent DCA, and 12 percent analog (Strom, 2005a). It is expected that the market share of DSP hearing aids will continue to increase. At this time, most of the hearing aid manufacturers have DSP models of hearing aids that can fit hearing losses from mild to profound. In addition, manufacturers typically offer different price point categories for their line of DSP hearing aids which allows patients with varying financial resources access to DSP hearing aids. These price point categories are typically referred to as entry level (also referred to as low end or value-oriented), mid-level, and high end. The advantages of DSP hearing aids over other technologies along with affordability should make this type of signal processing the choice for the majority of hearing aid users.

Style of Hearing Aid

There is an array of hearing aid styles available for consumers. From largest to smallest styles the major choices include: behind-the- ear (BTE), in-the-ear (ITE), in-the-canal (ITC), and completely-in-the-canal (CIC). Examples of the primary styles are illustrated in Figure 11–2. Body and eyeglass hearing aids are style options as well, but are infrequently recommended.

BTE

BTE hearing aids are the largest of all the major styles. They constitute just over one-quarter of hearing aid sales (Strom, 2005a). The electronic components in a BTE hearing aid are housed in a plastic case which fits behind the patient's ear. The hearing aid is connected to a length of tubing that terminates in a custom earmold. Given the size of a BTE instrument, they can accommodate a greater variety of components and controls. Because of this BTEs can be used for the majority of hearing aid candidates regardless of the degree or configuration of the hearing loss. BTE hearing aids have the added advantage of being able to further shape the signal processed by the hearing aid via the use of an earmold and its associated plumbing (e.g., tubing, earhook). Finally, BTE style aids are able to accommodate dovetailing of a wide variety of assistive listening devices.

ITE

ITE hearing aids represent the largest of the hearing aids that fit all in the ear. These aids are sometimes sub-categorized as full-shell or half-shell aids. The hearing aid circuitry in ITE aids is housed in a custom-fabricated shell that fits in the concha area of the external ear. These devices make up about 40 percent of the

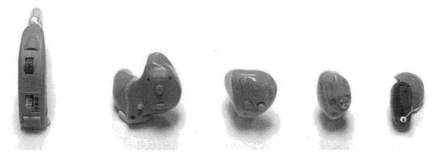

FIGURE 11–2.   Examples of various styles of hearing aids. From left to right: behind-the ear (BTE), full shell in-the-ear (ITE), half-shell ITE, In the canal (ITC), and Completely in the canal (CIC)

hearing aid sales (Strom, 2005a). Given their size, ITE aids can accommodate larger and more sophisticated circuitry than some of the smaller style aids that fit in the ear. This increases the fitting range of hearing loss, both degree and configuration, for these instruments. In addition, the controls of these instruments are larger and may be easier to manipulate for patients with reduced manual dexterity. For some, these aids have a greater cosmetic appeal than BTE hearing aids because there is no earmold or tubing attached to these instruments making them less noticeable. Those with severe or greater hearing losses (> 70 dBHL) are not likely candidates for ITE aids because of the greater risk for feedback due to the shortened distance between the microphone and the receiver. Due to their size, ITE aids may not be able to accommodate assistive listening devices which utilize electromagnetic induction technology because of telecoil size and strength. This can be a particular problem for telephone use. The potential problem of cerumen migrating into the receiver tubing and affecting the performance of the receiver is a concern for all styles of aids that fit into the ear. The cerumen problem is minimized with the use of a variety of cerumen guard systems that are placed in the receiver opening of the hearing aid and diligent daily cleaning by the patient.

ITC

ITC hearing aids constitute approximately 20 percent of the hearing aid sales (Strom, 2005a). What sets these aids apart from ITEs is their smaller size. These aids when inserted fill a smaller portion of the concha making them more cosmetically appealing to patients. An added advantage of filling a smaller portion of the concha is to enhance the high frequencies at the hearing aid microphone due to resonance effects of the outer ear. Patients may experience less difficulty from feedback using the telephone because of the increased separation between the telephone receiver and hearing aid microphone. ITC hearing aids by virtue of their size have smaller circuitry and fewer controls which limit their use to patients who have milder degrees of hearing loss. The geometry of the patient's ear is an important factor in determining what features and controls can be added to the ITC style aid. For those with smaller ears it may not be possible to add a volume control. Insertion and removal of the ITC hearing aid, manipulating the external controls of the aid and changing the battery will prove difficult for those with restricted manual dexterity.

CIC

The smallest style of hearing aids available is CIC. Currently, they comprise nearly 15 percent of hearing aid sales (Strom, 2000a). These aids were introduced on the hearing aid market in the early to mid 1990s. As the name indicates the instrument fits completely in the external ear canal. CIC aids have a removal wire attached to the faceplate to facilitate removal of the instrument from the ear. The field to microphone transfer function is enhanced even more with these instruments over ITCs, improving the transmission of the high frequencies as much as 10–12 dBSPL (Cornelisse & Seewald, 1997; Kent & Boney, 1997). Another acoustic effect of CICs is the added output SPL created in the ear canal due to the smaller volume between the medial tip of the hearing aid and the tympanic membrane. CIC aids provide a good style choice for those concerned with the cosmetic appeal of a hearing aid, assuming they are appropriate candidates for this style choice. With the small size of the hearing aid these instruments are most appropriate for those with losses in the mild to moderate hearing loss category. They can be used with hearing losses of a greater degree, however, feedback is a concern. Options for external controls are significantly limited in CICs due to size constraints. Telecoils and volume controls are rarely available in this style of instrument. Finally, the batteries for these instruments are smaller in size which leads to reduced battery life and increased operating cost. The smaller size also creates difficulty changing the battery for those with fine motor difficulties or visual problems.

There is a wide variety of hearing aid styles available to meet the needs of hearing aid consumers. Virtually all the styles can be utilized with any of the available signal processing options. Selecting the appropriate style of hearing aid is a collaborative decision made between the dispensing audiologist and consumer. Factors such as degree and configuration of hearing loss, cosmetic concerns, manual dexterity, visual problems, external ear geometry, and communication needs all enter into decision as to which style of instrument is best for the patient. This will be discussed later in the chapter.

Earmolds and Plumbing

Earmolds are custom fabricated devices which are used to channel sound from the hearing aid receiver to the listeners ear (Pirzanski, 2000). They serve a number of functions which include: coupling the hearing aid to the patient's ear, proving support for the BTE hearing aid, and modifying the amplified sound before it reaches the patient's ear. Earmolds can be fabricated in a variety of styles, materials and colors. A detailed description of earmolds and their acoustic effects is beyond the scope of this chapter. The reader is referred to Dillion (2001) or Valente et al. (2002) for a more detailed discussion of earmolds.

The National Association of Earmold Laboratories (NAEL) has standardized the nomenclature for basic earmold styles. Examples of these styles are shown in Figure 11–3. All earmold manufacturers offer these styles of earmolds along with other special-purpose designs. The special-purpose designs represent earmold options which are acoustically tuned to modify the frequency or amplitude characteristics of the signal from the hearing aid to better meet the needs of the patient. Since these special-purpose designs do not have standardized names, earmold manufacturers may use proprietary names; therefore the dispensing audiologist should be familiar with the line of earmolds available through the manufacturers that they use in their practice.

The BTE *earhook* and *tubing* used in connecting the earmold with the hearing aid represent the "plumbing" associated with the earmold to complete the transmission line from the hearing aid to the patient's ear. Earhooks connect the hearing aid with the earmold tubing. They have a curved half-moon shape to fit over

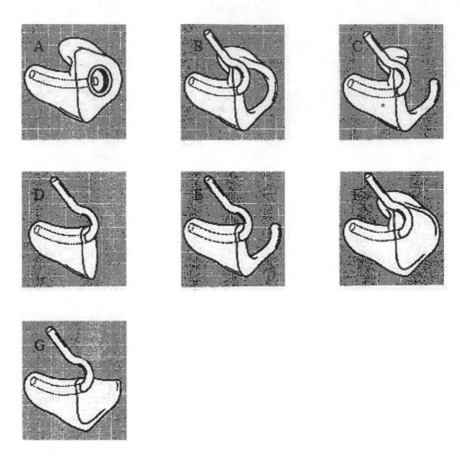

FIGURE 11–3.   Examples of basic earmold styles: (A.) Receiver/Regular. (B) Skeleton. (C) Semiskeleton. (D) Canal. (E) Canal lock. (F) Shell. (G) Canal shell. (With permission from Westone Laboratories, Inc.)

the patient's ear and typically have a length of 20–30 mm. Earmold tubing comes in various sizes which have been standardized by the NAEL. The tubing is secured into the earmold sound bore either with glue or a retention device. The internal diameter of the tubing can be varied to modify the frequency response of sound as it flows through the tubing. In general, increasing the internal diameter of the tubing will improve the transmission of the mid to high frequencies.

One of the most common modifications used in most earmolds and hearing aid shells is placement of a *vent*. A vent is hollow channel of varying configurations, lengths, and internal diameters in an earmold or hearing aid shell. Venting has been used for non-electronic acoustical control in hearing aids for over 60 years, primarily to allow for leakage of low frequency energy through the earmold. Reduction of the low frequencies often serves to help minimize the "full feeling" and "hearing in a tunnel" perceptions experienced by many hearing aid users due to the occlusion of the external ear. Vents can also be used for pressure release and improvement of sound quality and clarity. While there are several advantages to venting, there often exists the possibility of a feedback path being created via the vent. The vent provides a route whereby the amplified signal from the hearing aid leaks out of the ear canal and interacts with the hearing aid microphone. In general, the probability of feedback due to venting is proportional to the size of the vent. The reader is referred to Dillon (2001, p. 135) for a series of tables which can be used by the dispenser to maximize vent size and prevent feedback.

Earmolds and their plumbing provide an important transmission line in delivering the signal from the hearing aid to the patient's ear. The configuration of the transmission line can be useful in acoustic control of the hearing aid signal to better meet the needs of the patient. Proper use of earmold acoustics will result in a smoother and more comfortable sound to the patient.

CANDIDACY

The determination of whether or not a patient is a candidate for a hearing aid should be a multidimensional process consisting of both auditory-related and non-auditory factors. Further, there are no hard and fast rules, or a purely quantifiable approach that will work for all patients. The physiological consequences of sensorineural hearing loss cause not only changes in hearing sensitivity, but also create frequency (e.g., resolution and selectivity) and temporal changes which often affect speech perception. The speech perception changes, in turn, impact on conversational fluency in various situations, especially when the acoustics of the communication environment are compromised. Because of reduced communication secondary psycho-social difficulties may emerge. It's somewhat like a domino effect. Therefore, in determining hearing aid candidacy there are numerous interactive variables to consider. In examining these variables the audiologist must weigh both the *needs of* and *potential benefit* of amplification to the patient.

AUDITORY RELATED FACTORS

Degree and Type of Hearing loss

Consideration of the degree of hearing loss really becomes a question of how little pure tone hearing loss is necessary for a patient to benefit from a hearing aid, or what is the maximum hearing loss beyond which a patient can expect to receive limited benefit from a hearing aid. It should be noted that audiometric data alone are insufficient for determining hearing aid candidacy. Stabb (2000) makes a poignant observation that hearing aids are not necessarily fit on the degree of hearing loss, but on the degree of "hurt" experienced by the patient, and until this hurt is significant enough to the patient, they are not necessarily a hearing aid candidate.

In general, as the degree of hearing loss increases the expected benefit from amplification and successful use increases. Those with hearing losses of moderate or greater degree (average losses > 40 dBHL) are generally easy to discern as candidates. For these patients audibility of the long term spectrum of speech will be restricted, and lead to speech recognition difficulties in most listening situations. It is the patients with mild losses (average losses in the 25–35 dBHL range) that often are more difficult to identify as candidates. For these individuals it has been my experience that motivation, situational demands, and self-perceived disability are important factors which will need to be used in determining candidacy. These factors will be addressed later in the chapter. Many audiologists take the approach of examining the audiogram and if the patient's thresholds are < 25–35 dBHL through 4000 Hz, then patient is not likely to benefit from hearing aids. It is possible, however, with currently available signal processing to shape the response of the hearing aid to fit hearing losses restricted to 3kHz and above. In addition, with the current trend in using open ear acoustics in fitting hearing aids, it is possible have successful hearing aid users with these audiometric configurations. Dillon (2001) states that any hearing loss criteria that we set need to account for possible technology solutions that are currently available.

An alternative method to assess candidacy has been proposed by Mueller and Killion (1990). This method uses a simplified version of the Articulation Index and is called count the dot audiogram. In this method a shaded area representing the range of the long term spectrum of speech is placed on the audiogram. Within this area is a series of 100 dots. The dots are arranged with varying densities across frequencies, with greater density indicating greater frequency importance for speech recognition. An example is shown in Figure 11–4. The audiologist plots the patient's audiogram and simply counts the number of dots that are below the patients thresholds. This number is subtracted from 100, and represents the percentage of the average long term spectrum of speech audible to the patient. The authors suggest any value below 85 places the patient as a hearing aid candidate. They also suggest that motivation and communication disability need to be considered, as well. The count the dot audiogram is also an excellent counseling tool for explaining to patients the effects of hearing loss on the audibility of various parts of the speech signal.

Patients with severe and profound sensorineural hearing losses are certainly candidates for hearing aids, but may receive limited benefit from their use. Other types of sensory technologies, such as a cochlear implant or a frequency compression hearing aid, may be more appropriate. Currently, the audiological criteria for cochlear implant candidacy includes: a severe to profound bilateral sensorineural hearing loss (congenital or acquired) and aided speech recognition scores for sentence materials < 50 percent. Frequency compression technology is used to move the higher frequency components of speech, especially the voiceless fricatives, to lower frequencies where the patient has more residual hearing. This type of technology is used not only for those with severe to profound sensorineural hearing losses, but also for those with precipitous hearing losses above 500–1000 Hz.

In regard to the *type* of hearing loss, those with conductive and sensorineural hearing losses benefit from hearing aids. Generally, those with conductive hearing loss achieve greater improvement in speech recognition than those with sensorineural losses, due to the preservation of sensory structures in the cochlea.

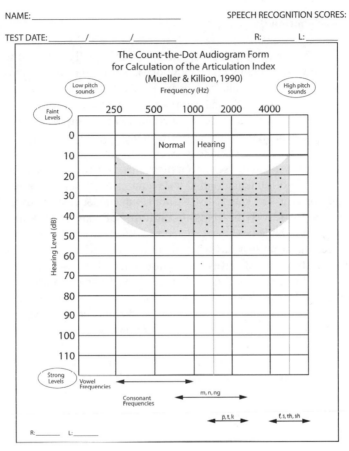

DEPARTMENT OF SPECIAL EDUCATION AND COMMUNICATION DISORDERS

NAME:_____   SPEECH RECOGNITION SCORES:

TEST DATE:_____/_____/_____   R:_____ L:_____

The Count-the-Dot Audiogram Form
for Calculation of the Articulation Index
(Mueller & Killion, 1990)

Low pitch sounds   Frequency (Hz)   High pitch sounds

Faint Levels

250   500   1000   2000   4000

Normal   Hearing

Hearing Level (dB)

Strong Levels   Vowel Frequencies

Consonant Frequencies   m, n, ng

p, t, k   f, s, th, sh

R:_____ L:_____

301 Barkley Memorial Center
P.O. Box 830738
Lincoln, NE 68583-0738
(402) 472-2145
FAX (402) 472-7697

FIGURE 11–4.

There are, however, certain conductive etiologies that contraindicate the use of conventional air conduction hearing aids such as congenital atresia, chronically draining ears, and ears that have been surgically modified. In these cases it is necessary for the audiologist to recommend an alternative form of amplification in the form of a bone conduction hearing aid or bone anchored hearing aid (BAHA). Decisions about these alternate forms of amplification should be made in consultation with the patient's physician.

On a final note, when using audiological test data for hearing aid fittings the test data should be current within the last six months, and within the last three months if there are concerns or evidence of a progressive hearing loss.

Speech Recognition

At one time the use of speech recognition scores, usually obtained with lists of monosyllabic words in quiet under earphones, was used as one of the criteria for predicting the expected benefit from hearing aids. Test scores obtained under these conditions are not predictable indicators of how well a person will perform in the types of everyday listening situations encountered by many adults. The problems associated with using monosyllabic words in hearing aid fittings have been documented by numerous researchers (e.g., Shore, Bilger & Hirsh, 1960; Walden et al., 1982). If clinicians want to use speech measures as part of the hearing aid candidacy process, use of sentential-based tests administered in a background of noise is more appropriate. The QuickSIN (Killion, Niquette, & Gudmundsen, 2004) and Hearing in Noise Test (HINT, Nilsson, Soli, & Sullivan, 1994) are examples of commercially available tests that can be used effectively to measure the difficulty a person with hearing loss has when listening to sentences in a background of noise. Both tests use an adaptive testing paradigm to determine the signal-to-noise ratio at which listeners can identify 50 percent of the speech material. A comparison of the aided and unaided performance on these measures can serve as part of the hearing aid validation process to determine the impact of intervention. It is recommended that these speech in noise measures not be used necessarily for candidacy decisions, rather they should be used to quantify the difficulty a person has in listening to speech in noise and as part of the validation process. In our center hearing aid patients are administered the QuickSIN both unaided and aided. This particular test was chosen because of ease of administration.

Loudness Discomfort Level (LDL)

The LDL is used to determine the upper level of comfort when measuring the patient's dynamic range: the range between threshold and LDL. The use of LDL in hearing aid fittings is to aid the audiologist in limiting the output of the hearing aid so that amplified signals that reach the listener's ear do not provide discomfort. Patients with sensorineural hearing losses often exhibit reduced dynamic ranges due to loudness recruitment. Those with reduced or limited dynamic ranges are more likely to be less successful hearing aid users than those with wider dynamic ranges. There is debate as to whether LDLs should be measured directly for each patient or predicted/estimated from threshold-based data obtained from listeners with varying degrees of sensorineural hearing loss. Those who argue for direct measurement cite the variability in LDL across subjects within various hearing loss categories (Kamm, Dirks, & Mickey, 1978; Valente et al., 1997). Hence, using predicted measurements could result in the hearing aid potentially delivering sound at an uncomfortable level in comparison to those with lower than predicted

LDLs. There are, however, patients who simply cannot make reliable loudness judgments in a clinical setting. Those who support using predicted LDLs based on thresholds indicate that there are large data sets like those of Pascoe (1988) which do suggest a relationship between threshold and LDL. This relationship, in turn, can be used for the majority of patients being seen for hearing aid fittings. Also, using threshold-based data reduces clinical testing time. The patients LDLs should not be used to determine candidacy for a hearing aid, rather they should be used for assessment of the potential benefit a hearing aid user can expect to get from a hearing aid, to set the output of the hearing aid during the fitting process, and ensure during the verification process that the hearing aid is not delivering uncomfortably loud sounds to the patient's ear.

Important auditory factors which contribute to determining if a patient is a hearing aid candidate includes: the type degree and configuration of the patients hearing loss, speech recognition ability, and the patient's dynamic range. While each of these factors contributes different auditory information to candidacy decisions, they interact and together to form a global auditory profile of the patien. It's important to remember that if the patient is deemed to be a hearing aid candidate, then there must be a technology available to meet their needs.

NON AUDITORY FACTORS

Key non-auditory factors in determining candidacy for a hearing aid are motivation, situational demands on hearing, and the patients' self-perceived handicap or disability associated with their hearing loss. These factors are not necessarily mutually exclusive. For example, a patient's motivation to pursue amplification may be, and often is, strongly influenced by the degree to which they perceive psycho-social difficulties related to their hearing loss.

Motivation

Perhaps the most important non-auditory factor related to hearing aid candidacy is the patient's motivation to obtain hearing aids. Dillon (2001) characterizes motivation as "the balance of all the advantages a patient expects hearing aids will provide offset by all the expected disadvantages, irrespective of whether all these positive and negative expectations are realistic" (p. 209). Hence motivation is a complex entity that is influenced by the interaction of a number of variables. As mentioned earlier, the penetration rate for hearing aids is 22 percent which suggests motivation to acquire hearing aids is low for those who could benefit from their use. Kochkin (1993) examined why so many adults in lack the motivation to use hearing aids. The top reasons included: the hearing loss was not severe enough to warrant hearing aids, aids were too expensive, stigma associated with wearing hearing aids, and the advice that they received from healthcare professionals.

Measuring motivation is difficult. In addition, there are no good standardized instruments available to measure motivation. How then do we assess a patient's motivation? Sauders (1997) suggested that motivation could be determined easily by asking two simple questions: What prompted you to come for a hearing test?; and What do you expect to gain from this visit? These or similarly phrased questions can be placed easily on a case history form for the patient to answer. The motivated patient will answer the first question by indicating that they came to get a hearing aid because they are experiencing difficulties hearing. The unmotivated patient will often report they came at the urging of friends, relatives or significant others. The second question provides information about acceptance of their hearing loss. The motivated patient will respond to this question with a statement indicating they are interested in pursing amplification. Those that are unmotivated might indicate that they are seeking a diagnosis of normal hearing; that is, a validation that there is no problem. These individuals have not yet accepted their hearing loss, and proactive measures on their part, such as trying a hearing aid, will not be considered until acceptance has taken place. It is the job of the audiologist to provide appropriate counseling to the unmotivated patient about the need for and benefits from amplification. The audiologist needs to realize, however, that there will always be those patients with negative attitudes toward amplification who will reject any form of auditory rehabilitation no matter how much counseling is provided. These individuals are not even willing to attempt a trial period with hearing aids. However, there are patients who reluctantly agree to a trial period (30–60 days) of amplification and with good counseling and frequent follow-up are able to perceive the benefits of hearing aids.

Situational Demands and Self-Perceived Disability/Handicap

I chose to combine the discussion of situational demands on hearing and self-perceived disability or handicap because of their interactive nature and the tools that we use to assess each of these are similar. Also, I use the terms disability and handicap even though the World Health Organization (WHO, 2000) has suggested the use of alternate designators to help standardize terminology world wide: activity limitation (disability) and participation restriction (handicap). The terms disability and handicap are better understood and used more frequently by various professionals.

Individuals who are more likely to pursue amplification tend to have more hearing loss and greater self-perceived disability and handicap (Fino, Bess, Lichtenstein, & Logan, 1992; Humphrey, Herbst, & Faurqi, 1981). Recent research also suggests that individuals who seek amplification have different personality profiles than the general population of adults (Cox, Alexander, & Gray, 2005). These investigators determined that those who seek amplification tend to be more pragmatic and less open to novel ways in dealing with hearing loss than the general population. In addition, there were differences in personality patterns between those seeking hearing aids at no cost through a government supported agency (Veterans Administration) and those seeking hearing aids though private practice facilities. Those seeking hearing aids through private practice facilities were more open in seeking solutions to problems, coped better with stress, and were more agreeable and trusting. These results have counseling implications for those that dispense hearing aids in different settings.

To determine the hearing-related communication difficulties patients are experiencing, the audiologist can use a well-designed case history, or a self-assessment inventory. The author prefers to use self-assessment inventories because they provide a quick and efficient way to assess the difficulties a patient is experiencing, and many of the inventories yield scores that the audiologist can use to quantify the patients degree of perceived difficulty. These inventories assess a broad range of areas including social/situational difficulties, emotional response to hearing loss, personality, and difficulties experienced in the workplace. Most inventories are constructed so that the patient records their perception on a likert scale to a series of specific questions. Table 11–2 provides a list of some of the available self-assessment inventories which are short enough to incorporate easily in a clinical setting. A more in depth review of these inventories is provided by Alpiner & Schow (2000) and Bray and Nilsson (2002).

The Hearing Handicap Inventory for Adults (HHIA; Newman et al. 1990, 1991) is completed by all adults who are seen for an audiological evaluation at our center. This particular inventory was chosen for use by our center for a number of reasons. First, it is appropriate for a large segment of the adult population (< 65 years age). Second, the psychometric properties of the HHIA are well established. Third, this instrument is easy to complete by patients and score by audiologists. Finally, the IIIIIA covers a wide range of situations experienced by many individuals who are hearing impaired.

TABLE 11–2
Examples of Short (≤25 items) Self-Assessment Inventories Used to Determine Communication Difficulties for Adults with Hearing Loss

Inventory	# Items	Age	Description
Abbreviated Profile of Hearing Aid Benefit (Cox & Alexander, 1995)	24	All adults ≥18	4 situational categories (6 questions in each); ease of communication, background noise, reverberation, and aversiveness. Individual category and global scores.
Hearing Handicap Inventory for Elderly (Ventry & Weinstein, 1983)	25	≥65	Social/situational ($n = 12$) & emotional ($n = 13$) difficulties associated with hearing loss. Overall & two subscale scores.
Hearing Handicap Inventory for Elderly-Screening (Newman et al., 1991)	10	≥65	Adapted version of HHIE. Five social/situational & emotional related questions.
Hearing Handicap Inventory for Adults (Newman et al., 1990)	25	18–64	Same as HHIE except for 3 items. Two items related to occupational effects and hearing loss & one related to time activities.
Hearing Handicap Inventory for Adults—Screening (Newman et al., 1991	10	18–64	Adapted version of HHIA. Five social/situational and emotional related questions).
Self-Assessment of Communication (Schow & Nerbonne, 1982)	10	All adults ≥18	Three sections with questions related to difficulty in various communication situations ($n = 6$), feelings about communication ($n = 2$), and reactions from others ($n = 2$)

The HHIA is a modified version of the Hearing Handicap Inventory for the Elderly (HHIE; Ventry & Weinstein, 1983; Newman and Weinstein, 1988), an inventory designed for a restricted range of adults > 65 years. Three replacement questions which focus on the occupational effects of hearing loss were placed in the HHIA. The HHIA consists of 25 questions which address social situational difficulties and emotional responses secondary to hearing loss. Patients answer questions by giving a yes, no or sometimes response. Responses in each of these categories are assigned a numerical value: yes = 4 points, sometimes = 2 points, and no = 0 points. Questions are worded such that a greater number of points indicate a greater self-perceived difficulty with, a total number of possible points being 100. Newman et al. (1990) reported an average total score of 37 for a population of sixty-seven adults with mild to moderate sensorineural hearing losses. Results from the HHIA provides the audiologist an idea of the types of situations in which the patient is experiencing difficulty, the degree of difficulty in these situations, and whether there are emotional responses attached to hearing loss. This instrument can also help in assessing patient motivation for a hearing aid. For example, if a patient with a moderate sensorineural hearing loss has an HHIA score of 10, it is unlikely that this person will be motivated to pursue amplification because they perceive a limited handicap associated with their hearing loss. Conversely, if a patient with a mild loss has a score of 50 on the HHIA, they most likely would be motivated to seek rehabilitation in the form of amplification due to their degree of self-perceived difficulty.

Medical Clearance

The FDA requires that patients who are fit with hearing aids receive medical clearance by a licensed physician, preferably an otolaryngologist, stating that the patient is a candidate for a hearing aid (FDA, Section 801.421, 1977). Patients 18 years or older may chose to waive their right to a medical evaluation. If the patient chooses to do this they need to sign a wavier form stating that do not wish to have a medical evaluation before purchasing a hearing aid. This should be kept in the patient's folder. In addition, the FDA (section 801.420) requires that hearing aid dispensers advise prospective users to seek a medical examination by a licensed physician if the prospective user presents with any of the following conditions: visible congenital or traumatic deformity of the ear, history of active drainage from the ear within the past 90 days, history of sudden or rapidly progressive hearing loss within the past 90 days, acute or chronic dizziness, unilateral hearing loss of sudden or recent onset within the past 90 days, air-bone gaps > 15 dBHL at 500, 1000, or 2000 Hz, visible evidence of significant cerumen or a foreign body in the external ear canal, or pain or discomfort in the ear. The above issues should be taken care of before the patient proceeds further in the process of procuring a hearing aid.

The decision as to whether a patient is a candidate for a hearing aid requires that the audiologist consider factors related to the patient's hearing loss in addition to the patient's motivation regarding amplification and self-perceived difficulties secondary to the hearing loss. Individuals with stronger motivation and self-perceived handicap or disability will be more likely to pursue amplification and ultimately be more successful hearing aid users. For those less motivated individuals, the use of a trial period in tandem with good counseling and guided experiences can be effective in helping the hearing aid candidate experience the benefits of amplification. The dispenser needs to realize, however, that there will be those patient's who are going to reject the notion of wearing hearing aids, even though they are clearly candidates.

SELECTION OF AMPLIFICATION

Once it has been determined that the patient is a candidate for a hearing aid, the audiologist needs to go through a systematic process of selecting the appropriate hearing aid style, earmold, and desired features. Some of the issues that the audiologist needs to consider when selecting a hearing aid for a patient are discussed below.

Style of Aid

The currently available styles of hearing aids and their advantages and disadvantages were presented earlier in the chapter. The choice of what style to choose depends on a number of factors such as degree and configuration of hearing loss, cosmetic concerns, patient's manual dexterity, visual ability, desired features, battery life, and external ear geometry. The audiologist and patient need to consider these factors, and together come up with an appropriate style choice. The final style choice may represent a compromise between the desire of the patient and recommendation of the dispensing audiologist. It should be clear, however, that the dispensing audiologist not compromise their professional opinion of what style to choose in order to make a sale. There are times when the audiologist must simply be assertive and indicate to the patient that the particular style is inappropriate. Representative models of the various style options should be available for the patient to view so they have a realistic idea of the shape, dimensions, and general appearance of the hearing aids. The patient can also have an opportunity to see how well they are able to manipulate and operate the instruments.

Monaural vs. Binaural Fitting

A recent survey of results from hearing healthcare providers who dispense hearing aids indicate that in 2004 binaural amplification was fit on approximately 75–80 percent of their patients (Kirkwood, 2005; Strom, 2005b). This is not surprising given the fact that the majority of patients who pursue hearing aids have a bilateral hearing loss. Even though the trend is to fit binaural instruments, the question remains: is this what we should be doing? In the authors opinion the answer is yes for most of the patients who have two aidable ears. The onus to discuss the advantages of binaural amplification with the patient falls on the shoulders of the audiologist. For those patients who are undecided about a monaural or binaural hearing aid arrangement, the use of a 30–60 day trial period will allow them to try both types of arrangements in a variety of listening situations. Frequent follow-up visits during this period can be effective in monitoring the patient's progress.

There are numerous advantages to listening with two ears rather than one. These advantages include: more accurate localization, better hearing in noise, loudness summation, elimination of the head shadow effect, and improved sound quality and speech intelligibility. Binaural amplification allows patients to experience many of these advantages. In addition, there are data to suggest that aiding one ear may cause a decrement in speech recognition performance in the unaided ear over time (Hurley, 1999; Silman et al., 1984; Silverman & Silman, 1990). This is referred to as auditory deprivation. Hence, fitting a patient with binaural instruments should be a consideration for the majority of hearing aid patients. There are, however, some disadvantages to consider.

A pragmatic concern with binaural amplification is that it simply costs more. Patients, especially those on fixed incomes, may not be able to afford the price of two hearing aids. There are persons, primarily elderly, who experience binaural interference, where there are interaural asymmetries when listening to dichotic speech which may result in better speech recognition when listening monaurally than binaurally (Chmiel et al., 1997; Jerger et al., 1993). It should be noted that audiometric asymmetries do not necessarily preclude individuals from experiencing the benefits from binaural listening. Some individuals feel that others may perceive that they have a greater handicap or disability if they wear two hearing aids. Appropriate counseling can be effective for these patients. Finally, some individuals may find it too difficult to manage two hearing aids, especially elderly patients.

Cost

Cost is an important consideration for many who are in the process of being fit with hearing aids. Estimates of the average cost of a hearing aid range from $1,800 to nearly $2,000 (Kirkwood, 2005; Strom, 2005b). There is considerable variability in price depending on the style of instrument and type of technology. Some high end digital hearing aids may cost $3,000–$4,000 per instrument. In any event, the purchase of hearing aids represents a major investment for many patients and there are few financial resources available for adult patients to help offset the cost of hearing aids. In reality, the patient is often left with making a decision as to what instrument will meet their communication needs at the best cost.

Directional Microphones

One of the most common complaints made by individuals with a hearing loss is that they have difficulty understanding speech in noisy environments. In addition, it is well documented that individuals with sensorineural hearing losses need more favorable signal to noise ratios (SNR) to achieve the same speech recognition performance as normal hearing listeners (Dirks et al., 1982; Killion, 1997; Suter, 1985). A recent survey of hearing aid users ranked limited benefit hearing in background noise as one of the top reasons why they no longer wore their hearing aids (Kochkin, 2000a). Directional microphones represent an effective hearing aid option to improve the SNR for those wearing hearing aids. These microphones are designed to have differential sensitivity to sound depending on the spatial origin of the sound. Directional microphones available in hearing aids can either have fixed or adaptive pattern characteristics. Many hearing aid manufacturers offer directional microphone options for a wide array of hearing aid styles; this option is not available on the smaller styles of hearing aids due to space limitations and inability to provide sufficient spatial separation between the microphone ports. Kochkin (2000b) documented improved customer satisfaction ratings with the use of digital hearing aids with directional microphones over conventional hearing instruments and digital hearing aids with single-microphone systems.

Manual Dexterity

Manual dexterity concerns impact most on the style choice of the hearing aid. Patients who have reduced fine motor skills or a diminished sense of touch will often find it difficult to manipulate the smaller style of hearing aids such as a CIC or ITC. Most likely they will also have difficulty changing batteries with these types of instruments. A larger style of hearing aid, raised volume controls, and use of remote controls (if available) are examples hearing aid options which can be selected to facilitate a patient's ability to manipulate their hearing aid.

Visual Status

Blindness or low vision affects approximately 1/28 Americans over the age of 40, and is expected to increase significantly over the next 20 years due to the aging of the U.S. population (Eye Disease Prevalence Research Group, 2004). Vision problems can create difficulties for the hearing aid user in orienting the hearing aid appropriately when inserting in the ear, cleaning the aid or earmold, changing batteries, or changing wax guards in ITE, ITC, or CIC instruments. For patients with reduced vision, consideration should be given to instruments that are large enough to see and manipulate. Allowing the patient to experiment with various styles of hearing aids before placing an order will be helpful in selecting which style of instrument is most appropriate.

FITTING PROCESS

This section will involve a discussion of the myriad of tasks associated with actually fitting the hearing aid on the patient. The discussion will include pre-fitting considerations, fitting and programming the hearing instrument, providing a hearing aid orientation for the patient, and follow-up visits. Verification and validation, although part of this process, will be dealt with separately in the following section.

Pre-Fitting Considerations

Before the patient comes in for their hearing aid fitting the audiologist should check to ensure that the proper hearing instruments have been sent from the manufacturer, and if fitting a BTE instrument make sure the correct earmolds have been received. In addition, at a minimum, the audiologist should do a listening check of the hearing aid(s) to verify an appropriate sound quality and at the same time ensure that the controls of the instrument are in proper working order. If time allows, the audiologist can complete an electroacoustic analysis of the hearing aid to verify that the instrument is functioning according to manufacturers specifications. Even though hearing instruments may go though a quality control check before being shipped from the manufacturer, there is always the possibility of damage during the shipping process. The audiologist can also fill out necessary paperwork associated with the dispensing of the hearing aid to save time at the actual fitting appointment.

Fitting and Programming the Hearing Instrument

At the time of the initial fitting of the hearing aid it is suggested that the patient bring along a significant other, relative or caregiver. The presence of these individuals at the fitting provides support for the patient, allows for an understanding of the problems the patient will experience while adjusting to the hearing aid, and if necessary, aid the patient in recalling the proper use, care and operation of the hearing aid.

The fitting should begin with ensuring the proper physical fit of the hearing aid. For ITE, ITC and CIC instruments this will entail making sure the shell of the hearing aid fits snugly into the patient's ear, and that the patient experiences no discomfort. For those fit with BTE instruments, the audiologist needs to make sure the earmold fits properly in the patient's ear. At this time the earmold tubing should be measured and cut for attachment to the earhook of the hearing aid. The use of a small amount of a lubricant on the earmold or shell of the hearing aid facilitates insertion into the ear canal for those being fit with hearing aids for the first time. First time users may want to continue this process during the initial stages of hearing aid use.

For digital and DCA hearing aids the next step in the fitting process is to program the hearing aid. Programming the hearing aid involves the use of a PC with installed software from the manufacturer and hardware devices to provide and interface between the hearing aid and the PC. NOAH, a common industry-wide integrative software system is used for storing and sending information between the hearing aid and PC. This system was developed by the Hearing Instrument Manufacturers' Software Association (HIMSA) in the early to mid 1990s. The next step in fitting analog hearing aids is to adjust the potentiometers on the instrument with a small screwdriver to set the appropriate electroacoustic parameters for the patient. Since only approximately 12 percent of the hearing aids fit are analog (Strom, 2005a), the remaining discussion will focus on the programming process.

When programming hearing instruments, specialized cables from the hearing aid manufacturer are typically attached to the hearing aid battery compartment, or on some BTE instruments to a programming port on the back of the hearing aid. The cables in turn are plugged into either a Hearing Instrument Programmer (HI-PRO) unit or a NoahLink. Both of these hardware units serve as an interface between the hearing aid and the computer. The HI-Pro unit attaches directly to the hard drive of the computer, while the NoahLink uses Bluetooth (wireless) technology to interface with the computer. Figure 11–5 shows the patient set up for both of these units. Once the above is completed, the audiologist opens the hearing aid manufacturers' software and begins the programming process. It should be noted the patient's audiometric information is linked to the software. The audiologist completes a series of prescribed programming procedures which set the operating parameters of the instrument based of the manufacturers fitting algorithm. When this is completed the programming data are stored in the hearing instrument, and can be retrieved and changed at a later date if fine tuning changes are needed. At this point the programming should be verified to ensure optimal functioning of the instrument for the patient. This process will be discussed separately in the following section.

With programming completed, the remaining time of the fitting process should focus on a hearing aid orientation. The hearing aid orientation involves discussing the parts of the hearing aid, proper use of the instrument, care and maintenance, and accommodating to the hearing aid. Sufficient time should be set aside to complete the orientation to make sure that all the necessary information is provided to the patient. Previous hearing aid users may need less time spent on a hearing aid orientation. Particular attention should be paid to insertion, removal, and

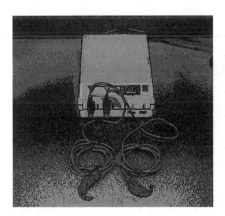
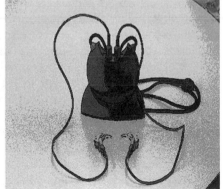

FIGURE 11–5.   Examples of units used to program analog programmable and digital hearing aids. In both units the hearing aids are connected via cables to the programming unit. The unit in the left panel is a HI-PRO (hearing instrument programmer). This unit is cabled to the hard drive of a computer to interface with the manufacturer's software. The unit on the right is a NOAH Link which operates using Bluetooth technology. During instrument programming this unit is placed around the patient's neck.

manipulation of the hearing aid controls since these are tasks that will be completed on a daily basis and need to be mastered early on in the fitting process. For some patients, especially those with cognitive challenges, it may be necessary to truncate the information provided during the orientation; the orientation should focus on use and care items which will allow the patient minimal competency in using their hearing aid. Other information can be provided at follow-up visits. There will also be patients who for physical or cognitive reasons may not be able to manage their hearing aids independently. For these individuals, the hearing aid orientation needs to be provided for someone (e.g. caregiver, relative, or spouse) who has daily contact with the patient. When completing the hearing aid orientation it is helpful for the audiologist to use a checklist of items to discuss with the patient as a way of ensuring the pertinent information is provided to the patient. Appendix A provides a copy of a checklist that is used in our hearing aid dispensary. Examples of specific hearing aid orientation programs are provided by Dillon (2001) and Mormer and Palmer (1999).

Even the most sophisticated hearing instruments are unable to provide normal hearing, or allow the listener the same degree of benefit in all listening situations. Hence, it is necessary at the hearing aid orientation for the audiologist to discuss realistic expectations with the patient. Sweetow and Valente (1998) have offered the following as a summary of realistic expectations from hearing aids: 1. aided performance in quiet and noise should be better than unaided performance under similar listening situations; 2. aided performance in noise will not be as good as aided performance in quiet; 3. soft speech should be audible, conversational speech should be comfortable, and loud speech should not be uncomfortable; 4. the earmold or shell of the hearing aid should be comfortable and allow an acceptable fit to preclude feedback; and 5. the patient's own voice should be acceptable.

The audiologist should discuss a wearing schedule and follow-up visits with the patient before they leave the fitting session. Patients should be encouraged to wear their hearing aids as often as possible throughout the course of the day. For most users it is not unrealistic to expect the patients to reach a point where putting on their hearing aid becomes part of their daily routine. Patients must also need to be aware that it will take time to get used to hearing amplified sound; this process is referred to as auditory acclimatization (Gatehouse, 1994). Acclimatization is thought to come about from the establishment of new neural pathways, a rewiring process, in the central auditory system from listening to amplified speech. Those that wear their hearing aids on a consistent basis will likely get through this process quicker. Gatehouse (1992) reported that this process is not immediate and may take a time course of at least 6–12 weeks. Hence, a trial period of amplification should be set at 45–60 days in lieu of the more typical 30 day period. For some patients who are having difficulties adjusting to their hearing aids the trial period may need to be extended to as long as 90 days. Extending the trial period to this length will not affect the dispenser's ability to return the hearing aids for credit if the patient decides not to continue with amplification because most manufacturers allow the hearing aid dispensary to return hearing aids for 100 percent credit up to 90 days post-invoice. Keeping a daily journal of hearing aid use and experiences in various listening situations is an excellent recommendation to the patient. This information will help the audiologist at follow-up visits determine problems the patient is experiencing and to see how the acclimatization process is progressing as well as helping the patient remember issues that they want to discuss with the audiologist.

It is a good idea to have patients return one-week post fitting for a follow-up visit, if possible. This allows the audiologist to address concerns that the patient may have about the hearing aids early on. Based on the patient's concerns, programming changes may need to be made. Also, it may be necessary to make earmold or shell modifications if the patient is experiencing discomfort. Often it is necessary at this visit to reinstruct the patient about use and care of the instrument. Further follow-up visits during the trial period should be established based on the difficulties the patient is experiencing. Some patients who are having difficulties adjusting to amplification may require weekly visits while others may only need to have one or two follow-up visits during the trial period.

VERIFICATION AND VALIDATION OF THE HEARING AID FITTING

Verification and validation are terms that are often used interchangeably, yet they have different meanings. The *verification* process is used for the physical assessment of the electroacoustic characteristics of the hearing aid and often involves determining if the proper gain and frequency response characteristics meet a set of expected target values. Also involved is determining if the physical fit of the hearing aid is appropriate for the patient. The *validation* process is used to measure the impact of intervention and involves the use of outcome measures which are often in the form of self-assessment inventories or speech recognition tests. In essence you are measuring the effectiveness of the hearing aid fitting. The ASHA Guidelines for Hearing Aid Fitting for Adults (ASHA, 1998) strongly recommends that both verification and validation procedures need to be part of the hearing aid fitting process. In addition, other authors have suggested that complete documentation of outcome from hearing aid fittings include electroacoustic verification, real-ear measurements, speech-recognition(quiet and noise), and measures of hearing aid benefit (Humes, 1999; Bray & Nilsson, 2002). The following section will provide information about clinical techniques that can be implemented to verify and validate hearing aid fittings.

VERIFICATION

There are several measurement techniques that can be used for the physical assessment of the electroacoustic characteristics of the hearing aid. These include measurements completed in a 2 cm^3 coupler, real ear probe-microphone measures (REPMs), and measurements made in a controlled sound field. The advantages and limitations of each of these techniques will be addressed. An important consideration when completing any of the above verification measurements is the spectral characteristics of the input signal at the hearing aid microphone. This is particularly important when verifying the electroacoustic characteristics of non-linear hearing aids.

As part of the verification process a variety of formal prescriptive methods are often used to set aided targets to determine if the frequency/gain and maximum output characteristics are set appropriately for the patients hearing loss. Prescriptive methods have been developed for both linear and non-linear hearing instruments. The methods for linear hearing instruments typically use pure tone audiometric thresholds as the basis to establish aided target gain values. Maximum output levels are established either by using individual loudness discomfort measures or predicted/estimated values from various data sets. Most prescriptive methods allow for frequency/gain targets and maximum output to be expressed as 2 cm^3 coupler or real-ear values. Several of the more popular linear-based prescriptive procedures include Prescription of Gain and Output (POGO; McCandless & Lyregaard, 1983; Schwartz, Lyregarrd & Lundh, 1988), Desired Sensation Level-linear (DSL[i/o]; Cornelisse, Seewald & Jamieson, 1995), National Acoustics Lab-Revised (NAL-RP; Byrne & Dillon, 1986; Byrne, Parkinson & Newall, 1990). Software is available for calculating targets for virtually all the linear and non-linear based prescriptive methods. It should be noted that the above procedures will likely establish a different set of target aided values for individuals with similar audiograms. The onus for deciding which fitting method to use most often depends on the audiologist's preference which is often based on clinical experience. Dillon (1999) states that "one can never say that a procedure is correct, just that it is better on some criterion than something else" (p. 12).

With the advent of DCA hearing aids in the 1980s and ultimately the fitting of more non-linear instruments, it became necessary to develop prescriptive methods which could be used to accommodate the more complex electroacoustic features of these types of hearing instruments. In these non-linear procedures gain at various frequencies is specified for various input levels; often for soft, conversational and loud inputs. Some procedures also suggest compression ratios and kneepoints. A number of non-linear based prescriptive procedures have been developed and include Fig. 11–6 (Killion, 1993), NAL-NL–1 (Byrne, Dillon, Ching, Katsch & Keidser, 2001), DSL[i/o] non-linear (Cornelisse, Seewald, & Jamieson, 1995), and Visual Input Output Loudness Algorithm (VIOLA; Valente & Van Vliet, 1997). The goal of the DSL[i/o], Fig. 11–6, and VIOLA procedures is to restore normal loudness perception; that is, they attempt to allow the listener with a hearing loss the same loudness perception that would be experienced by an individual with normal hearing listening to the same sound. DSL[i/o] and VIOLA require individual loudness measurements to be completed for calibrated auditory signals at various intensity levels. Figure 11–6 uses aggregate data from individuals with similar hearing losses, and hence only pure-tone thresholds are necessary. NAL-NL1 takes a different approach and attempts to maximize speech intelligibility and keep the overall loudness for any input level of speech similar to that experienced by an individual with normal hearing listening to the same sound (Dillon, 1999). As

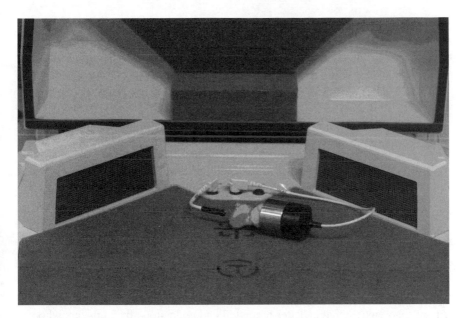

FIGURE 11–6.   An example of an ITE hearing aid attached to a 2 cm^3 coupler in an open test chamber. These types of measurements are designed to ensure quality control and to troubleshoot problems with the hearing aid.

with linear-based procedures, the decision as to which prescriptive method to use depends largely on the audiologist and their fitting philosophy. In consonance with the linear-based prescriptive methods, use of different methods will generate different prescriptive values for individuals with similar hearing losses.

At this time many of the hearing aid manufacturers use proprietary fitting algorithms specific to their line of hearing instruments. These algorithms are developed by the manufacturer to be used in conjunction with their circuitry. The audiologist needs to be knowledgeable and at the same time feel comfortable about the manufacturers fitting philosophy. The audiologist should also have a way to verify the hearing aid fitting if these proprietary procedures are used. Some manufacturers, in their fitting software, allow the audiologist to program the hearing instrument based on some of the non-proprietary non-linear based procedures mentioned above.

2 cm^3 Coupler Measurements

Coupler measurements are made in well-controlled acoustic environments. The hearing aid under test is attached to a standard device, a 2 cm^3 coupler, with a measuring microphone monitoring the output of the hearing aid in the coupler. Tests completed in this manner eliminate the patient from being present during testing. Figure 11–6 shows an ITE hearing aid attached to a 2 cm^3 coupler. While coupler measurements are highly reliable, the conditions under which the testing is completed bear little resemblance to the real world. It should be noted that the 2 cm^3 does not adequately account for the external ear characteristics, impedance of the middle ear, and head and body effects. Coupler measurements are used most effectively for quality control to determine if the hearing aid under test meets the specifications set forth by the manufacturer. The reader is referred to the following standards for a description of how to complete various electroacoustic measurements in a coupler: ANSI S3.22 (1996), Specification of hearing aid characteristics, and ANSI S3.42 (1992), Testing hearing aids with broad-band noise signal. The ANSI S3.22 (1996) standard was revised in 2003, however, it has yet to be officially adopted by the Food and Drug administration as the new labeling document for hearing aids (Frye, 2005).

With the majority of hearing aids utilizing non-linear processing, the type of acoustic signal that is used during the verification process in a coupler is important. For verifying non-linear hearing aid systems it would seem preferable to use a complex speech-like signal (also referred to as composite signals) rather than a pure-tone so that the results can be generalized to how the hearing aid will perform under real-life conditions. Pure tone signals do not represent the types of complex signals that hearing aids are expected to process, but the analysis from using a pure-tone input signal is better predicted and understood by engineers who design hearing instruments (Frye, 2005). Most hearing aid analyzers capable of completing coupler measurements allow for the option of using pure-tone or complex signals. However, the acoustic tests proffered in the ANSI S3.22 (1996) and 2003 standards are completed with the use of pure-tone signals. Therefore, coupler measurements are not well suited for determining how a hearing aid is likely to perform under typical real-life conditions. REPMs are better used for this purpose. There are, however, situations where REPMs cannot be completed. In this case, target levels can be verified in the coupler. Most testing equipment allows for setting target prescriptive levels based on 2 cm^3 coupler measurements. When doing this it is helpful to have measured the real-ear to coupler difference (RECD) for the patient. The RECD is the decibel difference across frequency between the output of the hearing aid in a 2 cm^3 and the real ear.

Real Ear Probe-Microphone Measurements

REPMs have become the standard and preferred method for verifying hearing aid fittings. They can be used clinically to measure the gain or output of the hearing instrument in the patient's ear. These measurements take into account the individual and unique characteristics of the patient's external ear as well as account for acoustic changes imposed by the head and torso, unlike 2 cm^3 measurements. REPMs are completed by inserting a small internal diameter silicone tube into the patient's ear, preferably within 5 mm of the tympanic membrane. This tube is attached to a measuring microphone which monitors the SPL in the patient's ear canal. A reference or control microphone, often placed either at the top of the pinna or under the earlobe, is used to calibrate the sound field and ensure the proper amplitude of the test signal. The test signal is delivered via a loudspeaker placed at a specific azimuth to the ear under test. A variety of test signals are available which range from simple pure-tones to more complex broadband signals which may be spectrally-weighted (often to approximate the long-term spectrum of speech). In addition, some test equipment allows the audiologist to choose recorded speech samples from male, female and child speakers. For verifying the fit of non-linear instruments clinicians should the more complex broadband signals at several input levels. The audiologist should be cognizant of the interaction between the spectral characteristics of the test signal and the instrument under test. The reader is referred to Kuk and Ludvigsen (2003) for a discussion of the issues surrounding the choice of stimuli to use when verifying hearing aid fittings.

There are a number of real-ear measures that can be completed and an accompanying plethora of terms and acronyms which have evolved for these measures. ANSI S3.46 (1997), *Methods of Measurement of Real-Ear Performance Characteristics of Hearing Aids*, provides a detailed description of the measures and terminology associated with REPMs. Ultimately, the audiologist chooses which tests to complete. This decision should be based on what particular fitting procedure (prescriptive method) you are using and the needs of the patient. Regardless of what tests the audiologist completes there are some preliminary steps that should be completed. These steps include: 1. an otoscopic examination; 2. calibration of the probe and control/reference microphones (re: manufacturers guidelines); 3. measurement of insertion depth for probe tube; 4. placement of patient in the proper position and adjustment of loudspeaker to appropriate azimuth; 5. setting the appropriate output limiting level for the eqipment; 6. choosing the desired prescriptive procedure and enter the patient's audiogram to set target values; and 7. instruct the patient. To ensure valid measures, especially for high frequencies, the probe tube should be inserted at least within 5–10mm of the patient's tympanic membrane (Hawkins & Mueller, 1986; Dirks & Kincaid, 1987). To achieve this for adults Hawkins, Alvarez, and Houlihan (1991) suggest a constant insertion depth of 27 mm past the intertragal notch. Applying small amount of lubricant on the probe will allow it to slide easier into the ear and help keep the probe in place. Care should also be taken to make sure that the probe is at least 5 mm beyond the medial tip of the hearing aid or earmold for BTE instruments to avoid the acoustic turbulence at the point where the sound enters the external ear canal from the hearing instrument (Burkhard & Sachs, 1977). Once the above steps have been completed the chosen REPMs can be completed.

The audiologist can choose to measure the more traditional real ear insertion gain (REIG) or measure the output SPL in the patient's ear or real ear aided response (REAR). The REIG is a relative measure and is the difference across frequencies between the natural gain provided by the external ear without the hearing aid in place (i.e. real-ear unaided gain; REUG) and the gain provided with the hearing aid in the ear and turned on (i.e. real-ear aided gain; REAG). Since the ear responds to output, rather than gain, it is preferable to quantify real-ear measurements in output in the ear canal at the tympanic membrane rather than in gain. As mentioned above, this can be done via the REAR. Measuring output also allows the audiologist to determine audibility of the speech spectrum in different frequency regions. The audiologist can also complete REAR measurements at various input levels to determine audibility for soft, conversational, and loud speech input levels. To measure the REAR (assuming the preliminary steps are completed) the audiologist places the hearing aid in the patients ear, turns the hearing aid on and adjusts the aid to the desired settings, selects the input level, and completes the test. The patient is passive during this procedure, and instructed to keep their head stationary during measurement. It is sometimes helpful to give the patient a point in the room or a picture to focus on during testing. The output levels measured in the patient's ear canal can be compared to the target prescriptive values displayed on the screen of the instrument. At a minimum the REAR levels need to be above the patient's unaided thresholds for sound to be audible. REARs measured with loud input levels of 85–90 dBSPL can be used to ensure that the hearing aid is not delivering sound that is uncomfortable to the patient. If targets values are not met then the audiologist can reprogram the hearing instrument and repeat testing. With digital hearing instruments it is possible to reach target values within + 5dB for many patients.

There are a number of other real-ear measures that can be completed; however, discussion of these measures is beyond the scope of this chapter. See Revit (2002) for a complete discussion of real-ear measures. It is also helpful to keep in mind that REPMs are only one component of the verification process. Subjective information about the sound quality and intelligibility of the hearing instrument need to be considered, as well. REPMs can be thought of as an initial step in the verification process.

Functional Gain

Before the commercial availability of REPM equipment in the early 1980s, functional gain measures were used extensively for verifying hearing aid fittings. The term functional gain was coined by Pascoe in 1975. It is defined as "the difference between unaided and aided sound-field thresholds in a specific frequency region" (Skinner, 1988; p. 141). Functional gain and REIG are the same when verifying linear hearing instruments; however, they may not be the same for non-linear instruments (Dillon & Murray, 1987; Mason & Poplka, 1986). Unlike REPMs, functional gain is a psychoacoustic task and requires a subjective response from the patient. To accurately measure functional gain it is necessary that the patient is able to provide valid and reliable responses, the examiner must use frequency-specific stimuli, the patient's head must stay in the same position during measurement, and participation of the non-test ear needs to be avoided by utilizing masking.

There are a number of disadvantages associated with measuring functional gain versus REIG. First, functional gain is time consuming, especially if you are verifying a binaural fitting. Second, only gain information is obtained at a single input level, the patient's threshold. This provides an inaccurate picture for non-linear instruments where gain varies as a function of input level. Functional gain can provide an estimate of gain for soft-level inputs. Third, the noise level in the sound room and internal noise level of the hearing aid may have a masking effect on the aided sound field threshold for those individuals who have regions of normal or near-normal hearing. This leads to an underestimation of functional gain. Fourth, for those with severe-to-profound hearing losses measurement of unaided sound field thresholds may be beyond the limits of the sound-field system. Fifth, functional gain measurements do not allow the audiologist to examine how the hearing aid functions when complex signals are used. Finally, investigators have highlighted the variability associated with functional gain measures, and have suggested that differences on the order of 10–15 dB are necessary to ensure true differences between test conditions (Hawkins, Montgomery, Prosek, and Walden, 1987; Humes & Kirn, 1990). Recently, Kuk et al. (2004) reported that the reliability of aided sound field thresholds obtained with for non-linear hearing instruments can be improved by using a modified ascending threshold procedure in lieu of the typical bracketing technique.

When available, REPMs are the preferred method to verify hearing aid fittings. There are some situations when functional gain may be the better choice. Stelmachowicz and Lewis (1988) argue that for those with severe-to-profound hearing losses REIG may indicate that the hearing aid is providing significant gain; however, the actual output of the hearing aid in the patient's ear may be below their threshold. In addition, since functional gain measures are a psychoacoustic task, formulation of a response by the patient requires involvement of the central auditory system and gives the audiologist an indication of how the patient perceives and uses sound. Still, all things considered, for the majority of patients REPMs will be the preferred choice for verifying hearing aid fittings, especially in the case of non-linear hearing aids.

Physical Fit of the Hearing Aid

As part of the verification process the audiologist needs to ensure that the hearing aid fits properly in the patient's ear and that the hearing aid is comfortable. Proper fit is verified via visual inspection. The hearing aid or earmold should fit snugly in the patient's ear, and there should be no sign of feedback. It should also be cosmetically appealing to the patient. Comfort of fit is addressed by patient report after they have been allowed to wear the hearing aid for several days. Appropriate modifications should be made as necessary. In some cases, even after modifications have been completed, hearing aid shell or earmold remakes need to be done.

VALIDATION

Validation of hearing aid fittings involves determining the impact of the hearing aid fitting via outcome measures. The outcome measures often used in validation generally fall into two categories: subjective measures which incorporate the use of self-assessment inventories and measures of speech recognition. The self-assessment inventories are designed to examine the benefit, performance and satisfaction perceived by the patient as a result of using the hearing aid. Hearing aid use is also an important variable to assess. Speech recognition measures are used to determine the extent to which the hearing aids facilitate understanding of speech in everyday life. A discussion of the various outcome measures and their use in the validation process follows.

Self-Assessment Measures

Self-assessment measures are used primarily to determine the extent to which hearing disability and handicap are reduced from wearing hearing aids. These measures give an indication of the benefit patients perceive from amplification. Benefit is related to the performance of hearing aid and reflects the degree to which the patients behavior and reaction to various situations has changed. Satisfaction, on the other hand, is affected by benefit but also includes things not related to the hearing aid such as the value of the hearing aid, dependability of the instrument, the competence of the person fitting the hearing aid, and residual communication competency. The following is an examination of measuring benefit and satisfaction as it related to hearing aid fittings.

Benefit

Researchers and clinicians have developed a number of self-assessment instruments designed to measure hearing aid benefit. Examples of shorter instruments which lend themselves to clinical use include the Abbreviated Profile of Hearing Aid Benefit (APHAB; Cox and Alexander, 1995), the Client-Oriented Scale of Improvement (COSI; Dillon, James, & Ginis, 1997), the Glasgow Hearing Aid Benefit Profile(GHABP; Gatehouse & Glasgow, 1999), and the HHIE (> 65 years) or HHIA (< 65 years).

A common feature shared by the APHAB, HHIE and HHIA is that the questions in the instruments are answered by the patient under two conditions: unaided and aided. A difference score between the unaided and aided conditions reflects the benefit that the patient perceives from wearing the hearing aid. From a clinical standpoint it is best and most efficient to have the patient complete the unaided administration at the time of the hearing aid consultation when the ear impressions are taken, or at the time of the hearing aid fitting. At these times the patient still has a good recollection of the difficulties they were experiencing before wearing the hearing aid. Sufficient wearing time of the hearing instrument in a variety of listening situations should be allowed before the aided administration is completed, at least 4–6 weeks.

The benefit measure we have chosen to use in our dispensary is the APHAB. The APHAB incorporates 24 items, which are grouped into 4 categories or subscales: Background Noise (BN), Reverberation (RV), Ease of Communication (EC), and Aversiveness of Sounds (AV). Each category has six items. The items in the APHAB are in the form of a statement, and the patient provides a response from seven alternatives ranging from always to never. Each alternative has an associated percentage value to aid the patient in interpreting each response alternative. The percentage value represents how often the particular statement is true. An example statement is "When I am in a crowded grocery store, talking with the cashier, I can follow the conversation." If a particular item is not relevant to the patient, they are instructed to either think of a similar situation they have experienced and answer accordingly for that situation, or simply leave that item blank. The APHAB can be completed using a paper-and-pencil format, or via the use of a software program developed by Cox (2000). The software program displays individual items on the computer screen and allows the patient to enter their responses by the use of a keyboard response or a mouse click. Elderly patients may have some difficulty with this approach if they lack computer literacy skills. A paper-and-pencil format is recommended for these individuals. Use of the software program for test administration is preferred, if possible, because the test data are analyzed by the program and benefit profiles can be displayed for viewing by the patient and audiologist on the computer screen.

Benefit scores for the APHAB are calculated by examining the difference between the responses for the unaided and aided conditions. It is also possible to use difference scores to compare differences between hearing aid fittings. Scores are calculated for each subscale, with particular attention paid to the EC, BN, and RV subscales. Benefit is indicated by the patient perceiving they experience fewer problems when wearing the hearing aid (aided condition) as compared to problems experienced prior to amplification (unaided condition). Cox (1997) has provided a set of rules to determine if a particular difference score is significant. Significant benefit at $p < 0.1$ is indicated as follows: 1. if the benefit score on the EC, BN, or RV is > 22 points; or 2. if the EC, BN, and RV are all > 5 points. For significance at $p < .02$ a benefit score of > 10 points is required on the three subscales EC, BN, or RV. The above critical difference scores were based on experienced hearing aid users fit with linear hearing aids. A recent study by Burns (2004) indicated that individuals fit with digital amplification scored similarly on the APHAB to those fit with linear instruments, and that similar critical difference scores were appropriate for users of both types of amplification. The AV scale is used more to determine if the patient experiences tolerance problems when listening to a variety of loud environmental sounds (e.g., construction work, screeching tires). An increase in problems on the AV scale (i.e., a negative benefit score) suggests that the output of the hearing instrument may need to be adjusted to better match the patient's dynamic range.

Satisfaction

There has been less emphasis on the measurement of satisfaction and thus there are fewer instruments that are available to measure satisfaction. This certainly does not diminish its importance as a validation measure in the hearing aid fitting process. Cox and Alexander (1999, 2001) have developed the Satisfaction with Amplification in Daily Life (SADL) Scale which allows clinicians the opportunity to measure hearing aid satisfaction with a short inventory, and can be easily adapted into the validation protocol for most hearing aid dispensaries. The SADL is comprised of fifteen questions which encompass four domains associated with hearing aid satisfaction: positive effect, service and cost, negative features, and personal image. There are seven responses alternatives available for each question which range from not at all to tremendously. As with the APHAB, the SADL can be administered with a paper-and-pencil or computer format. The SADL and scoring software can be obtained from Robyn Cox's Web site at www.ausp. memphis.edu/harl. Normative data (mean, SD, 20th and 80th percentile values) and 90 percent and 95 percent critical difference values are available for global scores and scores for each of the domain subscales. In our hearing aid dispensary we have incorporated the SADL as part of our verification protocol. The SADL is mailed to patients, along with a self-addressed stamped envelope, six months after their hearing aid fitting. There are limited data which have addressed when satisfaction stabilizes, however, in our clinical experience we have observed that satisfaction appears to be stable at least after wearing the hearing aid for 5–6 months. Data obtained from the SADL have been beneficial in making changes in some of our administration policies (e.g., pricing), and making follow-up contacts with patients who have experienced low satisfaction with their hearing aids.

Speech Recognition Measures

If the goal in fitting hearing aids is to ensure audibility for as wide a range of the speech spectrum as possible, then it seems appropriate that we incorporate some form of speech measures in our validation protocol. Measures of speech recognition can be used to measure not only hearing aid benefit (aided vs. unaided), but can also be used for patient counseling, hearing aid troubleshooting, and comparison of various hearing instruments and settings.

The speech measures chosen should incorporate the use of at least sentential-level materials and be able to evaluate the patient's ability to understand speech both in quiet and in noise, unaided and aided. Two commercially available speech recognition tests that meet these criteria are the HINT and QuickSIN. Both of these tests were discussed previously (see section on candidacy). Of the two measures, the QuickSIN is the most time efficient to administer, and the measure we have chosen to use as part of a validation protocol. The QuickSIN (on CD with an accompanying manual) can be purchased from Etymotic Research (URL: www.etymotic.com). The manual provides suggested sound field speaker arrangements, calibration procedures, and background information on the test. Also included are critical difference scores for the 80th and 95th confidence levels which can be used when comparing aided vs. unaided performance, and different hearing instruments and settings. Regardless of what speech measure is used, Bray and Nilsson (2001) state that the patients aided performance, both in quiet and noise, should show improvement over unaided performance. If this goal is not met, then changes need to be made either to the hearing aid settings, or in some cases consideration of a different hearing instrument that will achieve this goal and result in an acceptable hearing aid fitting.

FOLLOW-UP PROCEDURES

This section will focus on what happens with patient follow-up once the trial period is completed and the patient has purchased the hearing aid. In order to ensure continued satisfaction and use of amplification, a systematic follow-up program should be part of a comprehensive hearing aid fitting protocol. It is suggested that some sort of time-point procedures be implemented after the aid is purchased in order to monitor how the patient is progressing with their hearing aids. Industry figures indicate that 16.2 percent of hearing aid users report that they don't wear their hearing aids (Kochkin, 2000a); the aids are commonly referred to as "in-the drawer." The reasons given for non-use include poor benefit, background noise, fit and comfort, negative side effects, hearing aids broken or no longer working, and volume control adjustments. It seems reasonable that a number of these problems could be addressed and the number of potential in-the-drawer hearing aids reduced by seeing patients for follow-up at scheduled intervals. At six-months post-fitting, using the SADL can help identify those individuals who are experiencing low satisfaction with their instruments. These individuals are likely to discontinue hearing aid use. At one-year post-fitting, a follow-up visit to the dispensary is appropriate. This visit can be used to check hearing aid use, re-evaluate hearing to determine if there have been any progression in hearing which may require re-programming of the hearing aid, and evaluate the hearing aid to determine if it is functioning according to manufacturers specifications. Also, if the hearing aid warranty is to expire, this visit provides an opportunity to discuss options for extending the warranty along with loss and damage coverage. Most manufacturers provide a basic one-year warranty on most of their instruments, however, at the time of purchase there is an option to provide extended coverage. If this is the case, another follow-up visit can be scheduled before the warranty expires.

CONCLUDING REMARKS

The selection and fitting of hearing aids represents a dynamic process with the primary goal to provide audibility for as much of the speech spectrum as possible and, at the same time, ensure that sound is not uncomfortable. In order to achieve this goal the dispenser needs to be able to provide up to date hearing aid technology options to match the patient needs. In addition, the dispenser needs to use EBP to provide optimal clinical services; this requires the dispenser be a life-long learner and consumer of current research in the area of hearing aids and related fields.

This chapter has proffered a clinical framework for the process involved in fitting and selecting hearing aids on adults. This process begins by making the decision as to who is a candidate for a hearing aid, taking into account both auditory and non-auditory factors. Once candidacy is established, the dispenser needs to select, in consort with the patient, the appropriate hearing aid technology, style of aid and addition of any special features. Fitting the hearing aid follows. The fitting process involves ensuring the hearing aid fits comfortably, providing a comprehensive hearing aid orientation, and verifying the fit with REPMs. Validation measures may also be completed at this time. Finally, a comprehensive follow-up program needs to be established to monitor the patient's progress with amplification and make changes to the hearing aid, as needed. The reader needs to keep in mind that is no general consensus among dispensing audiologists as to who is a hearing aid candidate, and how the hearing aids should be selected, fit, verified, and validated. As mentioned previously, national organizations such as ASHA (1998) have provided general guidelines for hearing aid fittings for adults based on current research; however, these are merely suggested practice patterns which dispensers can opt to follow, or not.

Throughout the chapter the focus has been on the process of selecting and fitting hearing aids along with setting up a follow-up plan to monitor the patient's progress. For most adults, hearing aids will provide sufficient benefit in most situations. There will be those, however, who continue to experience difficulty in specific situations such as listening on the telephone, waking up to conventional alarm clocks, or hearing better in noise. For these individuals the dispensing audiologist need to consider the use of assistive listening devices whether they be stand-alone devices, or those that dovetail in some manner to the hearing aid. Use of these devices along with the hearing aids will afford the patient better access to a variety of important auditory signals across a wide range of listening situations. There are also some patients who will be candidates for aural rehabilitation programs. These programs, whether group or individual, may include intervention strategies aimed at enhancing conversational fluency through techniques which focus on strengthening the patient's ability to maximize the use of auditory and visual cues. In addition, the aural rehabilitation programs are often more effective when spouses and other family members are included in the intervention process. Patients might also be encouraged to join self-help groups for those with hearing loss such as Self-Help for Hard of Hearing (SHHH). SHHH is a nationally based organization with chapters at the state and local levels throughout the country.

It's difficult to accurately predict the future of hearing aids. As we acquire new information about how the impaired auditory system functions, new technologies can be incorporated in hearing aids to better address the auditory needs of those with hearing loss. Sometime in the future there may medical or surgical treatments designed to reverse the damage caused to auditory system by sensorineural hearing loss, until then hearing aids remain the best available sensory technology for the majority of adults who experience hearing loss.

REFERENCES

Alpiner, J., & Schow, R. (2000). Rehabilitative evaluation of hearing-impaired adults. In J. Alpiner & P. McCarthy (Eds.). *Rehabilitative audiology: Children and adults* (pp. 305–331). Baltimore: Lippincott Williams & Wilkins.

American National Standards Institute. (1992). *Testing hearing aids with a broad-band signal (ANSI S3.42–1992)*. New York: Author.

American National Standards Institute. (1996). *Specification of hearing aid characteristics (ANSI S3.22–1996)*. New York: American National Standards Institute.

American National Standards Institute. (1997). *Methods of measurement of real-ear performance characteristics of hearing aids (ANSI S3.46–1997)*. New York: American National Standards Institute.

American Speech-Language-Hearing Association. (1998). Guidelines for hearing aid fitting in adults. *American Journal of Audiology, 7*(1), 5–13.

American Speech-Language-Hearing Association. (2005). *Evidence-based practice in communication dsorders (Position Statement)*. Available at http://www.asha.org/members/deskref-journals/deskref/default.

Bray, V., & Nilsson, M. (2002). Assessing hearing aid fittings: An outcomes measures battery approach. In M. Valente (Ed.), *Strategies for selecting and verfying hearing aid fittings (2nd ed)*, (pp. 151–175). New York: Thieme.

Byrne, D., & Dillon, H. (1986). The National Acoustic Laboratories' (NAL) new procedure for selecting gain and frequency response of a hearing aid. *Ear and Hearing, 7*(4), 257–265.

Burkhard, M., & Sachs, R. (1977). Sound pressure in insert earphone couplers and real ears. *Journal of Speech and Hearing Research, 20*, 799–807.

Burns, N. (2004). *APHAB performance for individuals fit with digital amplification*. Unpublished master's thesis, University of Nebraska-Lincoln, Lincoln, NE.

Byrne, D., Parkinson, A., & Newall, P. (1990). Hearing aid gain and frequency response requirements for the severely/profoundly hearing impaired. *Ear and Hearing, 11*(1), 40–49.

Byrne, D., Ching, T., Katsch, R., & Keidser, G. (2001). NAL-NL1 procedure for fitting nonlinear hearing aids: characteristics and comparisons with other procedures. *Journal of the American Academy of Audiology, 12*, 37–51.

Chmiel, R., Murphy, E., Pirozzolo, F., & Tooley, Y. (1997). Unsuccessful use of binaural amplification by an elderly person. *Journal of the American Academy of Audiology, 8*(1), 1–10.

Cornelisse, L., Seewald, R., & Jamieson. (1995). The input/output formula: A theoretical approach to fitting of personal amplification devices. *Journal of the Acoustical Society of America, 97*(3), 1854–1864.

Cornelisse, L., & Seewald, R. (1997). Field-to-microphone transfer functions for completely-in-the-ear (CIC) instruments. *Ear and Hearing, 18*, 342–345.

Cox, R. (1997). Administration and application of the APHAB. *The Hearing Journal, 50*(4), 32–48.

Cox, R., & Alexander, G. (1999). Measuring satisfaction with amplification in daily life: The SADL scale. *Ear and Hearing, 20*, 306–320.

Cox, R., & Alexander, G. (2001). Validation of the SADL questionnaire. *Ear and Hearing, 22*, 151–160.

Cox, R., Alexander, G., & Gray, G. (2005). Who wants a hearing aid? Personality profiles of hearing aid seekers. *Ear and Hearing, 26*(1), 12–26.

Dillon, H., & Murray, N. (1987). Accuracy of twelve methods of estimating real ear gain of hearing aids. *Ear and Hearing, 8*(1), 2–11.

Dillon, H., James, A., & Ginis, J. (1997). Client oriented scale of improvement (COSI) and its relationship to several other measures of benefit and satisfaction provided by hearing aids. *Journal of the American Academy of Audiology, 8*(1), 27–43.

Dillon, H. (1999). NAL-NL1; A new procedure for fitting non-linear hearing aids. *The Hearing Journal, 52*(4), 10, 12, 14, 16.

Dillon, H. (2001). *Hearing Aids*. New York: Thieme

Dirks, D., Morgan, D., & Dubno, J. (1982). A procedure for quantifying the effects of noise on speech recognition. *Journal of Speech and Hearing Disorders, 47*, 114–123.

Dirks, D., & Kincaid, G. (1987). Basic acoustic considerations of ear canal probe measurements. *Ear & Hearing, 8* (supplement 5), 60S–67S.

Eye Disease Prevalence Research Group. (2004). Causes and prevalence of visual impairments among adults in the United States. *Archives of Ophthalmology, 122,* 477–485.

Fino, M., Bess, F., Lichtenstein, M., & Logan, S. (1992). Factors differentiating elderly hearing aid wearers vs. non-wearers. *Hearing Instruments, 43*(2), 6–10.

Frye, G. (2005). Understanding the ANSI standard as a tool for assessing hearing instrument functionality. *The Hearing Review, 12*(5), 22–27, 79.

Gatehouse, S. (1992). The time course and magnitude of perceptual acclimatization to frequency response: Evidence from monaural fitting of hearing aids. *Journal of the Acoustical Society of America, 92*(3), 1258–1268.

Gatehouse, S. (1994). Components and determinants of hearing aid benefit. *Ear and Hearing, 15*(1), 30–49.

Hawkins, D., & Mueller, G. (1986). Some variables affecting the accuracy of probe tube microphone measures of hearing aid gain. *Hearing Instruments, 37*(1), 8–12, 49.

Hawkins, D., Montgomery, A., Prosek, R., & Walden, B. (1987). Examination of two issues concerning functional gain measurements. *Journal of Speech and Hearing Disorders, 52,* 52–63.

Hawkins, D., Alvarez, E., & Houlihan, J. (1991). Reliability of three types of probe-tube microphone measurements. *Hearing Instruments, 42,* 14–16.

Humes, L., & Kirn, E. (1990). The reliability of functional gain. *Journal of Speech and Hearing Disorders, 55,* 193–197.

Humes, L. (1999). Dimensions of hearing aid outcome. *Journal of the American Academy of Audiology, 10,* 26–39.

Humphery, C., Herbst, K., & Faurqi, S. (1981). Some characteristics of the hearing-impaired elderly who do not present themselves for rehabilitation. *British Journal of Audiology, 15,* 25–30.

Hurley, R. (1999). Onset of auditory deprivation. *Journal of the American Academy of Audiology, 10*(10), 529–534.

Jerger, J., Silman, S., Lew, H., & Chmiel, R. (1993). Cases in binaural interference: Converging evidence from behavioral and electrophysiologic measures. *Journal of the American Academy of Audiology, 4*(2), 122–131.

Kamm, C., Dirks, D., & Mickey, M. (1978). Effect of sensorineural hearing loss on loudness discomfort level and most comfortable loudness judgments. *Journal of Speech and Hearing Research, 21,* 668–681.

Kent, D., & Boney, S. (1997). *Field-to-microphone transfer function for ITE and ITC hearing aid.* Paper presented at the annual convention of the American Academy of Audiology, Ft. Lauderdale, FL.

Killion, M. (1997). SNR loss: I can hear what people say, but I can't understand them. *Hearing Review, 4*(12). 8–14.

Killion, M., Niquette, P., & Gudmundsen, G. (2004). Development of a quick speech-in-noise test for measuring signal-to-noise ratio in normal hearing and hearing impaired listeners. *Journal of the Acoustical Society of America, 116*(4), 2395–2405.

Kochkin, S. (2000a). MarkeTrak V: Why my hearing aids are in the drawer: The consumers' perspective. *The Hearing Journal, 53*(2). 34–42.

Kochkin, S. (2000b). Customer satisfaction with single and multiple microphone digital hearing aids. *Hearing Review, 7*(11), 24–34.

Kochkin, S. (2001). MarkeTrak V: The VA and direct mail sales spark growth in hearing aid market. *The Hearing Review, 8*(12), 16–24, 63–65.

Kochkin, S. (2005). MarkeTrak VII: Hearing loss population tops 31 million. *The Hearing Review, 12*(7), 16–29, 22–29.

Kuk, F., & Ludvigsen, C. (2003). Changing with the times: Choice of stimuli for hearing aid verification. *The Hearing Review, 10*(8), 24–28, 56–57.

Kuk, F., Keenan, D., Lau, C., & Ludvigsen, C. (2004). The reliability of aided sound-field thresholds in non-linear hearing aids. *The Hearing Review, 11*(13), 22–27, 66.

Mason, D., & Popelka, G. (1986). Comparison of hearing-aid gain using functional, coupler, and probe-tube measurements. *Journal of Speech and Hearing Research, 29*(2), 218–226.

McCandless, G., & Lyregaard, P. (1983). Prescription of gain and output (POGO) for hearing aids. *Hearing Instruments, 3,* 16–21.

Mormer, E., & Palmer, K. (1999). A systematic program for hearing aid orientation and adjustment. In R. Sweetow (Ed.), *Counseling for hearing aid fittings* (pp. 165–201). San Diego, CA: Singular Publishing Group.

Mueller, G., & Killion, M (1990). An easy method for calculating the Articulation Index. *The Hearing Journal, 45*(9), 14–17.

National Center for Health Statistics. (2004). Summary of health statistics for U.S. adults: National Health Interview Survey, 2002. *DHHS Publication No. (PHS) 2004–1150.* Hyattsville, MD: U.S. Department of Health and Human Services; Center for Disease Control and Prevention.

Newman, C., & Weinstein, B. (1988). The hearing handicap inventory for the elderly. *Ear and Hearing, 9,* 81–85.

Newman, C., Weinstein, B., Jacobson, G., & Hug, G. (1990). The hearing handicap inventory for adults: psychometric adequacy and audiometric correlates. *Ear and Hearing, 11,* 430–433.

Newman, C., Jacobson, G., Hug, G., Weinstein, B., & Malinoff, R. (1991). Practical method for quantifying hearing aid benefit for older adults. *Journal of the American Academy of Audiology, 2*(2), 70–75.

Newman, C., Weinstein, B., Jacobson, G., & Hug, G. (1991). Test-retest reliability of the hearing handicap inventory for adults. *Ear and Hearing, 12,* 355–357.

Nilsson, M., Soli, S., & Sullivan, J. (1994). Development of the hearing in noise test for the measurement of speech reception thresholds in quiet and noise. *Journal of the Acoustical Society of America, 95,* 1085–1099.

Pascoe, D. (1988). Clinical measurements of the auditory range and their relation to formulas for hearing aid gain. In J. Jensen (Ed.), *Hearing aid fittings: Theoretical and practical views,* 13th Danavox Symposium. Copenhagen: Stongaard Jensen.

Piranski, C. (2000). Earmold acoustics and technology. In R. Sandlin (Ed.), *Textbook of hearing aid amplification (2nd ed.)* (pp. 137–170). San Diego, CA: Singular Publishing Group.

Revit, L. (2002). Real-Ear measures. In M. Valente (Ed.), *Strategies for selecting and verifying hearing aid fittings (2nd ed.)* (pp. 66–124). New York: Thieme Medial Publishers, Inc.

Saunders, G. (1997). Other evaluative procedures. In H. Tobin (Ed.), *Practical hearing aid selection and fitting* (Monograph 001103–119). Washington, DC: Department of Veterans Affairs.

Schow, R., & Nerbonne, M. (1982). Communication screening profile: Use with elderly patients. *Ear & Hearing, 3*(3), 133–147.

Schwartz, D., Lyregaard, P., & Lundh, P. (1988). Hearing aid selection for severe-to-profound hearing loss. *The Hearing Journal, 41*(2), 13–17.

Shore, I., Bilger, R., & Hirsh, I. (1960). Hearing aid evaluation: Reliability of repeated measurements. *Journal of Speech and Hearing Research, 25,* 152–170.

Silman, S., Gelfand, S., & Silverman, C. (1984). Late-onset auditory deprivation: effects of monaural versus binaural hearing aids. *Journal of the Acoustical Society of America, 76*(5). 1357–1362.

Silverman, C., & Silman, S. (1990). Apparent auditory deprivation from monaural amplification and recovery with binaural amplification: two case studies. *Journal of the American Academy of Audiology, 1*(4), 175–180.

Skinner, M. (1988). *Hearing Aid Evaluation.* Englewood Cliffs, NJ: Prentice Hall.

Stabb, W. (2000). Hearing aid selection: An overview. In R. Sandlin (Ed.), *Textbook of Hearing Aid Amplification* (pp. 55–137). San Diego, CA: Singular Publishing Group.

Stelmachowicz, P., & Lewis, D. (1988). Some theoretical considerations concerning the relation between functional gain and insertion gain. *Journal of Speech and Hearing Research, 31*(3), 491–496.

Strom, K. (2005a). Reasons for optimism: A look at the 2004–2005 hearing instrument market. *The Hearing Review, 12*(3), 18–25, 79.

Strom, K. (2005b). The HR 2005 dispenser survey. *The Hearing Review, 12*(6), 18–31, 34–36, 72.

Suter, A. (1985). Speech recognition in noise by individuals with mild hearing impairments. *Journal of the Acoustical Society of America. 78*(3), 887–900.

Sweetow, R., & Valente, M. (1998). *"I bought some digital hearing aids so I don't have to listen anymore."* Paper presented at the Annual Convention of the American Academy of Audiology, Los Angeles, CA.

Valente, M., Potts, L., & Valente, M., (1997). Differences and intersubject variability of loudness discomfort levels measured in sound pressure level and hearing level for TDH–50P and ER–3A earphones. *Journal of the American Academy of Audiology, 8,* 59–67.

Valente, M., & Van Vliet, D. (1997). The independent hearing aid fitting forum (IHAFF) protocol. *Trends in Amplification, 2,* 6–35.

Valente, M., Valente, M., Enrietto, J., & Layton, K. (2002). Earhooks, tubing, earmolds, and shells. In M. Valente (Ed.) *Hearing aids: Standards, options and limitations* (pp. 214–273). New York: Thieme.

Ventry, I., & Weinstein, B. (1983). The hearing handicap inventory for the elderly: A new tool. *Ear and Hearing, 3,* 128–134.

Walden, B., Schwartz, D., Williams, D., Holum-Hardegen, L., & Crowley, J. (1982). Test of assumptions underlying comparative hearing aid evaluations. *Journal of Speech and Hearing Disorders, 48,* 264–273.

World Health Organization (WHO). (2000). *International classification of functioning, disability and health.* Geneva: WHO.

CHAPTER 12

Noise-Induced Hearing Loss: Models for Prevention

Deanna K. Meinke
University of Northern Colorado

Mark R. Stephenson
National Institute for Occupational Safety and Health

Noise-induced hearing loss (NIHL) might be more accurately termed *sound-induced hearing loss*. This new nomenclature broadens the historical context of occupational noise exposure to include recreational sound sources of NIHL. Sound, if it is loud enough, has the potential to cause hearing loss, whether from everyday activities such as music we listen to and the toys children play with or from daily exposure to jackhammer noise of a construction worker. Traffic noise and recreational noise exposure from off-road recreational vehicles and power tools can cause hearing loss and tinnitus over time as effectively as any occupational noise hazard. Even the sound that is "music to our ears" has the potential to cause hearing loss.

Noise exposure primarily damages the delicate hair cells in the cochlea. This defines NIHL as a "sensory" hearing loss. Typically, excessive sound exposure results in hearing loss that is most extreme at 3-, 4-, or 6 kHz frequencies. This characteristic "dip" in hearing threshold that is usually seen on the audiogram at one of these frequencies is so typical, in fact, that it is often referred to as a "noise notch." Another characteristic of NIHL is that the loss is so insidious that affected individuals are unaware of their worsening hearing until a considerable loss is present. If the hazardous sound exposure continues without intervention, the notch will deepen and spread to adjacent frequencies. This change is greatest during the first 10 years of exposure. Although the rate of hearing loss may decelerate after 10 years, the fact that continued exposure may spread and begin to affect frequencies most critical for speech understanding (e.g., 2000 Hz and 1000 Hz) suggests an urgency to the intervention strategy. And, the presence of an audiometric "notch" in combination with a noise exposure history usually distinguishes NIHL from other causes of hearing loss.

NIHL is so frequently considered irreversible that it becomes synonymous with a condition known as 'noise-induced permanent threshold shift' (NIPTS), which does not always develop gradually. Sounds of sufficient energy can cause an immediate NIPTS, termed "acoustic trauma." There are numerous documented cases where one unprotected shot from a rifle, shotgun, or handgun resulted in a permanent hearing loss (Humes, Joellenbeck, & Durch, 2005). However, before noise causes a permanent hearing loss, it usually causes a reversible or recoverable level of hearing known as a "temporary threshold shift" (TTS). The determining factors in the potential hearing risk for any sound are exposure level or intensity, and the time duration of the exposure that are discussed in greater detail below.

Although NIHL is a common cause of hearing loss, it is difficult to determine the precise prevalence. Dobie (1993) referenced a Swiss study that estimated almost one in five hearing loss patients (20 percent) could attribute at least a part of their hearing loss to noise exposure. The Bureau of Labor statistics annually reports occupational hearing loss among the top three most common occupational illnesses. And, NIHL is not just a problem among adults. Niskar et al. (1998, 2001) report NIHL among children, which is being surveyed extensively in a national surveillance effort conducted jointly by the National Institutes of Health (NIH), the National Center for Health Statistics (NCHS) and the National Institute for Occupational Safety and Health (NIOSH). This effort is part of the National Health and Nutrition Examination Survey (NHANES), and is particularly relevant because each participant tested will be asked to report his/her history of occupational and non-occupational noise exposure. Initiated in 1998, the data from the first five years (approximately 1,000 hearing tests per year) will identify hearing levels and hearing loss patterns, including NIHL, of the 20–60+ year-old participants. It is anticipated that results of the NHANES survey will verify that NIHL is common across the lifespan.

Sadly, NIHL is so common that many people think it is normal to acquire a hearing loss in the course of earning a living. This fact is especially disturbing considering that NIHL is nearly always preventable. It is important that audiologists not become complacent, and treat NIHL as a hard-wired companion to presbyacusis. The fact is; a typical, healthy, non-noise exposed person should not have a hearing impairment before age 60. And NIHL can affect quality of life in many ways. For example, there is growing public awareness that NIHL reduces an ability to experience intimacy (Hetu & Getty, 1991). As such, NIHL creates problems for the person with the hearing loss as well as their significant others.

Tinnitus frequently accompanies NIHL and may be more severe in those with NIHL (Axelsson, 1995). An estimate of the prevalence of tinnitus in noise-exposed workers varies greatly, ranging from approximately 10–58 percent of individuals (Axelsson, 1995; Coles, Smith, & Davis, 1990; Cooper, 1994). Tinnitus is also implicated as an early warning indicator of NIHL (Griest & Bishop, 1998). As noted by Davis and Rafaie (2000), prevalence estimates are dependent upon several factors such as age of the study group, degree of hearing loss and the noise exposure sustained. One construction worker put it best when he said; "I expected to lose my hearing, but I thought it would be quiet; now, I never get a moment of peace and quiet" (M. R. Stephenson, personal communication, February 2001).

Occupational NIHL is particularly relevant to audiologists and physicians who, by law, are given responsibility for determining whether or not a hearing loss is work-related. Audiologists and physicians *will* see patients who are exposed to loud noise, and in large numbers. Medical professionals should manage these patients proactively by helping to prevent further NIHL while maintaining existing hearing levels. "Prevention of NIHL (by noise level reduction, exposure time reduction, and use of personal hearing protection devices) would probably do more to reduce the societal burden of hearing loss than medical and surgical treatment of all other ear diseases combined" (Dobie, 1993). Most medical professionals have a responsibility to play a leading role in efforts to prevent NIHL.

DEVELOPMENTAL RISK OF NIHL

The risk of NIHL encompasses the human lifespan; from fetus to geriatric. An awareness of potential noise sources and any applicable exposure recommendations for various age groups are fundamental to a preventive approach.

Fetal Exposures

Sound exposure levels delivered to the developing fetus occur from a variety of sources and evidence that the fetus experiences NIHL is not documented. Auditory stimulation of the developing fetus not only stimulates the auditory system after approximately 20 weeks gestation (Pujol & Lavigne-Rebillard, 1992) but also influences other physiological responses such as changes in heart rate, breathing and movements. The sounds that ultimately reach the fetal ear are much different from those generated externally. Environmental sounds are transmitted through the fluid and tissues of the womb and stimulation is not via the typical air-conduction route. In order for an environmental sound to stimulate the fetal auditory system it must contain sufficient energy to (1) penetrate the uterus (typically low-frequency $\geq$300 Hz), (2) exceed the intensity of the ambient noise levels within the womb, and (3) produce mechanical displacements in the middle ear and cochlea (Abrams and Gerhardt, 2000). Consequently, any noise related damage-risk criteria must take into account the intensity and frequency differences between air and fluid for the source measurements, the fetal auditory transmission pathway (which is non-air conduction) as well as the potential for other physiological responses to hazardous sound.

Little is known of the direct impact of environmental noise exposure on the development and function of the human fetal auditory system or if maternal noise exposure indirectly influences the fetus via neuroendocrine system effects (Morris, Philbin, & Bose, 2000). Animal studies provide the majority of evidence from which inferences are deduced relative to humans. Often such studies include extreme noise exposure (120 dB SPL) over extended periods, which are atypical of typical noise exposures. Such methodological issues aside, there appears to be fetal animal evidence that hazardous sound exposures can induce changes in hearing sensitivity and damage cochlear hair cells especially in the region stimulated by low-frequency sound energy (Gerhardt, Pierson, Huang, Abrams, & Rarey, 1999). The American Academy of Pediatrics (AAP) Committee on Environmental Health reviewed the hazards of noise on the fetus and newborn in a statement published in 1997 (AAP, 1997). This group concluded that: (1) exposure to excessive noise during pregnancy may result in high-frequency hearing loss in newborns, and may be associated with prematurity and intrauterine growth retardation, (2) exposure to noise in the neonatal intensive care unit (NICU) may result in cochlear damage, and (3) exposure to noise and other environmental factors in the NICU may disrupt the normal growth and development of premature infants.

Based on the available research, the American Conference of Governmental Industrial Hygienists (ACGIH, 2004) guidelines for employers currently state that "noise exposure in excess of 8-hour time-weighted average (TWA) of 115 dBC or a peak exposure of 155 dBC to the abdomen of pregnant workers, beyond the 5th month of pregnancy, may cause hearing loss in the fetus." The C-weighting scale referenced in this guideline is different from the typical A-weighted scale the Occupational Safety and Health Administration (OSHA) mandates in order to account for the greater influence of low-frequency acoustic energy on a fetus.

Neonatal Exposures

The first auditory experiences for a neonate are in part, dictated by the gestational age at birth since premature newborns may require care within a neonatal intensive care unit (NICU). Ambient noise levels within hospital nurseries have been measured between 57–90 dBA (Philbin, 2000) and prolonged exposures to loud sounds in the 70 to 80 dBA range with peak levels of 105 dB SPL are possible (Anagnostakis, Petmezakis, Messaritakis, & Matsaniotis, 1980; Gottfried, 1985). Incubators do not necessarily provide a more sheltered auditory environment. Incubator operation, objects striking the plastic walls and port doors snapping shut contribute additional noise sources. In addition, the reverberant closed container may function as a resonant chamber and amplifier when the infant cries. Unfortunately, a direct relationship between NICU sound levels and hearing loss has not been established for either infants or adult caregivers.

The physiological effects of sound on human neonates include the potential for increased heart rate as intensity is increased from 55–90 dBA, short-term increases in blood pressure in response to incubator alarms, sleep disruption, changes in respiratory rates and an increase in intracranial pressure when sudden loud noises (70 to 75 dBA) caused behavioral agitation and crying (Morris et al., 2000). Inference from animal and adult human studies suggests that high sound levels may have an effect on the neuroendocrine system, which may indirectly influence immunity (Morris et al., 2000). Ultimately, vigorous investigation into the direct pathological effects of sound on neonates is needed to identify the most protective and nurturing sound environment. In the meantime, readers may wish to review the recommendations for care that have been developed by the Physical and Developmental Environment of the High Risk Infant Center, Study Group on NICU Sound, and the Expert Review Panel (Graven, 2000).

Childhood and Adolescent Exposures

Children accompany their parents and caregivers to many more loud events and participate jointly in numerous "noisy" activities, which were previously restricted or unavailable to earlier generations. At some point in their young lives, 97 percent of 273 third graders surveyed had been exposed to hazardous sound levels (Blair, 1996). The World Health Organization (WHO) reports that North American children "may receive more noise at school than workers from an 8-hour work day at a factory" (1997). Common hazardous sound sources include toys, music, firearms, fireworks, power tools, motorized vehicles, racing events and arcades. These exposure risks are encountered in home, community, school and work environments and hearing protection is neither widely utilized nor made available to youth (Fig. 12–1). The appropriate damage-risk criteria to adopt for a young

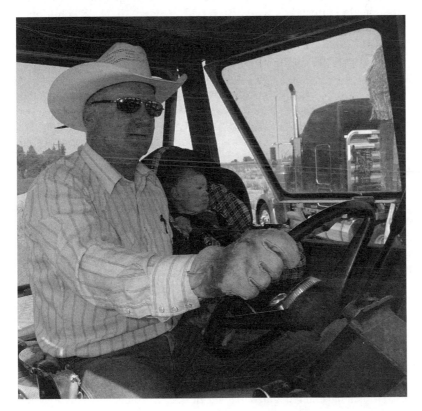

FIGURE 12–1.   Agricultural worker farming with young son in tractor cab. (Courtesy Deanna K. Meinke, PhD, University of Northern Colorado).

population with a lifetime of potential noise exposure ahead of them are not known. Permissible noise exposure levels created for regulatory purposes are not designed for application to children and need to be developed in the context of 24-hour exposures and auditory development. Current conservative approaches suggest that sound levels below 75 dBA are unlikely to cause hearing loss (WHO, 2002). This may be an adequate reference to utilize until more appropriate hazardous sound exposure criteria can be developed specifically for children.

The outcomes in terms of permanent hearing loss and tinnitus from unprotected noise exposures in children are better established in the literature. Niskar et al., (2001) has reported that 12.5 percent (approximately 5.2 million) of U.S. children aged 6 to 19 years are estimated to have noise-induced hearing loss in one or both ears. Other studies suggest that the prevalence of NIHL among children is markedly increasing (Chermack & Peters-McCarthy, 1991; Montgomery & Fujikawa, 1992). Wisconsin youth engaged in farm work experience twice the rate of NIHL as their peers not involved in farm work (Broste, Hansen, Strand, & Stueland, 1989). A unique public health research and educational outreach project called Dangerous Decibels® uses a science museum exhibit to measure hearing thresholds at 4 kHz of visitors aged 6 to 85 years. Results for 6 to 19 year old visitors revealed thresholds > 20 dBHL in 21 percent of 21,389 children as of March 2007 (http://www.dangerousdecibels.org/resultshearingloss.cfm).

Although, the prevalence study results cannot be directly attributed to noise exposure, the evidence of high-frequency hearing loss in youth is certainly worrisome. School hearing screening programs are not designed to identify the early onset of NIHL. Many school hearing screening programs do not include children in middle and high school when participation in noisy activities becomes more commonplace. This eliminates the opportunity to intervene at an early stage and minimize the hearing loss. Newer strategies might include the use of a high risk noise behavior questionnaire to identify youth most at risk for NIHL and using the mobile industrial hearing test model for monitoring hearing in high school students (Meinke, Meade, Johnson, & Jensema, 2005)

Approximately 5.1 percent of the 2001 workforce (6.9 million) was comprised of adolescent workers aged 16–19 years of age (NIOSH, 2004). Youth work in a variety of industries including retail, construction, manufacturing services and agriculture. Experts also suspect that these statistics may underestimate the actual number of teen workers. For example, youths working in an "underground economy" with unreported jobs might operate unregulated machinery and heavy equipment. These practices may be in violation of child labor laws that prohibit a teen from operating certain noisy equipment. Since adolescents may work informally and/or seasonally, they are not usually included in formal employer-provided hearing conservation programs. This creates a climate whereby poor hearing protector habits develop and the risks of NIHL are unregulated and hearing loss is unreported. Consider the possibility for occupational noise exposures of adolescent patients and recognize that a teen may be reluctant to divulge the true nature of their employment in some situations. Similarly, children may also be reluctant to identify the source of a sudden acoustic trauma (such as fireworks) in front of a parent or teacher due to a fear of disciplinary outcomes. Skillful clinicians will develop rapport with young patients and may need to enlist the cooperation of adults to provide a "safe" communication environment in order to obtain accurate noise exposure histories.

Effective clinical intervention for youth includes the following; (1) inclusion of case history questions regarding noise exposures, (2) audiometric threshold monitoring (including 3000 and 6000 Hz), (3) noise exposure assessment for at-risk youth, (4) adequate hearing protector fitting, and (5) education focused on changing knowledge, beliefs, attitudes and behaviors related to loud noise exposures.

Parental and community education is fundamental and essential for the implementation of hearing loss prevention strategies targeting youth. Audiologists can partner with school nurses, teachers, speech-language pathologists, employers and pediatricians to increase awareness and to encourage systematic public health programs aimed at preventing NIHL. A review of intervention programs by Folmer, Griest, and Martin (2002) will provide the clinician with established resources for such efforts. In the future, it is hoped that youth will view the routine use of hearing protection in noisy environments, the same as using a helmet while riding bicycles or seatbelts while riding in a car. Changing the fundamental behaviors related to hearing loss prevention at a young age will provide a stronger foundation for successful hearing loss prevention programs within the adult workplace and increase the opportunities for normal hearing throughout the lifespan.

Adult Exposures

Military.   Many adolescents move from school to the workplace via military service and find themselves potentially exposed to hazardous sound levels regardless of military branch (Army, Navy, Air Force, Marine Corps, and Coast Guard). Noise exposure in the military may begin as early as basic training and recruits will find themselves engaged in a variety of activities with highly variable levels of noise sources. Aircraft, jet engines, watercraft, heavy equipment and vehicles, communication systems, maintenance operations, weapons and combat environments are among the obvious sources of hazardous sound.

Military noise-exposures are somewhat unique from typical industrial noise exposures, in terms of the duration of the exposures and the nature of the noise sources (high intensity, intermittent, impulsive etc.). Personnel may be exposed continuously over long periods of time; for instance when deployed on an aircraft carrier for months at a time or to high-intensity blasts. The exposure issue becomes more complex when one considers that traditional hearing protectors may present unique challenges in the military context. These challenges include: unexpected exposures in field deployment, critical warning signal audibility and communication interference. Fortunately, the availability of level-dependent hearing protectors is becoming more widespread and these devices may afford protection while facilitating audibility in military listening environments. Recognizing the limitation of hearing protectors and looking toward the future, the military is also involved with pharmacological research efforts, primarily with regard to the potential for otoprotectants or dietary supplements to reduce NIHL.

Hazardous military noise exposures have contributed to auditory disabilities (including tinnitus) accounting for nearly 10 percent of the total number of disabilities claimed among veterans receiving disability compensation in 2003 (Humes et al., 2005). The report on Noise and Military Service (Humes et al., 2005) indicates that by the end of 2004 annualized payments of $660 million for hearing loss and $190 million for tinnitus claims were realized. The costs in this case extend beyond the obvious personal impact and extend to society as a whole. Civilian audiologists may very well be the first point of contact for many veterans and familiarity with veteran's benefits and referral resources will be advantageous.

Occupational. Approximately 10 million persons in the United States (Jackson & Duffy, 1998) and 25–30 million in Europe (Quaranta, Sallustio, & Quaranta, 2001) have permanent hearing loss from noise or trauma. Another 30 million people a day are exposed to injurious noise levels in the U.S. An awareness of the deleterious effects of noise from work has been known for centuries. Bernardino Ramazzini described noise-induced hearing loss suffered by coppersmiths in the 18th century and the advancements in technology during the Industrial Revolution have led to increased risks both in developed and developing countries. Yet, despite this historical awareness, there continued to be a 26 percent increase in hearing loss between 1971 and 1990 for 18–44 year olds (NIOSH, 2004). Godlee (1992) estimates that 4.5 percent of the general population has NIHL. This is in comparison to the 35–51 percent of the occupationally noise-exposed population that has NIHL. More recently, Hager (2006) summarized the U.S. Bureau of Labor Statistics data relative to OSHA 300 recordable hearing loss statistics for 2004, and reported that 11 percent of all OSHA recordable occupational injuries were due to hearing loss.

Some jobs are by their nature, more risky in terms of noise exposure than others. The most commonly recognized noise-exposed (or "at-risk") occupations include; agriculture (farming, forestry, commercial fishing), mining, construction, manufacturing, utilities, transportation (aircraft, railroad and marine) and military (Fig. 12–2). Other at-risk occupations include medical and emergency personnel such as firefighters, police officers, emergency medical technicians, surgeons, dentists and professional musicians. Additionally, combined exposures of noise with chemical agents such as solvents or pharmaceutical agents such as diuretics or aminoglycosides are thought to increase the risk of hearing loss.

When evaluating adults with potential NIHL, audiologists are encouraged to obtain a comprehensive noise and chemical exposure history including details not only related to occupation, but to specific duties, tools and tasks that are involved in the job. A patient may also work a quiet job in his/her primary employment setting but work under hazardous noise conditions in a second job. It is wise to obtain updated noise dosimetry studies on patients as work-related tasks and equipment may often change. Current noise measurements will facilitate appro-

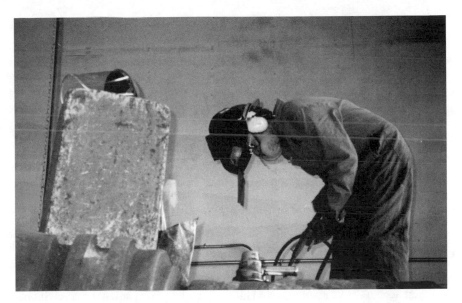

FIGURE 12–2.   Air arc welder at coal mine. Note the need for compatibility of safety equipment. (Courtesy Deanna K. Meinke, PhD, University of Northern Colorado.

priate clinical decisions and interventions, especially as they relate to hearing protectors.

Recreational.   Current government mandated work-related damage risk criteria are founded on the assumption that there is no noise exposure outside of the workplace and none beyond the traditional 40-year, 40-hour per week career timeframe. The social and recreational exposures from amplified music, motorized vehicles, firearms, public transportation and sporting events contribute to the noise burden on our ears and need to be considered in terms of the overall risk of NIHL for a given individual. The commute to and from work on the subway or the motorcycle trip to the plant at 80–114 dBA (U.S. EPA, 1974) may very well combine with a slightly < 85 dBA work-related exposure to create a hazardous impact on the ears. This may give workers a false sense of security when they assume they do not need to wear hearing protection at work because their noise exposures are minimal in terms of regulatory compliance. However, their overall noise exposures for a 24-hour period that includes any off-the-primary-job noise exposures may be hazardous, and hearing protector use at work would be beneficial. Patients may also fail to recognize the non-work related noise hazards because they are associated with the pleasure of recreation rather than the doldrums of work. Noise as a byproduct of entertainment may be perceived as relatively "quiet" compared to the sound levels experienced at work, although both are potentially hazardous. In addition, hearing protector use is seldom recommended or enforced during recreational activities. A NIOSH 1998 Healthstyles survey found that "32% of adults say that while they regularly use noisy equipment around the house (e.g., lawn mowers or vacuum cleaner), they do not believe that their use of this equipment could damage their hearing" (NIOSH, 1998a).

Even regular attendance at professional sporting events exposes attendees to noise levels and durations that exceed most North American federal guidelines (WHO, 1997). One noise dosimetry study on a sports fan for the duration of an indoor U.S. hockey game resulted in a L_{eq} of 99.5 dBA, while a World Series baseball game sports fan received an L_{eq} of 96.9 dBA (WHO, 1997). Cheering sports fans, foghorns, public address systems and amplified music all contribute to the overall noise environment.

Unprotected firearm use can cause acoustic trauma and permanent NIHL, especially with repeated exposures. Firearms are a common source of non-occupational noise exposure, especially for hunters and target shooters. Impulse noise levels from firearms vary from approximately 140 dB peak sound pressure level to 170 dB SPL_{pk} (Odess, 1972). It has been estimated that approximately one-third of households in the U.S. own firearms (Johnson, Coyne-Beasley, & Runyan, 2004). There are 28 million Americans who consider themselves hunters and 13 million hunted in 2000 (U.S. FWS, 2001). Additionally, there were 1.74 million children aged 6–15 years of age who hunted in 2000. The National Sports Shooting Foundation reports that there are 19.8 million Americans who are active sports shooters in the United States (NSSF, 2005). Hearing protection is more commonly used when target shooting and less frequently used during hunting activities.

Loud music is also a common source of both occupational and non-occupational noise exposure for both classical and contemporary music. Music levels at concerts have been documented above 100 dBA at rock concerts and discotheques (Clark, 1991). Short-term exposures such as received while attending live music events can result in a temporary NIHL. Longer duration exposures are possible when listening to loud music via personal MP3 or compact disk music players, especially from those with power supplies that enable a unit to run for 20 hours or more without recharging. Sound exposures in excess of 85 dBA TWA are possible when listening to compact disk players above a 70 percent volume setting for more than one-hour duration (Fligor & Cox, 2004). Reporting on data obtained with the iPod nano MP3 player, Fligor and Ivers (2006) found that the free-field equivalent sound levels exceed 85 dBA at approximately 60 percent of the volume control. Volume control settings are the primarily influence on the noise hazard risk. Fligor et al. (2006) suggest that 5–25 percent of iPod nano listeners exceed 85 dBA in terms of their chosen listening level. Additionally, the sound levels of the ambient noise environment, the attenuation characteristics of the headphones and the hearing status of the listener will all influence the preferred listening level and ultimately the listener's risk of NIHL. Although the potential for over-exposure is apparent, the research literature is weak in terms of directly linking recreational music exposure with permanent NIHL.

An adult's noise exposure profile extends beyond the primary employer. Noise exposure records are required to be available to workers and these records should be requested by clinical audiologists when seeing patients with NIHL. It is not uncommon for a job to be reported as "noisy" by the employee, but minimally hazardous when sampled for regulatory purposes. It is erroneous to assume there is a true noise hazard at work based solely on employee report, previous experience with co-workers or because hearing protector use is recommended by an employer. The integration of recreational, societal and occupational noise exposures into a true representation of an individual's personal risk is important, and will facilitate patient education, good clinical judgment and trusted medical-legal decision making.

Societal. A 1997 World Health Organization (WHO) report on "Prevention of Noise-Induced Hearing Loss" points out that for developed countries "both occupational noise and urban, environmental noise (especially traffic noise) are increasing risk factors for hearing impairment." As populations increase, the sources of noise increase and in some cultures "noise" is an accepted part of holidays, celebrations and life. While for other geographic regions, noise is an unacceptable consequence of war, terrorism, civil unrest and societal conflict. Hearing disorders, tinnitus, loudness sensitivity and balance disorders can result from traumatic blast injury. Following the 1995 Oklahoma City bombing, 76 percent of explosion survivors had a predominately sensorineural hearing loss at one or more conventional audiometric test frequencies and 24 percent required amplification (Van Campen, Dennis, Hanlin, King, & Velderman, 1999). Unfortunately, audiologists may very well find themselves caring for victims of tragedies such as the 2001 World Trade Center attack and the 1995 Oklahoma City bombing.

Developmentally, there is a risk of NIHL from the time our ears are formed until death. Sound sources, intensities and durations are continually changing. The relative contributions of recreational, societal and occupational noise exposures will change dependent upon available leisure time, work demands, transportation modes and geographical locations. An adolescent or geriatric patient may have more time for recreational noise exposures, and a middle-aged adult may have greater contributions from occupational noise sources. An adolescent on the farm may have greater exposures than an adolescent in suburbia. The variable nature of exposures across a lifespan requires that clinicians recognize potential hazards and educate their patients regarding the risks and the means to prevent hearing loss at all stages of life.

HEARING LOSS PREVENTION MODELS

At least four models exist for approaching the prevention of NIHL; (1) regulatory model, (2) educational model, (3) medical treatment model and (4) preventive medicine model. A regulatory model focuses on the scientific evidence for noise toxicity, dose-effect data and epidemiology as it applies to the workplace. This model is heavily influenced by technology, political climates and economics; it is time-locked to 1983 for the OSHA regulation and 2000 for the MSHA regulation. An educational model focuses on teaching children and adults to recognize common noise hazards and how to take appropriate individual and community actions to reduce the noise exposure to safe levels. It is a proactive approach that is readily adaptable to new knowledge and technology. A medical treatment model is based upon the pathophysiology of NIHL and any medical/nutritional treatments, which may intervene to prevent the occurrence of the disease or halt its progression. Lastly, a preventive medicine model incorporates a comprehensive sequential approach beginning with early detection and intervention, followed by appropriate diagnosis and if necessary, rehabilitation. The preventive medicine model incorporates an individual- or patient-centered approach based on their current hearing status. There is no one model that is preferable to another and many are complementary. Audiologists can draw from the strengths of all models when designing their hearing loss prevention services and emphasize the approach most appropriate for a particular setting.

REGULATORY PREVENTION MODEL

The regulatory model relies on government agencies gathering scientific evidence associated with NIHL and facilitating academic, private and public input on the legal requirements for employers to protect the hearing of their workers. These agencies also provide "best practice" documents to guide the public, especially in cases where the legal requirements may lag behind scientific, technological and methodological advancements.

Historically, audiologists have approached hearing loss prevention via the regulatory model through the implementation and professional supervision of hearing conservation programs (HCPs). In some cases, this approach prevents the application of contemporary knowledge, advanced technology and new interventions from being implemented due to the finite boundaries imposed by legal mandates. This perspective limits the role of the audiologist to that delineated in national standards (audiometric test provider and audiogram reviewer including work-related determinations) but is beneficial in that it provides a legal description of the audiologist's role. The legally-based regulatory model is often the only model known to employers. Consequently, it is essential that audiologists understand and monitor the legal mandates for various work sectors in both state and federal regulations.

Hearing Loss Prevention Programs

In the U.S., there are numerous federal and state regulatory requirements governing hearing loss prevention programs (HLPPs). For example, the Occupational Safety and Health Administration (OSHA) promulgated the Hearing Conservation Amendment, 29 CFR 1910.95, in 1983. It contains specific details for hearing conservation programs (HCP) to persons working in general industry and manufacturing. OSHA has a separate regulation 29 CFR 1926.52 that applies to construction workers, and the Mine Safety and Health Administration (MSHA) promulgated a federal regulation (30 CFR Parts 56 and 57 that applies to the mining industry. The Department of Defense (DoD) has established its own regulation governing hearing conservation for the military (DoD Instruction 6055.12). Additional program guidance is also available by reviewing OSHA "letters of interpretation" and technical manuals.

Not all noise exposures are related to work. The U.S. Environmental Protection Agency has established recommended exposure levels for the general public (EPA, 1973). Furthermore, not all hearing conservation guidelines are regulatory in nature. Professional organizations provide excellent sources for information on issues related to HCPs. For example, the National Hearing Conservation Association (NHCA) <www.hearingconservation.org> offers a wealth of resources that promote hearing loss prevention in the workplace. Both the American Academy of Audiology and the American Speech-Language-Hearing Association provide guidelines and recommendations for audiologists engaged in preventing NIHL. The Council for Accreditation in Occupational Hearing Conservation (CAOHC) provides certification for occupational hearing conservationists (OHC), and professional supervisors (i.e., audiologists and physicians) of HCPs. CAOHC also provides programs to certify Course Directors who teach audiometric technician classes leading to OHC certification and Professional Supervisor certification. The CAOHC Web site <www.caohc.org> is a valuable source of information. Many of these resources are provided for your reference in Table 12–1.

Because there is no single regulation governing all work sectors and noise exposures, audiologists should be careful to follow appropriate state and federal standards. Likewise, there is an array of guidelines, position statements and recommendations from many professional organizations. Thus, audiologists should also be familiar with professional standards of practice. All of the regulatory bodies and professional organizations maintain Web sites with information and links to other resources. However, if the audiologist is responsible for a hearing conservation program, he/she is encouraged to obtain CAOHC Professional Supervisor certification. The coursework leading to this certification will help the audiologist navigate through the maze of regulations, standards, and guidelines that apply to the hearing conservation field and network them to an ongoing resource for future changes in regulations and official interpretations used for regulatory compliance determinations.

Despite the plethora of regulations, standards, guidelines, and recommendations, there is a common thread that runs through almost every hearing loss prevention program. In 1972, the National Institute for Occupational Safety and Health (NIOSH) published recommended criteria for preventing occupational hearing loss (NIOSH, 1973). This document addressed the basis for, and laid out the elements of, an effective HCP. OSHA adopted the majority of the NIOSH recommendations as it developed the first general regulatory standard for HCPs in the workplace. Most subsequent HCPs were patterned after the NIOSH recommendations. In 1998 NIOSH updated its criteria for a recommended standard for occupational noise exposure and introduced the terminology of "hearing loss prevention program" as opposed to HCP (NIOSH, 1998). While the 1998 document shifted the emphasis from conserving remaining hearing to preventing *initial* as well as subsequent hearing loss, the basic elements of a HCP or HLPP remain essentially unchanged. These elements consist of (1) the program audit, (2) noise measurement (3) noise control, (4) hearing protection, (5) audiometric monitoring, (6) training, and (7) documenting program effectiveness. These elements are discussed below. Since it is beyond the scope of this chapter to adequately address each of these elements, a list of additional resources is provided in Table 12–1.

TABLE 12-1
INTERNET HLPP RESOURCES

American Academy of Audiology Position Statement Preventing Noise-Induced Occupational Hearing Loss	www.audiology.org/publications/documents/positions/Hearingconservation
American Speech-Language Hearing Association (ASHA) Division 8 Hearing Conservation & Occupational Audiology	www.asha.org/about/membership-certification/divs/div_8.htm
Council for Accreditation in Occupational Hearing Conservation (CAOHC)	www.caohc.org
Dangerous Decibels®	www.dangerousdecibels.org
Department of Defense (U.S.)	www.dtic.mil/whs/directives/corres/html/605512.htm
E-A-R® Hearing Conservation & EarLogs	www.e-a-r.com/hearingconservation/
Mine Safety & Health Administration (MSHA) 30 CFR Part 62	www.msha.gov/30CFR/62.0.htm
MSHA Compliance Guide Noise	www.msha.gov/REGS/COMPLIAN/GUIDES/NOISE/GUIDE303 COVER.HTM
National Hearing Conservation Association (NHCA)	www.hearingconservation.org
National Institute for Occupational Safety & Health (NIOSH) Criteria for a RecommendedStandard—Occupational Noise Exposure	www.cdc.gov/niosh/98-126.html
NIOSH Hearing Protector Compendium	www.cdc.gov/niosh/topics/noise/hpcomp.html
NIOSH Noise and Hearing Loss Prevention	www.cdc.gov/niosh/topics/noise/
NIOSH Preventing Occupational Hearing Loss—A Practical Guide	www.cdc.gov/niosh/96-110.html/
Noise Pollution Clearing House	www.nonoise.org

Occupational Hearing Loss—Kevin Kavanagh MD Online ANSI S3.44 calculator	www.occupationalhearingloss.com
Occupational Safety and Health Administration (OSHA) 29 CFR 1904.10 Recording criteria occupational hearing loss	www.osha.gov/pls/oshaweb/owadisp.show_document?p_table =STANDARDS&p_id=9641
OSHA 29 CFR 1910.95 Occupational Noise Exposure	www.osha.gov/pls/oshaweb/owadisp.show_document?p_table =STANDARDS&p_id=9735
OSHA 29 CFR 1926.52 Construction Occupational Noise Exposure	www.osha.gov/pls/oshaweb/owadisp.show_document?p_table =STANDARDS&p_id=10664
OSHA 29 CFR 1926.101 Construction Hearing Protection	www.osha.gov/pls/oshaweb/owadisp.show_document?p_table =STANDARDS&p_id=10664
OSHA eTool Noise and Hearing Conservation	www.osha.gov/dts/osta/otm/noise/index.html
OSHA Letters of Interpretations	www.osha.gov/pls/oshaweb/owasrch.search_form? p_doc_type=INTERPRETATIONS &p_toc_level=0&p_keyvalue=
OSHA Injury and Illness: Recordkeeping	www.osha.gov/recordkeeping/index.html
OSHA Recordkeeping Handbook	www.osha.gov/recordkeeping/handbook/index.html
OSHA Technical Manual	http://www.osha.gov/dts/osta/otm/otm_toc.htm

The Program Audit.   Before developing a hearing loss prevention program, and periodically thereafter, the HLPP manager should do some "management by walking around." Much can be learned by simple observation as well as by talking to employees and supervisors. What is the overall safety culture, i.e., is safety valued? What kinds of hearing protectors are provided to employees? Are workers wearing hearing protectors in noise hazard areas and using them correctly? What other personal protective equipment is being used? Are supervisors setting a good example? Are signs posted regarding hazardous noise areas? Have engineering controls been applied? If so, are they being maintained? What elements of a hearing loss prevention program are already operational? What are management's goals for preventing hearing loss? Having a feel for the general safety culture and the attitudes and beliefs about preventing occupational hearing loss can be of great value in helping the audiologist interact with workers and management. It can also help to efficiently address the remaining elements in an effective HLPP.

Noise Measurement.   Noise measurements serve one of three purposes: (1) identify the presence of a noise hazard, (2) monitor employees to be included in a HLPP, and (3) evaluate engineering noise control options. A general survey is used to determine whether or not hazardous noise is present. Noise monitoring identifies area and/or individual noise levels and doses. Sound level meters and dosimeters may be used for either of these purposes. When engineering controls are involved, it may be necessary to have detailed noise measurements of a piece of equipment or an area. This approach would require more sophisticated noise measurement procedures and equipment, including octave or 1/3 octave noise band measurement, real-time spectral analysis, as well as digital recordings for subsequent laboratory analysis. The audiologist is less likely to be involved with detailed noise measurements for noise control and more likely to conduct a general survey or to conduct employee noise monitoring measurements. While most regulations do not require specific credentials, the skills and knowledge needed to make valid noise measurements typically requires additional education, such as professional organization workshops, manufacturer training, and other academic courses outside of traditional audiology curricula.

Many variables must be considered when making a general survey. First, decide what equipment is needed: a sound level meter and noise dosimeter or if either one will suffice? What degree of accuracy is called for, i.e., do you need a Type 1 (approximately ± 1 dB accuracy) or Type 2 (approximately ± 2 dB accuracy) instrument? Where will you place the microphones, and how will they be oriented with respect to the noise? Before taking measurements decide how long to sample each event or area, and how many samples will be needed to adequately characterize the noise.

Sound measurement instrumentations have many settings and adjustments. Most measurements will be made using "slow" exponential averaging, as required by regulations. But there may be times when you may wish to use the "fast" setting. Likewise, most measurements will be made using A-weighting. However, there may be times when less filtering of the noise is desired or when you wish to filter out almost none of the noise. In such cases you would use C or Z weighted filter settings, respectively. Fortunately, many of today's sound measurement instruments are capable of simultaneously measuring sound events with multiple measurement protocols. Common uses of multiple protocols include simultaneous measurements of L_{OSHA} as well as L_{NIOSH} . The chief differences between these two are the exchange rate—OSHA uses a 5 dB exchange rate while NIOSH recommends a 3 dB exchange rate. OSHA uses a 90 dBA permissible exposure limit for an 8-hour exposure while NIOSH recommends an 85 dBA limit. The differences between the OSHA and NIOSH methods will yield substantially different results. Time weighted average (TWA) exposures based on the OSHA criteria will allow longer exposures to higher noise levels than do the NIOSH criteria. By taking samples with both protocols you will have much more information and be better able to make informed decisions about whether or not a given exposure is hazardous and what regulatory requirements must be met. Most manufacturers can provide excellent guidance on how to set up and use their instruments. Do some of these noise measurement terms sound confusing? Try doing an internet search. For example, Google <noise "exchange rate"> or < "A weighting">, or < "time weighted average" noise >. You may be surprised at the many sources of useful information that are at your fingertips.

Noise Control. Even though audiologists are less likely to be called upon to design, develop, and field control technologies, they should still be familiar with some basic concepts. There are often workshops specifically designed to introduce audiologists to the basics of noise control. Several organizations including the National Hearing Conservation Association (NHCA), the American Industrial Hygiene Association (AIHA) and CAOHC have periodically offered such workshops. In addition, the Institute of Noise Control Engineering (INCE) offers certification credentialing.

In reality, the best way to prevent NIHL is to eliminate the noise hazard. Noise control technology focuses on source controls—making the machine quieter, and path controls—inhibiting the noise from reaching the workers' ears. Design of heating and air conditioning ventilation, fan blade designs, impact isolators and dampers, and mufflers are all examples of source controls. Enclosures, vibration pads, and sound barriers (such as are often seen adjacent to highways) are examples of path controls. It is not difficult to gain a basic understanding of the principles associated with source and path control. Because of the primacy of engineering controls as a means of reducing or eliminating noise hazards, audiologists should be aware of basic control technology principles.

Hearing Protectors. Presently, there are over 300 different models of hearing protector devices (HPDs) available in the United States. But, they will only be effective if they are fit and worn properly. The most common types of hearing protection devices (HPD) are earplugs, earmuffs, and canal caps (sometimes called semi-aural insert devices). Earplugs come in many varieties. They may be a "pre-molded" (e.g. a fixed-shape flanged) or "formable" (e.g., an expandable foam) type. Earplugs are available in "one size fits most," multiple sized products, or custom molded to an individual's ear. Earmuffs vary by type of cushions (e.g., foam or "liquid" fillers) and by headband type (e.g., either fixed or variable position). For instance, earmuffs may have headbands that can be worn above the head, behind the neck and under the chin. Earmuffs may be designed to mount on hard hats or worn under welder helmets. Canal caps are essentially earplugs mounted on lightweight headbands. There are many sophisticated passive and active hearing protectors that can be utilized for unique listening (e.g., music) or specific communication demands. These include flat attenuator hearing protectors, active noise-reduction (ANR) circuitry, and electronic hearing protectors. The so-called "musicians earplugs" are a popular example of flat attenuation hearing protectors since they essentially diminish all frequencies equally and are a viable solution when fidelity is an important consideration for the listener. Audiologists are a key professional resource for patients interested in these specialty protectors.

Hearing protectors are only effective if care is taken to fit and wear them properly. Failure to wear hearing protectors correctly and appropriately is the single most important reason people develop noise-induced hearing loss. Why is this so? The barriers which inhibit proper HPD use can be lumped into five general categories, referred to as the five Cs: comfort, convenience, communication, compatibility and cost. Obviously, no one would wear something that is uncomfortable. Unfortunately, there is no way to predict comfort. When dispensing or fitting people with HPDs it is important to explain that finding a comfortable HPD is similar to finding a comfortable pair of shoes. It is a simple matter of trial and error—trying different HPDs to find one that is comfortable and then gradually adjusting to longer hours of wear. You wouldn't run a marathon in a new pair of shoes; so immediately expecting 8 to 12 hours of new HPD use may be unrealistic. Locating the HPD dispensers in close proximity to the noise source and making HPDs readily available to the user can usually resolve the issue of convenience. The third barrier, communication, refers not only to the need to hear speech, but also to the need to hear any sound that is important to the wearer (e.g., warning signal detection, engine rpm changes). Communication can be adversely affected by hearing too much noise (not enough hearing protection) or as a result of over-protection. It may sound strange, but the HPD, which offers the most attenuation, is not necessarily the best choice. Ideally, an HPD will reduce noise levels to between 70 and 80 dBA. HPDs that attenuate sounds to this range will reduce noise to a safe level while yielding the best chance of providing a satisfactory signal to noise ratio for audibility of other sounds such as speech (Fig. 12–3). When hearing protection is incompatible with other safety equipment or directly interferes with the task at hand, the fourth barrier is encountered. A worker should not have to choose between a face-guard that protects his/her eyes and earmuffs that protect hearing. There are options (e.g., earplugs), which afford protection to both eyes and ears. The fifth "C," cost, actually refers to two concepts. One is the direct financial cost of HPDs. Unfortunately, in some companies, purchasing decisions for personal protective equipment is based solely on the bottom line. The hearing loss prevention professional can enlighten the employer's HPD buyers to the reality that not all HPDs are alike, and that the cheapest device will be a waste of money if it is ineffective or not worn. The other cost-related barrier refers to social cost. Be aware that in many noisy situations, a person wearing hearing protectors may be considered a "wimp." Peer pressure can be a powerful barrier to overcome. A good education and motivation program may be the best place to start when hearing safety is not valued.

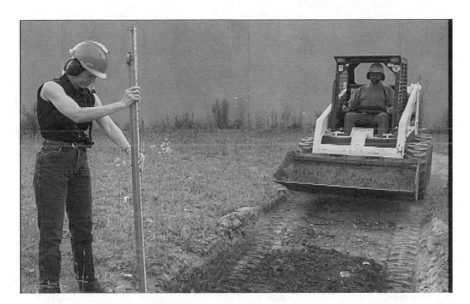

FIGURE 12–3.   Use of voice-activated two-way communication earmuffs facilitates the work activity and provides protection from hazardous sound levels. (Courtesy Mark R. Stephenson, PhD, CDC-NIOSH)

By law, manufacturers must specify how much attenuation their HPDs provide. Each box or package will have a Noise Reduction Rating (NRR). This NRR is a single number that represents the optimum attenuation an HPD will provide when it is fit by an expert and tested under pristine laboratory conditions. It should not be surprising that the NRR bears little relation to the attenuation users achieve in the workplace. In general, the "real-world" attenuation for pre-molded earplugs may be only 25 percent of their rated value. Formable foam earplugs and earmuffs may provide about 50 to 70 percent of their rated value, respectively. Some manufacturers are now providing NRR_{SF} values. The NRR_{SF} uses values based on subjects fitting their own HPDs during laboratory testing. The NRR_{SF} provides a more realistic estimate of the amount of attenuation that may be expected in the "real world." The web-based NIOSH HPD compendium is a good resource for centrally retrieving HPD specifications and evaluating options for particular noise exposures.

Audiometry.   By some accounts, monitoring audiometry represents the "gold standard" for determining whether an HLPP has been successful at preventing NIHL. Others have stated that audiometry simply documents the progression of hearing loss. Both perspectives have merit. The purpose for audiometry is to determine if hearing changes over time by comparing pre-exposure (baseline) hearing thresholds to annual hearing tests.

Ideally, audiometric monitoring begins before the hazardous noise exposure. When establishing baseline thresholds, persons should not have been exposed to loud noise for 14 hours. This will ensure a TTS does not interfere with establishing accurate thresholds for future test comparisons. Subsequent annual exams are then performed in order to monitor for threshold changes compared to a baseline exam. Regulations define the degree of hearing change, sufficient to trigger follow-up action, as a Standard Threshold Shift (STS). When conducting annual monitoring audiometry, it is best if the worker reports straight from his/her job. If a TTS is detected, this will provide the best chance of capturing it and ultimately initiating preventive strategies. Per regulations, intervention to prevent additional NIHL begins once a STS is identified. The audiologist becomes involved in notifying the employee and employer, investigating the potential sources of hazardous noise levels and assuring adequate hearing protector fit for the affected worker.

If the annual monitoring audiogram reveals a shift from a worker's baseline, it is then desirable to conduct a follow-up hearing test within 30 days and assure that the worker has been in quiet prior to the retest. This will determine if a shift was temporary or permanent. If the shift is permanent it may be necessary to formally record the hearing change and submit the record of this change to the agency that has jurisdiction over the work sector. For example, you would fill out an OSHA Log 300 for workers in the manufacturing sector. OSHA, MSHA, the DoD, etc., have individual requirements that specify how baseline and annual monitoring hearing tests must be conducted, how any follow-up tests should be conducted, as well as what hearing loss changes must be formally reported. Make sure you are familiar with the appropriate regulations that you must abide by. It would be a good idea to keep copies of these regulations handy. The OSHA, MSHA standards, and the DoD instruction may all be downloaded for free at each organization's web site. The CAOHC *Hearing Conservation Manual* (CAOHC, 2002) also provides useful comparisons of various HLPP standards.

Regulations stipulate that an audiologist, physician, or a qualified technician can conduct audiometric testing, and either an audiologist or physician must supervise the audiometric testing component to the HCP. If you are supervising audiometric technicians, you should ensure that they have been properly trained. OSHA and MSHA recognize CAOHC certification as an Occupational Hearing Conservationist (OHC) as constituting appropriate training for an audiometric technician. Some states may also require licensure for audiometric technicians. It is your professional responsibility to ensure that any technicians you supervise have appropriate certification and comply with local licensure requirements.

The early detection of NIHL using pure-tone audiometry is confounded by many factors in the practical world; age corrections to pure-tone thresholds may not be appropriate for all individuals, baseline tests may be contaminated with pre-test noise exposure, audiograms are not transferred to successive employers and not all audiograms are reviewed for validity. Ultimately, it is in the workers' best interest to maintain their own long-term personal audiometric records with support from audiologists.

Training.   Training is not just "nice to have." Effective training is possibly the most essential component of HLPPs. It empowers individuals to make good decisions about their hearing health and value their hearing. Most HLPP standards require training with timelines and content specified. For example, the OSHA Hearing Conservation Amendment (29 CFR 1910.95) requires initial and annual training for all employees whose time-weighted average exposure equals or exceeds 85 dBA. Furthermore, OSHA specifies the training must address: (1) the effect of noise on hearing, (2) the purpose of hearing protection, including the advantages, disadvantages, and attenuation of various types, as well as instructions on selection, fitting, use, and care of HPDs, and (3) the purpose of audiometric testing, and an explanation of the test procedures. An effective training program will both educate and motivate. It is safe to say that without effective training a HLPP program has minimal, if any, chance of success.

Effective training will result in supervisors taking the program seriously and motivate decision makers to provide a supportive climate and adequate resources. Effective group or individual training will help employees learn to value their hearing and convince them they can take control of their hearing health and prevent NIHL. It is very important that training be tailored to the specific audience. If you choose to employ "canned" training materials, you must be ready to tweak them to ensure relevance to your audience. While studies have demonstrated the best way to influence safety behaviors is to repeat the message, you should make every attempt to vary the educational materials from year to year.

Training is where you will have the best opportunity to address the barriers that prevent workers from using HPDs. Ask workers what prevents them from using HPDs and make every effort to provide information and HPDs that address workers' needs and resolve any reported problems. It may seem that passing out HPDs and asking workers to use the package instructions would be adequate to ensure HPDs are worn correctly. This is *absolutely not the case*! Workers *must* be shown how to fit and use HPDs. (Berger, 2000; Joseph, 2004). Both NIOSH and the NHCA have a wealth of information you can use to help you develop an effective HLPP training program: <www.cdc.gov/niosh/topics/noise/>, <www.hearingconservation.org>.

Program Effectiveness.   The goal of any HLPP is to eliminate NIHL. One way of monitoring the status of this goal is to track the incidence (i.e., new cases) of significant threshold shifts. OSHA and MSHA use the term "standard threshold shift" (STS) to describe a significant change from baseline hearing levels. As mentioned previously, they define STS as a change in either ear from a person's baseline that averages 10 dB or more (when averaged across 2000, 3000, and 4000 Hz). OSHA and MSHA also permit the use of age corrections when determining if standard threshold shift is present. There is not a professional or scientific consensus on what constitutes a significant threshold shift. NIOSH (1998) and the American Academy of Audiology (2003) recommend using a persistent change of 15 dB at any individual test frequency. The military has adopted a two-stage process: they use a 15 dB change at 1, 2, 3, and 4 kHz as an "early warning" indicator and the OSHA procedure for computing STS. However, the military does not allow the use of age corrections when computing STS (DoD, 2004). Other approaches to determining program effectiveness have utilized a comparison of the percentages of compensable hearing loss, or shift rate comparisons between job categories, departments or plant locations. There really is no definitive way of critiquing program effectiveness. It is a matter of how much hearing loss you are willing to accept before raising a flag that a hearing loss may have occurred. Ideally, it is desirable to have an STS incidence of 0 percent; realistically, this is unlikely. Currently, NIOSH recommends using a 3 percent STS incidence as a criterion for an effective HLPP. For more information, see section 5.9 "Evaluation of Program Effectiveness" in the NIOSH revised criteria for occupational noise exposure (NIOSH, 1998).

EDUCATIONAL MODEL

In terms of hearing loss prevention, two health educational models have been utilized: primarily: the "Health Belief Model" (HBM) and the "Stages of Change Model" (SCM). The HBM is a psychologically based model, which attempts to explain and predict health behaviors by focusing on the attitudes and beliefs of individuals. The key provisions of the HBM model applied to hearing loss prevention are (1) Perceived Susceptibility: one's subjective perception of the risk of developing a NIHL, (2) Perceived Severity: one's feelings about the seriousness of NIHL and opportunities for amelioration, (3) Perceived Benefits: how effective are the strategies to reduce the threat of NIHL, (4) Perceived Barriers: any negative consequences which result from taking particular actions to prevent NIHL such as the potential negative social implications of hearing protector use, the economics of purchasing hearing protectors etc., (5) Cues to Action: bodily symptoms (e.g., tinnitus) or environmental events (e.g., media publicity) that motivate people to take action, (6) Other Variables: such as cultural diversity that may affect an individual's perceptions and health-related behaviors, and (7) Self-Efficacy: the confidence that one can successfully execute the behavior required to prevent NIHL. (Janz & Becker, 1984).

The SCM outlines an individual's readiness to change, or attempt to change, unhealthy behaviors such as not wearing hearing protectors in hazardous noise environments. In this model, behavior change is viewed as a process, with groups of individuals functioning at different points in the process (Prochaska, Norcross, & DiClemente, 1994). The six stages of behavior change have been identified as (1) Precontemplation: A person is unaware of the risk of hazardous noise levels and has not thought about any behavior changes, (2) Contemplation: a person is seriously thinking about a behavior change (e.g., wear earplugs/earmuffs) in the near future, (3) Preparation: the person is planning to take action and making final adjustments (e.g., purchasing earplugs/earmuffs), (4) Action: the person implements some specific action plan to overtly modify behavior and surroundings (e.g., wears earplugs/earmuffs while doing noisy activities), (5) Maintenance: the person continues with desirable actions and works to prevent lapses and relapses back to unhealthy behaviors, and (6) Termination: the person has zero temptation and has the ability to resist relapse. This model is not sequential and a person may spiral through several cycles of the stages before permanently changing behavior. For instance, an individual may utilize hearing protection at work religiously, while the use of hearing protection for recreational pursuits such as hunting is at a different stage.

Audiologists can utilize their teaching skills to provide educational presentations in formal training programs provided to local employees/employers or in public forums. Marketing efforts such as private practice newsletters and websites provide educational opportunities to inform and motivate readers. Audiologists can facilitate an individual's journey through the behavior changes via counseling and professional support. For instance, when an audiologist provides a monitoring audiogram that reveals stable hearing thresholds, a perfect opportunity exists to praise the patient's behavior change and reinforce the continued use of hearing protectors in order to prevent relapse. When hearing protection is dispensed directly in clinical practices it easily accommodates an individual's progression to an "action" stage in the behavior change process.

Formal training content will be dependent upon the nature of the educational outreach, but in general will include the general topics of (1) how we hear, (2) how noise damages hearing, (3) the effects of hearing loss, (4) recognition of hazardous noise sources in terms of intensity and duration, (5) strategies to minimize noise exposures such as moving away from the noise source, purchasing quiet equipment and maintaining equipment for optimal performance, (6) the proper selection and fitting of hearing protection, and (7) the purpose and outcomes of audiometric testing. Training tailored to the sound experiences of the audience will be more relevant and useful than generic training programs (Royster & Royster, 1990). Although the research literature frequently reports an improvement in the knowledge gained from training endeavors, direct evidence of subsequent behavior change is lacking. Research is needed to better define who the most effective trainer is, what the critical content is and what delivery method(s) are most successful at changing behavior in persons of all ethnicities and cultures.

The HBM and the SCM have primarily been utilized to promote behavior change in adolescents and adults. For younger children, health education models primarily are grounded within the school environment. Health promotions in the schools generally incorporate three characteristic components or domains of activity; (1) Formal Health Curriculum that gives school-aged children the essential knowledge and skills that will allow them to make enlightened choices regarding the prevention of NIHL, (2) the School Environment, which refers to the quality of the physical environment and the school climate relative to health services and school policies (e.g. hearing protection is available in classrooms, noise levels are controlled and monitored), and (3) the School/Community interaction (e.g., parents expect the school environment to be acoustically safe for their children) (Parsons, Stears, & Thomas, 1996).

Unfortunately, it appears that our efforts to infuse hearing loss prevention within school curriculums, school environments and communities have had limited successes. Folmer (2003) outlined several reasons regarding the omission of basic hearing loss prevention information in the schools. These include a lack of public awareness regarding the risk of NIHL, the relatively less severe health consequences of NIHL when compared with more serious, potentially life-threatening health issues, poor dissemination of existing hearing conservation educational programs, the lack of perpetuation of educational programs once implemented and the lack of a legal mandate requiring HLPPs for children and schools. Each audiologist has a social and professional obligation to raise public awareness of hearing and the potential damage from noise by educating the general public, teachers, administrators and parents. Audiologists are encouraged to personally advocate for school curriculums (K–12 grades) that incorporate hearing loss prevention concepts. Audiologists can also advocate for local, state and/or federal mandates to require HLPPs for children, teachers and school district employees. Innovative, large-scale public health campaigns held at farm shows, state fairs, museums, sporting venues, governmental offices and community events are encouraged. These campaigns are feasible when implemented as a public outreach and/or marketing effort by local and regional audiology professional associations.

When one considers the potential for hazardous noise exposure of children who are not yet old enough to attend school, it becomes apparent that educational outreach needs to access a different domain other than schools, such as parent groups and pre-school teachers. Parenting classes can incorporate hearing loss prevention into their health and safety topics for expectant parents. Community child safety fairs are occasionally offered through local health departments or community agencies. Universal newborn hearing screening programs provide audiologists a unique opportunity to reinforce the value of good hearing and the need to protect a child's hearing throughout the years as they grow and experience new activities. Newborn hearing screening brochures might incorporate a message such as *"Repeated exposure to loud sounds without hearing protection may contribute to the development of noise-induced hearing loss in children."* This is similar to the approach used to alert parents to a possibility of otitis media and the need to monitor their child's hearing in the future.

Education may be the key to all that we hope to accomplish relative to hearing loss prevention for all age groups. Audiologists are encouraged to look for these educational opportunities and actively contribute their expertise.

MEDICAL TREATMENT MODEL

At the heart of the medical treatment model of hearing loss prevention is the belief that if the pathophysiology of NIHL can be unraveled, then medical treatments can prevent and/or cure the disorder. Advances in molecular biology, biochemistry, histopathological techniques and electron microscopy have contributed to our understanding of the pathologic changes in the auditory system from noise exposure and provide tools to evaluate the benefit of potential medical/nutritional treatments. Stockwell, Ades, and Engstrom (1969) were the first to propose that two different mechanisms might underlie NIHL: direct mechanical trauma to the Organ of Corti and metabolic stress from maintaining high levels of biological activity over prolonged periods of time. Advances in our understanding of these underlying mechanisms and their associated timelines afford an opportunity to intervene with proactive medical/nutritional treatments prior to noise exposure or rescue an ear from further degeneration following a hazardous noise exposure.

Pathophysiology of NIHL

Hazardous sound exposures cause anatomical, physiological and biochemical changes in the auditory system, primarily in the cochlea. The amount of damage is highly dependent upon both intrinsic (species, genetics, susceptibility) and extrinsic variables (intensity, duration, frequency characteristics of noise). Acoustic damage to the ear has both an initial dynamic phase and a subsequent static phase (Saunders, Cohen, & Szymko, 1991). Human research is limited by ethical considerations and the difficulties in obtaining human tissue with documented exposure histories. Human studies are typically limited to the use of indirect measures of auditory damage via audiometric pure-tone threshold testing, electrophysiologic tests and otoacoustic emissions. Animal studies afford the best research opportunity for control of these variables and for evaluating the auditory damage and their associated time course at specific stages of degeneration and repair. From these studies, it appears that there are critical levels of noise exposure for particular types of damage.

Irreparable damage to the cochlea may occur above this critical level due to permanent mechanical and structural damage. This is the case with acoustic trauma, whereby the tissues and structures of the outer, middle and/or inner ear(s) are literally torn apart. This type of damage is most often caused by impulse noise that is characterized by short duration (~< 100 ms), high intensity (~> 125 dB SPL) sound bursts. Often these exposures are unanticipated. Acoustic trauma has been reported as a consequence of a gas pipe exploding, a school bus tire blowing up while changing a flat, an automotive airbag exploding, a firework blast occurring nearby or telephone/communication headsets malfunctioning among others. Subjectively, the NIHL is evident immediately.

In terms of gradual onset NIHL due to moderate levels of continuous noise exposure, the auditory damage in the cochlea includes swollen and missing hair cells, stereocilia disarray, discontinuity between stereocilia and the tectorial membrane and obvious disruption of supporting cellular architecture. The auditory degeneration begins when the thin strands of protofilaments (tip links), which connect the tip of one hair cell to the shaft of the next tallest hair cell, are broken and the stereocilia rootlets may shorten (Liberman, 1987). This results in floppy or disarrayed stereocilia, which may recover through the regeneration or reattachment of tip links and afford a possible physiological explanation for temporary threshold shift (TTS) (Kurian, Krupp, & Saunders, 2003; Patuzzi, 2002). Irreversible changes begin to occur when the cilia become fractured and are scavenged. Beyond the stereocilia micromechanics, additional changes occur in outer hair cell (OHC) motility, cellular energy metabolism, pillar cells, inner ear blood flow, ion and fluid balances, cytoskeletal proteins and the structure and function of mitochondria and endoplasmic reticulum (Miller, Schacht, & Altschuler, 2001). Ultimately, outer hair cells become metabolically exhausted and undergo necrosis or apoptosis and scarring replaces previously healthy tissues.

Current pathophysiology theory of NIHL focuses on the underlying biochemical processes within the cochlea and proposes that NIHL is primarily due to excitoxicity and metabolic stress, especially as related to the outer hair cells and their stereocilia. Outer hair cells with normal functioning transduction channels are essential to normal cochlear function. They enhance and sharpen the mechanical basilar membrane displacement necessary for initiation of eighth nerve afferent signaling from inner hair cells. Metabolic stress occurs when outer hair cells are responding to high intensity noise sources over prolonged periods of time which results in biochemical and molecular changes within the cochlea which ultimately lead to cell damage and cell death. Normal metabolic activity is associated with the formation of reactive oxygen molecules (ROM) also called reactive oxygen species (ROS) or "free radicals." These metabolic byproducts are ordinarily scavenged by endogenous antioxidant systems that prevent their degenerative influence on the cochlea. As long as the ROS and antioxidant systems are in balance, cellular damage from ROS can be prevented. Excessive noise increases the production of ROS which damage phospholipids in cell and nuclear membranes and deoxyribonucleic acid (DNA), increase intracellular Ca++ and up-regulate apoptotic genes that lead to cell death (Miller et al., 2001). A review article by Henderson, Bielefeld, Harris, and Hu (2006) provides a more comprehensive review of the role of oxidative stress in NIHL for interested readers (Fig. 12–4).

Damage from noise is not limited to outer hair cells, but also destroys eighth nerve dendrites below the inner hair cells and results in dysfunction of the afferent auditory nerve synapses. The efferent feedback loop between outer hair cells and the central auditory system can also be disrupted when outer hair cells are damaged or destroyed. The damage may be temporary or permanent depending on the degree of trauma and the reconnection of inner hair cells to primary auditory neurons (Puel, Ruel, Gervais, & Pujol, 1998). In the central auditory system, spiral ganglion cells may degenerate in response to noise and damage may spread into the cochlear nucleus (Liberman and Mulroy, 1982).

Medical Intervention

Discovery of the biochemical and molecular changes underlying NIHL has led to efforts to control ROS formation and manipulate endogenous antioxidant systems through the use of otoprotectants. Under this model of hearing loss prevention,

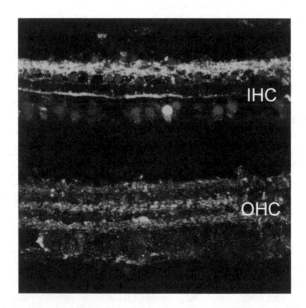

FIGURE 12–4.   Microphoto showing oxidative stress in a chinchilla organ of Corti observed 30 min after exposure to an impulse noise at 155 dB SPL. The specimen was stained with 5-(pentafluorobenzoylamino) dihydrofluorescein diacetate (PFB-H2FDA) which illustrated free radical generation. The generation of oxidative stress is illustrated by the brighter white fluorescence around both the inner hair cell (IHC) and outer hair cell regions. (Courtesy of Donald H. Henderson, PhD, and Bohua Hu, PhD, State University of New York at Buffalo)

increasing the cellular level of antioxidants in the inner ear either via naturally occurring nutritional supplements or pharmacological treatments prevents NIHL. Henderson, Bielefeld, Harris and Hu (2006) outline four interventions to reduce the damaging effects of noise, (1) restoring the normal balance of ROS with antioxidants or
substrates for antioxidant synthesis, (2) limiting the amount of lipid peroxidation, (3)
maintaining adequate cochlear blood flow during and after noise exposure, and (4)
preserving hair cells by inhibiting pathways to apoptotic cell death. Antioxidant
cellular levels can be increased by several techniques; (1) gene-therapy to increase
production of antioxidants (van de Water, Staecker, Halterman & Federoff, 1999);
(2) upregulating endogenous antioxidant enzyme levels (Hu, Zheng, McFadden,
Kopke & Henderson, 1997); (3) rapid restoration of glutathione (Yamasoba, Nuttall,
Harris, Raphael & Miller, 1998); and (4) administration of antioxidants (Henderson,
McFadden, Liu, High & Zheng, 1999). For example, increased levels of antioxidants
such as glutathione have been shown to reduce the effects of noise trauma in the
guinea pig ear (Yamasoba et al., 1998). Glutathione may also be an effective prophylactic intervention when given in advance of noise exposure (Ohinata, Yamasoba,
Schacht, & Miller, 2000). Treatment delivery systems incorporate a direct pharmacological infusion to the round window or indirectly through systemic application.
Treatments may be administered prior to the exposure, during the exposure or after
the exposure in an effort to rescue the ear from auditory damage.

Other attempts to protect the ear involve the use of dietary supplements known
to promote antioxidants such as vitamins A, C, E, ebselen, phenylisopropyladeno-
sine (R-PIA) and selenium or through dietary modifications to include foods rich
in other micronutrients such as magnesium found in fish, almonds, spinach, shrimp
and bran, D-Methionine (D-MET) found in cheese and yogurt, N-Acetylcysteine
(NAC) found in brussel sprouts and resveratrol found in red wine (Campbell, 2002;
Hu et al., 1997; Lynch, Gu, Pierce, & Kil, 2004; Pourkbakht & Yamasoba, 2003;
Rosen, Olin, & Rosen, 1970; Seidmman, Babu, Tang, Naem, & Quirk, 2003). The
micronutrients found in food can also be given as a dietary supplement.

Some otoprotectants show additional benefit when given in combinations or
when paired with salicylates (Kopke et al., 2000). In general, there is evidence that
at least partial prevention of NIHL from both continuous and/or impulse noise exposures in animals and/or humans is feasible, however none are totally protective. The
dose/effect relationships specific to various types and durations of noise exposures
and across individuals are not known. Additional limitations include possible side
effects such as nausea, vomiting or diarrhea and otoprotectants may be contraindicated for certain individuals such as those with schizophrenia or liver disease.

Currently, the Food and Drug Administration (FDA) has not legally approved
an otoprotectant agent for marketing as a means of preventing or treating NIHL. For
now, the details regarding clinical uses of otoprotectants remain under active investigation. In the future, audiologists will find themselves implementing otoprotectants
as a hearing loss prevention strategy and monitoring the effectiveness of otoprotectants in partnership with physicians. While it is predicted that the use of otoprotectants
will be considered under all hearing loss prevention models, otoprotectants are not expected to be mandated by a government agency under regulatory models. In other
words, a worker would not be required to take a dose of otoprotectant prior to work-

ing or being exposed to noise. In the future, there may be an exception to this for military noise exposures where hearing protection use is not easily implemented nor adequate for all noise hazardous situations, consequently otoprotectants might be administered prior to combat duty. Otoprotectants are not expected to replace hearing protection; however they may be used in conjunction with earplugs/earmuffs, especially when noise exposures are extreme. Educational models will incorporate the general topic of otoprotectants and health behavior changes may involve dietary modifications or supplement use. In the future, otoprotectants may prove to be an essential tool in the preventive medicine approach, especially in terms of treatment for NIHL.

PREVENTIVE MEDICINE MODEL

Preventive medicine is founded upon the belief that it is better to avoid the occurrence of disease or disability than to treat one. Preventive medicine is a blend of clinical skills and public health knowledge to reduce the risk of disease, death and disability in individuals and communities. A preventive medicine model approaches disease prevention on three levels: primary, secondary and tertiary. The primary prevention encompasses the efforts aimed at reducing the potential for disease or illness in someone who does not have the disease but might develop it in the future, such as immunizations in healthy children. Secondary prevention focuses on identifying and treating an asymptomatic person who has risk factors for the disease or early indications of the disease that are not readily identified by the patient, such as mammograms to detect early forms of breast cancer. Tertiary prevention involves the treatment of symptomatic individuals in an effort to decrease complication and minimize the severity and consequences of the disease, such as monitoring sugar control in a diabetic patient.

The preventive health model has been widely accepted in western medicine over recent years. We expect physicians to utilize blood tests, mammograms and other diagnostic tests for early detection of disease. We expect dentists and dental hygienists to instruct us in the use of dental floss and to monitor the health of our teeth. Healthcare providers are expected to not only treat diseases, but to prevent them. Audiologists are uniquely positioned to adopt a preventive medicine approach to NIHL by (1) preventing the occurrence of NIHL, (2) providing early detection and intervention to minimize the effects of NIHL, and (3) palliating the effects of NIHL by providing comprehensive diagnostic and rehabilitative services.

Primary Prevention: Eliminate the Risk

Primary prevention of NIHL can easily be incorporated into routine practices by embracing a proactive attitude. Employers and consumers can purchase quieter equipment and/or implement noise controls to reduce noise levels of existing equipment or products. Audiologists can use case history information to identify potential noise risks for patients of all ages, educational brochures and information can be provided in patient waiting areas and complimentary hearing protection samples and instructions can be distributed to all patients to teach them to avoid the noise risk. Audiologists can be community advocates for reduced noise exposures and become instrumental in promoting responsible listening habits and reasonable sound levels at public events. Similar to HLPP models; public speaking engagements, newsletter columns and modeling of healthy listening behaviors are all opportunities for the audiologist to promote their practice and support public health outreach efforts.

Secondary Prevention: Early Detection and Intervention

Traditionally, audiologists have practiced the secondary level of the preventive medicine model while working in the occupational setting under regulatory HCPs. The early warning sign of a subtle change in high frequency hearing is used to alert employees to their personal risk of permanent NIHL. When done correctly, pure-tone audiometry is the gold standard for the early detection of NIHL as incorporated into our regulatory requirements for HCPs. Using a preventive approach, a change in hearing or the occurrence of tinnitus following noise exposure becomes the trigger for action. The audiologist can then facilitate the necessary intervention by: obtaining detailed case histories, updating noise exposure data, evaluating hearing protectors and resolving communication issues that may be preventing the use of hearing protectors.

As important as audiometry, secondary intervention also includes a detailed case history incorporating a discussion of both occupational and non-occupational sources of noise exposure. Noise records may be requested from employers and a reassessment of current exposure levels may be indicated, especially if records are outdated. Measures of non-occupational noise exposures are also useful. Hearing protection attenuation may then be reconciled to the noise exposures and the fit checked to assure appropriate levels of protection. In cases of noise exposure above 100 dBA, dual hearing protection (earplugs worn in combination with earmuffs) may be recommended as well as more frequent audiometric monitoring. The patients can be asked to bring their earplugs/earmuffs to the office visit. This will permit the audiologist to inspect the condition of the HPD and evaluate the wearers' ability to insert their hearing protectors. The fit can be evaluated using a visual/physical inspection of the HPD and objective measures of sound-field attenuation. The latter is especially important when 100 percent compliance with hearing protector use is reported in persons with a STS. More than one type of hearing protection may be dispensed to patients with diverse noise exposures. At this stage, medical referral for a differential diagnosis may be indicated, especially in cases of asymmetrical or progressive sensorineural hearing loss or when hearing changes are accompanied by dizziness, ear pain, drainage or severe tinnitus.

Research continues to investigate other diagnostic tools that may provide early detection of NIHL such as otoacoustic emissions (OAEs). Spontaneous otoacoustic emissions (SOAEs), transient otoacoustic emissions (TEOAEs) and distortion product otoacoustic emissions (DPOAEs) all demonstrate a reduction in emission level as a result of hazardous noise exposure (Lonsbury-Martin & Martin, 2001). This is often called a noise-induced emission loss (NIEL). The relationships between noise exposure and OAEs are complex. Avan, Bonfils and Loth (1996) noted that TEOAE and DPOAE amplitudes are most useful for detection of NIHL in excess of 30 dBHL. Our ability to use OAEs to predict auditory sensitivity or monitor the cochlea for sub-clinical signs of NIHL is still under active investigation (Marshall, Lapsley Miller, & Heller, 2000). Clinically, OAEs serve to complement behavioral pure-tone audiometry. Researchers hope to advance our understanding of the underlying mechanisms of OAE generation and better understand how the choice of stimulus parameters might enhance our ability to detect NIHL in the future.

Audiologists have a tremendous opportunity to incorporate the secondary preventive level of care into standard clinical practice. The inclusion of 3- and 6 kHz thresholds as part of routine pure-tone test protocols will enable the early detection of NIHL in asymptomatic clients. Many patients (and potential clients) are exposed to recreational and occupational noise sources. They may not be part of a formal employer-based hearing conservation program. These individuals need a structured program of routine audiometric testing and analysis to provide for the early identification of NIHL and to monitor the effectiveness of their personal hearing protector choices. These potential patients need audiologists familiar with their diverse listening demands and audiologists who are capable of fitting and dispensing an assortment of hearing protectors. Audiology as a profession should not make the same mistake with hearing protection that was made with hearing aids decades ago. Prior to the time that audiologists directly dispensed amplification, they recommended a hearing aid and then sent the client elsewhere to purchase the device. This is a common approach relative to hearing protection in clinical practices today. Hearing protection should be directly dispensed in an audiology practice and our clients need not be sent elsewhere to find the devices necessary to protect their ears. A variety of hearing protectors may be stocked in the office and provide the client a choice based on the five C's. Custom earplugs are not necessarily the best choice for all patients. An audiologist's professional role and patient base can be expanded under a preventive medicine model especially when one considers the opportunities to incorporate comprehensive hearing loss prevention services and products.

Tertiary Prevention: Diagnosis and Treatment

Unfortunately, without an effective secondary level of preventive audiological care, there will be permanent NIHL, requiring the tertiary level of preventive medicine. At this point, the audiologist becomes involved in the diagnosis and treatment of individuals with symptomatic NIHL in an effort to maintain communication skills and minimize the effects of NIHL on the quality of life. Clients may seek audiology services independently, upon referral from employers for the determination of work-relatedness for regulatory recordkeeping requirements or as part of a worker's compensation evaluation. Job functions may become more difficult and workplace accommodations may be requested.

Differential Diagnosis.   The differential diagnosis of NIHL relies primarily on the gold standard of reliable audiometric threshold testing. The classic configuration of a notched high-frequency sensory hearing loss is often the most salient feature, especially for younger patients. Other diagnostic tests such as speech testing, immittance measures, acoustic reflex thresholds, OAEs and auditory brainstem response are consistent with a sensory impairment in the cochlea. Special test techniques may be required for cases of suspected functional hearing loss, especially when the visit is for the purposes of qualifying for financial compensation. Since age-related hearing loss occurs in the same high-frequency range as NIHL, it often is challenging if not impossible to differentiate the two pathologies, particularly for older patients. Serial audiograms completed before, during and after the period of hazardous noise exposures are most helpful in identifying whether noise exposure contributed to the hearing loss measured in an older person.

Work-relatedness.   Separate work-related determinations may be necessary for regulatory compliance (e.g., OSHA 300 Log Recordability) and for workers' compensation or disability claims. A team approach with the audiologist working in collaboration with physicians, industrial hygienists, occupational nurses, and industrial audiometric test providers is critical for accurate determinations. In terms of differentiating work-related hearing loss, a series of questions serve to guide professionals through the decision-making process: (1) Is a hearing loss evident? (2) Is the hearing loss consistent with NIHL? (3) Is there evidence of hazardous noise exposure(s)? (4) Was hearing protection utilized for each hazardous noise exposure? (5) Was the HPD attenuation adequate for the noise hazard(s)? (6) Was the hearing protector fit and worn correctly in order to provide adequate attenuation? and (7) Were there any combined exposures that might exacerbate the noise exposure? (adapted from Dobie & Megerson, 2000). It is imperative to conduct comprehensive patient interviews and to review detailed records from employers and other healthcare providers. Workers' compensation benefits are neither universal nor standardized across the U.S., nor are NIHLs treated equally in all states. In many states, the determination comes down to a "medical opinion", and in these instances variable determinations may be made based on the damage risk criteria and recommended exposure limits referenced by the medical provider. Additionally, many jurisdictions reference various hearing impairment formulae and different payment schedules. The applicable workers' compensation laws should always be consulted. In addition, audiologists will find the review provided by Dobie and Megerson (2000) most helpful in determining the issues relative to a specific practice area.

Damage Risk Criteria and Recommended Exposure Limits.   Audiologists are frequently asked if a given noise can cause hearing loss. To answer this question properly, you need to know a number of things. For example, the spectrum and rise-time of the noise, concomitant exposure to other noise, medications, exposure to ototoxicants such as solvents, asphyxiates, or heavy metals, history of smoking, gender, ethnicity, and individual susceptibility (to name a few) influence the characteristics, time-course and severity of NIHL. However, by far, the most important variables for any given exposure are the noise level and duration of the exposure, and the time period (e.g., days, weeks, years) over which the exposure(s) take place.

Sometimes you will want to know how much NIPTS can be expected after a number of years of occupational exposure to a given noise. There is an excellent source you can turn to for information about the amount of NIPTS as a function of exposure level and years of exposure: ANSI S3.44 1996, *Determination of Occu-*

pational Noise Exposure and Estimation of Noise-Induced Hearing Impairment. This document provides convenient tables that list the predicted NIPTS for the median, 10th and 90th percentiles of the population from daily TWA exposures to 80, 85, 90, 95, and 100 dBA for 10, 20, 30, and 40 years of exposure. It provides equations that enable you to calculate the NIPTS for other percentiles, durations, and levels. There are also a number of other reference values for normal hearing levels as a function of gender, ethnicity, age, and medical history. If you deal at all with noise-induced hearing loss, this document will be indispensable.

Other times, you will want to know whether or not a given noise event is potentially harmful. In the U.S. today, there are two approaches for determining whether or not a noise is hazardous. The first method uses a 90 dBA permissible exposure limit (PEL) and a 5-dB exchange rate. It has been adopted by the U.S. Department of Labor in the OSHA and MSHA hearing conservation regulations. Thus, OSHA and MSHA consider any noise exposure to be hazardous if it exceeds an 8-hour TWA of 90 dBA. A 5-dB exchange rate means that over the course of an 8-hour day, an 8-hour exposure to a 90 dBA noise would be equally hazardous as 4-hours of exposure to 95 dBA, 2 hours of exposure to 100 dBA, and so forth.

The second method is based on an 85 dB recommended exposure limit (REL) and a 3-dB exchange rate. This has been adopted by NIOSH (1998b), the Department of Defense, the American Academy of Audiology, the National Hearing Conservation Association, the American Conference of Governmental Industrial Hygienists, and the American Industrial Hygiene Association. Sometimes the 3-dB exchange rate is referred to as the "equal energy rule" because the energy in a noise doubles with every 3-dB increase. Thus, over the course of an 8-hour day, an 8-hour exposure to an 85 dBA A noise would be equally hazardous (and would have the same energy) as a 4-hour exposure to an 88 dBA, a 2-hour exposure to 91 dBA, and so forth.

There is no "right" or "wrong" exposure level. It is a matter of how you define "hearing loss" and how much hearing loss risk you feel is acceptable. For example, after a lifetime (i.e., 40 years) of daily exposure to 90 dBA, approximately 25 percent of those exposed will develop a material hearing impairment.[1] Those similarly exposed to time-weighted averages of 85 or 80 dBA could expect to have 8 percent and 1 percent incidences of material hearing impairment, respectively (NIOSH, 1998b). It is worth noting that impulsive sounds (e.g., gunfire, hammering) are considered to be more hazardous than continuous-type noises. To account for this, ANSI S3.44–1996 allows a +5 dB correction factor to be added to TWAs that are based on exposure to impulsive sounds. Thus a 90 dBA TWA exposure that was derived from impulsive events could be treated as a 95 dBA exposure. These damage-risk criteria have all been based on studies evaluating NIHL in adults. There are currently no specific criteria which have been developed for children or to consider the risk of NIHL across the entire lifespan and not just limited to a typical 40 year working career.

---

[1] Material hearing impairment is defined as an average of the hearing threshold levels for both ears at 500, 1000, and 2000 Hz that exceeds 25 dB hearing level.

Rehabilitation. NIHL may require amplification when it has progressed into the speech frequencies and begins to impact audibility. In such cases, the patient will need guidance relative to wearing the hearing aids in noise-hazardous environments and how best to communicate in environments where hearing protection is required. Specialized hearing protectors may need to be dispensed in addition to the hearing aid(s). Assistive listening devices may be useful in the workplace for group listening and/or training activities. Special consideration should be given to the worker's ability to hear critical warning signals and communication, especially while wearing hearing protectors. Pagers, visual signaling devices and other strategies may be beneficial to the worker. These items may be provided through workers' compensation benefits or through workplace accommodation requests by the worker as provided for by the Americans with Disabilities Act (ADA). Lastly, the worker may be concerned that the hearing loss has progressed to a point where he/she can no longer perform the essential functions of his/her job. In such cases, the audiologist will be called upon to review the applicable hearing criteria and evaluate the auditory skills necessary for job performance.

Summary

As mentioned previously, there is no single approach to hearing loss prevention that is ideal for all situations and persons. Opportunities to apply hearing loss prevention models will vary with the setting and the circumstances that audiologists work in. There may be times when one preventive model is an obvious choice and others whereby the HLPP will be customized to an individual using a combination of components from various models. Flexible approaches will ensure that HLPPs are adaptable to changes in the environment and utilize progressive interventions over time.

For patients of all ages, your audiology skills and expertise are critical to the prevention, early identification and treatment of NIHL. Embrace a prevention attitude and integrate prevention services into your professional practice. Take the time to explore the opportunities that exist in your communities, schools, recreational venues, and local employers to educate and motivate. The young deserve to hear when they get old.

ACKNOWLEDGMENTS

The findings and conclusions in this chapter are those of the author(s) and do not necessarily represent the views of the National Institute for Occupational Safety and Health.

REFERENCES

American Academy of Audiology. (2003). *Position statement: Preventing noise-induced occupational hearing loss.* Reston, VA.

American Academy of Pediatrics Committee on Environmental Health & Health. (1997). Noise: A hazard for the fetus and newborn. *Pediatrics, 100*(4), 724–727.

Abrams, R. M., & Gerhardt, K. J. (2000). The acoustic environment and physiological responses of the fetus. *Journal of Perinatology, 20,* S30–S35.

American Conference of Governmental Industrial Hygienists. (2004). *2004 TLVs and BEIs*. Cinncinati, OH: ACGIH.

Anagnostakis, D., Petmezakis, J., Messaritakis, J., & Matsaniotis, N. (1980). Noise pollution in neonatal units: A potential health hazard. *Acta paediatrica Scandinavica, 69*, 771–773.

ANSI. (1996). *American national standard: Determination of occupational noise exposure and estimation of noise-induced hearing impairment.* (ANSI S3.44–1996). New York: American National Standards Institute, Inc.

Avan, P., Bonfils, P., & Loth, D. (1996). Effects of acoustic overstimulation on distortion-product and transient-evoked otoacoustic emissions. In A. Axelsson, H. Borchgrevink, R. Hamernik, P. Hellstrom, D. Henderson & R. Salvi (Eds.), *Scientific basis of noise-induced hearing loss* (pp. 65–81). Stuttgart: Thieme.

Axelsson, A. (1995). Tinnitus epidemiology. In G. Reich, & J. Vernon (Eds.), *Proceedings of the fifth international tinnitus seminar* (pp. 249–254). Portland, OR: The American Tinnitus Association.

Berger, E. H. (2000). Hearing Protection Devices. In E. H Berger, L. H. Royster, J. D. Royster, D. D. Driscoll, & M. Layne (Eds.), *The noise manual* (pp. 379–454). Fairfax, VA: American Industrial Hygiene Association.

Blair, J. C., Hardegree, D., & Benson, P. V. (1996). Necessity and effectiveness of a hearing conservation program for elementary students. *Journal of Educational Audiology, 4*, 12–16.

Broste, S. K., Hansen, D. A., Strand, R. L., & Stueland, D. T. (1989). Hearing loss among high school farm students. *American Journal of Public Health, 79*(5), 619–622.

Campbell, K. C. M. (2002). Developing otoprotectant agents for ototoxic and noise induced hearing loss: D-methionine and other compounds. *NHCA Spectrum, 19*(2), 12–14.

CAOHC. (2002). *Hearing conservation manual*. Milwaukee, WI: Council for Accreditation in Occupational Hearing Conservation.

Chermack, G. D., & Peters-McCarthy, E. (1991). The effectiveness of an educational hearing conservation program for elementary school children. *Language, Speech and Hearing Services in Schools, 22*(1), 308–312.

Clark, W. W. (1991). Noise exposure from leisure activities: A review. *Journal of the Acoustical Society of America, 90*(1), 175–181.

Coles, R., Smith, P., & Davis, A. (1990). The relationship between noise-induced hearing loss and tinnitus and its management. I, B. Berglund & T. lundvall (Eds.), Noise as a Public Health Problem (vol. 4). *New Advances in Noise Research. Part I* (pp. 87–112). Stockholm: Swedish Council for Building Research.

Cooper, J. C. J. (1994). Tinnitus, subjective hearing loss and well-being. Health and nutrition examination survey of 1971–75: Part II. *Journal of the American Academy of Audiology, 5*, 37–43.

Davis, A., & Rafaie, E. A. (2000). Epidemiology of Tinnitus. In R. Tyler (Ed.), *Tinnitus Handbook* (pp. 1–23). San Diego: Singular Publishing Group.

Dobie, R. A. (1993). *Medical-Legal Evaluation of Hearing Loss*. New York: Van Nostrand Reinhold.

Dobie, R. A., & Megerson, S. C. (2000). Workers' Compensation. In E. H Berger, L. H. Royster, J. D. Royster, D. D. Driscoll, & M. Layne (Eds.), *The noise manual* (pp. 689–710). Fairfax, VA: American Industrial Hygiene Association.

Environmental Protection Agency. (1973). *Public Health and Welfare Criteria for Noise*. Washington, DC: U.S. Environmental Protection Agency, EPA Report No. 550/9-73-002.

Environmental Protection Agency. (1974). *Information on levels of environmental noise requisite to protect public health and welfare with an adequate margin of safety*. Washington, DC: U.S. Environmental Protection Agency. EPA Report No. 550/9-74-004.

Fligor, B. J., & Cox, L. C. (2004). Output levels of commercially available portable compact disc players and the potential risk to hearing. *Ear and Hearing, 25*(6), 513–527.

Fligor, B. J. & Ivers, T. E. (2006) *Does earphone type affect risk for recreational noise-induced hearing loss?* [Abstract]. Retrieved 3/24/2006 from <http://www.amauditorysoc.org/downloads/AAS_2006_Meeting_Abstracts.pdf>

Folmer, R. L. (2003). The importance of hearing conservation instruction. *The Journal of School Nursing, 19*(3), 140–148.

Folmer, R. L., Griest, S. E., & Martin, W. H. (2002). Hearing conservation education programs for children: A review. *Journal of School Health, 72*(2), 51–57.

Gerhardt, K. J., Pierson, L., Huang, X., Abrams, R. M., & Rarey, K. E. (1999). Effects of intense noise exposure on fetal sheep auditory brainstem response and inner ear histology. *Ear and Hearing, 20,* 21–32.

Godlee, F. (1992). Noise: breaking the silence. *British Medical Journal, 304*(6819), 110–113.

Gottfried, A. W. (1985). Environment of newborn infants in special care units. In A. W. Gottfried & J. L. Gaiter (Eds.), *Infant stress under intensive care* (pp. 23–54). Baltimore, MD: University Park Press.

Graven, S. N. (2000). Sound and the developing infant in the NICU: Conclusions and recommendations for care. *Journal of Perinatology, 20*(8, Pt. 2), S88–S93.

Griest, S. E., & Bishop, P. M. (1998). Tinnitus as an early indicator of permanent hearing loss: A 15 year longitudinal study of noise exposed workers. *American Association Occupational Health Nurses Journal, 46,* 325–329.

Hager, L. (2006). *Recordable hearing loss in the United States 2004.* Paper presented at the 31st Annual Conference of the National Hearing Conservation Association, Tampa, FL.

Henderson, D., Bielefeld, E. C., Harris, K. C., & Hu, B. H. (2006). The role of oxidative stress in noise-induced hearing loss. *Ear & Hearing, 27*(1), 1–19.

Henderson, D., McFadden, S. L., Liu, C. C., Hight, N., & X. Y., Z. (1999). The role of antioxidants in protection from impulse noise. *Annals of the New York Academy of Sciences, 884,* 368–380.

Hetu, R., & Getty, L. (1991). The nature of the handicaps associated with occupational hearing loss: Implications for prevention. In W. Nobel (Ed.), *Occupational noise-induced hearing loss—Prevention and rehabilitation* (pp. 64–85). Papers presented at a national seminar series, November 1990. Sydney, National Occupational Health and Safety Commission; Armidale, The University of New England, Australia.

Hu, B. H., Zheng, X. Y., McFadden, S. L., Kopke, R., & Henderson, D. (1997). Phenylisophyladenoside attenuates noise-induced hearing loss in chinchilla. *Hearing Research, 113,* 198–206.

Humes, L. E., Joellenbeck, L. M., & Durch, J. S. (2005). *Noise and military service: Implications for hearing loss and tinnitus.* Washington, DC: National Academies Press.

Jackson, L. D., & Duffy, B. K. (1998). *Health communication research: A guide to developments and directions.* Westport, CT: Greenwood Publishing Group.

Janz, N. K., & Becker, M. H. (1984). The health belief model: A decade later. *Health Education Quarterly, 11*(1), 1–47.

Johnson, R. M., Coyne-Beasley, T., & Runyan, C. W. (2004). Firearm ownership and storage practices, U.S. households, 1992–2002. *American Journal of Preventive Medicine, 27,* 173–182.

Joseph, A. R. (2004). *Attenuation of passive hearing protection devices as a function of group versus individual training.* Doctoral Dissertation Michigan State University, East Lansing, MI.

Kopke, R., Weisskopf, P. A., Boone, J. L., Jackson, R. L., Wester, D. C., Hoffer, M. E., et al. (2000). Reduction of noise-induced hearing loss using L-NAC and salycylate in the chinchilla. *Hearing Research, 149*(1–2), 138–146.

Kurian, R., Krupp, N. L., & Saunders, J. C. (2003). Tip link loss and recovery on chick short hair cells following intense exposure to sound. *Hearing Research, 181*(1–2), 40–50.

Liberman, M. C. (1987). Chronic ultrastructural changes in acoustic trauma: Serial section reconstruction of stereocilia and cuticular plates. *Hearing Research, 26*(1), 65–88.

Liberman, M. C., & Mulroy, M. J. (1982). Acute and chronic effects of acoustic trauma: Cochlear pathology and auditory nerve pathophysiology. In R. P. Hamernik, D. Henderson, & R. J. Salvi (Eds.), *New perspectives on noise-induced hearing loss* (pp. 105–135). New York: Raven Press.

Lonsbury-Martin, B. L., & Martin, G. K. (2001). Otoacoustic Emissions. In A. F. Jahn & J. Santos-Sacchi (Eds.), *Physiology of the Ear* (pp. 443–480). San Diego: Singular.

Lynch, E. D., Gu, R., Pirece, C., & Kil, J. (2004). Ebselen-mediated protection from single and repeated noise exposure in rat. *Laryngoscope, 114*(2), 333–337.

Marshall, L., Lapsley Miller, J., & Heller, L. (2001). Distortion-Product Otoacoustic Emissions as a Screening Tool for Noise-Induced Hearing Loss. In D. Henderson, D. Prasher, R. Kopke, R. J. Salvi, & R. P. Hamernik (Eds.), *Noise induced hearing loss: Basic mechanisms, prevention and control* (pp. 453–470). London: NRN Publications.

Meinke, D. K., Meade, S., Johnson, C., & Jensema, J. (2005). *Industrial model of audiometric testing for high school students.* Poster session presented at the National Hearing Conservation Association 30th Annual Convention, Tucson, AZ.

Miller, J. M., Schacht, J., & Altschuler, R. (2001). Prevention of noise-induced hearing loss. In D. Henderson, D. Prasher, R. Kopke, & R. P. Hamernik (Eds.), *Noise induced hearing loss: basic mechanisms, prevention and control* (pp. 215–230). London: NRN publications.

Montgomery, J. K., & Fujikawa, S. (1992). Hearing thresholds of students in the second, eighth, and twelfth grades. *Language, Speech and Hearing Services in Schools, 23*, 61–63.

Morris, B. H., Philbin, M. K., & Bose, C. (2000). Physiological effects of sound on the newborn. *Journal of Perinatology, 20*, S53–S58.

MSHA (1999). Health standards for occupational noise exposure; Final rule. U.S. Department of Labor, Mine Safety and Health Administration, 30 CFR Part 62, 64, Fed Reg. 49458–49634, 49636–49637.

National Sports Shooting Foundation (2005). *Shooting.* Retrieved 11/30/2005 from <http://www.nssf.org/shooting_idx.cfm?AoI = shooting>

NIOSH. (1973). *Criteria for a recommended standard: occupational exposure to noise* (No. NIOSH Publication No. 73–11001). Cincinnati: U.S. Department of Health, Education, and Welfare, Health Services and Mental Health Administration, National Institute for Occupational Safety and Health.

NIOSH. (1998a). *Noise-Induced Hearing Loss—Attitudes and Behaviors of U.S. Adults.* Retrieved 11/30/2005 from <http://www.cdc.gov/niosh/topics/noise/abouthlp/nihlattitude.html>

NIOSH. (1998b). *Revised criteria for a recommended standard: Occupational noise exposure* (No. NIOSH Publication 98–126). Cincinnati U.S. Department of Health and Human Services, Public Health Service, Centers for Disease Control and Prevention, National Institute for Occupational Safety and Health, DHHS

NIOSH. (2004). *Worker health chartbook 2004* (No. DHHS Publication No. 2004-146). Cincinnati: NIOSH.

Niskar, A. S., Kieszak, S. M., Holmes, A., Esteban, E., Rubin, C., & Brody, D. (1998). Prevalence of hearing loss among children 6 to 19 years of age. *Journal of the American Medical Association, 279*(14), 1071–1075.

Niskar, A. S., Kieszak, S. M., Holmes, A. E., Esteban, E., Rubin, C., & Brody, D. (2001). Estimated prevalence of noise-induced hearing threshold shifts among children 6 to 19 years of age: The Third National Health and Nutrition Examination Survey, 1988–1994, United States. *Pediatrics, 108*(1), 40–43.

Odess, J. S. (1972). Acoustic trauma of sportsman hunter due to gun firing. *Larygoscope, 82*(11), 1971–1989.

Ohinata, Y., Miller, J. M., Altschuler, R. A., & Schact, J. (2000). Intense noise induces formation of vasoactive lipid perosidation products in the cochlea. *Brain Research, 878*, 163–173.

OSHA. (1983). 29 CFR 1910.95, *Occupational Noise Exposure.* 29 CFR 1910.95, Washington, DC: U.S. Department of Labor, Occupational Safety and Health Administration. Fed. Reg. Vo. 48, pp. 9738–9744.

OSHA. (2002). *Occupational injury and illness recording and reporting requirements.* 29 CFR 1904.10: U.S. Department of labor, Occupational Safety and Health Administration. Fed. Reg., December 17, 2002, Vol. 67, No. 242, pp. 77165–77170.

Parsons, C., Stears, D., & Thomas, C. (1996). The health promoting school in Europe: Conceptualizing and evaluating the change. *Health Education Journal, 55,* 311–321.

Patuzzi, R. (2002). Non-linear aspects of outer hair cell transduction and the temporary threshold shifts after acoustic trauma. *Audiology and Neuro-otology,* 7, 17–20.

Philbin, M. K. (2000). The influence of auditory experience on the behavior of preterm newborns. *Journal of Perinatology, 20,* S76–S86.

Pourbakht, A., & Yamasoba, T. (2003). Ebselen attenuates cochlear damage caused by acoustic trauma. *Hearing Research, 2003*(181), 1–2.

Prochaska, J. O., Norcross, J., & DiClemente, C. (1994). *Changing for Good.* New York: William Morrow and Company, Inc.

Puel, J. L., Ruel, J., Gervais d'Aldin, C., & Pujol, R. (1998). Excitotoxicity and repair of cochlear synapses after noise-trauma induced hearing loss. *NeuroReport, 9*(9), 2109–2114.

Pujol, R., & Lavigne-Rebillard, M. (1992) Development of neurosensory structures in the human cochlea. *Acta Otolaryngologia, 112,* 259–264.

Quaranta, A., Sallustio, V., & Quaranta, N. (2001). Noise induced hearing loss: summary and perspectives. In D. Henderson, D. Prasher, R. Kopke, R. J. Salvi, & R. P. Hamernik (Eds.), *Noise induced hearing loss: Basic mechanisms, prevention and control* (pp. 539–557). London: Noise Research Network Publications.

Rosen, S., Olin, P., & Rosen, H. (1970). Dietary prevention of hearing loss. *Acta Otolaryngologia, 70,* 242–247.

Royster, J. D., & Royster, L. H. (1990). *Hearing conservation programs: Practical guidelines for success.* Chelsea, MI: Lewis Publishing.

Saunders, J. C., Cohen, Y. E., & Szymko, Y. M. (1991). The structural and functional consequences of acoustic injury in the cochle an dperipheral auditory system: A five year update. *Journal of the Acoustical Society of America, 90*(1), 136–146.

Seidman, M. D., Babu, S., Tang, W., Naem, E., & Quirk, W. S. (2003). Effects of resveratrol on acoustic trauma. *Otolaryngology Head and Neck Surgery, 129*(5), 463–470.

Stockwell, C. W., Ades, H. W., & Engstrom, H. (1969). Patterns of hair cell damage after intense auditory stimulation. *Annals of Otology, Rhinology and Laryngology, 78*(6), 1144–1168.

U.S. Department of the Interior Fish and Wildlife Service; U.S. Department of Commerce; U.S. Census Bureau. (2001). *2001 national survey of fishing, hunting and wildlife associated recreation.*

Van Campen, L. E., Dennis, J. M., Hanlin, R. C., King, S. B., & Velderman, A. M. (1999). One-year audiologic monitoring of individuals exposed to the 1995 Oklahoma City bombing. *Journal of the American Academy of Audiology, 10*(5), 231–247.

Van De Water, T. R., Staecker, H., Halterman, M. W., & Federoff, H. J. (1999). Gene Therapy in the Inner Ear: Mechanisms and Clinical Implications. *Annals of the New York Academy of Sciences, 884,* 345–360.

WHO. (1997). *Strategies for prevention of deafness and hearing impairment. Prevention of noise-induced hearing loss.* Geneva: World Health Organization.

WHO. (2002). *Technical meeting on exposure-response relationships of noise on health.* Bonn: World Health Organization.

Yamasoba, T., Nuttall, A. L., Harris, C., Raphael, Y., & Miller, J. M. (1998). Role of glutathione in the protection against noise-induced hearing loss. *Brain Research, 784,* 82–90.

CHAPTER 13

Hearing Loss in Later Life

Scott J. Bally and Janet L. Pray
Gallaudet University

The U.S. Census identifies 31 million Americans with significant hearing loss. Due to the effects of the aging process and increasing environmental noise, a disproportionate number are adults over 60. The Centers for Disease Control and Prevention (1995) reported that in 1991, 31.7 million adults were 65 years or older, with a projection of 52 million by 2020, and 70 million by 2040 (Brock, Guralnick, & Brody, 1990). These statistics reflect the results of the baby boom—individuals born between 1945–62. Hearing loss is expected to affect 26 percent of those ages 65–74, 36 percent between 75 and 84, and approximately 50% for persons 85 and older (National Center for Health Statistics, 1987). The latter is the fastest growing segment of the U.S. population and is expected to triple between 2000 and 2040 (Brock et al., 1990). Three independent studies provide evidence that 70–80 percent of institutionalized older adults have measurable hearing loss, the loss being greater with advancing age. (Garahan, Waller, Houghton, Tisdale, & Runge, 1992; Schow and Nerbonne, 1980; Voeks, Gallagher, Langer, and Drinka, 1990). The growing body of literature since 1980 focusing on psychological and social aspects of hearing loss provides evidence that hearing loss is a biological/physiological phenomenon that occurs within a psychological and social context (Gilhome-Herbst & Humphrey, 1980; Glass, 1991; Laufer, 1985; Meadow-Orlans, 1991; Myers, 2000; Orlans & Meadow-Orlans, 1991; Pray, 1989, 1992; Weinstein & Ventry, 1982). Effects of the hearing loss and adaptation are determined by the interplay of biological, psychological, and social factors, or biopsychosocial dynamics (Pray, 1996). Thus, the nature and severity of the hearing loss, effects of other health conditions or disabilities, psychological makeup of the individual, response of family and friends, and attitudes in society all have a role in the complex process of adaptation.

The literature is abundant with research relating to the functioning of the hearing mechanism, related testing and rehabilitation. By contrast, there is meager research or professional writing that specifically examines the biological effects of hearing loss, or rehabilitation for culturally Deaf older adults. Given that significant hearing loss is a defining characteristic of the culturally Deaf population, it is reasonable to conclude that the effects of presbycusis and noise exposure may further decrease thresholds of residual hearing. The change of audiometric thresholds is cause for hearing reassessment by audiologists and otologists. The literature which addresses these concerns for the older adult population, in general, may provide insights regarding members of the Deaf culture.

Traditionally, hearing loss has been viewed from two competing paradigms: the cultural perspective and the medical/legal perspective. The cultural perspective views self-identified Deaf persons as part of a cultural and linguistic minority whose most distinguishing factor is the use of American Sign Language. Hearing loss is viewed as a normally occurring *difference* rather than a disability. In the United States, this cultural minority numbers about 500,000 persons and has a rich background of history, tradition, art, and values. Membership is determined by a complex interplay of the self-definition of the individual and acceptance by the cultural group.

The medical-legal perspective defines the physiological differences and considers them as pathologies and as disabilities. Primary objectives of the medical community are to return both hearing and communicative functioning to as near a normal state as possible. Intervention may include prostheses including hearing aids and other communication technology, surgical procedures, medication, as well as aural habilitation and rehabilitation. Hearing Loss is measured using objective standardized formulas. These provide a legal basis for determining among other things, who will be protected by disability-related laws and have access particular educational programs.

Bally (1999) presents aural rehabilitation models for professionals working with older adults with hearing loss (Figures 13–1 & 13–2) which incorporate and reconcile the competing paradigms through use of a systems approach. An ecological perspective views a person within the context of his or her environment (Kirst-Ashman & Hull, 1993; Rogers, 1979). The Nested Systems-Ecological Model (Fig. 13–1) utilizes this perspective to provide a context for looking at the affects of hearing loss across and between life systems and depicts the biological, affective, behavioral, cognitive and spiritual systems of the individual in the context of micro-, meso-, and macro-social systems. For example, a hearing loss in an older adult may affects communication with others (social system). This may result in frustration (affective system), avoidance of family communication situations (behavioral, meso-social systems) and a belief that successful communication is no longer possible (cognitive system). The frustration may cause blood pressure to rise (biological). The nested-systems ecological model also identifies several external influences which may affect human systems. These may include cultural, ethical, political and economic influences as well as those brought about by social policy and laws, healthcare and human services and the physical

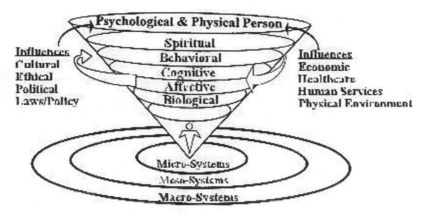

FIGURE 13–1.   Nested Systems-Ecological Model.

environment. For successful adaptation to hearing loss, Bally posits that the effects on all systems must be addressed. The Bally Aural Rehabilitation Model (Fig. 13–2) is a choronosystemic model which provides professionals with a template for an inter-system analysis and for planning assessment and intervention across systems. Based on this approach we will examine biopsychosocial effects of hearing loss, their assessment and intervention from both cultural and medical-legal perspectives.

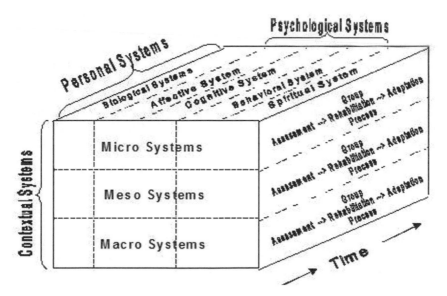

FIGURE 13–2.   The Bally Aural Rehabilitation Model.

CAUSES OF HEARING LOSS IN OLDER ADULTS

Each of the physiological systems change as part of the aging process. In addition to changes which have a direct affect on hearing, other changes occur which compound hearing loss e.g. vision loss. Some of these changes may interfere with adjustment by limiting expressive communication ability. There is an extensive literature describing such changes. This chapter addresses only those changes which have a direct bearing on hearing loss, receptive communication ability and adaptation.

Presbycusis and noise exposure (Gates, Cobb, D'Agostino, & Wolf, 1993; Gulya, 1991) are the primary causes of hearing loss among older adults. "Presbycusis is a global term used to refer to hearing loss associated with age" (Tye-Murray, 1998, p. 302). Although age-related degeneration and genetic make up are probably key factors, the precise cause or causes of presbycusis are unknown (Tye-Murray). Noise exposure is a consequence of living in an industrialized society and increases or compounds presbycusis.

All parts of the auditory system undergo change as part of the aging process. Comprehensive descriptions of these changes are provided by Gulya (1991), Strouse, DeChicchis and Bess, (1997), Soucek and Michaels, (1990), Weinstein (2000) and Willott (1991). While some of the changes have a direct affect on auditory receptive communication, others may affect hearing testing and the use of amplification.

Changes in the outer ear (pinna and external auditory canal) including a loss of elasticity and thinning and dryness of the skin of the pinna, leaving it less resilient to the manipulation needed for hearing testing, ear mold fitting and cleaning (Nerbonne, 1988; Schuknecht, 1993; Weinstein, 2000). Ear canals of older adults have a higher likelihood of collapse when using traditional earphones. Similar changes occur in the middle ear including thinning and loss of elasticity of the tympanic membrane. In addition, eustachian tube functioning may be affected by atrophy of the supporting musculature and calcification of the cartilaginous support of the tube (Weinstein, 2000). These changes along with the decreasing abilities of the immune system increases the risk of middle ear infections, especially in adults 65 or older (White & Regan, 1987). Although these changes have minimal affect on hearing thresholds and communication, they may affect auditory testing and influence outcome measures, hearing aid fitting and use and health care management (Ballachanda, 1995; Gleitman, Ballachandra, & Goldstein, 1992, Oliveria, 1995).

Inner Ear and Auditory Neural Pathways

"The most important changes in the aging auditory system occur within the sensory and neural structures" (Weinstein, 2000, p. 77). The most significant age-related changes occur in the Organ of Corti of the cochlea and in the afferent auditory portion of the eighth nerve and are reflected in both pure-tone thresholds and speech audiometry. Landmark research by Schuknecht and Gacek (1993) resulted in the categorization of prebycusis types as sensory, neural, strial, and cochlear conductive and may help to explain the varying ways in which this disorder manifests itself as well as guiding intervention approaches. Each is reflected in a differential diagnosis of pure tone results and speech audiometry; each has its particular effects on receptive communication, and each presents unique challenges for provision of appropriate amplification.

Other significant effects on hearing which have increased incidence in older adults and have been explored by researchers and practitioners include ototoxicity related to medications used for chronic conditions also related to aging (Abrams, Beers, & Berkow, 1995; Boettcher, Gratton, Bancroft, & Sprongr, 1992; Schwartz, 1999), acoustic neuroma (Schuknecht, 1993), cardiovascular disease (Gates, Cobb, D'Agostino, & Wolf, 1993; Brant, Gordon-Salant, Pearson, Klein, Morrell, Metter, & Fozard, 1996), metabolic disease including diabetes mellitus (Gates et al., 1993; Willott, 1991), hyperlipoproteinemia (Spencer, 1973), renal disorders (Beck & Burkhart, 1994), and dementia (Abrams et al., 1995; Russell & Burns, 1999; Gates, Cobb, Linn, Rees, & Wolf, 1996). Although some of these physiological changes may be rectified with medical or technical intervention, others may not. These studies suggest that a better understanding of these etiologies may result in more effective assessment and intervention approaches.

Weinstein (2000) and Ryugo, Limb, and Redd (2000) note important neurological changes which may affect audition and adaptation to hearing loss including changes in the duplication of neurons and the plasticity of the brain. Of particular significance to communication is a 30 percent decline in the speed of the action potentials through the nerve fibers (Kenney, 1988). Kenny states "reaction time (that is, the time which elapses between a signal being given and the required motor responses being undertaken) is prolonged with aging." This may explain, for example, why an older adult hears a message, responds by saying "huh?," and then demonstrates by a non-verbal or verbal reaction or response indicating that he understood. This delayed reaction alone has vital implications for successful assessment of auditory parameters as well as intervention approaches and adaptation.

Neurological Changes

The most common forms of neurological impairments which occur in older adults include stroke-related communication impairments, (aphasia and right hemisphere communication deficits) progressive neorological disease (dementia), head trauma, motor speech disorders and laryngeal cancer (Lubinski, 1995, 1997; Mueller & Goeffrey, 1987, 1991; Shadden & Toner, 1997; Weinstein, 2000). Given the prevalence of such phenomena, as well as that of hearing loss in aging, it is reasonable to assume that some of these conditions will superimpose themselves on hearing loss, further compromising communication function and complicating assessment and intervention approaches. Shaddon (1988) asserts that chronological age is likely to influence the nature and severity of these disorders as well as the prognosis for rehabilitation.

OTHER PHYSIOLOGICAL CHANGES IN AGING WHICH IMPACT HEARING OR COMPOUND THE AFFECTS OF HEARING LOSS

Vision and Receptive Communication

Receptive communication involves the ability to integrate auditory and visual input. Hearing loss results in a greater dependence on receptive visual communication and is, therefore, critical to the information provided in this chapter. Brock, Guralnik and Brody, (1990) report that, in the United States, vision impairment affects approximately 10 percent of individuals from age 65 to 74, 16 percent from age 75 to 84, and 27 percent of adults 85 and older. Such vision difficulties are likely to affect receptive communication, specifically the ability to lipread and monitor non-verbal communication from facial expression, gesture and body language. Changes in vision may be more significant to culturally Deaf individuals than to their hearing counterparts because of the reliance on the visual mode for communication including the reception of sign language, non-verbal communication, and lipreading.

Wainapel (1994) and Rumney (1998) describe several specific morphologic and functional changes which occur to vision as part of the aging process. As a result of thickening, the lens becomes less elastic and more rigid resulting in *presbyopia* or the inability to change focus between near and far images. In addition, the lens begins yellowing and becomes more opaque resulting in less ability to distinguish some color fields. Pinpoint opacities develop within the lens which make bright lighting less tolerable. These changes may limit the range of lighting conditions in which an older individual may be successful in facilitating lipreading or the reception of sign language. In addition, ocular diseases such as cataracts, macular degeneration, diabetic retinopathy, and glaucoma are more prevalent in older adults. Wainapel (1994) reports that these account for 90% of vision loss in persons over the age of 70.

Additional Physiological Factors Influencing Hearing Loss

Older adults also have higher incidences of other chronic diseases including arthritis, balance disorders, hypertension, heart disease and orthopedic problems, all of which, although not immediately life-threatening may contribute to functional limitations (Lubinski, 1997). Because the incidence of all these conditions increases with advancing age, individuals may sustain more than one condition, thereby compounding the psychosocial effects of hearing loss. For example, the affects on communication for an older deaf adult who develops cataracts or rheumatoid arthritis may be devastating because of the impact on speechreading and/or the reception of sign language. A study by Smith-Worrall, Hickson and Dodd (1990) concludes that an estimated 90 percent of older adults in residential care will have one or more conditions which impact on communication.

Older adults have a greater likelihood to experience other conditions which affect cognitive processes as well as communication including dementia, aphasia and apraxia, and head trauma, as well as progressive neurological diseases such as Alzheimer's, Huntington's, Korsakoff's, Parkinson's, or Pick's Disease, (Lubinski, 1995, 1997; Schow, Christensen, Hutchinson, & Nerbonne, 1978; Tonkovich, 1988). Each of these conditions impacts communication uniquely and each may result in a variety of communication disorders. Based on a review of related studies, Chartrand (2001) concluded that there is "a strong correlation between unmitigated hearing loss and dementia in older adults." However, this increase may be attributed to increased longevity of older adult rather than an increase of the actual pathologies and, likely, rather than a causal effect between those two factors, age being the controlling factor. Some types of dementia may be caused by ototoxicity and the effects, in some cases, may be reversed. A cautionary note is that older adults with deficits in hearing and vision or those experiencing depression may present symptoms which may be confused with neurological disorders. Symptoms such as disorientation, memory loss, speech irrelevance, increased auditory processing time, and difficulties with new learning should be regarded carefully (Tonkovich, 1988). Finally, these etiologies may increase the difficulty of hearing assessment, and the design and facilitation of effective aural rehabilitation.

PSYCHOSOCIAL FACTORS CONTRIBUTING TO THE EFFECTS OF HEARING LOSS AND ADAPTATION PROCESS

There is substantial evidence in the literature that numerous factors have a bearing on the effects of hearing loss and the way in which individuals and their families cope. Perhaps the most obvious of these are the nature and degree of hearing loss, whether the loss is progressive, and the rate of progression (Kaplan, 1991). Other significant factors include the age of onset and the degree to which the hearing loss effects communication (Webb, Schreiner, & Asmuth, 1995). Changes in mobility associated with other disabilities or health conditions may also affect the adaptation process (Cacciatore, Napoli, Abete, Marciano, Triassi, & Rengo, 1999; Webb, Schreiner, & Asmuth, 1995).

Many personal and psychological factors come into play. There is evidence that certain health conditions have effects on personality (strokes, multiple sclerosis, among others). Issues of personality and aging are addressed by many including Hooker and Shifren (1995) and Pray, (1992). Other personal characteristics include the capacity of the individual to cope with stress (Palmer, 1995), adaptability (Gould, 1978), self-concept (Erikson, Erikson, & Kivnick, 1986), realistic expectations (Maurer & Rupp, 1979), perspectives on hearing loss (Glass, 1991; Schlesnger, 1985), motivation (Kaplan, 1985), technophobia (Perlstein, 1990; Ross, 1992). Spirituality and religion are areas that research has consistently shown to be important in people's lives and how they cope with stress (Hooyman & Kiyak, 1999).

The context of the family and support system is important for understanding adaptation to hearing loss. Family issues include: changes in the family through death or divorce, change in family functioning due to illness of disability of a family member, retirement of a spouse (or self), change in economic circumstances, relocation of the family or individual family members, family perspectives about hearing loss (Hession, 1991; Meadow-Orlans, 1991; Pray, 1989, 1996; Weinstein & Ventry, 1982).

There is also evidence in the literature that hearing loss affects the spouse and other family members in significant ways (Beck, 1991; Pray, 1996). Beck, a clinical social worker with a severe hearing loss, identified feelings of helplessness, frustration, and hopelessness in families. Pray identified "parallel reactions" to the difficulties in communicating experienced by the person with hearing loss, family members, and virtually anyone attempting to communicate effectively. Some studies found spouses affected, but to a lesser extent than the person with hearing loss (Newman & Weinstein 1986; Quinn, 1986).

Societal context cannot be ignored when considering factors that influence adjustment to hearing loss. There is a body of literature that posits that disability is defined not by the physical condition or "impairment," but instead by the "spoiled identity" resulting from stigma and alienation (Calhoun & Lipman, 1984, Goffman, 1963). Watson and Maxwell (1977) maintain that social criteria and not physical criteria determine disability and are based upon the person's ability to function in the group. Harvey (1989) observes that "hearing loss per se need not be a handicapping deficit; rather, this disability may be molded to become such a deficit in the context of the ecology" (xii).

For an older person with hearing loss there is the added issue of attitudes in society towards aging. Butler (1975) coined the term "ageism" to describe stereotyping of persons who are old and drew comparisons with racism and sexism. Rosow (1974) noted the devalued position of older persons in society. Orr (1982) hypothesized that older persons, like children and youth, are treated with paternalism and are disenfranchised. Wax (1982) suggested the concept of double and multiple jeopardy for older persons with hearing loss. It should be noted, though, that Markides (1983) found mixed support in empirical studies for the concept of double jeopardy.

Effects of Major Life Events on the Adaptation of Older Persons to Hearing Loss

There is a common assumption that certain major life events—sometimes classified as crises—are barriers to successful aging. If this assumption is correct, it has relevance to understanding the effects of hearing loss since a person experiencing one of these major life events could be presumed to have particular difficulty with adaptation. The literature does not consistently support the assumption. The second longitudinal study conducted by the Duke Center for the Study of Aging and Human Development included data on five major life events: participant's retirement, spouse's retirement, widowhood, departure of last child from home, and occurrence of an illness severe enough to require hospitalization. Few effects on social-psychological adaptation were found as a consequence of spouse's retirement, widowhood, and the departure of the last child. Even major medical events were found to have little lasting impact. The most negative effects were related to the participant's retirement and even they were considered to be relatively minor (Palmore, 1985).

Earlier writings reported these events to have negative outcomes such as unhappiness, loss of self-esteem, withdrawal, and general decline (Butler, 1975; Datan & Ginsberg, 1975; Rosow, 1973, 1974). Other literature predating the 25-year longitudinal study at the Duke Center suggested that such life events were stressful but resulted in successful readjustment and new growth (Gould, 1978; Maas & Kuypers, 1974). Such results are consistent with favorable outcomes associated with crisis and crisis intervention models (Aguilera, 1994).

The extent to which major life events are stressful or create crisis is the subject of ongoing study and is covered well in encyclopedic works that report on research on: aging and mental health (Lomranz, 1998), aging and the family (Blieszner & Bedford, 1995), the psychology of aging (Birren & Schaie, 2001), theories of aging (Bengtson & Schaie, 1999), intellectual development in adulthood (Schaie, 1996), normal aging (Palmore, 1984, 1985), and research on aging internationally (Palmore, 1993).

ASSESSMENT AND INTERVENTION FOR THE BIOPSYCHOSOCIAL EFFECTS OF HEARING LOSS IN AGING

Assessment and Intervention for Auditory Differences and Disorders

Two generally accepted characteristics which distinguish humans from other species are language and technology. Intervention approaches for adaptation to hearing loss in older adults have two primary components: biopsychosocial rehabilitation/habilitation and use of technology. Both target the end result of functional communication. The objective of communication technology may be to restore communication function or to enhance an individual's ability to interact with the environment. Habilitation or rehabilitation may focus on adaptation to communication differences or disorders, enhancement of communication skills and the use of technology.

Assessment of Auditory Differences and Disorders

Gordon-Salant (1987, 1991) and Raiford (1988) describe modified audiologic test procedures, including interviewing, pure tone, speech recognition, suprathreshold speech threshold, central auditory function and acoustic immittance measures for use with older adults. More specialized electropyhsiological testing comprises a highly specialized and significant battery of tests to study functioning of the auditory and vesitibular pathways. The value of these assessment approaches is in learning about signal transmission through the central nervous system which may change as part of the aging process. Specific assessment protocols for auditory potentials and balance-related disorders in older adults and supportive data are presented by Jacobson (1997) and Jacobson and Calder (1998).

Communication Enhancement Through Technology

Pichora Fuller (1997a, b) and (Ross, 1992) identify factors that predispose as well as enable older adults to use assistive listening devices including physiological, environmental and psychosocial factors including culture, technophobia, lifestyle and economic factors. In a state-of-the-art professional text on aging, Lubinski and Higginbotham (1997) preside over a team of leading professionals who present current research and practical assessment and intervention approaches for vision, hearing and speech technology for older adults.

Hearing aid technology, fueled by the competitiveness of the hearing aid industry, has made enormous strides in the past decade. Older adults are prime consumers of amplification devices and much of the extensive literature in this area has been focused on this population. Researchers have examined:

> candidacy issues (Garstecki & Erler, 1998; Jahn & Cook, 1997; Jerger, Chmeil, Florin, Pirozzolo & Wilson, 1996; Mueller & Carter, 2002; Ross, 1992; Sweetow & Shelton, 1996), assessment techniques (Jerger, Silman, Lew & Chmeil, 1993), selection and fitting considerations (Agnew, 1996, Danhauser & Danhauser, 1997; Keidser, Dillon & Byrne, 1996; Kochkin, 1996; Kuk, 1998; Mueller & Carter, 2002; Palmer, 1995; Primeau, 1997; Ross, 1995a, 1995b; Sweetow & Shelton, 1996) and orientation procedures (Chmeil & Jerger, 1995; Kochkin, 1997; Kochkin, 1997; Mulrow, Michael & Aquilar, 1992; Nerbonne, Christman & Fleschner, 1995. Trends for hearing aid fitting and development are explored in research by Christensen (1999) and Sweetow (1999).

Subjective measures of hearing aid satisfaction which may suggest approaches for fitting candidacy, fitting, auditory training and orientation include the Abbreviated Profile of Hearing Aid Benefit (APHAB) (Cox & Alexander, 1995), Client Oriented Scale of Improvement (COSI) (Dillon, James & Ginis (1997) and the Hearing Aid Performance Inventory (HAPI) (Weinstein, 1991). Hearing aid information from such scales provides information for professionals in addressing the low incidence of reported hearing aid use (Ross, 1992). Comprehensive approaches to hearing aid fitting for older adults are described by Lesner and Kricos (1995), Novak (2000), Stach and Stoner, (1991) and Weinstein (1997, 2000).

Paul Rao (1997) provides an important overview of the broad issues of functional assessment relative to older adults and describes the implications of these issues in assessment protocols. These include the manner in which professionals approach functional communication in older adults, the influences of the World Health Organization's classification system of disability, impairment and handicap on our perspectives, and assessment and intervention approaches, the focus of functional communication assessment, and how to evaluate the purpose, scope, measurement domains and scoring properties of assessment measures. Chafetz and Wilson (1988) describe approaches for communicating effectively with older adults. Given the neurological and physiological changes discussed earlier, Groher (1988) and Weinstein (2000) provide useful test modifications for older adults including adaptations of test complexity, test directions and administration as well as criteria for interpretation of test results. They present guidelines which have application for audiometric, aural rehabilitation as well as all other psychosocial assessment and interventions for all individuals with communicative disorders hearing as well as when working with Deaf older adults.

Cochlear implants are discussed in Chapter 8. Waltzman, Cohen and Shapiro (1993) describe the benefits of cochlear implants for the geriatric population. Holmes notes, "there is no upper age limit for cochlear implantation"(2002, p. 88), although other health conditions may contraindicate the surgery. Ryugo, Limb, and Redd (2000) provide strong evidence that continued plasticity of the brain well into old age provides support for successful adaptation to cochlear implantation.

Neurological Assessment in Older Adults with Hearing Loss

There is an increasing interest in assessment and intervention approaches for working with individuals who have both hearing loss and forms of dementia, including groundbreaking work by Durrant, Gilmartin, Holland, Kamerer, and Newall (1990), Palmer (1995), Palmer, Adams, Durrant, Bourgeouis, and Ross (1998), Peters, Potter, and Scholar (1988) and Ulmann, Larson, Koepsell, and Duckert (1989). Chartrand (2001) describes the role of hearing healthcare professionals as well as critical, but removable barriers to effective service in treating patients with Alzheimers. Ripich (1991) describes language and communication assessment protocols for global communication, pragmatics, discourse, semantics, syntax, phonology, and language memory (p. 269). Lubinski (1995) provides professionals with a comprehensive compilation of research and current thinking on assessment and intervention approaches for professionals working in the area of communication and dementia.

Assessment and Intervention Approaches for Aural Rehabilitation

Lesner and Kricos (1995) describe criteria for an holistic audiologic rehabilitation assessment when working with older adults and provide a series of Tables which compare and contrast tests of auditory speech reception (p. 34–35) speechreading (p. 37), audiovisual speech reception (p. 38) and conversational fluency (p. 39), providing the professional with criteria for selecting among the assessment protocols included. An integrated approach for aural rehabilitation assessment for culturally Deaf populations is described by authors in Moseley and Bally (1996). Rather than approaches which isolate and compartmentalize global and communication based skills and abilities (i.e., communication strategies, auditory training, speechreading), they are addressed together in context-based integrated rehabilitation protocols.

Self-report scales may be used to examine psychosocial issues including adaptation to hearing loss. Such scales provide subjective information and draw on the perspective of the person with hearing loss to explore the impact and attitudes associated with hearing loss, the use of communication strategies, hearing aid use and assistive technology as well as adaptation to hearing loss. Information from these scales may foster more effective biopsychosocial intervention approaches. Erdman (2001) provides criteria and rationale for selection and use of self-report scales. The Communication Scale for Older Adults (CSOA) (Kaplan, Bally, Brandt, Busacco, & Pray, 1994) examines attitudes related to communicative functioning, use of communication strategies and identifies difficult communication situations and their importance to the individual. The Hearing Handicap Inventory for the Elderly (HHIE) (Ventry & Weinstein, 1982; Weinstein, Spitzer, & Ventry, 1986) looks at the emotional and social/situational effects of hearing loss in older adults. There is a spouse version (HHIE-SP) designed to screen the impact of an individual's hearing loss on his or her spouse or significant other (Armero, 2000, Ventry & Weinstein, 1982). The Communication Scale for Deaf Adults (CSDA) (Kaplan, Bally, & Brandt, 1991) is unique in that it is designed for the culturally Deaf population and provides information about difficult communication situations, their importance to the individual, use of communication strategies and attitudes related to communication.

Aural Habilitation and Rehabilitation for Older Deaf Adults

Tye Murray (1998), Kricos and Lesner (1995), Schow and Nerbonne (2001), Waynor and Abrahamson (1996) and a seminal work by Weinstein (2000) provide assessment and rehabilitation approaches for hard of hearing populations which focus on the enhancement of oral/aural communication through the use of technology and communication skills and strategies. Although these authors do not address the specific needs of older adults specifically, many of the approaches may be adapted for use with older adults.

Chartrand (2001) reports that there is persuasive evidence by Durrant et al. (1990), Hardick (1977), and Ratcliffe (1992) that hearing instrument use combined with proper aural rehabilitation (in a multi-disciplinary setting), can be cost-effective approach to alleviating many AD-identified symptoms in patients who have AD and hearing loss.

Traditionally, habilitation and rehabilitation provided by audiologists and speech pathologists focuses on the communicative function of individuals. Social workers, counselors and psychologists may work with both populations in addressing the psychosocial impact of deafness or hearing loss. Professional intervention may include work with spouses and family members and use family-centered or person centered approaches. With hard of hearing and late-deafened individuals the primary objective is functional oral-aural communication. Culturally Deaf clients may access such services to increase their ability to function more successfully when they are in environments predominated by hearing people, such as a workplace or place of worship. Speech pathologists, audiologists, social workers, and aural rehabilitationists describe an integrated aural rehabilitation approach to communication therapy with deaf and hard of hearing adolescents and adults in an edited work by Moseley and Bally (1996). The text provides a comprehensive model for intervention designed for culturally Deaf populations, but may be generalized to all adults with hearing loss.

Research and intervention strategies for specific skill areas of aural rehabilitation is plentiful. This body of literature includes information on speechreading (Kaplan, Bally, & Garretson, 1987, Kaplan, 1996, Tye-Murray, 1998) auditory training (Redinger, 1996, Tye-Murray, 1998) and communication strategies (Kaplan, Bally, & Garretson, 1987, Kaplan, 1996, Tye-Murray, 1998). Despite the abundance of research showings the positive effects of such training, there as a general lack of aural rehabilitation services. The scarcity of programs was studied by Oyer et al., (1976) who identified contributing factors including, physical limitations of participants, cost effectiveness, transportation, lack of motivation, scheduling difficulties, and lack of awareness of programs.

Several integrated programs have been reported in the literature in an effort to provide a more holistic approach to aural rehabilitation (Jennings, 1995; Kricos, 1997; Kricos & Lesner, 1995; Moseley & Bally, 1996; Tye-Murray, 1998; Wayner & Abrahamson, 1996). However, when reviewed, models from the hearing health field of audiology, speech-language pathology and aural rehabilitation continue to focus on use of amplification, the development of speechreading skills and communication strategies and, only superficially, focus on psychosocial issues. Newer models from some counseling professions provide intervention constructs for psychosocial aspects of hearing loss based on cultural perspectives, while ignoring, minimizing or dismissing the pathological aspects of hearing loss (Kyle, Jones, & Wood, 1991; Harvey, 1989). Holistic approaches which attempt to address all life systems remain on a multidisciplinary basis, although the Gallaudet model (Wilson & Scott, 1996) espouses a more interdisciplinary approach.

Psychosocial Assessment and Intervention

Hearing loss in the older population has been found to be associated with depression and other psychological conditions (Cacciatore et al., 1999; Carabellese et al., 1993; Maggi et al., 1998; Strawbridge et al., 2000). Commenting on the strong association that Cacciatore and others found between hearing loss and depression, Bazargan, Baker, and Bazargan (2001) cite studies that have documented a significant reduction of psychotic activity and improvement in mood, self-sufficiency in instrumental activities of daily living, and social relationships after the fitting of hearing-aids (Almeida, 1993; Appollonio, Carabellese, Frattola, & Trabucchi, 1996; Kreeger, Raulin, Grace, & Priest, 1995). Bazargan and Barbe (1994) found self-reported memory problems. A number of studies have identified reduced cognitive capacity (Cacciatore et al., 1999; Lindenberger & Baltes, 1994). Other studies in older adults have indicated a significant relationship between hearing impairment and self-sufficiency (Carabellese et al., 1993), quality of life and well-being (Mulrow et al., 1990; Scherer & Frisina, 1998), social integration (Resnick et al., 1997), and social isolation (Strawbridge et al., 2000; Weinstein & Ventry, 1982).

Culturally Diverse Populations

There is a limited amount of research on hearing loss among aging minority populations. Bazargan, Baker, and Bazargan (2001) conducted a study of 988 older African Americans, age 62 and older, and evaluated the relationship between vision and hearing loss and psychological well-being. Fair to poor vision was reported by 36.5 percent of the sample and 26 percent reported fair to poor hearing. Eighty-four percent of the participants used eyeglasses to improve their vision, but only 4.3 percent of those who described their hearing as poor reported using hearing aids. In contrast, Popelka and colleagues (1998) reported that 10 percent to 21 percent of people with hearing loss in the general population used amplification. Poor vision and poor hearing were each found to be associated with a lower level of psychological well-being among older African Americans. They conclude that their findings indicate that there is potential for improving the psychological well-being of older African Americans through both visual and audiological rehabilitation.

Bazargan, Baker, and Bazargan also cited results from other studies of older African Americans. They noted that in a small sample, Marcus-Bernstein (1986) documented a relationship between hearing handicap and overall rating of mental health as well as with key aspects of psychological function including lethargy, life satisfaction, and paranoia. In addition, Bazargan, Bazargan, and King (2001) found that hearing loss had a significant impact on paranoid ideation in older African Americans.

In a qualitative study of eight deafened adults (ages 31–68) in Ontario Canada, Aguayo and Coady (2001) found that none were referred to counseling services despite severe emotional trauma associated with becoming deaf; severe family problems including exclusion, isolation and even abuse within the family; and social oppression and exclusion outside of the home. The participants in the study expressed dissatisfaction with rehabilitation services, in part because their psychosocial needs were not addressed. They indicated interest in both formal counseling (individual, family, and group) and informal help (individual or group peer support). There is other evidence that there are substantial psychosocial effects on the deafened individual and others (David & Trehub, 1989; Kyle & Wood, 1987; Luey, 1980) and that intervention with these kinds of problems can be beneficial (Rothschild & Kampfe, 1997).

Koretz and Moore (2001) recommends a comprehensive screening for older patients at the time of their initial visit to a health care provider. This screening includes a screening for hearing loss and Koretz notes that referral should be made to an audiologist if hearing loss is detected. Koretz notes further that amplification can enhance the quality of life of an older person with hearing loss. Koretz suggests using the Hearing Handicap Inventory for the Elderly—Screening Version, a 10-item questionnaire that evaluates the effect of hearing loss on the patient's social and emotional well-being (Ventry & Weinstein, 1983). Not mentioned in the discussion is the risk of assuming an older person has dementia if hearing loss is overlooked as a possibility if the person misunderstands or does not participate appropriately in conversation. It is, of course, possible that a person could have both a hearing loss and dementia and that too needs to be understood. Gomez and Madey (2001) proposed a coping-with-hearing-loss model that explains how hearing loss, psychosocial factors (i.e., attitudes about aging, personal adjustment to hearing loss, and perceived social support), and perceived strategy effectiveness affect the use of adaptive and maladaptive strategies. They tested the model with 33 men and 28 women, ages 61–85, and found that nonaudiological variables were more important than physical hearing loss in predicting coping behaviors. They concluded that psychosocial issues as well as results of audiological evaluations may need to be addressed in order to help older adults cope effectively with hearing loss. Their conclusion is consistent with Andersson, Melin, Lindberg, and Scott's (1996) finding that the hearing loss as measured by an objective audiological assessment is not necessarily the only predictor, or even the most important predictor, of how a person will cope with hearing loss. Pray (1992) conducted a qualitative study of 28 individuals with hearing loss (ages 60–90) and their spouses/significant others (ages 56–86). The coping strategies identified by participants in this study were often grounded in psychosocial factors unrelated to strategies that might be most effective to address the communication problems stemming from the nature and severity of the hearing loss. Discomfort with being assertive and relationship with significant other people were two major factors in choice of coping strategies.

Gomez and Madey (2001) used a number of scales to measure psychosocial variables:

- Anxiety about Aging Scale (Lasher & Faulkender, 1993).
- Social and Emotional Impact Scale and the Lack of Acceptance and Adjustment Scale from the Attitude Toward Loss of Hearing Questionnaire (ATLHQ; Saunders & Cienkowski, 1996) and the Personal Adjustment Scale from the Communication Profile for the Hearing Impaired (CPHI) (Demorest & Erdman, 1987) to measure personal adjustment to hearing loss.
- Perceived social support with the Perceived Absence of Support Scale from the ATLHQ (Saunders & Cienkowski, 1996)
- Attitude of Others and the Behavior of Others subscales from the CPHI (Demorest & Erdman, 1986, 1987)

Garstecki and Erler (1999) conducted a study to examine gender difference in self-perceived hearing handicap among women and men age 65 years and older.

The intent was to increase understanding of differences in communication effectiveness and personal adjustment to hearing loss among individuals who represent the fastest growing segment of society with impaired hearing. The subjects were 301 members of organizations for seniors in the metropolitan Chicago area. All took the Communication Profile for the Hearing Impaired. Some gender-based differences were found. Compared with the men in the study, older women:

- Assign greater importance to social communication
- Rely more on nonverbal repair strategies
- Report more frequent feelings of anger and stress related to their hearing loss
- Are more willing to report communication problems and negative reactions due to hearing impairment.

Palmer et al (1999) reported on a study of eight patients with Alzheimer's Disease who were evaluated for hearing aid fitting and were successfully using the hearing aids between five and fifteen hours a day by the end of the study. Participants were recruited from the Alzheimer Disease Research Center, University of Pittsburgh; the Benedum Geriatric Center, University of Pittsburgh; the Alzheimer Association of Pittsburgh; and the Aging Research and Education Center of Lutheran Affiliated Services. Eight caregiver/subject dyads were able to complete this investigation and one to four problem behaviors were significantly reduced for all of the participants after hearing-aid treatment. In addition, nearly all of the caregivers indicated that hearing handicap had been significantly reduced, according to the significant other's version of the HHIE. These results have important implications for those working with persons with Alzheimer's Disease for a number of reasons. Palmer et al. (1999) note, for example, that there are notable similarities between the effects of hearing loss and Alzheimer's Disease on life activities and feelings. These include communication problems, social isolation, feelings of helplessness, depression, passivity, and negativism. They note further that among individuals with dementia of various etiologies, hearing loss has been associated with an accelerated and rapid cognitive decline (Peters et al. 1988; Uhlmann, Larson, & Koepsell, 1986; Uhlmann, Larson, et al., 1989). This suggests the possibility that hearing loss may indirectly contribute to cognitive dysfunction. There are data indicating that there is a high incidence of hearing loss among persons with Alzheimer's. Moreover, Palmer et al. cite Durrant (1991) who reported that only one out of ten persons with Alzheimer's disease and hearing loss had hearing aids, whereas 6 out of 10 hearing-loss matched individuals used amplification. Self-perceived hearing handicap was reported as being very similar for both groups. Palmer et al. (1999) note that persons with Alzheimer's are typically considered difficult or impossible to test. The results of their study, as well as two other studies they cite (Uhlmann, Rees, Psaty, & Duckert, 1989; Durrant, Gilmartin, Holland, Kamerer, & Newall, 1991) suggest otherwise. The findings of these studies suggest that "conventional wisdom" may need to be reconsidered in the interest of enhancing the quality of life of persons with both Alzheimer's Disease and hearing loss and those with responsibility for their care.

Despite the literature in the fields of audiology and speech language pathology about the psychosocial dimensions of hearing loss in aging, there is scant attention in the literature of the professions of social work and psychology to working with older persons with hearing loss to address the many issues raised in this chapter. Luey, Glass, and Elliot (1995) wrote for social workers of the complex and interrelated dimensions of assessing and providing services to deaf and hard of hearing people in general. Although Glass has done a major study on characteristics of successful coping with late onset hearing loss, the results have not yet been published. Desselle and Proctor (2000) wrote of the need for social workers to advocate for the older hard of hearing population, "the deaf people we ignore." Dalecki (1988) identified the importance for social workers of having older persons evaluated by an audiologist for hearing loss because of concern that older persons are being misdiagnosed as having cognitive impairments when the problem may be hearing loss.

CONCLUSION

Examination of the literature on aging and on hearing loss in aging identifies a complex set of issues that suggests the need for an interdisciplinary perspective on assessment and intervention. Hearing loss should not be addressed outside the context of the total biopsychosocial system. Nor should other aspects of the older person's life be assessed and treated without considering the possibility of hearing loss and the problems and challenges that frequently are associated with it. The models (Bally, 1999) described in this chapter provide one framework for an approach that enables professionals across disciplines to focus on the whole person in a way that enhances the likelihood that older persons with hearing loss and those who are culturally Deaf will be afforded opportunities to function at their full potential. The two perspectives described earlier in the chapter do not have to be competing paradigms but can be respectively addressed when integrated approaches are used. As described in this chapter, there is an extensive literature which addresses each of the systems affected by hearing loss in later years. This interdisciplinary body of work provides the professional with a basis for conceptualizing and executing successful integrated assessment and intervention.

REFERENCES

Abrams, W., Beers, M., & Berkow, R. (2000). *Merck manual of geriatrics* (3rd ed.) Whitehouse Station, NJ: Merck & Co.

Agnew, J. (1996). Hearing aid adjustments through potentiometer and switch options. In M. Valente (Ed.), *Hearing aids: Standards, options and verification* (pp. 210–251). New York: Thieme.

Aguayo, M. O., & Coady, N. F. (2001). The experience of deafened adults: Implications for rehabilitative services. *Health and Social Work. 26*(4), 269–277.

Aguilera, D. C. (1994). *Crisis intervention: Theory and methodology.* St. Louis: C. V. Mosby.

Almeida, O. P. (1993). *Clinical and cognitive diversity of psychotic states arising in late life (late paraphrenia).* Unpublished doctoral thesis, University of London, England.

Anderson, R. G., & Meyerhoff, W. L. (1982). Otologic manifestation of aging. *Otolaryngologic Clinics of America, 15*, 353–370.

Andersson, G., Melin, L., Lindberg, P., & Scott, B. (1996). Elderly hearing-impaired persons' coping behavior. *International Journal of Behavioral Medicine, 4*, 303–320.

Appollonio, I., Carabellese, C., Frattola, L., & Trabucchi, M. (1996). Effects of sensory aids on the quality of life and mortality of elderly people: A multivariate analysis. *Age and Aging, 25*, 89–96.

Armero, O. E. (2000). The six stages of grieving a hearing loss. *The Hearing Review, 7* (6), 28–33.

Ballachanda, B. (1995). Cerumen and the ear canal secretory system. In B. Ballachanda (Ed.), *The Human ear canal: Treatment considerations and clinical applications including cerumen management* (pp. 181–201). San Diego, CA: Singular Publishing Group.

Bally, S. J. (1999). *A self-help group aural rehabilitation model for older adults with hearing loss.* Unpublished doctoral thesis, Cincinnati, OH: The Union Institute.

Bazargan, M., Baker, R. S., & Bazargan, S. H. (2001). Sensory impairments and subjective well-being among aged African American persons. *The Journals of Gerontology, 56B*(5), 268–278.

Bazargan, M., & Barbe, A. R. (1994). The effects of depression, health status, and stressful life- events on self-reported memory problem among status, and stressful life-events on self-reported memory problem among aged Blacks. *The International Journal of Aging and Human Development, 38*, 351–362.

Bazargan, M., Bazargan, S. H., & King, L. (2001). Paranoid ideation among aged African American persons. *The Gerontologist, 41*, 366–373.

Beck, R. L. (1991). The forgotten family. *SHHH. 12*(1), 7–9.

Beck, L., & Burkhart, J. (1994). The renal system and urinary tract. In W. Hazzard, R. Andres, E. Bierman, & J. Blass (Eds.), *Principles of geriatric medicine and gerontology* (2nd Ed.). New York: McGraw Hill.

Bess, F. (1995). Applications of the Hearing Handicap Inventory for the Elderly - Screening Version (HHIE-S). *The Hearing Journal, 48*, 51–57.

Birren, J. E., & Schaie, K. W. (Eds.) (2001). *Handbook of the psychology of aging.* San Diego, CA: Academic Press

Blieszner, R., & Bedford, V. H. (Eds.) (1995). *Handbook of aging and the family.* Westport, CT: Greenwood Press.

Boettcher, F., Gratton, M., Bancroft. B., & Sprongr, V. (1992). Interaction of noise and other agents: Recent advances. In A. Dancer, D. Henderson, R. Salvi, & R. Hammerik (Eds.), *Noise induced hearing loss* (pp. 175–187). St. Louis, MO: Mosby.

Brant, L., Gordon-Salant, S., Pearson, J., Klein, L., Morrell,C., Metter, E., & Fozard, J. (1996). Risk factors related to age-associated hearing loss in the speech frequencies. *Ear and Hearing, 7*, 152–161.

Brock, D., Guralnick, J., & Brody, J. (1990). Demography and epidemiology of aging in the United States. In E. Schneider & J. Rose (Eds.), *Handbook of the biology of aging* (3rd Ed., pp. 3–23). San Diego, CA: Academic Press.

Butler, R. N. (1975). *Why survive? Being old in America.* New York: Harper & Row.

Cacciatore, F., Napoli, C., Abete, P., Marciano, E., Triassi, M., & Rengo, F. (1999). Quality of life determinants and hearing function in an elderly population: Osservatorio Geriatrico Campano Study Group. *Gerontology, 45*, 323–328.

Calhoun, D. W., & Lipman, A. (1984). The disabled. In E. B. Palmore (Ed.), *Handbook on the aged in the United States* (pp. 311–322). Westport, CT: Greenwood Press.

Carabellese, C., Appollonio, I., Rozzini, R., Bianchetti, A., Frisoni, G. B., Frattola, L., & Trabucchi, M. (1993). Sensory impairment and quality of life in a community elderly population. *The American Geriatrics Society, 41*, 401–407.

Centers for Disease Control and Prevention. (1995). *Vital and health statistics trends in the health of older Americans: United States, 1994*. Washington, DC: U.S. Department of Health and Human Services.

Chafetz, P. K., & Wilson, N. L. (1988). Communicating effectively with elderly clients. *Seminars in Speech and Language, 9*, 177–182.

Chartrand, M. (2001). Hearing health care and Alzheimer's Disease. *The Hearing Review, 8*(11), 26–29.

Chmeil, R., & Jerger, J. (1995). Quantifying improvement with amplification. *Ear and Hearing, 16*, 166–175.

Christensen, L. (1999). Future hearing aid technology. *Audiology Today, 11* (Special Issue), 32–33.

Cox, R.M. & Alexander, G.C. (1995). The Abbreviated Profile of Hearing Aid Benefit. *Ear and Hearing*, 16, 176–183.

Dalecki, L. (1988). Hearing versus cognitive impairment in the elderly: Implications for social work practice. *The Social Worker—Le Travailleur Social*. 56(4), 158–160.

Datan, N., & Ginsberg, L. H. (1975). *Life span developmental psychology: Normative life crises*. New York: Academic Press.

David, M., & Trehub, S. (1989). Perspectives on deafened adults. *American Annals of the Deaf, 134*, 200–204.

Demorest, M. E., & Erdman, S. A. (1986). Scale composition and item analysis of the Communication Profile for the Hearing Impaired. *Journal of Speech and Hearing Research, 29*, 515–535.

Demorest, M. E., & Erdman, S. A. (1987). Development of the communication profile for the hearing impaired. *Journal of Speech and Hearing Disorders, 52*, 129–142.

Desselle, D. D., & Proctor, T. K. (2000). Advocating for the elderly hard-of-hearing population: The deaf people we ignore. *Social Work, 45*(3), 277–281.

Erdman, S. A. (2001). How to select a self-assessment instrument: What is it you want to know and why? *Aural Rehabilitation and Its Instrumentation, 9*(1),7–8.

Erikson, E. H., Erikson, J. M., & Kivnick, H. Q. (1986). *Vital involvement in old age*. New York: W. W. Norton.

Garahan, M., Waller, J., Houghton, M, Tisdale, W., & Runge, C. (1992). Hearing loss prevalence and management in nursing home residents. *Journal of the American Geriatrics Society, 40*, 130–134.

Garstecki, D. C., & Erler, S. F. (1998). Hearing loss, control and demographic factors influencing hearing aid use among older adults. *Journal of Speech, Language and Hearing Research, 41*, 527–537.

Garstecki, D. C., & Erler, S. F. (1999). Older adult performance on the communication profile for the hearing impaired: Gender difference. *Journal of Speech, Language, and Hearing Research, 42*(4), 785–796.

Gates, C., Cobb, J., D'Gostino, R., & Wolf, P. (1993). The relationship of hearing in elderly to the presence of cardiovascular disease and cardiovascular risk factors. *Archives of Otolaryngology Head and Neck Surgery, 119*, 156–161.

Gates, C., Cobb, J., Linn, R., Rees, T., & Wolf, P. (1996). Central auditory dysfunction, cognitive dysfunction and dementia in older people. *Archives of Otolaryngology Head and Neck Surgery, 122*, 161–167.

Gilhome-Herbst, K., & Humphrey, C. (1980). Hearing impairment and mental state in the elderly living at home. *British Medical Journal, 282*, 903–905.

Glass, L. E. (1991). Psychosocial aspects of hearing loss in adulthood. In H. Orlans (Ed.), *Adjustment to adult hearing loss* (pp. 167–178). San Diego, CA: Singular Publishing Group.

Gleitman, M. M., Ballachandra, B. B., & Goldstein, D. P. (1992). Incidence of cerumen impaction on the general adult population. *The Hearing Journal, 45*(5), 28–32.

Goffman, E. (1963). *Stigma: Notes on the management of spoiled identity*. Englewood Cliffs, NJ: Prentice-Hall.

Gomez, R., and Madey, S. (2001). Coping-with-hearing-loss model for older adults. *The Journals of Gerontology, 56B*(4), 223.

Gordon-Salant, S. M. (1991). The audiologic assessment. In D. Ripich (Ed.), *Handbook of geriatric communication disorders* (pp. 367–393). Austin, TX: Pro-Ed.

Gordon-Salant, S. M. (1987). Basic hearing evaluation. In H. G. Mueller & V. C. Goeffrey (Eds.), *Communication disorders in aging: Assessment and management* (pp. 301–333). Washington, DC: Gallaudet University Press.

Gould, R. L. (1978). *Transformations.* New York: Simon & Schuster.

Groher, M. (1988). Modifications in speech-language assessment procedures for the older adult. In B. B. Shadden (Ed.), *Communication behavior and aging: A Sourcebook for clinicians* (pp. 248–260). Baltimore, MD: Williams & Wilkins.

Gulya, J. (1991). Structural and physiological changes of the auditory and vestibular mechanisms with aging. In D. Ripich (Ed.), *Handbook of geriatric communication disorders* (pp. 39–54). Austin, TX: Pro-Ed.

Harvey, M. A. (1989). *Psychotherapy with deaf and hard of hearing persons.* Hillsdale, NJ: Lawrence Erlbaum Associates.

Hession, C. M. (1991). Hearing loss and aging: Psychosocial aspects and implications for rehabilitation. *Texas Journal of Audiology and Speech Pathology, 17*(2), 10–13.

Holmes, A. E. (2002). Cochlear Implants and other rehabilitative areas. In R. L. Schow & M. A. Nerbonne (Eds.), *Introduction to audiologic rehabilitation* (4th Ed., pp. 81–100). Boston: Allyn and Bacon.

Hooker, K., and Shifren, K. (1995). Psychological aspects of aging. In R. A. Huntley & K. S. Helfer (Eds.), *Communication in later life* (pp. 99–126). Boston: Butterworth-Heinemann.

Hooyman, N., & Kiyak, H.A. (1999). *Social gerontology: A multidisciplinary perspective,* (5th Ed.). Boston: Allyn and Bacon.

Jacobson, G. (1997). Ten tips (give or take a couple) for balance function testing. *Hearing Journal, 50,* 10–19.

Jacobson, G. P., & Calder, J. H. (1998). A screening version of the Dizziness Handicap Inventory (DHI-S). *American Journal of Otology, 19,* 804–808.

Jahn, A. F., & Cook, E. W. (1997). Medical issues related to CIC fitting. In M. Chasin (Ed.). *CIC handbook* (pp. 53–67). San Diego, CA: Singular Publishing Group.

Jennings, M. B. (1995). Service delivery models for older adults with hearing impairments: Individual sessions. In P. B. Kricos & S. A. Lesner, *Hearing care for the older adult* (pp. 227–266). Boston: Butterworth-Heinemann.

Jerger, J., Chmeil, R., Florin, E., Pirozzolo, F., & Wilson, N. (1996). Comparison of conventional amplification and assistive listening devices in elderly persons. *Ear and Hearing, 17,* 490–504.

Jerger, J., Silman, S., Lew, H., & Chmeil, R. (1993). Case studies in binaural interference: Converging evidence from behavioral and electrophysiologic measures. *Journal of the American Academy of Audiology, 4,* 122–131.

Kaplan, H. (1991). Benefits and limitations of amplification and speechreading for the elderly. In H. Orlans (Ed.), *Adjustment to adult hearing loss,* 85–98. San Diego, CA: College-Hill Press.

Kaplan, H., Bally, S. J., & Brandt, F. (1991). Communication self-assessment scale for deaf adults. *Journal of the American Academy of Audiology, 2*(3), 164–182.

Kaplan, H. (1996). Speechreading. In M. J. Moseley, & S. J. Bally, (Eds.), *Communication therapy: An integrated approach to aural rehabilitation with deaf and hard of hearing adolescents and adults* (pp. 229–250). Washington, DC: Gallaudet University Press.

Kaplan, H., Bally, S. J., Brandt, F., Bussaco, D. A., & Pray, J. L. (1994). Effects of the Gallaudet University Elderhostel programs on the lives of older adults with hearing loss: The Communication Scale for Older Adults. Presentation to the American Academy of Audiology Summer Institute, June 1994, Salt Lake City, UT.

Kaplan, H., Bally, S. J. & Garrettson, C. (1987). *Speechreading: A way to improve under-standing.* (2nd Ed.) Washington, DC: Gallaudet University Press.

Keidser, G., Dillon, H. & Byrne, D. (1996). Guidelines for multiple memory hearing aids. *Journal of the American Academy of Audiology, 7,* 404–418.

Kenney, R. A. (1988). Physiology of aging. In B. B. Shadden (Ed.), *Communication be-havior and aging: A sourcebook for clinicians* (pp. 58–78). Baltimore, MD: Williams & Wilkins.

Kochkin, S. (1997). Customer satisfaction and subjective benefit with high-Performance hearing aids. *The Hearing Review, 3*(12), 16, 18, 22–24, 26.

Kochkin, S. (1997). MarkeTrak IV norms: Subjective measures of satisfaction and benefit. Establishing norms. In B. Weinstein (Ed.), *Seminars in Hearing, 18*(1), 37–48.

Koretz, B., & Moore, A. A. (2001). Assessment of the geriatric patient: A practical ap-proach. *Journal of Clinical Outcomes Management, 8*(7), 35–40.

Korper, S. P. (1989). Epidemiologic and demographic characteristics of the aging popula-tion. In J. Goldstein, H. Kashima, and C. Koopman (Eds.), *Geriatric otorhinolarn-gology* (pp. 19–28). Philadelphia: B. C. Decker.

Kreeger, J. L., Raulin, M. L., Grace, J., & Priest, B. L. (1995). Effect of hearing enhance-ment on mental status ratings in geriatric psychiatric patients. *American Journal of Psychiatry, 152,* 629-631.

Kricos, P. B., & Lesner, S. A. (1995). *Hearing care for the older adult.* Boston: Butterworth Heinemann.

Kricos, P. B. (1997). Audiologic rehabilitation for the elderly: A collaborative approach, *The Hearing Journal, 50*(2), 1–3, 18–19.

Kuk, F. K. (1998). Rationale and requirements for a slow acting compression hearing aid. *The Hearing Journal, 51*(6), 45–53, 79.

Kurtz, L. F. (1990). The self-help movement: review of the past decade of research. *Social Work with Groups, 13*(3), 101–115.

Kurtz, L. F. (1997). *Self-help and support groups: A handbook for practitioners.* Thou-sand Oaks, CA: Sage Publications.

Kyle, J., & Wood, J. (1987). *Adjustment to acquired deafness.* London: British Associa-tion of Deafened People.

Kyle, J. G., Jones, L. G., & Wood, P. L. (1991). Adjustment to acquired hearing loss: A working model. In H. Orlans (Ed.), *Adjustment to adult hearing loss* (pp. 119–138). San Diego, CA: Singular Publishing Group.

Lane, H. (1993). *The mask of benevolence.* New York: Vintage Books.

Lane, H., & Bahan, B. (1998). Ethic of cochlear implntation in young children: A review and reply from Deaf-World perspective. *Otolaryngology-Head Neck Surgery, 119*: 297–313.

Lasher, K. P., Faulkender, P. J. (1993). Measurement of aging anxiety: Development of the Anxiety About Aging Scale. *International Journal of Aging and Human Development, 37,* 247–259.

Laufer, M. B. (1985). *The influence of hearing impairment as a transition event on the life satisfaction of adults aged* 65–74. Unpublished doctoral dissertation, University of Maryland, College Park.

Lesner, S. A., & Kricos, P. B. (1995). Audiologic rehabilitation assessment: A holistic ap-proach. In P. B. Kricos & S. A. Lesner (Eds.), *Hearing care for the older adult* (pp. 21–58). Boston: Butterworth-Heinemann.

Lomranz, J. (Ed.) (1998). *Handbook of aging and mental health: An integrative approach.* New York: Plenum Press.

Lubinski, R. (Ed.) (1995). *Dementia and communication.* San Diego, CA: Singular Pub-lishing Group.

Lubinski, R., & Higginbotham, D. J. (1997). *Communication technologies for the elderly: Vision, hearing and speech.* San Diego, CA: Singular Publishing Group.

Luey, H. S. (1980). Between worlds: The problems of deafened adults. *Social Work in Health Care, 5,* 253–265.

Luey, H. S., Glass, L., & Elliot, H. (1995). Hard of hearing or deaf: Issues of ears, language, culture, and identity. *Social Work, 40*(2), 177–182.

Maas, H. S., & Kuypers, J. A. (1974). *From thirty to seventy.* San Francisco: Jossey-Bass

Maggi, S., Minicicuci, N., Martini, A., Langlois, J., Siviero, P., Pavan & Enzi, G. (1998). Prevalence rates of hearing impairment and comorbid conditions in older people: The Veneto study. *Journal of the American Geriatrics Society, 46*, 1069–1074.

Markides, K. S. (1983). Minority aging. In M.W. Riley, B. B. Hess, and K. Bond (Eds.), *Aging in society: Selected review of recent research*, 115–137. Hillsdale, NJ: Lawrence Erlbaum Associates.

Maurer. J., & Rupp, R. R. (1979). *Hearing and aging: Tactics for intervention.* New York: Grune and Stratton.

Meadow-Orlans, K. P. (1991). Social and psychological effects of hearing loss in adulthood: A literature review. In H. Orlans (Ed.), *Adjustment to adult hearing loss* (pp. 35–57). San Diego, CA: Singular Publishing Group.

Moseley, M. J., & Bally, S. J. (Eds.) (1996). *Communication therapy: An integrated approach to aural rehabilitation with deaf and hard of hearing adolescents and adults.* Washington, DC: Gallaudet University Press.

Miyamoto, R., & Miyamoto, R. (1995). Anatomy of the ear canal. In B. Ballachanda (Ed.), *The human ear canal: Treatment considerations and clinical applications including cerumen management* (pp. 21–26). San Diego, CA: Singular Publishing Group.

Mueller, H. G., & Carter, A. S. (2002). Hearing aids and assistive devices. In R. L. Schow & M. A. Nerbonne (Eds.), *Introduction to audiologic rehabilitation* (4th Ed., pp. 31–80). Boston: Allyn and Bacon.

Mueller, H. G., & Goeffrey, V. C. (Eds.) (1987). *Communication disorders in aging: Assessment and management.* Washington, DC: Gallaudet University Press.

Mulrow, C. D., Aguilar, C., Endicott, J. E., Velez, R., et al. (1990). Association between hearing impairment and the quality of life of elderly individuals. *Journal of the American Geriatrics Society, 38*(1), 45–50.

Mulrow, C., Michael, T., & Aquilar, C. (1992). Correlates of successful hearing aid use in adults. *Ear and Hearing, 13*, 108–113.

Myers, D. G. (2000). *A quiet world: Living with hearing loss.* New Haven, CT: Yale University Press.

National Center for Health Statistics. (1987). *Aging in the eighties: Functional limitations of individuals age 65 years and over. Advance data from vital health statistics* (No.133, DHHS Publ. No. PHS 87-1250.) Hyattsville, MD: Public Health Service.

Nerbonne, M. A. (1988). The effects of aging on auditory structures and functions. In B. B. Shadden (Ed.), *Communication behavior and aging: A sourcebook for clinicians* (pp. 137–161). Baltimore, MD: Williams & Wilkins.

Nerbonne, M., Christman, W., & Fleschner, C. (1995). *Comparing objective and subjective measures of hearing aid benefit.* Presentation at AAA Convention, Dallas, TX.

Newman, C., & Weinstein, B. (1988). The Hearing Handicap Inventory for the Elderly as a measure of hearing aid benefit. *Ear and Hearing, 9*, 81–85.

Newman, C. W., & Weinstein, B. E. (1996). Judgments of perceived hearing handicap by hearing-impaired elderly men and their spouses. *Journal of the Academy of Rehabilitative Audiology, 19*, 109–115.

Niparko, J. K., Kirk, K. H., Mellon, N. K., Robbins, A. M., Tucci, D. L., & Wilson, B. S. (2000). *Cochlear implants: Principles and practices.* Philadelphia, PA: Lippincott, Williams & Wilkins.

Niparko, J. K., Cheng, A. K., & Francis, H. W. (2000). In J. K. Niparko, K. H. Kirk, N. K. Mellon, A. M. Robbins, D. L. Tucci, & B. S.Wilson (Eds.), *Cochlear implants: Principles and practices*, 269–288. Philadelphia: Lippincott, Williams & Wilkins.

Nixon, J., Glorig, A., & High, W. (1962). Changes in air and bone conduction thresholds as a function of age. *Journal of Laryngology and Otology, 74*, 288–299.

Novak, R. E. (2000). Considerations for selecting and fitting of amplification for geriatric adults. In R.E. Sandlin (Ed.), *Textbook of hearing aid amplification* (2nd Ed., pp. 571–606). San Diego, CA: Singular Publishing Group.

Orlans, H., & Meadow-Orlans, K. P. (1985). Responses to hearing loss: Effects on social life, leisure, and work. *SHHH Journal 6*(1), 4–7.

Orr, J. B. (1982). Aging, catastrophe, and moral reasoning. In P. L. McKee (Ed.), *Philosophical foundations of gerontology* (pp. 243–260). New York: Human Sciences Press.

Oyer, J., Freeman, B., Hardick, J., Dixon, K., Donnelly, K., Goldstein, D., Lloyd, L., & Mussen, E. (1976). Unheeded recommendations for aural rehabilitation: Analysis of a survey. *Journal of the Academy of Rehabilitative Audiology, 9*(1), 20–30.

Palmer, C. V. (1995). Improvement of hearing function. In R. A. Huntley & K. S. Helfer (Eds.), *Communication in later life* (pp. 181–224). Boston, MA: Butterworth-Heinemann.

Palmer, C., Adams, S., Durrant, J., Bourgeouis, M., & Ross, M. (1998). Managing hearing loss in patients with Alzheimer's Disease. *Journal of the American Academy of Audiology, 9*, 275–284.

Palmer, C. V., Adams, S. W., Bourgeois, M., Durran, J., and Rossi, M. (1999). Reduction in caregiver-identified problem behaviors in patients with Alzheimer disease post-hearing-aid fitting. *Journal of Speech, Language, and Hearing Research, 42*(2), 312–328.

Palmore, F. B. (Ed.) (1993). *Developments and research on aging: An international handbook*. Westport, CT: Greenwood Press.

Palmore, E. B. (Ed.) (1984). *Handbook on the aged in the United States*. Westport, CT: Greenwood Press.

Palmore, E. B. (1985). *Normal aging III: Reports from the Duke longitudinal studies, 1975–1984*. Durham, NC: Duke University Press.

Perlstein, R. (1990). *Mature market report*. Atlanta, GA: Mature Market Report, Inc.

Peters, C., Potter, J., & Scholer, S. (1988). Hearing impairment as a predictor of cognitive decline in dementia. *Journal of the American Geriatrics Society, 36*, 981–986.

Pichora-Fuller, M. K. (1997a). Assistive listening devices for the elderly. In R. Lubinski & D. J. Higginbotham (Eds.). *Communication technologies for the elderly: Vision, hearing & speech* (pp. 161–201). San Diego, CA: Singular Publishing Group.

Pichora-Fuller, M. K. (1997b). Comparison of conventional amplification and assistive listening devices in elderly persons. *Ear and Hearing, 17*, 490–504.

Pichora-Fuller, K., & Schow, R. L. (2002). Audiologic rehabilitation for adults and elderly adults: Assessment and management. In R. L. Schow & M. A. Nerbonne (Eds.), *Introduction to audiologic rehabilitation* (4th Ed., pp. 335–402). Boston: Allyn and Bacon.

Popelka, N. M., Cruickshanks, K. J., Wiley, T. L., Tweed, T. S., Klein, B. E., & Klein, R. (1998). Low prevalence of hearing aid use among older adults with hearing loss: The epidemiology of hearing loss study. *Journal of the American Geriatrics Society, 46*, 1075–1078.

Pray, J. L. (1989). Older persons with hearing loss: A neglected minority. *Disability Studies Quarterly, 9* (3), 15–17.

Pray, J. L. (1992). *Aging and hearing loss: Patterns of coping with the effects of late onset hearing loss among persons age 60 and older and their spouses/significant others*. Unpublished doctoral dissertation, Cincinnati, OH: The Union Institute.

Pray, J. L. (1996). Psychosocial aspects of adult aural rehabilitation. In M. J. Moseley & S. J. Bally (Eds.), *Communication therapy: An integrated approach to aural rehabilitation with Deaf and hard of hearing adolescents and adults* (pp. 128–148). Washington, DC: Gallaudet University Press.

Primeau, R. (1997). Hearing aid benefit in adults and older adults. In B. Weinstein (Ed.), *Seminars in Hearing, 18*, 29–36.

Quinn, K. S. (1986). *Self, spouse and audiologist evaluation of hearing impairment and hearing handicap in a sample of older people.* Unpublished doctoral dissertation, University of Michigan.

Raiford, C. A. (1988). Modifications in hearing assessment procedures for the older adult. In B. B. Shadden (Ed.), *Communication behavior and aging: A sourcebook for clinicians* (pp. 227–236). Baltimore, MD: Williams & Wilkins.

Rao, P. (1997). Functional communication assessment and outcomes. In B. B. Shadden & M. A. Toner (Eds.), *Aging and communication* (pp. 197–225). Austin, TX: Pro-Ed.

Redinger, B. (1996). Auditory skills. In M. J.Moseley, & S. J. Bally (Eds.), *Communication therapy: An integrated approach to aural rehabilitation with deaf and hard of hearing adolescents and adults* (pp. 195–228). Washington, DC: Gallaudet University Press.

Resnick, H. E., Fries, B. E., & Verbrugge, L. M. (1997). Windows to their world: The effect of sensory impairment on social engagement and activity time in nursing home residents. *Journal of Gerontology: Social Sciences, 528*, S135–S144.

Ripich, D. N. (1991). Language and communication In dementia. In D. Ripich (Ed.), *Handbook of geriatric communication disorders* (pp. 255–283). Austin, TX: Pro-Ed.

Rosenwasser, H. (1964). Otitic problems in the aged. *Geriatrics, 19*, 11–17.

Rosow, I. (1973). Social contacts of the aging self. *The Gerontologist, 13*, 82–87.

Rosow, I. (1974). *Socialization to old age.* Berkeley, CA: University of California Press.

Ross, M. (1992). Why people won't wear hearing aids. *Hearing Rehabilitation Quarterly. 17*(2), B 11

Ross, M. (1995a). Developments in research and technology, *SHHH 16*, 32–34.

Ross, M. (1995b). Developments in technology, *SHHH 16*, 25–26.

Rothschild, M. A., & Kampfe, C. M. (1997). Issues associated with late onset deafness. *Journal of the American Deafness and Rehabilitation Association, 31*, 1–16.

Ruby, R. (1986). Conductive hearing loss in the elderly. *Journal of Otolarngology, 15*, 245–247.

Rumney N. (1998). The aging eye and vision appliances. *Ophthalmic Physiol-Opt, 18*, 191–196.

Russell, E., & Burns, A. (2003). Presentation and clinical management of dementia. In R. Tallies, H. Failed, & J. Brocklehurst (Eds.), *Brocklehurst's textbook of geriatric medicine and gerontology*, 801–817. London: Churchill-Livingstone.

Saunders, G. H., & Cienkowski, K. M. (1996). Refinement and psychometric evaluation of the Attitude Toward Loss of Hearing Questionnaire. *Ear & Hearing, 17*, 505–519

Schaie, K.W. (1996). *Intellectual development in adulthood: The Seattle longitudinal study.* New York: Cambridge University Press

Scherer, M. J., & Frisina, D. R. (1998). Characteristics associated with marginal hearing loss and subjective well-being among a sample of older adults. *Journal of Rehabilitation Research and Development, 35*, 420–426.

Schow, R., & Nerbonne, M. (Eds.) (2002). *Introduction to audiologic rehabilitation.* (4th ed.), Boston: Allyn and Bacon.

Schuknecht, H. F. (1993). *Pathology of the Ear* (2nd ed.). Philadelphia, PA: Lea & Febiger.

Schuknecht, H., & Gacek, M.(1993). Cochlear pathology in presbycusis. *Annals of Oto-Rhino-Laryngology, 102*, 1–16.

Schwartz, J. B. (1999). Clinical pharmacology, pp. 303–332. In W. Hazzard, R. Andres, E. Bierman, & J. Blass (Eds.), *Principles of geriatric medicine and gerontology* (2nd ed.), 303–331. New York: McGraw Hill.

Shadden, B. B., & Toner, M. A. (1997). *Aging and communication.* Austin, TX: Proed.

Smith-Worrall, L., Hickson, L., & Dodd, B. (1990). Communication disorders and the elderly in residential care. In R. B. Lefroy (Ed.), *Proceedings of the 25th Annual Conference of the Australian Association of Gerontology* (pp. 65–68). Canberra, Australia: Australian Association of Gerontology,

Soucek, S., & Michaels, L. (1990). *Hearing loss in the elderly.* London: Springer-Verlag.

Spencer (1973).

Stach, B. A., & Stoner, W. R. (1991). Sensory aids for the hearing impaired elderly. In D. Ripich (Ed.), *Handbook of geriatric communication disorders* (pp. 421–438). Austin, TX: Pro-Ed.

Strawbridge, W. J., Wallhagen, M. I., Shema, S. J., & Kaplan, G. A. (2000). Negative consequences of hearing impairment in old age: A longitudinal analysis. *The Gerontologist, 40*, 320–326.

Strouse, A. L., DeChicchis, A. R., & Bess, F. H. (1997). Changes in hearing with aging. In R. Lubinski & D. J. Higginbotham (Eds.). *Communication technologies for the elderly: Vision, hearing & speech* (pp. 123–128). San Diego, CA: Singular Publishing Group.

Sweetow, R. W. (1999). Things that are likely and unlikely to happen. *Audiology Today, 11*(Special Issue), 31.

Sweetow, R. W., & Shelton, C. W. (1996). Programmable vs. Conventional hearing instruments: Time/cost and satisfaction factors. *The Hearing Journal, 49*(4), 51–52, 54, 56–57.

Tye-Murray, N. (1998). *Foundations of aural rehabilitation.* San Diego, CA: Singular Publishing Group.

Tonkovich, J. D. (1988). Communication disorders in the elderly. In B. B. Shadden, *Communication behavior and aging: A sourcebook for clinicians* (pp. 197–215). Baltimore, MD: Williams & Wilkins.

Uhlmann, R., Larson, E., Koepsell, T. (1986). Hearing impairment and cognitive decline in senile dementia of the Alzheimer's type. *Journal of the American Geriatrics Society, 34*, 207–210.

Uhlmann, R., Larson, E., Rees, T., Koepsell, T., & Duckert, L. (1989). Relationship of hearing impairment to dementia and cognitive dysfunction in older adults. *Journal of the American Medical Association, 261*, 1916–1919.

Uhlmann, R. F., Rees, T. S., Psaty, B. M., & Duckart, L. G. (1989). Validity and reliability of auditory screening tests in demented and non-demented older adults. *Journal of General Internal Medicine, 4*, 90–96.

Ventry, I., & Weinstein, B. (1982). The hearing handicap inventory for the elderly: A new tool. *Ear and Hearing, 3*(3), 128–134.

Voeks, S., Gallagher, C., Langer, E., & Drinka, P. (1990). Hearing loss in the nursing home: An institutional issue. *Journal of the American Geriatrics Society, 38*, 141–145.

Wainapel, S. (1994). Visual impairments. In G. Felsenthal, S. Garrison, & F. Steinberg (Eds.) *Rehabilitation of the aging and elderly patient*, 327–337. Baltimore, MD: Williams & Wilkins.

Waltzman, S. B., & Cohen, N. L. (Eds.). (2000). *Cochlear implants.* New York: Thieme.

Waltzman, S., Cohen, N., & Shapiro, B. (1993). The benefits of cochlear implants in the geriatric population. *Otolaryngology—Head and Neck Surgery, 108*, 329–333.

Watson, W. H., & Maxell, R. J. (1977). *Human aging and dying: A study in sociocultural gerontology.* New York: St. Martins Press.

Wax, T. M. (1982). The hearing impaired aged: Double jeopardy or double challenge? *Gallaudet Today, 12*(2), 3–7.

Wayner, D. S., & Abrahamson, J. E. (1998). *Learning to hear again with a cochlear implant: An audiologic rehabilitation curriculum guide.* Austin, TX: Hear Again.

Wayner, D., & Abrahamson, J. E. (1996). *Learning to hear again.* Austin, TX: Hear Again.

Webb, L. M., Schreiner, J. M., & Asmuth, M. V. (1995). Maintaining interaction skills. In R. A. Huntley & K. S. Helfer (Eds.), *Communication skills in later life*, 159–179. Boston: Butterworth Heinemann.

Weinstein, B. E. (2000). *Geriatric audiology.* Thieme: New York.

Weinstein, B. E. (1997). Hearing aids and older adults. In R. Lubinski & D. J. Higginbotham (Eds.), *Communication technologies for the elderly: Vision, hearing & speech* (pp. 129–159). San Diego, CA: Singular Publishing Group.

Weinstein, B. E., Spitzer, J., & Ventry, I. M. (1986). Test-retest reliability of the Hearing Handicap Inventory for the Elderly. *Ear and Hearing, 7*, 295–299.

Weinstein, B. E., & Ventry, I. M. (1983). Audiometric correlates of the Hearing Handicap Inventory for the Elderly. *Journal of Speech and Hearing Research, 26,* 148–151.

Weinstein, B. E. & Ventry, I. M. (1982). Hearing impairment and social isolation in the elderly. *Journal of Speech and Hearing Research. 25,* 593–595.

White, J., & Regan, M. (1987). Otologic considerations. In H. G. Mueller & V. C. Goeffrey (Eds.), *Communication disorders in aging: Assessment and management* (pp. 37–71), Washington, DC: Gallaudet University Press.

Willott, J. F. (1991). *Aging and the auditory system.* San Diego, CA: Singular Publishing Group.

Yorkston, K. M., Beukleman, D. R., & Bell, K. R. (1988). *Clinical management of dysarthric speakers.* Austin, TX: Pro-Ed.

Yorkston, K. M., & Garrett, K. L. (1997). Assistive technology for elders with motor speech disability. In R. Lubinski & D. J. Higginbotham (Eds.), *Communication technologies for the elderly: Vision, hearing & speech,* 235–261. San Diego, CA: Singular Publishing Group.

Yorkston, K. M., Miller, R. M., & Strand E. A. (1995). *Management of speech and swallowing disorders in degenerative disease.* Tuscon, AZ: Communication Skill Builders.

Yorkston, K. M., & Waugh, P. F. (1989). Use of augmentative communication devices with apractic individuals. In P. Square-Storer (Ed.), *Apraxia of speech,* 267–283. London: Taylor & Francis.

Zwolan, T. A. (2000). Selection criteria and evaluation. In S. B. Waltzman & N. L. Cohen (Eds.), *Cochlear implants,* 63–71. New York: Thieme.

CHAPTER 14

Business Essentials In Audiology Private Practice

Robert M. Traynor

Audiology Associates of Greeley, Inc., Greeley, CO

So you want to be in private practice? Work for yourself? Drive the same car as the physicians? Take lots of time off? Be your own boss? If so, you will soon find out, that graduate school prepared you rather well to see the patients, but poorly for business management. Management, as in Audiology, has its own fundamentals, vocabulary, and practicum that are necessary to be successful in business. While audiologists are learning ABR, VNG, Audiometry and other procedures; our business and commercial counterparts are studying, Marketing, Customer Service, Human Resources, Accounting, Finance, Operations, Information Technology, Management Theory and other business skills. The purpose of this chapter is to present some business and management essentials to offer a picture of the skills necessary to manage a practice and encourage aspiring private practice audiologists to obtain more business and management skills. Although it is a good idea to have some business and management courses as part of the regular Doctor of Audiology program, obtaining these skills by practicing professionals in an Internet world is much easier than in the past. There are many business schools that are available to practicing professionals online and it is not essential to attend classes at the community college or university to become a wise practice manager.

DEVELOPMENT OF THE PRIVATE PRACTICE AUDIOLOGY

The field of Audiology developed in hospitals to treating World War II veterans from hearing losses encountered during the perils of war. The realities of hearing impairment created by bombs, rifle fire, airplane noise, trauma, and countless other noisy situations are the basic pillars of our profession. Bergman (2002) detailed the military origins of our profession in a monograph that outlines this era. He states that many aspects of early Audiology in the United States had been developed in the civilian leagues for the hard-of-hearing at the beginning of the 20th century. These early aspects of what is now known in general as "Audiology" involved new services for adults to complement the ongoing educational programs that were directed at hearing impaired children in previous decades. These new services were introduced mainly by adults who were themselves suffering from hearing impairment, and by teachers of hearing impaired children who were recruited by the former to teach them alternate communication skills. There was also a growing awareness of the increasing numbers of the aging population, many of them with hearing problems. In short, there was a realization that any noticeable hearing loss was a potential impediment to a comfortable and productive life. Clear also, was the threat of hearing loss accompanying modern war caused by its noisy machines and greatly enhanced firepower.

Since the late 1970s, more audiologists have chosen independent private practice as a setting to offer diagnostic and rehabilitative services including the dispensing of hearing instruments. A major criticism of audiologists by employers, manufacturers, insurance companies, bankers, accountants and others is that most clinicians are oblivious to the perils and promises of private business. Although owning an Audiology practice is impossible without the correct clinical skills, ultimately providing audiological products and services becomes a business and must be managed efficiently to initiate and continue the lifestyle to which clinicians aspired when they entered the profession.

From its earliest origins, Audiology was a "helping profession" doing what was necessary to facilitate the rehabilitation of our patients. The focus was on patients and how to best facilitate their auditory interaction with the environment, but not necessarily making a living as part of the process. Audiologists often find themselves at the crossroad of doing what is right for our patients without compromising our incomes and/or goals for ourselves and families. As clinicians, audiologists have the professional responsibility to provide the best possible care and think of their patients first. This does not, however, imply the necessity to compromise income, and subsequently lifestyle, to offer our patients high quality care. If the practice is simply there to "help people" the owner is donating time and, unless independently wealthy, will soon be a destitute "helping professional."

Consider that physicians, attorneys, accountants, and other professionals are also "helping professions" as these professions assist people in overcoming various difficulties. For example, as part of this process of assisting their patients, physicians may be required to "sell" their patient a follow up office visit or a surgical procedure as part of the cure. Similarly, an Attorney works as a "helping professional" to assist their clients with legal difficulties. As part of helping their client, it is often necessary to "sell" their clients legal services or representation in court as part of the process. Audiologists are also providing valuable services by either diagnosing hearing difficulties or providing rehabilitative treatment and/or appropriate products to the hearing impaired.

One of the complexities of audiology practice is actually getting paid for your services. At this point, audiologists are at the mercy of a system that was designed for physician reimbursement and not for audiologists or other non-physician specialties. Duncan (1999) indicates that audiologists have opted to provide both the professional services and the sales of equipment (hearing aids) and this has created an interesting problem in that it is difficult for consumers to tell the difference between an Audiologist and business people that simply sell inefficient, unreliable equipment (hearing aid dealers). This confusion by the general population has historically created difficulty in obtaining third party reimbursement for services audiology products. Audiology has had a significant identity problem fueled by the fact that audiologists were not well represented by organizations until the late 1980s. This lobbying difficulty coupled with the fact that we were not a doctoral level profession has complicated the reimbursement picture substantially.

By the end of 2006 over 30 percent of audiologists will be at the doctoral level. In the mid 1990s only about 3 percent of audiologists were educated at the doctoral level. The Doctor of Audiology (Au.D.) degree has substantially upgraded the profession and the skills available to our patients. This transformation of the profession has been accomplished by the modification of traditional training programs to the Au.D. model and the availability of online working professional programs allowing practicing audiologists to upgrade their level with little or no time away from the office. Since all new audiologists are doctors, the profession's promise for direct access to hearing care paid by government and private health insurers is now a very real possibility and makes private practice audiology quite attractive (Pessis, 2001).

LEGAL STRUCTURE OF AUDIOLOGY PRACTICE

No matter if the practice is brand new or if the practice has existed for years a major business decision is the legal structure of the practice. The major types of organizational structures are obvious to all of us as we see them throughout our environment. We live with sole proprietors, corporations (INC, PC) and more recently the Limited Liability Corporation (LLC) or Limited Liability Practice (LLP) for professionals. Let's review these various business structures and investigate their meaning.

SOLE PROPRIETORSHIP

Brealy, Myers, and Marcus (2002) cite the story of Charles Walgreen who, in 1901, bought the drugstore in which he worked on the south side of Chicago. Today Walgreen's is the largest drugstore chain in the United States. If, like Charles Walgreen, a person starts their own Audiology practice, with no partners or stockholders, they are said to be a sole proprietor. In a sole proprietorship format the owner bears all of the expense of equipment, office supplies, employees, marketing, billing, collections and other costs; but they are entitled to all of the after tax profits as income. The major advantages of a sole proprietorship structure is the ease with which it can be established, the lack of regulations governing this type of practice, and that the revenue is only taxed one time as personal income. It makes this style ideally suited for informal small businesses, such as an Audiology practice.

The downside of the sole proprietorship is that the owner is totally responsible for all of the business's debts and other liabilities. If the practice owes the bank and it does not pay, the owner of the practice is personally liable for the total amount of the loan. If the debts are large enough, the bank can force the owner into a personal bankruptcy since sole proprietors are the responsible party for all debts and liabilities of the business. Thus, as a sole proprietor, the owner has unlimited liability for not only their own actions, but the also the actions of their employees.

PARTNERSHIP

A partnership is formed when the choice not to establish the business on your own. Often money and expertise are pooled to facilitate practice with a colleague, friend, or relative. If the practice has others involved in the business structure, the sole proprietorship is inappropriate and a partnership is formed. An attorney draws a partnership agreement that sets out how the management decisions are to be made and the portion of profits to which each partner is entitled. The disadvantage of a partnership is that although the partners may keep all of the after tax profit, there is still unlimited liability of the partners for debts and malpractice. The real difference from a sole proprietorship is that the liability is now spread across the partners, rather than just on the shoulders of one person. Since the partners are associated for both debt and malpractice, it is imperative that the partners know each other very well. The best practical advice on partnerships is to "know thy partner" as this format has been likened a marriage in that it can be a very positive business relationships or a significant liability creating a difficult personal and business climate within the practice.

CORPORATIONS

As the practice grows and/or personal liability increases, it may be necessary to incorporate. A corporation is a distinct legal entity and, unlike the sole proprietorship or the partnership, it is totally separate from it owners. The corporation is somewhat costly to form when compared to sole proprietorships or partnerships as the formation is based upon articles of incorporation drawn up by an attorney and filed with the state. These articles are a legal document drawn and filed by an attorney within the state in which the corporation will operate and the owner(s) incurs numerous fees when the corporation is created such as attorney fees, filing fees, minute books, corporate seals, etc. These state determined, legal articles set out the purpose of the business, how many shares of stock can be issued, the number of directors to be appointed. A corporation, according to Brealey, Myers, and Marcus (2002), is considered a resident of its state, can borrow or lend money, can sue or be sued and pay its own taxes. The major benefit in establishing a corporation, usually designated by an Inc. after its name, is the shelter from personal liability for the owner(s) in terms of financial obligations and malpractice lawsuits referred to in business circles as "limited liability". In our industry most product manufacturers will require the owner(s) of a corporation to be personally liable for accounts; suits against the corporation are usually not a personal obligation. If the corporation goes bankrupt, the suit does not usually affect the owners beyond the limits of the stock that they own.

Although large corporations have boards that are responsible to a great number of stockholders, it is not uncommon for an incorporated Audiology practice to be wholly owned by one person. In this situation, the Board of Directors are the owner and relatives whose charge is to manage the corporation. In these "closely held corporations" the owner controls all of the stock and therefore makes all of the decisions. Sometimes it is necessary to sell some stock to others for expansion purposes, then depending upon how much stock is sold it may be necessary to pacify a controlling and a minority interests according to the percentage of stock owned. The major disadvantage of a C type corporation format is that double taxation. Since the corporation is a tax entity, it is taxed at a corporate rate. So, not only does the C corporation pay taxes on its profit, but the employees (including the 100 percent stockholder of the corporation) will pay taxes on their income received from the corporation. Thus, as a sacrifice for the shelter of the corporation, the 100 percent shareholder/owner of the corporation will pay taxes on the income generated by the corporation and taxes again the same income obtained by the shareholder as an employee. If the person was a sole proprietor they would only be taxed once on the income generated.

HYBRID FORMS OF BUSINESS ORGANIZATION

Many businesses do not fall into neatly into any of the three main types of categories and require legal modification of the structure to meet their needs. Brealey et al., (2002) describe these other versions of corporations as "hybrids" since corporate formats are combinations of the sole proprietorship, the partnership, and a corporation. A special hybrid type of corporation that does not have double taxation is the S corporation. Also designated with Inc after the name, the "sub S corporation" as it is known has all of the legal characteristics of a corporation except that the S corporation is not taxed, income is treated like a partnership and the partners and the shareholders are taxed according to their share of the profits from the S corporation on their individual tax returns. In many states there are Professional Corporations (PC), a designation usually reserved for physicians, dentists, lawyers, accountants and other professionals. Many states would like to separate professional corporations from other types of corporations and expose them to more liability than those in other types of businesses. In the PC, the business component has limited liability, but the professionals within the business can still be sued personally for malpractice, even if their malpractice occurs in their role as an employee of the corporation. Another hybrid example is the relatively new limited liability company (LLC) or the liability partnership (LLP) used by professionals. These LLC/LLP formats combine the tax advantages of a partnership and the limited liability advantage of a corporation.

Corley, Reed, Shedd, and Morehead (2002) indicate general advantages and disadvantages of corporations in the following table:

TABLE 14–1.
Advantages and Disadvantages of Business Structures

Sole Proprietorship		Partnership		Corporation	
Advantages	Disadvantages	Advantages	Disadvantages	Advantages	Disadvantages
Easily Established	Owner must bear all costs of business set up and maintenance	Relatively easy to establish	Each Partner has unlimited liability for debts	Corporation may be closely held.....owner may own all stock	Requires an Attorney and incurrence of other costs to establish
No Partners or Shareholders	No others to share burden or add expertise	Pooled Expertise	Each Partner has unlimited liability for Malpractice	Limited Liability for Debts	Responsible to shareholders
Only pay taxes once on income generated	Unlimited Liability for Debts	Pooled Resources	Need to be careful of partners, personalities, spending habits, etc	Limited Liability for Malpractice	Generally, profits are taxed twice...once in the corporation once in salary
All the after tax profits stay with the owner	Unlimited Liability for Malpractice	All the after tax profits stay with the Partners	Must share profits with partners	Some Hybrid formats have benefits of limited liability and taxed only once	
Lack of government regulations				A distinct legal entity	

HUMAN RESOURCES

Most private practices, at least at first, start with a clinician serving patients. By necessity, the clinician is the audiologist, business manager, receptionist, insurance clerk, finance officer, janitor, and the Director of Human Resources. As long as these clinician-managers have no employees, they are dealing with a highly motivated individual that will do whatever it takes to make the practice successful. Fortunately or unfortunately, practices inevitably grow and the clinician that initially had time to work all of these positions must now spend more of their time seeing patients to generate the practice income. Thus, these various jobs become filled by employees that may or may not share the same values and motivation for the ultimate success of the practice. These employees become the voice of the practice to the outside world, from the initial telephone contact to scheduling appointments, greeting the patients, and interacting with colleagues, suppliers and referral sources. Employees have a major influence on virtually every component of the practice and it is essential that they are well motivated and feel good about their contribution to the team effort that provides services to the hearing impaired. Since these expensive ambassadors will become the personality of your practice, representing you and/or your unit to the outside world, the process of hiring and maintaining good employees while terminating unproductive or bad employees is paramount to success.

HIRING

Employees are the single most expensive overhead component of the practice, considering that withholding, benefits, salary and commissions can cost much more than the ABR unit or that new VNG system. Burrows (2004) indicates that it is impossible for audiologists to understand all of the implications and laws pertaining to employment, especially when employment law does not always comply with common sense, fairness, and logic.

Robbins (2001) indicates that managers are individuals that get things done through other people, and therefore, the real key to success in a practice or the management of an Audiology entity is successful hiring. As new managers, we often idealistically assume that our employees will be loyal, qualified, dress appropriately, always be polite and courteous, seldom take breaks, never be absent, never complain, have no psychological disorders, and totally share our vision of the company. Ellison (1999) points out that, in reality, employees may not share our goals for the ultimate success of the practice or profit center. They may not be honest about their credentials, may or may not be loyal, may or may not enjoy their job, probably do not want to work to make the doctor or hospital rich, may not be computer literate, may be discriminatory toward certain types of patients and unfortunately create a significant management challenge. Since both administrative and professional employees have a major impact upon the care of patients, careful selection of employees is good patient care. Further, the additional effort expended in the hiring process can reduce difficulties encountered during the employees' tenure and reduce possible legal ramifications upon their departure.

ADVERTISING THE POSITION

Good hiring begins with the advertisement of the position opening. The better the position is described, either professional or administrative, the better the pool of candidates available for selection. Obviously, the advertisement for the position should include relevant information such as work history/experience, education/training (if actually job related) and specific skills required. It should further describe the necessary components of the position such as travel required, if relocation is necessary, and other specifics. Although questions about citizenship are allowed, personal characteristics can be included only if they are actually job related. Personal job requirements such as, age, sex, racial traits or characteristics, national origin, religious preference, and physical characteristics are extremely risky unless they are a component of a Bona Fide Occupational Qualification (BFOQ) and these BFOQs are not usually a component of an Audiology or administrative position. The advertisement should in no way offer the appearance of discrimination or exclusion of certain individuals or groups (Burrows, 2004).

THE INTERVIEW

Obviously, the purpose of the interview is to determine if the applicant meets the job requirements outlined in the advertisement and if they are able to provide the required work for which they are being hired. Of course, just as in the advertisement, interview questions about race, religion, sex, disability, national origin or ancestry are generally illegal, particularly if they are designed to exclude applicants based on these issues. Although we are usually determined to obtain the best-qualified person for the position from the pool of candidates, Hunt (2005) indicates that hiring decisions often focus too much on technical skills and expertise, overlooking the "soft skills." If individuals are hired on technical skills alone, it can result in personnel that have the cognitive firepower for success, but lack the social skills to effectively use what they know. Hunt suggests that this is a bit like having a car with a powerful engine, but lacking the steering and brakes necessary to make it win at the racetrack. Thus, during the interview process you should also note qualities such as self-awareness, sensitivity to others, social intelligence or method of influencing the behaviors and perceptions of others, and self control under stressful situations. These are not easy to assess in the interview process but should actually be the main considerations once the basic skills to perform the job are established.

EMPLOYEE HANDBOOK

Once an employee is hired, it is essential from the beginning of the employer/employee relationship that the practice rules for employees are presented in a clear and concise manner. Ellison (1999) indicates that if you do not make the rules for the employees, they will make them for you. Thus, to protect the practice and the employee it is a good idea to obtain an agreement from the employee to abide by the company's rules and regulations as well as other issues, such as the company's right to use pictures or photographs of employees, confidentiality and non-compete agreements, and drug and alcohol use policies and specifics. These and other issues can all be presented in an employee handbook. The employee handbook allows the employee access to the expectations and conditions of their employment while answering many of the common questions. Concerns such as, "How much vacation time and sick leave do I get?"; "What are the raises, benefits, holidays?"; "Do I get Family Medical Leave, Maternity Leave, and Leaves of Absence?"; "What are the hours of this job?"; "Do I have to dress up?"; and others, can easily be answered in writing with an employee handbook. In the absence of an employee handbook, the interpretation of specific items can become vague and ambiguous, allowing the employees to make up their own rules. Sample employee handbooks can be obtained from the Internet and modified according to the needs of the practice (e.g., www.certifiedemployeehandbook.com). Even with the expertise offered by "professional" or template employee handbooks, it is a good idea to have an attorney review the final version to insure that the practice complies with all state and federal regulations.

THE NON-COMPETE AGREEMENT

If your Audiology practice employs one or more additional audiologists, these professionals over time will build their own clientele and referral network. Thus, as these employees become more and more important in the generation of practice income, it will become clear that they could threaten the clinic's success if they were to leave and work for the competition or set up their own clinic in close proximity to the practice. Therefore, to reduce the likelihood of employee competition, non-compete agreements are often necessary for professional staff as insurance for the practice that the audiologist will not build up a loyal clientele and then quit and move "up the street" and take "their" practice with them. These non-compete agreements are similar to the non-disclosure agreements that are often required between manufacturers of products and employees or consultants and vary greatly in their capability of enforcement from state to state. Typically, these non-compete agreements limit the ability of an employee to work for or become a competitor for a set period of time after leaving employment. Johnson (2000) presents five specific components of non-compete agreements:

1. Employer must have a legitimate interest to protect, such as trade secrets, customer lists, marketing strategies, and other proprietary information. Preventing ordinarily competition is not considered a legitimate interest to protect.
2. The agreement must include a statement describing how long the employee must not compete against the employer. Usually this should not exceed 1 year, but varies from one state to another.
3. A statement is necessary as to the geographic area in which the non compete clause will be effective. The geographic area must not be any larger than absolutely necessary, usually the same area in which the employee has worked for the employer.
4. The employer must pay something extra for making the non-compete agreement. This extra compensation may be virtually anything as long as it is valuable to the employee and is documented as extra compensation for the non-compete agreement.
5. The non-compete agreement must be in writing and signed by both parties or it does not exist.

Specifically, these agreements restrict the employee from calling on or soliciting business from the customers (patients, referral sources) or seeking to hire away employees of the former employer.

MAINTENANCE OF EMPLOYEE RELATIONSHIPS

Commonly there is a "honeymoon" period for new administrative or professional employees. This is a time when some mistakes and interpersonal interactions are overlooked and simply considered a part of getting to know the new person and the new employee getting to know the practice. Eventually, it is necessary to evaluate employee performance, another problem area of the audiologist owner/manager. Although in small practices this is often done informally, Corley et al. (2004) suggest that these appraisals can pinpoint employee skills and competencies that need improvement while outlining possible methods to improve performance. These evaluations can also provide feedback as to how the employee sees the organization and facilitates the justification for rewards such as, further training and career development. Although performance evaluations are usually conducted once per year, the process may be done at other necessary intervals to insure that practice goals for patient care are met as well as the possible development or documentation of problem employees. There are many performance evaluation methods available on the Internet. The specifics of the chosen performance evaluation are often determined by the practice owner and should reflect performance in many areas. It should include a good job description, as presented in the original advertisement, a clear communication of expectations, and a review of the written policies as presented in the employee handbook.

FIRING

Termination is a challenging experience for both the employee and the employer. As Nemo (2005) reports from a Gallup poll of 60,000 top managers, if you have made a hiring mistake it is best to fire the employee as quickly as possible as weak employees rarely become strong ones. Usually employers can terminate an employee's employment at any time, for any reason, and will not become liable to the employee for any harm this may cause **unless** their termination violates the provisions of an employment contract. Johnson (2000) lists some of the power that employers may exercise over their employees:

1. Employers can hire and fire virtually at will.
2. Employers set all policies and procedures that employees must follow.
3. Employers set wages, benefits, and raises based upon any standard they choose (within legal guidelines).
4. Employers have free access to all property on their premises, such as employee lockers and lounges, bulletin boards, and computer systems.
5. Employers own and control access to employee files.
6. Employers generally understand the employer-employee relationship better than the employee.
7. Most employees are not likely to make a formal complaint about any grievances or problems they have with their employer
8. Many employees feel intimidated by their employer.

AT-WILL EMPLOYMENT

The basis of this tremendous employer power is "at-will" employment. Johnson (2000) and legaldefinitions.com (2005) state that "at-will" employment occurs when an employee is not under contract. They further indicate that an employer can dismiss an at-will employee hired for an indefinite term at any time for any non-discriminatory reason. Likewise, the at-will employee is free to terminate their employment at any time. Although most states have "at-will" employment, these at-will employment doctrines are being significantly eroded. Some of the legal challenges and exceptions to at-will employment include breach of implied contracts through an ill-conceived employee handbook, public policy violations, reliance on a written offer of employment, and intentional infliction of emotional distress. Employers must be careful not to imply a contract or employment duration in any verbal or written communications to meet the spirit of at-will employment. Unfortunately, for at-will employees, you can get fired for any number of job-related, and non-job related reasons; for instance, your supervisor can fire you if he or she doesn't like the clothes you wear, of if you tell lame jokes, or even if you simply rub your employer the wrong way.

BEFORE YOU TERMINATE THE EMPLOYEE—ASK THESE QUESTIONS

Burrows (2004) suggests some specific questions that employers should answer before firing an employee. Note that they may change significantly from state to state. Although it is a good idea to discuss your options with an attorney, generally the manager should consider the following items when terminating an employee:

1. Is the employee a member of a protected class?
2. Has the policy for discipline and performance improvement been followed?
3. Is the termination for valid business reasons? If so, are the procedures for determining who is to be fired fair and non-discriminatory?
4. Is there an employment contract—written or implied?
5. Do published manuals limit the scope of action?
6. Is the decision the result of a fair, proper procedure?
7. Would termination prevent vesting of benefits in the near future?
8. Did the employee engage in activity that may be protected?
9. Have other alternatives been considered?

Good employees result in good patient care. Obviously, it is essential to hire the correct person for each job, one that can get along with the rest of the staff as well as conduct the administrative or clinical procedures. Once hired, employees should be given an employee handbook to insure a mutual understanding of the

TABLE 14–2.
Do's and Don'ts of Hiring and Firing

Hiring		Firing	
Do's	**Don'ts**	**Do's**	**Don'ts**
Write the position advertisement carefully with detailed specifics	Be evasive in the position description	When a hiring mistake is made, terminate the employee as soon as possible	Assume that the employee will get better with time
Check Recommendations	Assume that a good job was done for the former employer	Check with an attorney as to the At-Will employment in your state	Make the firing decision on the basis of a single situation
Look for "soft skills" or interpersonal capabilities	Just consider intellectual and Clinical skills in the interview	Keep employee performance evaluations to justify the termination	Use written employee contracts
Have an Employee Handbook	Let your employees make up their own rules	Consider the alternatives to termination as part of the process	Create unpleasant situations hoping the person will quit
Watch out for the protected areas of discrimination	Assume that all employees are honest and psychologically healthy	Be careful of implied contracts	Give employees the impression that they will work for you forever

position, its responsibilities and benefits. As in other management considerations of the practice, it is always a good idea to consult your attorney before conducting any questionable activities regarding hiring and firing.

MANAGERIAL ACCOUNTING FOR AUDIOLOGISTS

Soon after the practice opens there will be a need for bookkeeping and accounting of the business to document the transactions that are made by the practice. Audiology practice managers should be familiar with accounting principles, financial statements and basic terminology so they can understand the differences between income and cash flow (two different things) as well as the impact of expenses on overall profit. Dunn (2000) feels that audiologists need to be conversant with common accounting terms and basic concepts to better manage their practices and protect their assets. While professionals need to use basic accounting to make decisions, Tracy (2001) indicates that they just need the fundamentals, not the technical stuff. Armed with this information, the audiologist manager can decide if it is a good idea to continue providing certain services or to initiate new techniques to add additional profit. Accounting data is typically used for trend analysis, capacity planning, billing, auditing and cost allocation. The transactions are documented for business, tax and other purposes in the form of managerial accounting.

Specifically, managerial accounting is the review of accounting data to make business decisions. Although the forms and specifics of the information vary somewhat these statements provide information that allows the manager to account for the thousands of details about the business. If the manager is inclined to do a budget, these managerial accounting statements are important for establishing the budget, and essential for maintaining a budget.

The very health of a practice is indicated by its financial statements, which include the balance sheet, income statement and the statement of cash flows. These statements present how much is earned, where the earnings came from, and what it cost to earn it. Financial statements and accounting information are so important that bankers and other lenders depend heavily upon them to support their decisions to grant credit.

Once the various totals are obtained within the financial statements, they can then be utilized to track the success or failures of certain specific procedures or products to make a profit. For example, if the ENG unit has become outdated and requires replacement; knowledge of how to read a balance sheet, income and cash flow statements become extremely important in the decision to purchase a new VNG unit. If, when reviewing data, the balance referrals had slowly dwindled to 1 or 2 per month, the profitability of new equipment may be questionable. On the other hand, if there are still 10–15 referrals per month, the information offered by financial statements can be extremely helpful in reviewing the profitability of the balance component of the practice based upon the current referral base.

The totals on these financial statements are the basis of the calculation of business ratios that can be utilized to demonstrate how current practice performance compares to past performance. Ratios, tracked over time, offer important business information as to debt, liquidity, and profitability. Kasewurm (2000) feels that practice financial documents are a road map designed to serve as a guide for the life of the business. Audiology managers need a fundamental capability to read these road maps or they may find themselves lost with little knowledge as to how they got off the main road with minimal skills to return. Thus, audiology practice managers should care about reviewing financial statements and accounting information because it is not only good practice management but also facilitates good, efficient patient care.

BALANCE SHEET

A balance sheet presents a snapshot of the financial condition of a practice at a specific moment in time usually at the close of an accounting period such as the end of the month (Brealey, Myers, and Marcus, 2002). Businesstown.com (2004) indicates that its purpose is to quickly view the financial strength and capabilities of the business as well as answer important questions such as: Is the business in a position to expand? Can the business easily withstand the normal financial ebbs and flows of revenues and expenses? Or should the business take immediate steps to strengthen cash reserves?

Specifically, a balance sheet (Fig. 14–1) presents assets, liabilities, and owners' or stockholders' equity. It displays the assets of the practice on the left side and liabilities and owners' equity on the right side. Assets, of course, are anything the business owns that has monetary value, while liabilities are the claims of credi-

ACME AUDIOLOGY, INC.
Balance Sheet
December 31, 2004

Assets		Liabilities & Owners' Equity	
Current assets.		Current liabilities.	
Cash	34,000.	Short Term Debt	20,000.
Accounts Receivable	30,000.	Accounts Payable	25,000.
Merchandise Inventory	170,000.	Other Accrued Liabilities	12,000.
Total Current Assets	234,000.	Total current liabilities	57,000.
Plant and equipment.		Long term debt	50,000.
Equipment	40,000.	Total Liabilities	107,000.
Less Accumulated depreciation	(4,000.)	Owners' Equity	202,000.
Total assets	220,000.	Total liabilities and owners' equity	220,000.

FIGURE 14–1. Balance Sheet.

tors against the assets of the business. In Figure 14–1, the assets column typically consists of some general categories such as, current assets, fixed assets, intangible assets, and total assets, these are the items owned by the practice. These categories are then delineated into subcategories to further describe them and offer enough detail so as to understand the specifics of the assets. For example, current assets may be divided into categories such as, cash, accounts receivable, and merchandise inventories. Fixed assets include the subcategories of building, equipment, and depreciation on fixed assets. The total of all of the assets are then labeled as total assets.

On the right side of the balance sheet, liabilities are a listing of the amounts owed to lenders and suppliers, usually separated between those due in the short term and those due in the long term. As with the asset categories, liabilities are delineated into subcategories such as short term debt, accounts payable and accrued liabilities (warranty servicing, etc). These are referred to as current liabilities while a separate category is for long term debt, such as bank or other loans. All current and long term liability amounts are then totaled collectively to reflect the total liability of the practice. Also, sharing the right side of the balance sheet is the owners' equity. This represents funds that were initially invested by the owner as well as the profit that was earned but retained in the practice.

The balance sheet gets its name from the fact that the two sides of the statement must numerically balance. Assets (A) must equal Liabilities (L) plus the Owners' Equity (OE) as presented in the basic accounting formula A = L+OE.

INCOME STATEMENT

Tracy (2001) refers to the income statement as "all-important" since it gets the most attention from practice managers and investors as well as other stakeholders. Although the other financial statements are very important, the income statement is reviewed by bankers with the most scrutiny, as it discloses information that directly relates to the practices' capability to pay back loans. The income statement (Fig. 14–2), sometimes called a profit and loss (P & L) statement, provides a summary of a company's profit or loss during any given period of time (Marshall, 2004). As with other financial statements, the income statement may be prepared for any financial reporting period. Income statements are used to track specific revenues and expenses so that the operating performance of the practice can be evaluated over a specific the period of time. Businesstown.com (2000) suggests that managers can use income statements to find out whether there are areas of the practice that are over budget or under budget and identify those areas that are causing unexpected expenditures. Additionally, income statements track increases or

ACME AUDIOLOGY, INC.
Income Statement
Year the Ended December 31, 2004

Net sales	1,200,000.
Cost of goods sold	850,000.
Net profit	350,000.
Selling, general and administrative expenses	311,000.
Income from operations (EBIT)	39,000.
Interest expense	9,000.
Income before taxes (EBT)	30,000.
Income taxes	12,000.
Net income	18,000.

FIGURE 14–2. Income Statement.

decreases in product returns; cost of goods sold as a percentage of sales and gives an indication regarding the extent of income tax liability. Since it is very important to format an income statement appropriate to the type of business being conducted, the structure of income statements may vary from one practice to another, depending on the particular mix of business conducted in the various areas of diagnostics, products, and/or rehabilitative services.

Specifically, Marshall (2004) states that net sales on the income statement consist of sales figures representing the actual revenue generated by the business. This figure is the total of all the sales, less any product returns or sales discounts. Directly below the net income (Fig. 14–2) is the cost of goods sold, that is, costs that are directly associated with making and/or acquiring the products. These costs include products, such as hearing aids or assistive devices, from outside suppliers as well as materials and internal expenses related to the manufacturing process, such as faceplates and shells, if products are manufactured within the practice. Net profit, sometimes referred to as gross profit, is then derived by subtracting the cost of goods sold from net sales. Net profit, however, does not include any operating expenses, interest expenses, or income taxes. Just below the net profit is a category for selling and general administrative expenses. This subcategory is described by Tracy (2001) and Marshall (2004) as a broad catch-all category for all expenses except those reported elsewhere in the income statement. Examples of expenses that go in the selling and general administrative section of the income statement are legal expenses, the president's salary, advertising costs, travel and entertainment, and other such costs. The income from operations, sometimes called earnings before interest and taxes (EBIT), is the result of deducting the sales, administrative, and general costs from the net profit. At this point, the interest expense is deducted and then the taxe amounts are subtracted to arrive at the net income (or loss).

STATEMENT OF CASH FLOWS

Tracy (2001) refers to business as a "two-headed dragon" in that profit and cash flow are inter-related. The practice can have significant profit but if there is no cash flow, it will bankrupt rapidly and, conversely, if there is cash flow but no profit, financial difficulties are also encountered. Cash flow problems can occur, for example, if the practice is very profitable but most of the services and products are sold on the accounts receivable. This results in minimal flow of cash left to pay the employees and other business bills. To illustrate how cash flows in and out of the practice, Marshall (2004) indicates that the statement of cash flows is used to identify the sources and uses of cash for a practice during a particular financial period, which can be compared to the current period for analysis.

Specifically, the statement of cash flows is broken down into three general sections (Fig. 14–3), cash flows from operating, investing, and financing activities. The operating activities area starts with the net income from the income statement and includes all transactions and events that normally enter into the determination of operating income. This includes cash receipts from selling goods or providing services, as well as income from income earned as interest and divi-

ACME AUDIOLOGY, INC.
Statement of Cash Flows
Year the Ended December 31, 2004

Cash Flows for Operating Activities:

Net Income ....$ 18,000.

Add (deduct) items not affecting cash:

Depreciation expense ....   +000.

Increase in accounts receivable ....   (30,000)

Increase in merchandise inventory ....(170,000)

Increase in current liabilities ....   67,000.

Net cash used by operating activities ....$(161,000)

Cash Flows from Investing Activities:

Cash paid for equipment..$(40,000)

Cash Flows from Financing Activities:

Cash received from issues of long term debt................$ 50,000.

Cash received from sale of common stock................190,000.

Net cash provided by financing activities................$ 240,000.

Net cash increase for the year................$ 39,000.

FIGURE 14–3. Statement of Cash Rows.

dends. Operating activities also include cash payments such as inventory, pay-roll, taxes, interest, utilities, and rent. The net amount of cash provided by (or used) by operating activities is the key figure on a statement of cash flows. Of course, the operations section of the cash flow statement is of the most interest as this will present the specific components of the practice where cash was utilized. The second section of a statement of cash flows, investing activities, includes transactions and events involving the purchase and sale of securities, land, build-ings, equipment, and other assets not generally held in the practice for resale. It also covers the making and collecting of loans, if the practice finances products and services these loans to consumers internally. Investing activities are not clas-sified as operating activities because they have an indirect relationship to the cen-tral, ongoing operation of the practice.

Transactions in the third category, cash flows from financing activities, deal with the flow of cash between the practice, the owners (stockholders) and creditors as well as cash proceeds from issuing capital stock or bonds. For example, if there was a need to transfer profit from the practice to the owners, it would be reflected in the financing activities section.

Often clinicians who run their own practices are so preoccupied with seeing patients and generating income that they do not take the time to review accounts or financial statements. Audiologists often do not keep their own books and simply hire a bookkeeper or a Certified Public Accountant (CPA) to handle their accounting needs. A common opinion is that these business fundamentals are "not Audiology" and the business component of the practice is better analyzed by an expert. These experts report the positive and negative directions of the practice and offer suggestions as to necessary changes for continued success. This is not a bad strategy for the routine day-to-day bookkeeping activities, but may leave you in the dark about specifics. Thus, it is beneficial, if not essential, to learn as much about the basic accounting process as possible to facilitate tracking of financial successes and failures and to arrive at timely management decisions.

FINANCIAL ACCOUNTING FOR AUDIOLOGISTS

Financial Accounting actually analyzes the data that is generated by managerial accounting and analyzes the information using ratios and calculations so that the success or failure can be tracked, trends noted and decisions made. Freeman et al. (2000) describes two forms of financial analysis ratio comparisons, cross sectional and a time series analysis. A cross sectional analysis compares the practice team industry standard, though probably more appropriate recent years, is still difficult to make these comparisons as there are not good data available within our industry to make these comparisons for Audiology practices. Thus, it is the time series analysis that becomes the most important by comparing the practice to itself over periods of time, usually month to month, quarter to quarter or year to year.

Financial statements are full of numbers that, by themselves, simply present how the practice performed at a particular point in time and do not have too much significance in isolation. Since the statements alone do not provide information on the efficiency or profitability of the practice, they require analysis and comparison to generate real information. When these numbers in the current statements are compared to financial statements conducted at other times (monthly, quarterly or yearly) they come alive with informative data that paints a true picture of how success or failure has developed. Financial statements with the correct calculations and comparisons can reveal a wealth of information to the stockholders about earnings over time, soaring or stagnated sales, and even the practice's capability to pay back a loan to the bank. Within the same practice comparing financial statement totals to others taken at the some point in time is very helpful, for example, comparing the 1st quarter 2004 with the 1st quarter or 2005 or 2004 with 2005, year to date. Marshall et al. (2002) indicate that these calculations assist in the determination of a practice's financial position and the result of their operations by reporting on liquidity, activity, and debt, and profitability analysis of financial statements. It is the calculation of various ratios for balance sheets and income statements that facilitate in comparison of practice success at various points in time, no matter what the size of the operation. These relatively simple measures can be calculated and tracked by spreadsheet then reviewed over time to demonstrate the health of practice for obtaining loans or supplier credit, reviewing success and failure for management decisions, or simply general information.

BALANCE SHEET CALCULATIONS

CLS already indicated the balance sheet is a report of assets, liabilities and owners equity at a particular point in time. These statements provide information regarding the capability of the practice can meet obligations to suppliers, employee salaries, product returns, loans, leases, and other expenses are presented in these balance sheet calculations. Managers use liquidity, activity and leverage ratios to analyze the balance sheet to demonstrate the strengths and weaknesses of the practice. Liquidity ratios are used to measure the short-term ability of practice to generate cash to pay currently maturing obligations while activity ratios measure how effectively the organization is using its assets, analyzing how quickly some assets can be turned into cash. Debt or leverage ratios reflect the long term solvency or overall liquidity of the practice and are of interest to the investors and/or the bankers that have loaned money.

LIQUIDITY RATIOS

A common liquidity ratio is the Current Ratio (CR). The CR is sometimes called a Working Capital Ratio as it is a calculation of how many times the practice's current assets cover its current liabilities and specifically looks at if the practice has sufficient resources to meet current liabilities. Put another way, the Current Ratio asks the questions, can the practice pay its bills or not? The Current Ratio is figured as follows:

$$\text{Current Ratio} = \frac{\text{Current Assests}}{\text{Current Liabilities}}$$

If the result of a CR calculation is less than 1, the practice will not be able to meet its current liabilities and if the CR is 2 or more, the practice can pay its bills with money left over. Usually most bankers and practice managers like to see this ratio at least between 1 and 2. The CR includes prepaid expenses (such as insurance, etc.) and the inventory it sometimes offers a cloudy view of the real picture. In these days of custom hearing instruments ordered upon demand, most Audiology practices do not have much inventory. Thus, a very common modification of the CR is the Quick Ratio (QR), also known as the Acid Test Ratio (ATR). The ATR evaluates the practice's liquidity without considering the inventory and prepaid expenses and, in doing so, presents a more accurate indication of the liquidity of an Audiology practice. The ATR is figured as follows:

$$\text{Acid Test Ratio} = \frac{\text{Cash + Marketable Securities+ Accounts Receivable}}{\text{Current Liabilities}}$$

As with the CR, Acid Test Ratio values less than 1 demonstrates that the practice has serious difficulty meeting everyday expenses.

Another useful liquidity calculation is the Defensive Interval Measure (DIM) which is a ratio that measures the time span that the practice can operate without any external cash flow or how long can the practice operate if there is no business. As our personal investments, wise practice managers keep an emergency fund in the case that business drops off or ceases for some reason. In Accounting these emergency funds are called Defensive Assets (DA). The DA are those assets that can be turned into cash within 3 months or less, such as cash (savings), marketable securities, or accounts receivable. To figure the DIM it is first necessary to know the Projected Daily Operating Expenses (PDOE) or how much it costs to keep the practice open each day. To find the PDOE, simply add up the cost of goods sold in a year, the selling and administrative expenses in a year and other ordinary cash expenses for the year then divide by 365:

$$\text{Project Daily Operating Expenses} = \frac{\text{Total yearly Expenses}}{365}$$

Once the daily operating expenses (PDOE) are known, the DIM is found by dividing the DA by the PDOE:

$$\text{Defensive Interval Measure} = \frac{\text{Defensive Assests}}{\text{Project Daily Operating Expenses}}$$

The DIM calculation gives the manager of the practice knowledge of the length of time the business could survive if revenue was substantially reduced or absent as present.

ACTIVITY RATIOS

Activity Ratios are calculations that allow the manager to review how efficiently the practice uses its assets to generate cash. Although there are a number of Activity Ratios that can present the efficiency of the practice, the Accounts Receivable Turnover Ratio (ART), The Inventory Turnover Ratio (IT), and the Total Assets Turnover Ratio (TAT) are useful to managers.

It is a good policy to insure that all patients to pay when services are delivered. In fact, most practices have a sign to that effect in the waiting room and collect as much as possible when the services and/or products are delivered. Reality is, however, that insurance companies are slow at paying; sometimes 60–120 days after the services are rendered and may often not even pay the first time the claim is submitted. Additionally, some patients that need time to pay for goods and services require credit to facilitate the sales of hearing aids, batteries and other goods or services. Although credit given to patients is another topic, the receivable account should be closely monitored to determine how much is due to the practice and how long, on the average, it takes to collect for these credit sales. The Accounts Receivable Turnover Ratio (ART) looks at how many times the receivable account is turned into cash each year. To obtain the ART ratio it is necessary to first find the average amount that is due the practice from the receivable account at any one time or average Accounts Receivable (AR) balance. This is obtained by adding the accounts receivable balance at the end of last year and balance of the accounts receivable at the end of the current year and dividing it by 2:

$$\text{Average Accounts Receivable} = \frac{\text{AR (Year 1)} + \text{AR Year 2}}{2}$$

Once the average AR is computed, the time it takes to convert this account into cash or the ART ratio is conducted by taking the Net Sales (sales after discounts and returns) and divided by the average accounts receivable balance:

$$\text{Accounts Receivable Turnover Ratio} = \frac{\text{Net Sales}}{\text{Average Accounts Receivable}}$$

Once known, the ART can tell the manager how long it takes, on the average, to collect the amounts that in the accounts receivable, thus, the higher the ratio the better. For example, if the ART ratio is = 5.3, the practice turns over the accounts receivable 5.3 times per year or every 2.26 months. To obtain more detail, the calculation of the number of days it takes to turn the accounts receivable can be obtained by simply dividing the average accounts receivable into 365.

Until the recent increase of open billings, Audiologists did not keep much inventory, a few loaners, some demonstration instruments, batteries, accessories and some assistive devices. Particularly these days, it still may be beneficial to understand how fast this inventory turns over. The Inventory Turnover (IT) Ratio is the calculation that measures how fast the inventory is sold. As in the calculation of the ART, to figure the IT ratio it is necessary to obtain the average inventory on hand in the practice in terms of value. Thus, the average inventory is found by taking the beginning inventory and then ending inventory and dividing by 2. Thus, the average inventory is found by taking the beginning inventory and then ending inventory and dividing by 2.

$$\text{Average Inventory} = \frac{\text{Beginning Inventory} + \text{Ending Inventory}}{2}$$

Once the average inventory is known, the IT ratio is computed by dividing the cost of the goods sold by the average inventory. If the IT ratio was 5.9 this indicates that the inventory will turn almost 6 times each year. As with other activity ratios, the turning of the inventor can be further delineated to reflect how long it takes the inventory to sell out in days by simply dividing 365 by the IT ratio. In this example, if the inventory turns about 6 times per year then it takes about 61 days for the inventory to sell out. These data assist the manager in taking advantage of discounts for more efficient ordering of products, insuring that there is always sufficient supply.

$$\text{Inventory Turnover Ratio} = \frac{\text{Average Inventory}}{\text{Cost of Goods Sold}}$$

Another Activity measure that presents how many times the practice assets turn over per year also indicates how effectively assets are turned into cash is the Total Assets Turnover (TAT) Ratio. The TAT looks at the sales for good and services and divides by the total assets to arrive at how many times the practices assets turnover per year.

$$\text{Total Asset Turnover Ratio} = \frac{\text{Sales}}{\text{Total Assets}}$$

Of course, the higher the ratio the better as this is an indication that the assets turn over more times per year, suggesting an efficient practice that uses it assets to the most benefit.

LEVERAGE OR DEBT RATIOS

There are two beneficial ratios that provide the practice manager with information as to how much debt is in the practice and how debt can be safely incurred. These are the Debt to Assets (DA) Ratio and the Times Interest Earned (TIE) Ratio. These ratios can give indications if the practice has enough capability to support more debt to add equipment or open another location and other expansion activities.

The DA presents how many liabilities the practice has for every dollar of assets and provides the creditors with information about the ability of the practice to withstand losses without impairing the interest of the creditors. The DA is simply the Total Assets divided by the Total Liabilities:

$$\text{Debt to Assets Ratio} = \frac{\text{Total Assets}}{\text{Total Liabilities}}$$

A desirable DA is a low number since the higher the number indicates that the practice is more dependent on borrowed money to sustain itself. If the DA is high it suggests that small changes in cash flow may cause serious difficulties in the capability to repay their debt.

Times Interest Earned ratio is an indication of how many times the practice earns the amount of interested that it is charged on the money that it has borrowed. The TIE is computed by taking the earnings before interest and taxes and dividing it by the interest

$$\text{Times Interest Earned Ratio} = \frac{\text{Earning Before Interest and Taxes}}{\text{Interest Charges}}$$

Freeman indicates that in audiology practice the TIE should be somewhere between three and five as it indicates that the earnings are at least three to five times greater than the interest payments. A TIE that is less than 1 indicates that the practice cannot pay its interest commitments.

INCOME STATEMENT CALCULATIONS

Sometimes the ratios that often tell the most about a practice are the profitability ratios that are conducted on the income statement. These profitability ratios are clues to how well the company performed and looks at if the company's net income is adequate, what rate of return was achieved and profit margin as a percentage of sales. The ratios considered in this group are the Profit Margin On Sales (PMOS) and the Asset Turnover (AT) Ratio presented earlier, that uses information from both the income statement and the balance sheet.

The Profit Margin On Sales presents the profit margin achieved after all of the expenses are subtracted and presents how much of every dollar of sales are profit. To compute the PMOS, Net Profit is divided by Sales:

$$\text{Profit Margin On Sales} = \frac{\text{Net Profit}}{\text{Sales}}$$

PMOS results are presented in a percentage that reflects the amount of each dollar that is profit. For example, if the calculation yields 20 percent then $0.20 cents of every dollar collected is profit. These values can be tracked to determine if there are changes in profitability that require attention.

TRACKING THE RATIOS

An easy method of tracking these ratios can be the use of a spreadsheet. By simply creating a spreadsheet and entering data each month, the data can be analyzed at a glance as presented in Figures 14–4 and 14–5. In Figure 14– 4, it is easy to see that the Quick Ratios for the years 2000 and 2001 indicate that the ability to pay the bills was easily achieved. In 2002, however, there were problems paying everyone, but in 2003, the situation was much better and 2004 was also rather good. This allows the manager to search further for differences between 2002 and the other years to insure that these difficulties do not repeat for 2005.

Another example of tracking is the ART ratio as presented in Figure 14–2. Presented is how long in days it takes for the practice to turn credit sales into

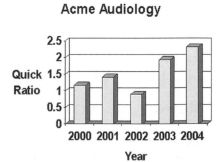

FIGURE 14–4.   Quick Ratios 2000–2004.

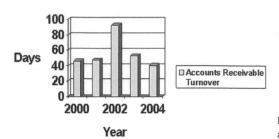

FIGURE 14–5. Accounts Receivable Turnover 2000–2004.

cash. It is obvious from these data that in most years it only takes 40–50 days to clear the accounts receivable. In 2002, however, it took over 90 days to clear the accounts receivable.

By reviewing Figures 14–1 and 14–2 together, the practice manager can see at a glance, one possible reason for the problems in 2002. At the same time (2002) it was difficult to pay the bills, the Accounts Receivable turnover Ratio indicated that it took over 90 days to turn credit sales in to cash. Tracking the various ratios and reviewing them interactively over time facilitates great knowledge for practice managers and allows them to see the problems and to fix them before they have had too much impact. Although this information is of great benefit, it must be remembered that all financial statements and the ratios conducted upon them is information from the past. These data reflect how business has been in the past and, due to competition, market pressures and other significant factors, may or may not be a predictor of the health of the business in the future.

Although ratios can be very helpful in the evaluation of a practice, Freeman et al., (2000), Tracy (2001) and Marshall et al. (2002) all offer cautions on the use of ratio analysis. They indicate that the best information about a company's health is determined from comparison and analysis of a group of ratios, not a single ratio, and that these comparisons need to be made from like-times of the year to arrive at accurate data on the practice's performance. Additionally, Freeman (2000) offers that these ratios may be distorted somewhat due to the reimbursement policies of insurance companies. In the tracking example offered in Figures 14–4 and 14–5, it could be that the insurance companies paid slowly during 2002 and that was the reason the Accounts Receivable Turnover was 90 days and the Quick Ratio indicated that there was difficulty paying the practice liabilities.

The development of an assessment technique to track various important components of your particular practice should be developed with the help of a Certified Public Accountant or other trained professional. Once set up, these calculations can be tracked using a spreadsheet analysis to facilitate managerial decisions.

PUTTING IT ALL TOGETHER

To be a successful private practitioner it is essential that you work within the correct corporate structure, know the rules of human resources and accounting basics.

These essentials are but surface knowledge that is required of the audiologist that engages in private practice. Johnson (2000) presents 20 basic fundamental questions a business (practice) owner must answer to establish and maintain goals. Some of these essential questions have been answered here and others are beyond the cope of this presentation. Those practitioners that can answer Johnson's 20 questions will survive in practice (Johnson, 2000):

1. What is the purpose of your Business?
2. What are the short and long term goals of the business?
3. Why is your business organized as it is?
4. What is the job description of each and every employee (from the CEO to part time help).
5. What state and federal employment laws apply to the business?
6. What local, state, and federal taxes, licenses and other registration requirements must your business meet?
7. How will you deal with employment issues, such as: hiring procedures; promotion; discipline; wages, benefits, and compensation issues; termination; absences; grievances; and just generally having and maintaining productive relations with employees?
8. How will you deal with customers and customer issues?
9. How will you deal with competition?
10. How will your business participate as a member of the local community?
11. Do you have a good, competent resources for handling legal matters?
12. Do you have good, competent resources for handling accounting issues?
13. Do you have a good relationship with at least one bank?
14. How will you handle collections?
15. How will you handle lawsuits?
16. How will you handle illness and injuries of employees, customers, and others that could have an effect on the business?
17. How will you handle creditors?
18. How will you handle surprises?
19. How will you handle stress?
20. Will key personnel (including yourself) have and actually take enough vacation time?

CONCLUSION

Being aware of the above 20 questions in the context of "putting it all together" will help the private practitioner succeed in a business and financial environment that is foreign to many practicing clinicians. Assuming overall clinical competence and good patient rapport, the business end of the practice can be managed successfully by following the principles outlined in this chapter.

REFERENCES

Appold, K. (2005). You're fired. *Advance for Audiologists, 7*(1), 14–15.

Bergman, M. (2002).The origins of audiology: American wartime military audiology (Monograph 1). *Audiology Today*. Reston, VA: American Academy of Audiology.

Brealey, R., Myers, S., & Marcus, A. (2002). *Fundamentals of corporate finance* (3rd edition). New York: McGraw Hill Publishers.

Corley, R., Reed, L., Shedd, P., & Morehead, J. (2002), The legal and regulatory environment of business (11th edition). New York: McGraw Hill Publishers.

Duncan, P. (1999). Paying for hearing care: An American experience. In R. Traynor (Ed.), *CAS 7308-Business and professional issues in hearing healthcare*. University of Florida Working Professional Doctor of Audiology Program.

Burrows, D. (2004). Human resources in audiology practice. In *CAS 7308, Business and professional issues*. University of Florida Working Professional Doctor of Audiology Program.

Businesstown. (2004). *The balance sheet*. Retrieved March 25, 2005, from http://www.businesstown.com/accounting/basic-sheets.asp

Businesstown. (2004). *The income statement*. Retrieved March 25, 2005, from http://www.businesstown.com/accounting/basic-sheets.asp

Corley, R., Reed, L., Shedd, P., & Morehead, J. (2002). *The legal & regulatory environment of business* (11th Edition). New York: McGraw Hill Publishers.

Dunn, D. (2000). Managerial Accounting for Daily and Long-Term Practice Success. In Hosford-Dunn, H., Roeser, R., & Valente, M. (Eds). *Audiology practice management* (pp. 337–349). Thieme: New York.

Ellison, K. (1999). Human resources. In *CAS 7308, Business and professional issues in hearing healthcare*. University of Florida Working Professional Doctor of Audiology Program.

Freeman, B., Barimo, J., & Fox, G. (2000). Financial management of audiology practices and clinics. In H. Hosford-Dunn, R. Roeser, & M. Valente (Eds.), *Audiology practice management* (pp. 351–362). Thieme: New York.

Hunt, S. (2005). Monster hiring guide. Retrieved February 2, 2005, from http://media.monster.com/id/hiring/58/marketing/pdf/MonsterGuide.pdf

Johnson, K. (2000). *Business owners legal guide*. Ft. Worth, Texas: Knowles Publishing.

Kasewurm, G. (2000). Business plan and practice accounting. In H. Hosford-Dunn, R. Roeser, & M. Valente (Eds.), *Audiology practice* management (pp. 313–336). Thieme: New York.

Legal Definitions.com. (2005). Retrieved February 2, 2005, from http://www.legal-database.com/at-will.htm

Nemo, M. (2005). Worlds shortest management course. Retrieved February 2, 2005, from http://www.bankrate.com/aolcrs/news/career/20050124a1.asp

Marshall, D. H. (2004). Accounting: What the numbers mean (6th ed., pp. 238–247.). New York: McGraw-Hill.

Pessis, P. (2002). Keystone Address: Ohio Academy of Audiology. Columbus, OH, February 27, 2007.

Tracy, J. (2001). Accounting for dummies (2nd ed.). Hoboken, NJ: Wiley Publishing.

Traynor, R. (2005). The business of audiology: A series of articles. *Audiology Today, 17*.

CHAPTER 15

Professional Issues: Ethics, Methods of Practice, and Conflicts of Interest

Michael J. Metz

University of California-Irvine, Irvine California

A text pertaining to clinical practice will, if relatively complete, contain more information than can be assimilated quickly or completely. Such a text necessarily will contain information about costs, equipment, patient management, state-of-the-art (science) protocols, as well as various recommendations, directions, predictions, and warnings. If such a text were compiled by a number of contributors, one might expect that the core topic would be approached in different manners and with different emphases, dependent upon the "leanings" of the various authors. As a contributor of one chapter to such a text, I would be astounded to have the topics of this particular chapter placed anywhere near the top of the hierarchy of topics essential to practicing clinical Audiology.

Nevertheless, the consideration of, and the adherence to, the concepts contained in this chapter may be more important than many other considerations that confront a clinician, especially in the sense of establishing good clinical foundations for a practice serving the hearing impaired public. Any clinical practice that offers professional services to the public become involved in many considerations beyond those generally accepted principles and protocols that constitute good business practices. Indeed, the public trust in the professional services offered is at the conceptual, fundamental, practical, and ethical center of clinical audiology. And, without adherence to these clinical concepts and ethical ideals, the services of audiology may not survive the close scrutiny of the public. In other words, if audiologists are to be considered as autonomous clinical entities, the cost for that belief, stature, and functional level lies in audiology performing in the very best of professional manners. Part and parcel of professional behavior is the adherence not only to a professional standard of care, but also to a standard or code of professional ethics.

It is not the intention of this chapter to discuss the elements that comprise morals and legalities, and the similarities and differences between these and professional ethics. But rather, we will try to focus on the ethical provision of services in such a manner that constitute the highest level of practice to the hearing impaired in a manner consistent with the public trust we desire as a profession.

ATTEMPTS TO DEFINE MODELS, TERMS, AND APPROACHES

As a consumer of insurance products—auto, health, life insurance, etc.—one may search out an independent insurance agent for help in selecting a policy for home and auto. This agent, who states that he/she is an independent expert in the insurance arena, suggests certain policies for purchase. What were/are your assumptions? Do you expect a certain degree of neutrality in the decisions this agent made on your behalf? For whom does this "independent" agent work?

As reported in the Wall Street Journal on November 29, 2004 (Davies, 2004), both the states of New York and California were investigating the actions of such insurance agents on the grounds of possible ethical violations. It seems that many of these agents appear to function in a manner that would be perceived as not in the best interests of their customers as they are paid commissions by the insurance companies they represent. That's to be expected, but sometimes they are paid in ways that are not fully disclosed to those who purchase insurance from them or the companies they represent. That is, they appear to be paid not only on a commission basis, but additionally by methods that are hidden from the public they serve.

Why would such insurance agents be investigated on potential violations of ethical standards? Are such agents—retailers—held to different standards when compared to automobiles salespeople, physicians, attorneys, or audiologists? If they call themselves "Independent," does that constitute the difference?

Let us consider an example that may perhaps be a little more illustrative. Also reported in the Wall Street Journal on November 24, 2004 (Solomon, 2004) was a story involving the Security and Exchange Commission investigating excessive gifts given to some security firms. It seems that, subject to the SEC investigation, some security retailers may have been informed of the intentions of certain mutual funds to buy or sell securities, and that this information was given to those firms that had provided gifts to the mutual fund advisors. The issue appeared to be whether the security firms reaping huge commissions were functioning in the best manner for the holders of these securities (investors) or more on behalf of the security firms who had supplied the gifts. Of course, the ethical questions posed and investigated ask the question: does this type of activity violate the fiduciary role of the fund or the security firm?

A third example of the impact of ethical constructs occurred in conjunction with an episode involving a member of the United States Supreme Court in 2003 and 2004. A Supreme Court Justice went to dinner and on a hunting trip with a high-ranking elected official. The elected official was involved in a legal matter that was in the process of being heard by the Supreme Court. The question of the appearance of a conflict of interest arose over these actions of the Justice, who stated that a Supreme Court Justice's opinion could not be purchased at such a low price. The Justice did not offer to recuse, and participated in the case. Was the Justice wrong not to recuse? Does the appearance of a conflict of interest constitute enough reason for action (or inaction in this case)? What's so important about appearance if there was really no conflict in the first place? Does the public have an inherent right to hold such a person in such a position to a higher standard?

These types of questions, albeit of lesser financial and legal impact, have faced Audiologists and other professional associations for the past few years. And, it would appear unlikely that audiologists and their organizations will be able to resolve such issues quickly or easily. In the profession, there are audiologists who believe that as long as they function in what they consider a "good" or "appropriate" manner, they are acting within the accepted ethical boundaries. As we shall see, individuals do not determine ethical behavior. Standards of behavior for those who function in a professional field should and will be set to a different level by the entire professional group's standard—and that standard is usually different from any standard set by any one individual.

It has long been argued by many who discuss business and ethics that the concept of business ethics may be oxymoronic. That is, if the purpose of business is profit, how can any legal method that produces profit be questioned. Or, less bluntly, if the bottom line is the major consideration of business, how much leeway can businesses exercise in maximizing the bottom line? Does a business have any sort of responsibility to its customers in terms of honesty and disclosures? Does a business have any ethical responsibility other than to the motive of profit and shareholders?

Too many times, health care providers make a comparison of a medical or pseudo-medical practice to this business model. It is appropriate to do so only in a very limited manner. The ethical principles of business are considerably different than the ethical principles of medicine, law and audiology. In fact, while most will admit that profit is a critical and therefore central motive for all professional practices, the public trust placed in the professional practitioner requires placing the public good even before the profit of the professional practice. Additionally, this order of placement is a global principle and, as such, the requirement for public protection cannot be offset by any professional through multiple or distant ownership, rationalizations of long-term benefit, or by any individual rationalizations of need of whatever type. That is, for those bound by professional ethics, these standards may not be forsaken by arguments of corporate, business, or personal policy. One may not shun ethical constraints by placing responsibility on "the general managers of the company," "the stockholders," "the group that does the purchasing," or any other party. In a professional sense, "the buck" always stops at the practitioner.

As audiology has progressed toward a status of autonomy, the field in general has struggled over concepts of ethical behavior. All too often this struggle involves the differences between what one would consider to be good business practice, compared to the professional requirements of health care providers.

The examples above of brokers, judges, and agents, taken from a very public media, are illustrative of a number of public misconceptions concerning ethical behavior, especially as it is applied to professional function. It would appear, on the surface, that the independent insurance agent did nothing illegal in recommending insurance policies from companies that offered the best commission. However, such maximizing of the agent's profit would appear to be hidden from the consumer. Does the ethical concern stem from the hidden nature of the commissions, or rather from the implication that the "independent" agent should be more objective on behalf of the purchaser—more independent from such profit motive?

The second example is a little more flagrant in that it involves increased profits which resulted from information obtained, or at least appearing to have been obtained, through lavish gifts. Most observers would argue that this example does contain reasons for questioning the ethical behavior of those involved. (It appeared that the Attorneys General in the first case and both the Securities and Exchange Commission and the National Association of Securities Dealers in the second case, had questions about these respective activities and the inability of the insurance agents or security firms to regulate themselves—to function in the best interest of others—and therefore stepped into these investigations for the protection of those others—the public.) This example has significant ramifications when compared to the audiology issue of gifts, rebates, trips, etc. that have been offered by hearing aid manufacturers and accepted by audiologists who dispense hearing aids.

The third example of the Supreme Court Justice was offered as an example that perhaps even those in quite high places or with considerable power and influence sometimes perhaps do not appear to be fully aware of the impact of their behavior on the general public. It seems not only are discussions of ethics common and popular, but also that many others have concerns similar to those in the field of audiology.

The over-riding principle here, as in the case of all those who deal with the public in a professional manner, involves the public trust. Attorneys, physicians, and other healthcare providers, including audiologists, enjoy elevated status in the public forum, and the price for this status is an increased responsibility to those who are served. When there is question regarding behavior that is, or appears to be, contrary to the public good, the public has a right to question this behavior, the individual, and the profession itself. Such is the price of higher public position and increased privilege. Elevated public trust likely caused the Attorneys General to investigate insurers, and certainly the presumed elevated position of those in the securities business—the managers of both public and private money—prompted the SEC investigations.

These same principles, encoded for the most part in the appended American Academy of Audiology Code of Ethics, apply to audiology even more so. As audiology employs elements of public trust, the profession has established codes of conduct in order to protect and justify that trust.

AUDIOLOGY: A BUSINESS OR A PROFESSIONAL MODEL?

As audiology rose from the "start-up" phases in the 1950s and 1960s, audiologists came to enjoy the licensed status of other health care providers. Audiologists were granted licensing statues in most states under the health care umbrella. We applied for, and many times received, the ability to be reimbursed from health insurance organizations. Almost without exception, audiology was considered para-medical. The professional organization to which most audiologists belonged, had a strict code of ethics which prohibited any member from receiving fees from the sale of any prosthetic instrument.

A major change took place in the late 1970s, as a Federal Court (National Society of Professional Engineers v. United States, 1978) ruled that professional organizations could not act in such a manner that restricts professional services to consumers. This ruling was judged to have implications in the then-prohibited delivery of hearing aids by audiologists to their patients, and thus opened the door to dispensing of these devices by audiologists. Prior to this case, audiologists were barred from selling hearing aids by the professional organizations which were in place at that time.

With this mandated change in the audiology profession's approach to dispensing hearing instruments, the movement of many private practices into this area of hearing care evolved rather rapidly. However, as both other medical providers and audiologists struggled with methods of implementing their practices and therapies by selling hearing aids, there existed no professional model, incorporating both professional services and professional products, which facilitated this transition. The only model available was the standard business model that was in place and being used by other retailers, including hearing aid dispensers.

The hearing aid dispenser model was, necessarily, a business model. Billing for professional health care related services is denied to those who do not hold a professional license allowing such professional service. As audiologists began dispensing, ease of practice, tax laws (demanding that prosthetics for hearing improvement bear the burden of a sales tax), models in place (business-based models involving mark-up pricing, etc.), as well as other considerations usually lead to following the easiest pathway. That is, audiologists began selling hearing aids using the business model that was the most convenient—that of the classic, retail hearing aid dispenser. While taking profit from goods rather than services had been previously banned by the profession, it suddenly became acceptable to combine prosthetic goods and therapeutic services.

Like most things in life as well as business, there were costs and benefits resulting from this relatively easy course of action. The most obvious benefit was that audiologists stepped into a business model that most customers understood. In functioning as a retailer, the dispensing audiologist quickly became competitive with other retailers of goods. However, one cost for the quick adaptation of this model has become a little more obvious over the ensuing years: many consumers cannot differentiate between audiologists and other sellers of hearing aids.

A more insidious and recent cost of the retail hearing aid model is that aspects of this retail-business model have come to be in conflict with the code of ethics of professional associations (sic: the American Academy of Audiology-AAA-and American Speech-Language and Hearing Association-ASHA).

By way of illustration, in most professional ethical codes, principles of conduct are enumerated. These Principles constitute aspirations to which professionals in an organization aspire. Principle 4 of the AAA Code of Ethics states:

> **Principle 4:** Members shall provide only services and products that are in the best interest of those served.

Members of AAA, in their joining the Academy, agree to abide by the Principles of the Code of Ethics of the Academy. They agree, by virtue of membership, to these principles.

The Principles having been stated, the Rules of the AAA Code of Ethics specify requirements for behavior. And, associated with Principle 4, Rule 4a and Rule 4c of the AAA Code of Ethics state:

> **Rule 4a:** Individuals shall not exploit persons in the delivery of professional services.
>
> **Rule 4c:** Individuals shall not participate in activities that constitute a conflict of professional interest

Members of the AAA must adhere to these rules for behavior or they may be subject to disciplinary actions imposed by the AAA.

Once principles and rules have been incorporated into the code, interpretations of these principles and rules may be required in order to clarify the intentions of the Academy or Association. Such interpretations and clarifications have led the AAA and ASHA to their position that even the appearance of a conflict of interest is a violation of Rule 4c. The idea that "appearance implies conflict" is neither new to the field of audiology nor unique to professional codes of behavior.

> The acceptance of even small gifts has been documented to affect clinical judgment and heightens the perception (as well as the reality) of a conflict of interest …. While following the Royal College of Physicians' guideline, "Would I be willing to have this arrangement generally known?", physicians should also ask, "What would the public or my patients think of this arrangement?" (American College of Physicians, 1998)

In general, there are a number of issues involving conflicts, appearances of conflicts, business practices, and the like that have caused, and continue to cause, concern and intervention by the various professional academies pertaining to audiology. Many of these issues involve the inherent conflict that exists between a professional model (placing patient or client interest above all else) and a business model whose profit motives generally do not require such placement of the customer's interests.

WHICH MODEL IS BEST?

In the professional meetings surrounding the discussion of ethics during the past few years (2001–2006), a great deal of confusion appears to exist regarding the conflict of interest requirements that the AAA has propagated. Many audiologists believe that, if they have the patient's best interest in mind, all activities that have to do with serving that interest and intention are ethical. While serving the patient requires that the patient's best interests are paramount, the ethical rationalizations surrounding some behaviors obviously arise from a lack of distinction or understanding between what should be called the professional model and the contrasting business model. The differentiating factor between the models is the standard of care that exists, or should exist in all professional models—medicine, law, dentistry, and audiology.

When one compares the professional modes of business to the typical business model, the first point of difference is the goal of the model. The medical model—all professional models for that matter—places the good of those served above all else, including the profit of the company. It is the ability of the professional to place him or herself in this position that typically commands the public respect, as well as their money, as these professional services are typically the result of higher learning, advanced knowledge, and/or special skill. The public expects that professional providers will earn a sufficient living—commensurate with the skill level of each—but they demand that public needs be served for this price.

On the other hand, the business model places profit above the needs of the customer. This is not as self-serving as it initially sounds. There are many examples of businesses that function for the public good. However, the typical and usual model of a business involves owners or shareholders whose investments are solicited by promises of profit of some sort. In a large sense, the business exists for the purposes of providing this profit to its shareholders and employees.

In the business arena, where business functions, as opposed to the professional arena, where law, medicine and medicine-like professionals function, the requirement for honest actions still exists. But, consumers expect that businesses exist for a profit and this profit will come at an expense to the consumer. Customers seldom expect a business to function in their best interest, especially when it comes to profit. Customers expect honesty, but not above all else. In general, consumers expect more from a professional than from a retail business. It is this difference in public expectations that provides the basis for professional ethics.

While important to a degree, maintenance of the public trust is not essential to a business. Such maintenance is both essential and required for a profession.

In discussing the differences between a business and a profession providing services such as audiology, it is always fruitful to consider some examples. In the business world, it is not uncommon for a wholesaler of products to offer incentives for increased sales from the retailers who buy through his or her company. Airplanes and resorts are commonly occupied with salespeople who have "won" a trip by completing a sales quota. Rewarding competitive efforts in retailing is a common practice, which has no (or very few) ethical considerations.[1] Such behavior on the part of a company supplying medical goods to the public, through a physician, dentist, or audiologist, has been judged a conflict of interest (American College of Physicians, op cit., American Academy of Audiology, 2005).

Other forms of incentives attempting to induce and increase in sales have also been ruled a conflict or potential conflict of interest by the American Academy of Audiology. These include, but are not necessarily limited to:

1. financial rewards of any kind in return for present or past sales of any product
2. rebates on products sold in the form of reduction of cost for number of sales (This includes the after-the-fact reduction of product cost through any third party purchasing group or account.)
3. gifts of money or in kind
4. trips, even if a certain portion of the trip involves education

Furthermore, it behooves any profession to police itself with respect to these types of ethical deviations. It is commonly stated that, if the profession will not police itself, the public and their legal methods will.

RELATIONSHIP BETWEEN STANDARD OF CARE (A MEDICAL MODEL) AND A BUSINESS MODEL

There are advantages to the medical model when it comes to matters of patient care that may not be obvious at first glance. These advantages accrue to the patient, as is appropriate, and involve the concept of "standard of care." It is not always an issue of great concern, but when brought forth in any sort of debate, it is generally easier to support a service provision model that treats the patient in a fashion that is most conducive to the medical model.

Within the medical model lie the concepts of best practice protocols and using diagnostic tests and rehabilitative treatments that correspond to the standards set by the majority of similar professional practitioners. In contrast, a business model takes into consideration efficiency, cost control, maintenance of profit, and competition with similar businesses as the central tenants. Clearly, these business aspects, while important in many arenas, do not always insure that the patient is treated in a manner that has patient benefit as the ultimate good.

---

1. Occasionally in the retail arena, the public good can be placed at risk and investigations into the "ethical" behavior of sales people is instigated, as already cited in the Wall Street Journal on Nov. 24, 2004—the article concerned with the giving of gifts to securities agents who sold investment vehicles to the public. The Securities and Exchange Commission begin an investigation into the giving of "lavish trips and other gifts" to a fund advisor in exchange for advice to buy that particular fund. One has little difficulty determining the violation of trust that purchasers place in these agents.

Interestingly, the American Academy of Audiology, the American Speech-Language and Hearing Association and the Veterans Administration joined in defining and publishing a standard for clinical practice in 1999/2000 (See ASHA, 1999; AAA, 2000.) In this statement, three large, professional organizations concerned with audiology came to agreement on what the standard of care in audiology should be. While there are obvious omissions in the document, especially in regard to the newer, specialized tests that are not used by the majority of audiologists, this statement establishes, for the most part, the types and extent of services that ought to viewed as the minimum battery that patients should expect.

Due to a number of confounding issues, these protocols seemed to have difficulties being fully integrated into many clinics. Perhaps, many audiologists believe that the use of these procedures is simply recommended and not meant to describe the protocols that should constitute a "best practices" approach to patient care. That there is a significant difference between these standards for care and the actual procedures in many clinics is a topic that also has been addressed for many years. The criticism leveled is that many universities respond to the demands of the employment sector of the field and have placed emphasis on the descriptions, manipulations, and fitting of hearing aids during the past 10–15 years.

In any event it would seem that many graduates entering the field of audiology are not trained in the full scope of diagnostic audiologic tests, nor do these graduates receive much training in many internship or clinical fellowship experiences. Lack of experience with such tests as outlined in the joint statement would certainly place the standard of care in jeopardy, if the standard is indeed set by these levels of evaluation.

DIRECTIONS EACH MODEL IS LIKELY TO TAKE US

Audiology as a field is poised to take either one of two pathways into the future. There are a significant number of members in the professional associations who believe that the retail/sales model of business will allow for the most flexibility and growth in the field. Those who advocate this direction reference the statistics and figures to indicate that the future would be better set if all audiologists in private practice adhered to a good business model.

The Business Model direction is certainly a viable method if audiologists are to achieve success in business. If the past is any indication, and it usually is a fairly good predictor at least in the near term, a large portion of the success of private practice audiology is due to the business profit involved in the sale of hearing aids. Indeed, in the opinion of many, it is this one aspect of audiology that has allowed for the establishment and growth of private audiology practices in this country. One has but to review the numbers involving annual salaries, sale of practices, etc. to see the potential profit involved in the sales model.

On the other hand, the alternative path involves the adherence to a medical model for the provision of audiology services to the public. This model does not eschew the sales aspects of hearing aids and other products, but rather it embraces these sales in a more service-oriented model. This Medical Model would have private providers billing third party payers, and, in general, functioning more like a typical medical, dental, or legal office. This model does not depend so exclusively on the profit of devices and/or products as it places these items more in the prosthetic realm.

There are many who see a great deal of overlap of the two models. Indeed, one cannot run a private practice without paying attention to the tenants of good business practices. But, the underlying philosophy that drives the practice eventually leads to the methods in which patients or customers are treated. And, as the underlying philosophies dictate, the two models produce considerably different ethical standards to which the hearing care providers must adhere. In the case of the Business Model, the underlying philosophy is that of business, tempered by concern for the customer. In the Medical Model, the underlying philosophy is concern for the patient, tempered by the modified practices of business.

Thus, the choice of models that audiology will follow will likely define the required ethical principles. These choices will involve:

1. Professional ethics vs. business ethics
2. Conflicts in ethical structures (business v. medical)
3. Legal, moral, and ethical differences

Once one considers these concepts, one's thoughts generally turn eventually back to a consideration of the standard of care that is presumed in healthcare in general and audiology in particular. If the public trust is placed in a professional, what does the public expect from this professional provider? Will the public require that their interest be placed before the profit of the provider? Does this placement require disclosure of all professional connections, reasons, rationales, and treatments? Is the perception of the public that professional care is up to date and consistent with the standards of the profession? Don't these expectations establish the concept of Standard of Audiologic Care in the minds of most providers? Perhaps they should, if they don't.

There will always be a conflict between the Medical Model of service provision and the requirements of running a business. A search on any web engine will uncover more references for Business Ethics that the average reader can assimilate. The discussion of "business ethics" is a confusing topic with which many undergraduates struggle. And, the typical topics of business ethics involve topics quite different from those facing a professional provider such as an audiologist, dentist, attorney, or physician.

Audiology is faced with some interesting decisions involving its professional future. These decisions will necessarily dictate the ethical structures under which the profession will function. As with laws and morals, these ethical principles most often evolve to meet the needs of the profession.

REFERENCES

American Academy of Audiology. (2000). Audiology clinical practice algorithms and statements. *Audiology Today*, (Special issue), August.

American Academy of Audiology. (2004). *Code of ethics & procedures, rules & penalties.* Retrieved November 1, 2004 from http://www.audiology.;org/about/code.php

American Academy of Audiology. (2006). *Ethics in audiology: Guidelines for ethical conduct in clinical, educational, and research settings.* Reston, VA: American Academy of Audiology.

American Speech-Language and Hearing Association. (1999). Joint audiology committee on clinical practice. *Clinical practice statements and algorithms.* Rockville, MD: American Speech-Language and Hearing Association.

American College of Physicians. (1998). Financial conflicts of interest. *Ethics Manual* (4th ed.). Also available online at: http://www.acponline.org/ethics/manual.htm

Council on Ethical and Medical Affairs. (2004). *Code of medical ethics.* American Medical Association Press.

Davies, P. (2004). *Consumers question "kickbacks."* Wall Street Journal, November 29, 2004.

National Society of Professional Engineers v. United States. (1978). 435 U.S. 679, 697–98.

Solomon, D. (2004). *Probe focuses on gifts to advisors.* Wall Street Journal, November 24, 2004.

APPENDIX 1

American Academy of Audiology

Code of Ethics & Procedures, Rules & Penalties April, 2004

PREAMBLE

The Code of Ethics of the American Academy of Audiology specifies professional standards that allow for the proper discharge of audiologists' responsibilities to those served, and that protect the integrity of the profession. The Code of Ethics consists of two parts. The first part, the Statement of Principles and Rules, presents precepts that members of the Academy agree to uphold. The second part, the Procedures, provides the process that enables enforcement of the Principles and Rules.

PART I: STATEMENT OF PRINCIPLES & RULES

PRINCIPLE 1: Members shall provide professional services and conduct research with honesty and compassion, and shall respect the dignity, worth, and rights of those served.

> **Rule 1a:** Individuals shall not limit the delivery of professional services on any basis that is unjustifiable or irrelevant to the need for the potential benefit from such services.

PRINCIPLE 2: Members shall maintain high standards of professional competence in rendering services, providing only those professional services for which they are qualified by education and experience.

Rule 2a: Individuals shall use available resources, including referrals to other specialists, and shall not accept benefits or items of personal value for receiving or making referrals.

Rule 2b: Individuals shall exercise all reasonable precautions to avoid injury to persons in the delivery of professional services or execution of research.

Rule 2c: Individuals shall not provide services except in a professional relationship, and shall not discriminate in the provision of services to individuals on the basis of sex, race, religion, national origin, sexual orientation, or general health.

Rule 2d: Individuals shall provide appropriate supervision and assume full responsibility for services delegated to supportive personnel. Individuals shall not delegate any service requiring professional competence to unqualified persons.

Rule 2e: Individuals shall not permit personnel to engage in any practice that is a violation of the Code of Ethics.

Rule 2f: Individuals shall maintain professional competence, including participation in continuing education.

PRINCIPLE 3: Members shall maintain the confidentiality of the information and records of those receiving services or involved in research.

Rule 3a: Individuals shall not reveal to unauthorized persons any professional or personal information obtained from the person served professionally, unless required by law.

PRINCIPLE 4: Members shall provide only services and products that are in the best interest of those served.

Rule 4a: Individuals shall not exploit persons in the delivery of professional services.

Rule 4b: Individuals shall not charge for services not rendered.

Rule 4c: Individuals shall not participate in activities that constitute a conflict of professional interest.

Rule 4d: Individuals using investigational procedures with patients, or prospectively collecting research data, shall first obtain full informed consent from the patient or guardian.

PRINCIPLE 5: Members shall provide accurate information about the nature and management of communicative disorders and about the research projects, services and products offered.

Rule 5a: Individuals shall provide persons served with the information a reasonable person would want to know about the nature and possible effects of services rendered, products provided or research being conducted.

Rule 5b: Individuals may make a statement of prognosis, but shall not guarantee results, mislead, or misinform persons served or studied.

Rule 5c: Individuals shall conduct and report product-related research only according to accepted standards of research practice.

Rule 5d: Individuals shall not carry out teaching or research activities in a manner that constitutes an invasion of privacy, or that fails to inform persons fully about the nature and possible effects of these activities, affording all persons informed free choice of participation.

Rule 5e: Individuals shall maintain documentation of professional services rendered.

PRINCIPLE 6: Members shall comply with the ethical standards of the Academy with regard to public statements or publication.

Rule 6a: Individuals shall not misrepresent their educational degrees, training, credentials, or competence. Only degrees earned from regionally accredited institutions in which training was obtained in audiology, or a directly related discipline, may be used in public statements concerning professional services.

Rule 6b: Individuals' public statements about professional services, products, or research results shall not contain representations or claims that are false, misleading, or deceptive.

PRINCIPLE 7: Members shall honor their responsibilities to the public and to professional colleagues.

Rule 7a: Individuals shall not use professional or commercial affiliations in any way that would limit services to or mislead patients or colleagues.

Rule 7b: Individuals shall inform colleagues and the public in a manner consistent with the highest professional standards about products and services they have developed or research they have conducted.

PRINCIPLE 8: Members shall uphold the dignity of the profession and freely accept the Academy's self-imposed standards.

Rule 8a: Individuals shall not violate these Principles and Rules, nor attempt to circumvent them.

Rule 8b: Individuals shall not engage in dishonesty or illegal conduct that adversely reflects on the profession.

Rule 8c: Individuals shall inform the Ethical Practice Board when there are reasons to believe that a member of the Academy may have violated the Code of Ethics.

Rule 8d: Individuals shall cooperate with the Ethical Practice Board in any matter related to the Code of Ethics.

APPENDIX 2

Procedures for the Management of Alleged Ethical Violations

Introduction

Members of the American Academy of Audiology are obligated to uphold the Code of Ethics of the Academy in their personal conduct and in the performance of their professional duties. To this end it is the responsibility of each Academy member to inform the Ethical Practice Board of possible Ethics Code violations. The processing of alleged violations of the Code of Ethics will follow the procedures specified below in an expeditious manner to ensure that violations of ethical conduct by members of the Academy are halted in the shortest time possible.

Procedures

1. Suspected violations of the Code of Ethics shall be reported in letter format giving documentation sufficient to support the alleged violation. Letters must be addressed to:
   Chair, Ethical Practice Board
   c/o Executive Director
   American Academy of Audiology
   11730 Plaza America Dr.
   Reston, VA 20190

2. Following receipt of a report of a suspected violation, the Ethical Practice Board will request a signed Waiver of Confidentiality from the complainant indicating that the complainant will allow the Ethical Practice Board to disclose his/her name should this become necessary during investigation of the allegation.

   a. The Board may, under special circumstances, act in the absence of a signed Waiver of Confidentiality. For example, in cases where the Ethical Practice Board has received information from a state licensure or registration board of a member having his or her license or registration suspended or revoked, then the Ethical Practice Board will proceed without a complainant.

   b. The Chair may communicate with other individuals, agencies, and/or programs for additional information as may be required for Board review at any time during the deliberation.

3. The Ethical Practice Board will convene to review the merit of the alleged violation as it relates to the Code of Ethics.

   a. The Chair of the Ethical Practice Board shall remove identifying information from the complaint and forward it to the members of this Board.

   b. The Ethical Practice Board shall meet to discuss the case, either in person or by teleconference. The meeting will occur within 60 days of receipt of the waiver of confidentiality, or of notification by the complainant of refusal to sign the waiver. In cases where another form of notification brings the complaint to the attention of the Ethical Practice Board, the Board will convene within 60 days of notification.

    c.   If the alleged violation has a high probability of being legally actionable, the case may be referred to the appropriate agency. The Ethical Practice Board may postpone member notification and further deliberation until the legal process has been completed.

4.   If there is sufficient evidence that indicates a violation of the Code of Ethics has occurred, upon majority vote, the member will be forwarded a Notification of Potential Ethics Concern.

    a.   The circumstances of the alleged violation will be described.

    b.   The member will be informed of the specific Code of Ethics rule that may conflict with member behavior.

    c.   Supporting AAA documents that may serve to further educate the member about the ethical implications will be included, as appropriate.

    d.   The member will be asked to respond fully to the allegation and submit all supporting evidence within 30 calendar days.

5.   The Ethical Practice Board will meet either in person or by teleconference:

    a.   within 60 calendar days of receiving a response from the member to the Notification of Potential Ethics Concern to review the response and all information pertaining to the alleged violation, or

    b.   within sixty (60) calendar days of notification to member if no response is received from the member to review the information received from the complainant.

6.   If the Ethical Practice Board determines that the evidence supports the allegation of an ethical violation, then the member will be provided written notice containing the following information:

    a.   The right to a hearing in person or by teleconference before the Ethical Practice Board;

    b.   The date, time and place of the hearing;

    c.   The ethical violation being charged and the potential sanction;

    d.   The right to present a defense to the charges.

At this time the member should provide any additional relevant information. As this is the final opportunity for a member to provide new information, the member should carefully prepare all documentation.

7.   Potential Rulings.

    a.   When the board determines there is insufficient evidence of an ethical violation, the parties to the complaint will be notified that the case will be closed.

b.   If the evidence supports the allegation of a Code violation, the rules(s) of the Code violated will be cited and sanction(s) will be specified.

8.   The Board shall sanction members based on the severity of the violation and history of prior ethical violations. A simple majority of voting members is required to institute a sanction unless otherwise noted. Sanctions may include one or more of the following:

   a.   Educative Letter. This sanction alone is appropriate when:

      1.   The ethics violation appears to have been inadvertent.

      2.   The member's response to Notification of Potential Ethics Concern indicates a new awareness of the problem and the member resolves to refrain from future ethical violations.

   b.   Cease and Desist Order. The member signs a consent agreement to immediately halt the practice(s) which were found to be in violation of the Code of Ethics.

   c.   Reprimand. The member will be formally reprimanded for the violation of the Code of Ethics.

   d.   Mandatory Continuing Education

      1.   The EPB will determine the type of education needed to reduce chances of recurrence of violations.

      2.   The member will be responsible for submitting documentation of continuing education within the period of time designated by the Ethical Practice Board.

      3.   All costs associated with compliance will be borne by the member.

   e.   Probation of Suspension. The member signs a consent agreement in acknowledgement of the Ethical Practice Board decision and is allowed to retain membership benefits during a defined probationary period.

      1.   The duration of probation and the terms for avoiding suspension will be determined by the Ethical Practice Board.

      2.   Failure of the member to meet the terms for probation will result in the suspension of membership.

   f.   Suspension of Membership.

      1.   The duration of suspension will be determined by the Ethical Practice Board.

      2.   The member may not receive membership benefits during the period of suspension.

      3.   Members suspended are not entitled to a refund of dues or fees.

   g.   Revocation of Membership. Revocation of membership is considered the maximum punishment for a violation of the Code of Ethics.

      1.   Revocation requires a two-thirds majority of the voting members of the EPB.

2. Individuals whose memberships are revoked are not entitled to a re-fund of dues or fees.

3. One year following the date of membership revocation the individual may reapply for, but is not guaranteed, membership through normal channels and must meet the membership qualifications in effect at the time of application.

9. The member may appeal the Final Finding and Decision of the Ethical Practice Board to the Academy Board of Directors. The route of Appeal is by letter format through the Ethical Practice Board to the Board of Directors of the Academy. Requests for Appeal must:

   a. be received by the Chair, Ethical Practice Board, within 30 days of the Ethical Practice Board's notification of the Final Finding and Decision,

   b. state the basis for the appeal, and the reason(s) that the Final Finding and Decision of the Ethical Practice Board should be changed,

   c. not offer new documentation.

The EPB chair will communicate with the Executive Director of the Association to schedule the appeal at the earliest feasible Board of Director's meeting.

The member may attend the portion of the Board of Directors meeting that addresses the appeal, but will be prohibited from providing new information. The deliberation must be on the facts presented to the EPB, as introduction of new evidence would compel the Board of Directors to act as the adjudicating body, rather than the appeals body.

The decision of the Board of Directors regarding the member's appeal shall be final.

10. In order to educate the membership, upon majority vote the Ethical Practice Board, the circumstances and nature of cases shall be presented in Audiology Today and in the Professional Resource area of the AAA website. The member's identity will not be made public.

11. No Ethical Practice Board member shall give access to records, act or speak independently, or on behalf of the Ethical Practice Board, without the expressed permission of the members then active. No member may impose the sanction of the Ethical Practice Board, or to interpret the findings of the Board in any manner which may place members of the Ethical Practice Board or Board of Directors, collectively or singly, at financial, professional, or personal risk.

12. The Ethical Practice Board Chair shall maintain a Book of Precedents that shall form the basis for future findings of the Board.

Confidentiality & Records

Confidentiality shall be maintained in all Ethical Practice Board discussion, correspondence, communication, deliberation, and records pertaining to members reviewed by the Ethical Practice Board.

1. Complaints and suspected violations are assigned a case number.
2. Identity of members involved in complaints and suspected violations and access to EPB files is restricted to the following:
   a. EPB Chair
   b. EPB member designated by EPB Chair when the chair recuses him or herself from a case
   c. AAA Executive Director
   d. Agent/s of the AAA Executive Director
   e. Other/s, following majority vote of EPB
3. Original records shall be maintained at the Central Records Repository at the Academy office in a locked cabinet.
   a. One copy will be sent to the Ethical Practices Board chair or member designated by the Chair.
   b. Redacted copies will be sent to members.
4. Communications shall be sent to the members involved in complaints by the Academy office via certified or registered mail, after review by Legal Counsel.
5. When a case is closed,
   a. The chair will forward all documentation to the Academy Central Records Repository.
   b. Members shall destroy all material pertaining to the case.
6. Complete records generally shall be maintained at the Academy Central Records Repository for a period of 5 years.
   a. Records will be destroyed five years after a member receives a sanction less than suspension, or five years after the end of a suspension, or after membership is reinstated.
   b. Records of membership revocations for persons who have not returned to membership status will be maintained indefinitely.

CHAPTER 16

Valuing Patients as Individuals: The Role of Culture

Jodell Newman-Ryan

Northern Illinois University

A woman schedules a child for a hearing evaluation. On the day of the evaluation, she brings that child, along with two of its siblings, to the clinic. The only pediatric audiologist on duty is a male. She refuses to take the child into the test area because it is "improper to be in a room alone with a man" and refuses to leave the other two children in the waiting room because it contains books "unsuitable" for children.

Parents bring a toddler to the clinic; while waiting for earmold impressions to set, they mention to the audiologist that the family will go skeet shooting next weekend.

A student clinician introduced herself to a patient who is a laborer with eight children as "I'm a doctoral student."

Do these scenarios have anything to do with culture? This chapter will argue, yes, when culture is defined broadly.

Culture shapes how we explain and value the world, and provides us with the lens through which we find meaning (Nuñez, 2000). Traditional chapters on cultural diversity warn that failure to consider sociocultural factors may lead to stereotyping, or biased or discriminatory treatment of patients based on race, culture, language proficiency, or social status (van Ryn & Burke, 2000; Donini-Lenhoff & Hedrick, 2000). Those that specifically mention audiology state that audiologists and those whom they serve may not share a common language or worldview (Scott, 2002), and that consideration of culture is needed today more than ever because of growing diversity in North America (Andrews, 1999a); for example, 45.2 percent of children who are deaf or hard-of-hearing in the United States (U.S.) are racial and ethnic minorities (Gallaudet Research Institute, 1999). The authors of these chapters urge clinicians to consider individuals in a broad societal context, in the context of their cultural upbringing, and as members of families who have varying strengths, resources, and capacities for care of family members. But they then proceed to define culture in such a way that tends to emphasize racial/ethnic categories while ignoring class, cohort or age, and other aspects of culture that do not fit neatly into the traditional narrow categories. For example, Battle (2002) includes an introductory chapter, then a chapter each devoted to African-Americans, Asian-Americans, Middle-Eastern and Arab-Americans, Native-Americans, and Latino Culture. Note that using the hyphenated terms excludes North Americans from locations outside the U.S., and that race/ethnicity is the predominant category while ignoring class, religion, or any other aspect of culture. In addition, these same books tend to devote the vast majority of content to speech and language implications while essentially ignoring any effects of culture on hearing or serving people who have hearing impairments. For example, influences of culture on standard pure-tone audiometry are ignored. Other than for directions, it is hard to argue that there would be influences of culture on pure-tone audiometry. But what about influences of cultural differences on hearing handicap scales, speech audiometry, audiological rehabilitation, etc.?

If our goal as audiologists is to improve hearing health outcomes and quality of care, does culture influence these outcomes? Although audiology is both a scientific and a humanistic endeavor, the humanistic aspect of care has received less attention (DeBonis & Donohue, 2004). Can audiologists separate humanistic from technical aspects of care? Does culture influence either or both?

Both the American Academy of Audiology (AAA) and the American Speech-Language-Hearing Association (ASHA) state that audiologists have a duty to provide services to *all* individuals:

> Individuals shall not discriminate in the provision of services to individuals on the basis of sex, race, religion, national origin, sexual orientation, or general health. (AAA Code of Ethics, 2003, Rule 2d)

> Individuals shall not discriminate in the delivery of professional services or the conduct of research and scholarly activities on the basis of race or ethnicity, gender, age, religion, national origin, sexual orientation, or disability (ASHA Code of Ethics, 2003, Principle 1, Rule C).

> Audiologists provide comprehensive diagnostic and treatment/rehabilitative services for auditory, vestibular, and related impairments. These services are provided to individuals across the entire age span from birth through adulthood; to individuals from diverse language, ethnic, cultural, and socioeconomic backgrounds; and to individuals who have multiple disabilities (ASHA, 2004b, p. 1).

> Audiologists serve diverse populations. The patient/client population includes persons of different race, age, gender, religion, national origin, and sexual orientation. Audiologists' caseloads include individuals from diverse ethnic, cultural, or linguistic backgrounds, and persons with disabilities. Although audiologists are prohibited from discriminating in the provision of services based on these factors, in some cases such factors may be relevant to the development of an appro-

priate treatment plan. These factors may be considered in treatment plans only when firmly grounded in scientific and professional knowledge (ASHA, 2004b, p. 1).

The goal of this chapter is to urge audiologists to consider many different aspects of culture while simultaneously viewing each patient as an individual.

CLINICIAN VALUES

Values are a freely chosen set of personal beliefs or attitudes about truth, the worth of any thought, object, person or behavior (Kozier, Erb, & Blais, 1997). Values form the core of a culture: time orientation, family obligations, communication patterns (including etiquette, space/distance, touch), interpersonal relationships (including long-standing historic rivalries), gender/sexual orientation, education, socioeconomic status, moral/religious beliefs, hygiene, clothing, meaning of work, and personal traits exert powerful influences on how individuals feel, behave, react within health-care settings (Andrews, 1999d).

Personal values underlie the perspectives from which health-care providers and patients attempt to interact. It is expected that clinicians promote an environment in which the values, customs and spiritual beliefs of patients will be respected. But anthropologists argue that every human being is ethnocentric, meaning that people subconsciously tend to view other people by using their own group or their own customs as the standard for all judgments. People consider their own way of life to be natural and good, and subconsciously tend to view others' ways as inferior their own. Value differences based on age, caste, class, education, gender, geographic location, political and religious beliefs, and traditions (Nasr, 1981) could exist between cultures, but also exist among different groups within the same culture. Consequently, health-care professionals need to be aware of their ethnocentric tendencies and develop strategies for avoiding cultural imposition of their values on patients while disregarding or trivializing those of the patients (Andrews, 1999a).

As clinicians become more mindful of managing their own diversity, questions initiated by "Why don't they … ?" are gradually balanced with "Why do we … ?" often prompting discussion of various approaches and perspectives (Kavanagh, 1999). With whom do you feel strange and uncomfortable, and why? How do your concerns and biases affect who gets care and what type of care you give? It is well known that there are cultural preferences among mental health providers for patients who are young, attractive, verbal, intelligent, and successful (also known as YAVIS) (Wilson & Kneisl, 1983), while those who are considered quiet, unattractive, old, indigent, different, and stupid (that is, the QUOIDS) often get less attention (Kavanagh, 1999). Are audiologists similarly guilty?

Self-awareness on the part of the audiologist is another requirement of a humanistic education. This refers primarily to clinicians developing an understanding of their own values, beliefs, history, and needs, and how these can influence emotional responses evoked in their interactions with patients (DeBonis & Donohue, 2004). What follows is an exercise to reveal biases (adapted from Randall-Davis, 1989). Describe your level of response to the groups below in Table 16–1.

TABLE 16–1
Bias-Revealing Exercise.

Qualifier	Unable to Greet	Greet	Accept	Help	Advocate
Haitians					
Jews					
Protestants					
Muslims					
Illegal Cocaine Users					
Alcoholics					
Neo-Nazis					

Are you emotionally prepared to interact with them? Do you have the background to help them? Are you able to greet, accept, and help them? Are you able to advocate for them?

Levels of Response:

I feel I am unable to greet: I feel I cannot greet nor have any positive regard for them.

I feel I am able to greet—I feel I can greet them warmly and welcome them sincerely.

I feel I could accept—I feel I can honestly accept them as they are and be comfortable enough to listen to their problems.

I feel I could help—I feel I would genuinely try to help them with their problems.

I feel I could advocate—I feel I could honestly be an advocate for them.

That exercise may have been relatively easy, but now try the following with specific application to patients and audiologists (Table 16–2). Are you able to

TABLE 16–2.
Bias-Revealing Exercise: Hearing-Related Issues.

Qualifier	Unable to Greet	Greet	Accept	Help	Advocate
Member of Deaf Culture					
Parent who purchases hearing aids for son but refuses same for daughter					
Public aid (Medicaid) recipient					
Rush Limbaugh					
Former U.S. President Clinton					

embrace members of Deaf culture? Are you able to respect parents who have different worldviews about gender roles? Are you able to separate political views and treat patients equally in some ways while also acknowledging the unique qualities that should be considered in caring for these individuals? (Note that both Rush Limbaugh and former U.S. President Clinton are known to have hearing impairments—they could be *your* patients).

After honestly reflecting on your values, review the "isms" under definitions (Appendix 1). Do your answers reflect any biases? Are they biases you wish to keep or are they biases you would like to reduce? For example, *ableism* is a bias that audiologists could consciously or unconsciously display, such as when making decisions for patients that they could make for themselves.

To summarize, just as it is critical in a humanistic approach to audiology to acknowledge that clinicians provide services to individuals, it is equally important to acknowledge that care providers are individuals with unique traits (DeBonis & Donohue, 2004). Only through this self-understanding of values are audiologists able to use that uniqueness for the benefit of the patient-clinician relationship.

PATIENT VALUES

Whenever clinicians interact with patients, there is a complex web of interrelated factors that influence the relationship (Andrews & Herberg, 1999). The challenge that audiology services be provided to diverse individuals requires audiologists to have broad understanding of, and comfort with, the range of characteristics possessed by human beings. People differ not only in their age, ability, and cultural background but also in such variables as temperament, motivation, ability to change, family dynamic, and reaction to hearing impairment (DeBonis & Donohue, 2004).

In order to be respectful of values, beliefs, rights, and practices, clinicians must first have knowledge of those values. Determining values, noticing perceptions, asking opinions, and watching behaviors and reactions could assist audiologists in providing optimal care. Clinicians should realize that cultural perspectives may have profound influences on how patients make decisions, conceptualize options, and conduct themselves in healthcare settings; also remember that the practitioner-patient relationship is often compromised by the status and power differentials of the participants (Hern et al., 1998). Refrain from considering these factors *only* in patients who belong to certain identified cultures; instead, consider that these values are important to consider for *all* patients.

Note that it is impossible to know everything about every culture just as it would be impossible in most clinical situations to gather information about more than a few of these items that appear below. Try to identify those which might be expected to have the greatest influence on the most cogent clinical decisions necessary for a given clinical encounter. Be aware of some basic cultural and religious differences that may result in a delay in seeking care, use of traditional cultural methods of healing, attitudes about impairments and disabilities, or even refusal of some medical procedures such as immunizations (Norton, 1999).

Audiologists are encouraged to develop skills that meld those of medical interviewing with the ethnographic tools of medical anthropology (Shapiro & Lenahan, 1996; Carrillo et al., 1999) in order to assess patient values which influence diagnostic and treatment decisions. Curiosity, empathy, respect, and humility are some basic attitudes that have the potential to help the clinical relationship and to yield useful information about the patient's individual beliefs and preferences. An approach that focuses on inquiry, reflection, and analysis throughout the care process is most useful for acknowledging that culture is just one of many factors that influence an individual's health beliefs and practices (Bonder, Martin, & Miracle, 2001). Goals for assessment of values include eliciting patient's explanatory models (i.e., how they conceptualize and understand their illnesses) and agendas, identifying and negotiating different styles of communication, assessing social contexts during which communication occurs (and during which hearing is necessary), assessing decision-making preferences and the role of family, determining each patient's perception of hearing health care, recognizing sexual and gender issues, and being aware of issues of mistrust, prejudice, and racism (Betancourt, 2003; Hill et al., 1990; Zweifler & Gonzalez, 1998; Gonzalez-Lee & Simon, 1987).

COMMUNICATION

Beginning with the first encounter the patient has with the hearing-health-care setting (which may be via telephone to schedule an appointment), there are opportunities to foster good communication or, conversely, to erect barriers to effective communication. Given that audiologists' patients already have communicative problems by definition, clinicians must be especially vigilant to monitor understanding. Difficulties understanding questions asked during interviews and difficulties understanding verbal or written instructions can lead to erroneous results and subsequently to misdiagnosis, followed by mismanagement. Language and communication problems may lead to patient dissatisfaction, poor comprehension and adherence, and lower quality of care. Ballachanda (2001) noted three areas of audiological assessment when language barriers are especially challenging: 1) gathering case history information; 2) selecting and administering audiological test materials; and 3) counseling.

Areas of communication include both verbal communication (language, greetings, titles) and nonverbal communication (time, space, distance, modesty, touch, gestures, posture, tone of voice, facial expressions). Frequently overlooked is the environmental context in which communication occurs and how it is influenced by the setting, purposes of the communication, and perception of time, distance, touch, and other factors (Andrews & Herberg, 1999).

General recommendations for successful communication include those of Lipson and Steiger (1996), who advocate flexibility in verbal and nonverbal communication style, ability to speak slowly and clearly without excessive slang, ability to encourage to others to express themselves, ability to communicate sincere interest and empathy, patience, and ability to observe and intervene when there is misunderstanding.

Modes of Communication

One of the first decisions made by the clinician (or someone else at the facility) is to decide whether to speak with someone face-to-face, send an electronic or paper memorandum, contact by telephone, or opt not to communicate about a particular matter at all. Although communication problems multiply in telephone communications because important nonverbal cues are lost and accents may be difficult to interpret (Andrews, 1999d), making appointments via telephone may be the patient's first choice about communication. After an initial appointment, clinicians should ask patients about preferred modes of communication. Throughout clinical interactions, clinicians should observe and monitor patients' verbal and nonverbal communications and communication styles.

Through both verbal and nonverbal means, clinicians collect information about factual matters as well as about the patient's emotional state. Use open-ended questions or questions phrased in several ways to obtain information, but be aware that some people do not consider direct questions to be polite (Kavanagh, 1999). Audiologists listen actively when patients share information about their emotional response, understanding that listening can be part of the healing process for the patient. In addition, audiologists attempt to evoke such information because ultimately this insight will assist in the process of diagnosis and rehabilitation. Humanist audiologists recognize their role as not only providing content counseling in the form of factual information, but also engaging with the patient, and the patient's parent/family, in support counseling as patients adjust to the life changes resulting from their communication disorder (DeBonis & Donohue, 2004). Audiologists also observe family interactions, and understand that the family, as well as the other important people in the patient's life, could play an important role in any effort to reduce the degree of communication deficit (DeBonis & Donohue, 2004).

Nonverbal Communication

There are five types of nonverbal behaviors that convey information about patients: vocal cues, such as pitch, tone, and quality of voice; action cues, such as posture, facial expression, and gestures; object cues, such as clothes, jewelry, and hair styles; use of personal and territorial space in interpersonal transactions and care of belongings; and touch, which involves the use of personal space and action (Lapierre & Padgett, 1991).

Wide cultural variation exists when interpreting *silence*. Consider messages conveyed by proverbs: "tell it like it is" which emphasizes values of direct confrontation and honesty at all costs as opposed to a zen proverb of "one who knows does not speak and one who speaks does not know" which emphasizes values of listening and silence. Some individuals find silence extremely uncomfortable and make every effort to fill conversational lags with speech, while others consider silence essential to understanding and respecting the other person (Andrews & Herberg, 1999). Silence may mean that the speaker wishes the listener to consider the content of what has been said before continuing could signal respect for another's privacy, a sign of agreement, or contempt for what is perceived as an inappropriate question. When monitoring for patients' unspoken reactions to difficult information, consider the role of silence in these emotional reactions.

Greetings, Titles, and Social Amenities

When audiologists first meet patients, they should use proper titles of respect: "Doctor," "Reverend," Mister," "Miss." Quickly follow by asking patients how they wish to be addressed, then indicate to them how you prefer to be called (Andrews & Herberg, 1999). If audiologists are working with others, decide if all team members should be introduced, or whether it would be better for the patient to interact with one clinician. Note that some women will be offended by being addressed as "Miss" or "Mistress" (Mrs.) while others will be offended by being addressed as "Ms." or any neutral salutation that does not acknowledge their marital status. Refrain from calling patients by their first names unless requested to do so by patients, since this practice may be considered rude, particularly if the patients are older than the clinician.

Space, Distance

Hall (1963) pioneered the study of *proxemics*, which focuses on how people in various cultures relate to their physical space. Although there are intercultural variations, the intimate distance in interpersonal interactions ranges from touching (or no distance) to about half a meter. At this distance, people experience visual detail and each other's smell, heat, and touch. Personal distance varies from about a third of a meter to over one meter, the usual space within which communication between friends and acquaintances occurs. Clinicians frequently interact with patients within the intimate or personal distance zones (Andrews & Herberg, 1999), but can minimize discomfort by respecting patients' preferences for distance during portions of clinical encounters where touching is not essential for diagnostic or treatment purposes. For example, audiologists need to touch patients to attach earphones or electrodes, but should arrange chairs in the counseling area to reflect distances comfortable for both the patient and the clinician. Allow patients to choose seating for comfortable personal space and appropriate eye contact (Kavanagh, 1999).

Jargon

In promoting effective communication, avoid technical jargon, slang, colloquial expressions, abbreviations, complex sentences, and excessive use of medical terminology (Andrews & Herberg, 1999). This advice seems obvious, but clinicians occasionally should audio-record their conversations with patients, replay them, and listen for how often words such as "audiogram" and "bilateral" slip in.

Using Translators and Interpreters

Obviously, clinicians should identify the patient's preferred language (including sign language) and communicate in that language whenever possible: ask "Which language do you prefer?" In the absence of bilingual clinicians, use interpreters. Even a person who has a basic command of English but for whom English is a second language (limited English proficiency) may need an interpreter when faced with the anxiety-provoking situation of entering a health-care setting. Ideally, a trained medical interpreter should be used who knows interpreting techniques, has a health-care background, and understands patients' rights (Andrews & Herberg, 1999), but the prevalence of this practice in audiology settings is unknown.

It is tempting to ask relatives, friends, or even other patients to interpret because they are readily available and may be anxious to help. But doing so would violate confidentiality for the patient; furthermore, the friend or relative, though fluent in ordinary language usage, is likely to be unfamiliar with terminology, clinic procedures, and health-care ethics (Andrews & Herberg, 1999). Interpreters and bilingual staff should demonstrate bilingual proficiency and receive training that includes the skills and ethics of interpreting, and should demonstrate knowledge in both languages of the terms and concepts relevant to clinical or non-clinical encounters (Chin, 2000); family or friends are not considered adequate substitutes because they usually lack these abilities.

The type of interpretation service provided to patients is an important factor in the level of satisfaction. When comparing various methods of interpretation, patients who used professional interpreters were found to be equally as satisfied with the overall health care visit as patients who used bilingual providers but patients who use family interpreters or non-professional interpreters, such as nurses, clerks, and technicians, were less satisfied with their visit (Lee, Batal, Maselli, & Kutner, 2002).

Summarized below in Table 16–3 are suggestions for the selection and use of an interpreter and for overcoming language barriers when an interpreter is unavailable.

So although use of an interpreter is the ideal, clinicians need strategies for promoting effective communication when none is present. Desperate measures include asking who among the patient's family and friends could serve as an interpreter, using AT&T Language Line Services (offering translations in nearly 150 languages; 800-752-6096 in the U.S.), or using co-workers who may not be fluent in another language but may know more of the language than the primary clinician.

Apparently it is relatively common to lack interpreters; among non-English speakers who needed an interpreter during a health care visit, less than half—48 percent—report that they always or usually had one (Collins, Hughes, Doty, Ives, Edwards, & Tenney, 2002).

Within the Latino community, the use of *promotoras*, also known as peer educators who are liaisons between their community and the world of health care, is becoming increasingly popular. Using *promotoras* is not only cost-effective, but also has been shown to be more effective in terms of reaching populations who find the information more credible coming from someone with a familiar background (Kolker, 2004).

TABLE 16–3.
Using Interpreters (adapted from Andrews, 1995; Newman-Ryan,
Northrup, & Villarreal-Emery, 1995).

Use of an Interpreter—General Recommendations

Contact local agencies and hospitals for lists of interpreters, and use both formal and informal networking to locate suitable interpreters.

When using an interpreter, expect that the interaction with the patient will require more time than caring for verbal-English-speaking clients and schedule accordingly.

Before locating an interpreter, be sure that the language the patient speaks at home is known, since it may be different from the language spoken publicly (e.g., French is sometimes spoken by Asians).

Avoid interpreters from a rival culture.

Be aware of gender differences between interpreter and patient. In general, same gender is preferred.

Ask the interpreter to translate as closely to verbatim as possible.

Speak directly to the patient, even if an interpreter is present.

Recommendations for Institutions

Maintain a computerized list of interpreters who may be contacted as needed.

Network with area hospitals, colleges, universities, and other organizations that may serve as resources.

Allocate funds for interpreting.

What to Do When There is No Interpreter

Be polite and formal.

Greet the person using the last or complete name. Gesture to yourself and say your name. Offer a handshake or nod.

Proceed in an unhurried manner. Pay attention to any effort by the patient or family to communicate.

Speak in a low, moderate voice. Avoid talking loudly. Remember that there is a tendency to raise the volume and pitch of your voice when the listener appears not to understand. The listener may perceive that you are shouting and/or angry.

Use any words known in the patient's language. This indicates that you are aware of and respect the patient's culture.

Use simple words, such as *pain* instead of *discomfort*. Avoid medical jargon, idioms, and slang. Avoid using contractions. Use nouns repeatedly instead of pronouns. Example: Do not say, "He has been wearing his hearing aid, hasn't he?" Do say, "How many hours each day does he wear his hearing aid?"

Pantomime words and simple actions while verbalizing them.

Instruct clearly in the proper sequence. Example: Do not say, "Before you change the battery, take it out of your child's ear." Do say, "First, remove the hearing aid from your baby's ear. Second, change the battery. Third, put the hearing aid back in your baby's ear." And provide written information stating these same recommendations.

Discuss one topic at a time. Avoid using conjunctions. Example: Do not say, "Is that too loud, such that you couldn't listen to it for 10 minutes?" Do say, "Is that too loud?" Wait for answer, then verify by asking "could you listen to it for 10 minutes?"

Validate if patients understand by having them repeat instructions, demonstrate the procedure, or act out the meaning.

Write several short sentences in English, and determine the person's ability to read them.

Try a third language.

Buy phrase books, make or purchase flash cards. Directions and terms useful for assessing balance are available (e.g., Newman-Ryan et al., 1995).

Ideally, clinicians should be able to choose from a variety of interpreters. Reasons to terminate services from an interpreter include interpreters who take the meaning of the word literally as one who explains or expounds instead of merely translating (Kavanagh, 1999).

Finally, to avoid communication mismatches, be alert to behaviors considered possibly indicative of low health literacy (from Weiss, 2003): forms that are incomplete or inaccurately completed, frequently-missed appointments, lack of compliance with referrals and recommendations, and statements such as "I forgot my glasses; I'll read this when I get home." Table 16–4 offers suggestions for improving understanding in patients with low-literacy skills.

AUDIOLOGICAL IMPLICATIONS

Consider the following examples from materials on hearing-related topics prepared for patients.

Example One (from Grundfast & Carney, 1987).

If a parent is aware that a child is not hearing well because of middle-ear fluid, she can spend extra time emphasizing speech and playing word games with the child to help compensate for speech that the child may not be hearing.

This message assumes that the parent is aware of hearing impairment resulting from otitis media with effusion, which may or may not be the case. The sentence is quite long and begins with a conditional clause. One way to reduce

TABLE 16–4.
Suggestions for Bridging a Literacy Gap: Oral Communication
(adapted from Weiss, 2003).

Create a shame-free environment.
Offer to help: "Is there anyone in your family who helps you read?" "May we help you complete these forms?"
Involve family members.
Speak slowly.
Use plain, non-medical "living room" language.
Try to determine the patient's learning style (whether the patient prefers to learn by using written materials, pictures, verbal counseling, or some other technique; Kiefer, 2001) and adjust accordingly.
Show pictures and models (if appropriate; see above).
Limit amount of information provided and repeat it.
Use "teach-back" or "show-me" technique (don't ask "do you understand?" but instead ask "how would you tell your friends about this?")
Avoid jargon and use the simplest terms possible; e.g., instead of *referral*, say "you need to go to _____."
Stage a literacy office evaluation: evaluate and modify if necessary signs, forms, patient education materials, etc.
Identify community resources that offer literacy and adult education programs.

miscommunication is to use direct language. For example, Margolis (2004) recommends saying "use earplugs when you use your power tools" rather than "keep your noise exposure to a minimum." Applying this principle, a more direct recommendation would be:

- Your child may have a hearing loss when there is fluid in the ear (earache, otitis media).
- Get close to your child and speak clearly.
- Keep reading to your child.
- Watch for signs that your child doesn't hear what you say. Repeat if necessary.

**Example Two (from Auditory Neuropathy: Quick Facts
by the National Institute on Deafness and Other
Communication Disorders, 2003).**

Although outer hair cells—hair cells adjacent to and more numerous than the inner hair cells—are generally more prone to damage than inner hair cells, outer hair cells seem to function normally in people with auditory neuropathy.... Outer hair cells help amplify sound vibrations entering the inner ear from the middle ear. When hearing is working normally, the inner hair cells convert these vibrations into electrical signals that travel as nerve impulses to the brain, where the impulses are interpreted as sound.

This message assumes that people know there are different types of hair cells, that it is important to know there are different types of hair cells, and that this information is important in understanding auditory neuropathy. Note that this passage includes long sentences and embedded phrases, making it difficult to follow. Newman-Ryan (2004) calculated reading levels for seven consumer sections of hearing-aid manufacturer-sponsored Web sites using the Flesch-Kincaid Grade Level Reading program through Word®. Only two, *Oticon Useful Tips for Friends and Relatives* (grade 7) and *Widex Maintenance* (grade 8.5), were written at levels below a tenth-grade reading level. The other five were above grade 10.5. These preliminary data indicate that at least some of the information available to patients regarding their hearing and hearing aids may not be understood by average patients, let alone those who struggle with reading.

The tests and forms must be readable to people with low literacy. Examine case histories, hearing handicap scales, consent forms, purchase agreements, user instructions, etc. Revise clinic-specific forms if necessary. Two possible problems exist with reducing reading levels of audiological materials. First, consider that while the market is flooded with materials written "for dummies" (e.g., *Windows for Dummies*, *French for Dummies*), there is a potential for people with high literacy skills to be insulted by materials written at levels substantially below their abilities. Second, making buyer's agreements and consent-for-treatment forms sophisticated enough to withstand legal challenges while still understandable to patients is next to impossible. Perhaps having multiple versions of the same materials but geared towards different reading levels would be the best solution. That way, the first problem is solved by having people comfortably choose materials aimed at their particular reading levels and the second problem is solved by satisfying the legal requirement of providing people materials with complete information but adding supplemental materials written at levels they can understand.

ASSESSMENT

Audiologists need to consider whether there are biologic variations that are important to consider in different populations (Boyle, 1999b). The influence of age on hearing-related abilities is well established, but are there other demographic or cultural differences such as racial/ethnic differences that should be known in order to provide appropriate care? Incidence/prevalence among groups and historical factors that might shape health behaviors could impact on audiological and other health outcomes. If normative data for standardized tests are gathered from a population that is primarily middle class, English speaking, and of European background, clinicians must be aware of the possibility that test validity and reliability are compromised if applying these norms to other populations (Kayser, 2001).

Certain conditions known to cause hearing impairments are known to be more prevalent in particular groups than others. The prevalence of otitis media in American Indian and Eskimo populations is well documented (e.g., Brody, Overfield, & McAlister, 1965; Shaw, Todd, Goodwin, & Feldman, 1981) and will not be reviewed here. Instead, consider racial differences that could result in misdiagnosis if not recognized. Scott (2002) states that sickle cell disease (SCD) is recognized as a world health problem predominantly affecting people originally descended from of areas in Africa and areas surrounding the Mediterranean Sea and Indian Ocean. The prevalence of sensori-neural-central hearing impairment in sickle cell disease has been reported as 41 percent in adults (Crawford, Gould, Smith, Beckford, Gibson, & Bobo, 1991; Gould, Crawford, Smith, Beckford, Gibson, Pettit, & Bobo, 1991) and 3.5 percent (MacDonald, Bauer, Cox, & McMahon, 1999) to 12 percent (Friedman, Luban, Herer, & Williams, 1980) in children. When audiometric results suggest sensori-neural-central hearing impairment of unknown origin in young children, the possibility of SCD needs to be explored.

The assessment process, consisting of gathering history, interviewing, observing, and performing tests, should be conducted with some deference to culture. Case history and interviewing suggestions were reviewed earlier, especially in the section on Patient Values. Other factors to consider appear below.

Informed Consent

The first step in assessment is obtaining permission to assess and treat. When and how should audiologists ask for informed consent to assess patients? Clinicians should recognize that concepts such as *informed consent* are not universally shared, even within the U.S. During the 1960s and 1970s in North America, a process of patients' emancipation gave rise to the patients' rights movement promoting a respect for patient autonomy and the principle of informed consent (Norton, 1999). During this time physicians were persuaded not only to share information with patients about their illnesses, but also to ensure that patients had sufficient understanding of the information to give an informed consent for treatments, procedures and participation in research. Thus, the role of the patient evolved from one of dependence on the physician to make clinical decisions to one of mutual participation in designing treatment plans (Szasz & Hollender, 1956). The process found expressions in the language of rights, such as the right to informed consent. It was a language quite familiar in the Western cultural context that arose from the various rights movement of the decade such as the civil rights movement and the women's rights movement (Norton, 1999). In addition, the human rights movement supported the patient's rights movement and the bioethical movement in general (Viafora, 1996). As a result, it was the language of rights that influenced the development of bioethics in the West in contrast to the language of virtues and duties, which characterized ethical traditions in other parts of the world.

Hearing Screening

Screening, meant to identify people who need further testing to identify conditions, is an activity performed by audiologists and others to identify people who have hearing impairments and/or hearing disabilities. When designing programs that may include people with limited English proficiency, the following considerations are recommended by Lavizzo-Mourey, Smith, Sims, and Taylor (1994) based on their experiences.

- Write using translations that are consistent with everyday speech.
- Have drafts reviewed by samples of the target population and revise if necessary.
- Consult a literacy expert.
- Incorporate local scenes and include target population in photographs.

Lavizzo-Mourey et al. (1994) designed two large-print, large-size (8.5 x 11-inch) booklets depicting people of color presenting causes, signs, symptoms and functional consequences of hearing impairment; one version had English and Spanish text at a fifth-grade reading level. The booklets were mailed directly to 19,000 households targeted as having high concentrations of black or Latino households in Philadelphia. Free hearing screenings were offered. Approximately three-quarters of those tested failed screening, yet only 26 percent pursued assessment, reportedly due to financial reasons (15 percent), lack of transportation (8 percent), and illness (13 percent). Clearly, effectiveness of screening programs could be improved.

Distance and Proximity in Audiology

Performing many audiological procedures such as pure-tone audiometry, earmold impressions, and electrophysiological tests requires the audiologist to be physically close to patients. Yet many individuals may be uncomfortable with having strangers so close. In particular, some cultures adhere to strict rules relating to touching children. For example, many Asians believe that touching the head is a sign of disrespect because the head is thought to be the source of a person's strength or the residence of the soul (Devine & Braganti, 1986). Audiologists need to be aware that placing earphones or electrodes on infants and toddlers should be done only with parental permission; non-essential activities such as patting a child on the head should be avoided. Similarly, patients' attire especially around the area of the head could pose challenges to audiologists. Consider how the following people could be accommodated for auditory evoked potential testing or pure-tone audiometry (see Newman-Ryan, 2001): Hindu women dressed in the *sari*, Sikh men who wear a turban, Amish and Mennonite women who wear bonnets and men who wear straw or black felt hats, Muslim women wearing a *chador*, Catholic nuns wearing wimples, Arab men who wear a *khafia*, an Orthodox Jewess, and anyone with jewelry or accessories in their hair.

Pure-Tone Audiometry

The effects of culture on pure-tone audiometry are not known; i.e., where there are differences in motivation that could affect results, whether different directions are needed (other than for limited English-proficiency patients), etc. There is some indication that blacks have better hearing sensitivity than other groups in the U.S. (e.g., Berger, Royster, & Thomas, 1977; Royster & Thomas, 1979), but more data are needed. Differences in rates of hearing impairment based on gender and race have been found in industrial noise-exposed populations in the U.S.: black women showed the least effects of noise on auditory thresholds, followed by white women and black men, and then white men (Jerger, Jerger, Pepe, & Miller, 1986).

Speech Audiometry

Scott (2002) cautions audiologists to carefully consider whether it is appropriate to use English-language speech audiometric materials on non-native English speakers. But she does not advise audiologists as to how to make that decision. For example, should audiologists ask patients if they would like to have tests administered in other languages, or should patients be expected to ask if they would prefer non-English-language tests? Should patients undergo screening tests for English proficiency? Although statements such as those made by Scott (2002) seem intuitively obvious, research is lacking to confirm these claims: for example, Scott states that the languages (or dialects) of audiologists and patients should match or test results could be altered by differences in vocabulary and pronunciation. Research is lacking to support whether audiologists are able to predict, from a few minutes of conversation, English proficiency, the impact of administering word recognition tests in English to non-native-English speakers, and the effect of regional dialects on word recognition scores. Audiologists are advised to always use recorded speech audiometric materials, with good reason, but recorded materials in a variety of regional dialects are lacking. Furthermore, recorded materials of phonetically-balanced words common to adults learning English are not available.

Although more research is needed in this area, one suggestion is to use digits as speech stimuli. Miller, Heise, and Lichten (1951) recommended the use of digits, which are among the 500 most frequently used words in English (Rudmin,1987), for speech-recognition audiometry and more recently Ramkissoon, Bilger, and Proctor (2000) developed a digit-speech reception test for individuals acquiring English as a second language.

Vocabulary and the way vocabulary words are depicted should be reviewed for whether they would be known to people from different regions, different classes and backgrounds, and possibly different age groups or cohorts. For example, nowadays, children have difficulty identifying a bar of soap if they have only had experience with liquid soap; consider the influence of this effect on tests such as the Northwestern University-Children's Perception of Speech Test (NU-CHIPS; Elliott & Katz, 1980).

Electroacoustic Immittance

There is limited information suggesting that there are racial differences in electroacoustic immittance values. Tympanometric peak pressure (TPP), peak, compensated acoustic admittance (Peak Y_{tm}), tympanometric width (TW), and ear-canal volume (V_{ea}) values for white non-Hispanic adults (Roup, Wiley, Safady, & Stoppenbach, 1998; Wiley, Cruickshanks, Nondahl, Tweed, Klein, & Klein, 1996) were compared to those in Southern Chinese adults (Wan & Wong, 2002). The Southern Chinese subjects were found to have lower Peak Y_{tm}, lower V_{ea}, wider TW, and more positive TPP values than the white subjects. Note that whether these differences are due to true racial differences or size differences (or conceivably, some other difference) is unknown; i.e., it has not been established whether non-Chinese people with lower-than-average ear-canal volumes might present with findings similar to the Chinese subjects in this study.

Oto-Acoustic Emissions

There is limited information suggesting that there are racial differences in oto-acoustic emissions (OAEs). In comparing spontaneous oto-acoustic emissions (SEOAs) and transient oto-acoustic emissions (TEOAEs) in Chinese and white subjects, Chan and McPherson (2001) found significantly more SOAEs were found in the higher frequencies in Chinese subjects than in white subjects; they also found minor signal-to-noise differences for TEOAEs.

Asssessment Summary

Finally, more data are needed to establish or exclude the possibility of cultural differences in hearing-related abilities. Clearly, much research is needed in the area of audiological assessment and effects of culture, particularly in the area of speech audiometry, motivation and its effect on audiometric tests, etc. Whether modifying test instructions such as when using translated instructions affects results has not been researched extensively for audiological tests. At this time, there is no compelling reason to establish different normative databases for hearing sensitivity or OAEs according to race, but more data are needed. Note that some of the differences discussed here are described by the original authors as racial/ethnic differences, but are not necessarily since whites from Mediterranean areas are known to be susceptible to SCD, and the immittance differences may be due to ear-canal volume differences, not to race per se. If racial differences (or differences on some other basis) are established, then audiologists must be aware of these differences in establishing normative databases, deciding presence or absence of impairments or disabilities, judging the effectiveness of hearing conservation programs (Scott, 2002), or in making other clinical decisions. In order to determine which differences are due to genetic differences and which are due to social factors such as disparities in health care, international data need to be examined, or perhaps more correctly, need to be collected, as few studies are known to exist currently. As always, the genetic influences of belonging to a certain race need to be differentiated from the social factors of living in a certain location (i.e., the general genetic composition of being black needs to be differentiated from being black and living in the U.S., as the general genetic composition of being white needs to be differentiated from being white and living in Finland).

DEAF CULTURE

Any audiologist who was still unaware of the growing influence of Deaf culture might have been surprised at the 2002 news that a family wanted to increase its "chances of having a baby who was deaf;" Sharon Duchesneau and Candace Mc-Cullough found a sperm donor who was congenitally hearing impaired with this goal in mind (Mundy, 2002).

It may seem a shocking undertaking: two parents trying to screen *in* a quality, deafness, at a time when many parents are using genetic testing to screen *out* as many disorders as science will permit. Though most cases of congenital hearing impairment cannot be identified before birth, Mundy suggests that many parents would seek to eliminate it if they could. Mundy (2002) quotes R. Alta Charo: "I think all of us recognize that deaf children can have perfectly wonderful lives, but the question is whether the parents have violated the sacred duty of parenthood, which is to maximize to some reasonable degree the advantages available to their children."

But members of the Deaf community see hearing impairment (actually, they would say deafness) as an identity, not a medical affliction that needs to be fixed. And yet, while deafness may be a culture, in the U.S. it is also an official disability, recognized under the Americans with Disabilities Act (Mundy, 2002). What about the obligation of parents to see that their child has a better life than they did? Then again, what does a better life mean? Does it mean choosing a hearing donor so your baby, unlike you, might grow up hearing? Does it mean giving birth to a deaf child, and raising it in a better environment than the one you experienced? What if you believe you can be a better parent to a deaf child than to a hearing one? Is taking action to have a baby who is deaf a natural outcome of the pride and self-acceptance the Deaf movement has brought to so many, or a crime against humanity?

At least for Duchesneau and McCullough, because they do not view deafness as a disability, they do not see themselves as bringing a disabled child into the world; rather, they see themselves as bringing a different sort of normal child into the world (Mundy, 2002). How do audiologists react to this action, or to members of Deaf culture in general?

Because many members of Deaf culture reject amplification, they would have limited contact with audiologists. Some states, however, require annual hearing tests in order to maintain eligibility for state-supported services, so like it or not, they would have to see a hearing health-care professional.

In order to facilitate smooth communication with supporters of Deaf culture, audiologists should involve people other than audiologists, scientists, and the medical community in making decisions that affect members of the Deaf community. Include community members and leaders in programs such as public information panels concerning newborn-hearing screening or cochlear implants. Include bicultural providers, translators, and others who are knowledgeable about the value systems of other cultures including Deaf culture. When developing policies and forms such as informed consent procedures, include members of the Deaf community to assist with developing such procedures, or at least ask members of the Deaf community to review such policies if they are already in place.

TREATMENT INCLUDING AUDIOLOGICAL REHABILITATION

There are many reasons to consider cultural influences in planning audiological rehabilitation programs. For example, the role of culture in motivation, communication styles, judgments of treatment success or failure, just to name a few. Not only are data lacking regarding possible differences in hearing sensitivity and hearing impairment in different groups, but hearing disability among racial and ethnic minority groups has received even less attention. Different definitions of disability and different reactions to impairments and disabilities may mean that normative data for hearing handicap scales are not appropriate for certain individuals. But which cultural factors are important to include are unknown. Further research is needed in this area.

Some other factors to consider appear below.

First, identify those people who need to be involved in treatment decisions (preferably those identified by the patient) and then include them in planning for care.

Then, consider views regarding independence and autonomy. While some patients value individualism, self reliance, and independence, others may not value independence in themselves or in their family members; advocating that hearing aid use will encourage independence may not be well received.

Next, when establishing goals for treatment, consider whether the patient is oriented to the present or the future. Making plans may not be valued because the future is seen as neither uncertain nor preordained but as something that one accepts with fatalistic grace (Jalali, 1982). Decide whether to work with patients in establishing goals, or to be more directive in prescribing treatments (more parentalistic).

It is also important to consider behaviors relating to compliance. Terms such as *compliance* and *noncompliance*, while commonly used in healthcare, have a negative connotation, and their use is problematic. The underlying assumption in labeling a patient *noncompliant* is that health-care providers know what is best for patients and have effectively communicated their advice. It also assumes that patients understood the advice and agree that the recommendation will be efficacious (Andrews & Herberg, 1999). When patients fail to do what was suggested, recommended or ordered, clinicians are tempted to label the behavior as *noncompliant*. But when patients seem to disregard advice, it would be useful to examine communication and other aspects of the interaction critically for an explanation, and ask, Why *should* the patient comply? Have clinicians clearly explained *why* patients should follow recommendations to achieve their health-related goals? Are personal preferences, mental/cognitive status, or other variables including cultural factors contributing to the person's refusal to follow advice?

Patients who gradually discontinue visits to health-care providers when they perceive that "nothing is happening" (i.e., not being restored to "normal") could be considered noncompliant or neglectful, but reasons for this behavior including its cultural context need to be examined carefully (Andrews, 1999b). Consider the expected time course for treatment to show improvement: are patients indeed patient, or do they expect immediate improvement? Patients may be dissatisfied with treatment that they see as only treating the symptoms but not solving the underlying problem, including hearing aids.

Another factor to consider regarding components of audiological rehabilitation involves the role of speechreading. Consider whether eye contact is valued or minimized for the patient. If minimizing eye contact is considered respectful, caring behavior, it hardly seems appropriate to recommend intensive speechreading. Even a simple recommendation of "watch other people when they talk to you" may not be appropriate.

Although the value of a positive role model has merit, research demonstrates that patients are likely to experience a level of comfort when in company of others who are like themselves (Andrews, 1999c). This advice could be useful in establishing support groups or audiological rehabilitation groups, but on what basis do patients want others to be like them? Which qualities are most salient: race? income? gender? geographic location? shared interests? The influence of these qualities on audiological rehabilitation groups and hearing disability support groups needs further examination.

When evaluating effectiveness of a treatment protocol, ask probing questions regarding how to further improve services if goals were met, and also ask probing questions to determine reasons for failure if outcome goals were not met. Consider any cultural influences on outcomes. Were extended family members included in the plan? Did the person responsible for making decisions participate in the care plan?

Consider the role of culture, broadly defined such as to include hobbies and lifestyle, when making recommendations to change behavior. When recommendations include advice to change a behavior, for example, limit exposure to power tools, remember that knowledge that a practice is harmful does not necessarily promote change in that behavior, as is commonly seen in people who are obese yet continue to overeat (Andrews, 1999c). This behavior is seen regardless of the patient's cultural background, educational level, socioeconomic status, or religious affiliation. Clinicians must balance the patients' rights to determine their own future against the clinician's need to promote change. The goal should be to provide advice and recommendations in a positive and culturally appropriate manner that encourages learning and promotes behavioral change in the desired direction. The decision to change behavior based on this advice is up to the patient.

Compatibility with current beliefs refers to the degree to which the recommended change is perceived as consistent with the existing norms and practices of the patient. In general, changes that do not conflict with existing traits are more readily accepted. Remember the skeet-shooting family mentioned in the introduction; how would audiologists prioritize recommendations? Is there a way to find a balance between eliminating exposure to high-intensity sounds and allowing this family to continue with an activity enjoyed by all? Is skeet-shooting the only activity the family shares such that recommending the family not take the child who is hearing impaired for risk of increasing the degree of hearing impairment means that positive experiences associated with this outing are not realized? Note that the family visits the audiologist to obtain earmolds, not to obtain hearing protectors. If they decline to spend the additional funds needed to obtain the hearing protectors the audiologist recommends, is the audiologist comfortable with continuing to treat this family? If not, does the audiologist have referral sources available?

Lastly, the above recommendations hold true for all patients, but there are special considerations for people of various races, those who have low incomes, and for members of the Deaf community. Regarding dispensing hearing aids, are there models that reflect a variety of hair and skin tones or are all samples and publications "pink?" Many audiologists recoiled in horror a few years ago when a recurring black character on the American television series *ER* was shown wearing pink hearing aids.

Access to hearing services in low-income communities, perhaps especially in low-income racially and ethnically diverse communities, is an important issue. Bazargan, Baker, and Bazargan (2001) evaluated the relationship between vision impairment, hearing impairment, and psychological well-being among a sample of almost 1000 elderly blacks living in New Orleans, Louisiana. Only 7 percent reported no chronic illnesses; the most frequently-cited chronic illnesses were arthritis (66 percent), hypertension (62 percent), eye problems (47 percent), heart trouble (33 percent), diabetes (24 percent), and circulation problems (23 percent). Note hearing problems were not mentioned; conversely, despite data showing many should have hearing impairments, over 60 percent described their hearing as good and only 3 percent wore hearing aids (yet over 84 percent of the sample reported using corrective lenses). Perhaps not surprisingly, only 4 percent of those people who described their hearing as poor were using hearing aids. Making simple suggestions to increase services to these people and to become familiar with community resources for referrals ignores the challenges in doing so: are the reasons these subjects did not wear hearing aids any different than the reasons that white, middle-class Americans do not wear hearing aids? Do audiologists have a duty to provide services to people who cannot pay for hearing aids? Are transportation difficulties partly to blame for these subjects not wearing aids? If patients from particular culture groups express desires to see certain providers in their own culture groups, consider those wishes, but could doing so be considered discriminatory? If audiologists truly want to improve services, more research is needed to determine the best ways to treat low-income patients.

As mentioned earlier, treatments designed to integrate people who are hearing and hearing-impaired may be met with resistance from members of the Deaf community. Cochlear implants have been a source of discord between the Deaf community and the hearing community. The Deaf community's concerns regarding cochlear implants focus around Deaf education, identity of the Deaf community, and the possibility of "cultural genocide"—the gradual and eventual elimination of Deaf culture and language (Bagli, 2002). Include the Deaf community in cochlear implant programs, as advocated by Holcomb (1999), among others, but be aware of difficulties and risks in doing so.

CONCLUSION

Audiology cannot be a purely data-driven or technology-driven discipline; it must also be a patient-driven one (DeBonis & Donohue, 2004). Audiologists must be knowledgeable about the cultures of the people they serve, because culture may affect the way people accept a diagnosis of hearing impairment, cope with the emotional impact of hearing disability, interact with professionals, implement treatment, allow the clinician to participate with the family, and tolerate what may be perceived as intrusion from the clinician (Bagli, 2002). Audiologists need to acknowledge the diversity that occurs *within* as well as *between* and *among* groups. And to achieve successful outcomes, audiologists will have to become more conscious about culture, develop cultural competence, and design, develop, and implement assessment and treatment protocols that reflect the diversity of the individuals they serve.

Commentator George Will has stated that multiculturalism attacks individualism by defining people as mere manifestations of groups (racial, ethnic, sexual) rather than as self-defining participants in a free society (Will, 1994). This chapter has attempted to help audiologists understand some group tendencies, but also appreciate patients as individuals.

Audiologists likely will, throughout their lifetimes, have several jobs and live in several places. An understanding of and respect for those different from themselves should enable them to provide better care to the patients they serve and to be more productive members of their communities. Cultural competence is a process rather than an ultimate goal. Hopefully this chapter provides an introduction to the many facets of culture which need to be considered when treating any patient.

REFERENCES

American Academy of Audiology (AAA). (2003). *Code of ethics.*

American Speech-Language-Hearing Association (ASHA). (2003). Code of ethics, revised. *Asha Supplement, 23,* 13–15.

American Speech Language Hearing Association (ASHA). (2004a). Knowledge and skills needed by speech-language pathologists and audiologists to provide culturally and linguistically appropriate services. *Asha Supplement, 24,* 152–158.

American Speech Language Hearing Association (ASHA). (2004b). Scope of practice in audiology. *Asha Supplement, 24,* 1–9.

Andrews, M. (1995). Transcultural considerations in health assessment. In C. Jarvis (Ed.), *Physical examination and health assessment.* Philadelphia: W. B. Saunders.

Andrews, M. M. (1999a). Theoretical foundations of transcultural nursing. In M. M. Andrews & J. S. Boyle (Eds.), *Transcultural concepts in nursing care*, 3rd ed. (pp. 3–22). Philadelphia: Lippincott.

Andrews, M. M. (1999b). Transcultural perspectives in the nursing care of children. In M. M. Andrews & J. S. Boyle (Eds.), *Transcultural concepts in nursing care*, 3rd ed. (pp. 107–159). Philadelphia: Lippincott.

Andrews, M. M. (1999c). Culture and nutrition. In M. M. Andrews & J. S. Boyle (Eds.), *Transcultural concepts in nursing care*, 3rd ed. (pp. 341–377). Philadelphia: Lippincott.

Andrews, M. M. (1999d). Cultural diversity in the health care workforce. In M. M. Andrews & J. S. Boyle (Eds.), *Transcultural concepts in nursing care*, 3rd ed. (pp. 471–506). Philadelphia: Lippincott.

Andrews, M. M., & Boyle, J. S. (1999). *Transcultural concepts in nursing care*, 3rd ed. Philadelphia: Lippincott.

Andrews, M. M., & Herberg, P. (1999). Transcultural nursing care. In M. M. Andrews, & J. S. Boyle (Eds.), *Transcultural concepts in nursing care*, 3rd ed. (pp. 23–77). Philadelphia: Lippincott.

Asch, A. (1998). Distracted by disability. *Cambridge Quarterly of Healthcare Ethics, 7,* 77–87.

Bagli, Z. (2002). Multicultural aspects of deafness. In D. E. Battle (Ed.), *Communication disorders in multicultural populations*, 3rd ed. (pp. 361–414). Boston: Butterworth-Heinemann.

Ballachanda, B. B. (2001). Audiological assessment of linguistically and culturally diverse populations. *Audiology Today, 13*(4), 34–35.

Battle, D. E. (2002). *Communication disorders in multicultural populations*, 3rd ed. Boston: Butterworth-Heinemann.

Bazargan, M., Baker, R. S., & Bazargan, S. H. (2001). Sensory impairments and subjective well-being among aged African American persons. *Journal of Gerontology, 56B,* 268–278.

Beauchamp, T. (1978). Distributive justice and morally relevant differences. In: *The National Commission for the Protection of Human Subjects of Biomedical and Behavioral Research.* The Belmont Report, Appendix I. Washington, DC: GPO, DHEW publication #(OS) 78-0013, 6–10.

Berger, E. H., Royster, L. H., & Thomas, W. G. (1977). Hearing levels of nonindustrial noise exposed subjects. *Journal of Occupational Medicine, 19,* 664–670.

Betancourt, J. R., Green, A. R., & Carrillo, J. E. (2002). *Cultural competence in health care: Emerging frameworks and practical approaches.* New York: The Commonwealth Fund.

Blacksher, E. (1998). Desperately seeking difference. *Cambridge Quarterly of Healthcare Ethics, 7,* 11–16.

Bobo, L., Womeodu, R. J., & Knox, A. L., Jr. (1991). Principles of intercultural medicine in an internal medicine program. *American Journal of Medical Sciences, 302,* 244–248.

Bonder, B., Martin, L., & Miracle, A. (2001). Achieving cultural competence: The challenge for clients and healthcare workers in a multicultural society. *Generations, 25,* 35–42.

Boyle, J. S. (1999a). Transcultural perspectives in the nursing care of middle-aged adults. In M. M. Andrews & J. S. Boyle (Eds.), *Transcultural concepts in nursing care,* 3rd ed. (pp. 161–188). Philadelphia: Lippincott.

Boyle, J. S. (1999b). Culture, family and community. In M. M. Andrews & J. S. Boyle (Eds.), *Transcultural concepts in nursing care,* 3rd ed. (pp. 308–337). Philadelphia: Lippincott.

Branch, W., Kern, D., Haidet, P., Weissmann, P., Gracey, C. F., Mitchell, G., & Inui, T. (2001). The patient-physician relationship. Teaching the human dimension of care in clinical settings. *Journal of the American Medical Association, 286*(9), 1067–1074.

Brock, D. (1993). Quality of life measures in health care and medical ethics. In M. Nussbaum, A. Sen (Eds.), *The quality of life* (pp. 95–132). New York: Oxford University Press.

Brody, J. A., Overfield, T., & McAlister, R. (1965). Draining ears and deafness among Alaskan Eskimos. *Archives of Otolaryngology, 81,* 29–33.

Carrillo, J. E., Green, A. R., & Betancourt, J. R. (1999). Cross-cultural primary care: A patient-based approach. *Annals of Internal Medicine, 130,* 829–834.

Chan, J. C. Y., & McPherson, B. (2001). Spontaneous and transient evoked otoacoustic emissions: A racial comparison. *Journal of Audiological Medicine, 10,* 20–32. Available at http://www.otoemissions.org/whitepapers/clinical/racial_dif.html

Chin, J. L. (2000). Culturally competent health care. *Public Health Report, 115,* 25–33.

Collins, K. S., Hughes, D. L., Doty, M. M., Ives, B. L., Edwards, J. N., & Tenney, K. (2002). *Diverse communities, common concerns: Assessing health care quality for minority Americans.* New York: The Commonwealth Fund.

Crawford, M. R., Gould, H. J., Smith, W. R., Beckford, N., Gibson, W. R., & Bobo, L. (1991). Prevalence of hearing loss in adults with sickle cell disease. *Ear and Hearing, 12,* 349–351.

Cross, T., Bazron, B. J., Dennis, K. W., & Issacs, M. R. (1998). *Towards a culturally competent system of care.* Vol. 1: Monograph on effective services for minority children who are severely emotionally disturbed. Washington, DC: Georgetown University Child Development Center, CASSP Technical Assistance Center.

Davis, T. C., Dolan, N. C., Ferreira, M. R., Tomori, C., Green K. W., Sipler, A. M., & Bennett, C. L. (2001). The role of inadequate health literacy skills in colorectal cancer screening. *Cancer Investigation, 19,* 193–200.

Davis, T. C., Holcombe, R. F., Berkel, H. J., Pramanik, S., & Divers, S. G. (1998). Informed consent for clinical trails: A comparative study of standard versus simplified forms. *Journal of the National Cancer Institute, 90,* 668–674.

DeBonis, D. A., & Donohue, C. L. (2004). *Survey of audiology: Fundamentals for audiologists and health professionals.* Boston: Allyn & Bacon.

Devine, E., & Braganti, N. L. (1986). *The traveler's guide to Asian customs and manners.* New York: St. Martin's Press.

Donini-Lenhoff, F. G., & Hedrick, H. L. (2000). Increasing awareness and implementation of cultural competence principles in health professions education. *Journal of Allied Health, 29,* 241–245.

Elliott, L. L., & Katz, D. R. (1980). Development of a new children's test of speech discrimination. St. Louis, MO: Auditec.

Fletcher, J. C., Hite, C. A., Lombardo, P. A., & Marshall, M. F. (Eds.) (1995). *Introduction to clinical ethics.* Frederick, MD: University Publishing Group.

Friedman, E. M., Luban, L. L. C., Herer, G. R., & Williams, I. (1980). Sickle cell anemia and hearing. *Annals of Otology, Rhinology, and Laryngology, 89,* 342–349.

Gallaudet Research Institute. (1999). Regional and national summary report of data from 1998–1999. *Annual Survey of Deaf and Hard-of-Hearing Children and Youth.* Washington, DC: Gallaudet University.

Gausman Benson, J., & Forman, W. B. (2002). Comprehension of written health care information in an affluent geriatric retirement community: Use of the Test of Functional Health Literacy. *Gerontology, 48,* 93–97.

Gonzalez-Lee, T., & Simon, J. H. (1987). Teaching Spanish and cross-cultural sensitivity to medical students. *Western Journal of Medicine, 146,* 502–504.

Good, B. J., & Good, M. J. (1980). The meaning of symptoms: A cultural hermeneutic model for clinical practice. In L. Eisenberg & A. Kleinman (Eds.), *The relevance of social science for medicine.* Boston: D. Reidel.

Gould, H. J., Crawford, M. R., Smith, W. R., Beckford, N., Gibson, W. R., Pettit, L., & Bobo, L. (1991). Hearing disorders in sickle cell disease: Cochlear and retrocochlear findings. *Ear and Hearing, 12,* 352–354.

Grundfast, K., & Carney, C. J. (1987). *Ear infections in your child.* Hollywood, FL: Compact Books.

Hall, E. (1963). Proxemics: The study of man's spatial relationships. In I. Gladstone (Ed.), *Man's image in medicine and anthropology* (pp. 109–120). New York: International University Press.

Hanson, M. J. (1998). The religious difference in clinical healthcare. *Cambridge Quarterly of Healthcare Ethics, 7,* 57–67.

Henderson, G. (1994). *Cultural diversity in the workplace.* Westport, CT: Praeger.

Hern, H. E., Jr., Koenig, B. A., Moore, L. J., & Marshall, P. A. (1998). *Cambridge Quarterly of Healthcare Ethics, 7,* 27–40.

Hill, R. F., Fortenberry, J. D., & Stein, H. F. (1990). Culture in clinical medicine. *Southern Medical Journal, 83,* 1071–1080.

Hoffmaster, B. A. (1994). *Cross cultural approach to health are ethics: A research agenda and statement of methodology.* Unpublished manuscript. Westminster Institute, London, Ontario.

Holcomb, T. (1999). Early intervention/late results: The need to "depathologize" the service model. *Seminars in Hearing, 20,* 269–276.

Jalali, B. (1982). Iranian families. In M. McGoldrick, J. K. Pearce, & J. Giordano (Eds), *Ethnicity and family therapy* (pp. 289–309). New York: Guilford Press.

Jerger, J., Jerger, S., Pepe, D., & Miller, R. (1986). Race difference in susceptibility to noise-induced hearing loss. *American Journal of Otology, 7,* 425–429.

Kavanagh, K. H. (1999). Transcultural perspectives in mental health. In M. M. Andrews & J. S. Boyle (Eds.), *Transcultural concepts in nursing care* (3rd ed., pp. 223–261). Philadelphia: Lippincott.

Kayser, H. (2001). Service delivery issues for culturally and linguistically diverse populations. In R. Lubinski, & C. Frattali (Eds.), *Professional issues in speech-language pathology and audiology,* (2nd ed. pp. 389–399). San Diego, CA: Singular Thomson Learning.

Kleinman, A. (1982). The teaching of clinically applied anthropology on a psychiatric consultation liaison service. In N. J. Chrisman and T. W. Maretzki (Eds.), *Clinically applied anthropology* (pp. 83–115). Dordrecht, Holland: Reidel.

Kolker, C. (2004). "Familiar faces bring health care to Latinos." *The Washington Post*, January 5, 2004, p. A03.

Kozier, B., Erb, G., & Blais, K. (1997). *Professional nursing practice: Concepts and perspectives* (3rd ed.). New York: Addison-Wesley.

Lapierre, E. D., & Padgett, J. (1991). How can we become more aware of culturally specific body language and use this awareness therapeutically? *Journal of Psychosocial Nursing, 29*(11), 38–41.

Lauderdale, J. (1999). Childbearing and transcultural nursing care issues. In M. M. Andrews & J. S. Boyle (Eds.), *Transcultural concepts in nursing care* (3rd ed., pp. 81–106). Philadelphia: Lippincott.

Lavizzo-Mourey, R., Smith, V., Sims, R., & Taylor, L. (1994). Hearing loss: An educational and screening program for African-American and Latino elderly. *Journal of the National Medical Association, 86,* 53–59.

Lebacqz, K. (1998). Difficult difference. *Cambridge Quarterly of Healthcare Ethics, 7,* 17–26.

Lee, L. J., Batal, H. A., Maselli, J. H., & Kutner, J. S. (2002). Effect of Spanish interpretation method on patient satisfaction in an urban walk-in clinic. *Journal of General Internal Medicine, 17,* 641–646.

Levin, B. W., & Schiller, N. G. (1998). Social class and medical decisionmaking: A neglected topic in bioethics. *Cambridge Quarterly of Healthcare Ethics, 7,* 41–56.

Lipson, J. G., & Steiger, N. J. (1996). *Self-care nursing in a multicultural context.* Thousand Oaks, CA: Sage Publications.

Lock, M. (1993). Education and self reflection: Teaching about culture, health and illness. In R. Masi et al. (Eds.), *Health and cultures: Exploring the relationships.* Oakville, Ontario: Mosaic Press.

Ludwig-Beymer, P. (1999). Transcultural aspects of pain. In M. M. Andrews & J. S. Boyle (Eds.), *Transcultural concepts in nursing care* (3rd ed., pp. 283–307. Philadelphia: Lippincott.

McCaffery, M. (1979). *Nursing management of the patient with pain,* (2nd Ed.). Philadelphia: J. B. Lippincott.

McFadden, D., & Pasanen, E. G. (1998). Comparison of the auditory system of heterosexuals and homosexuals: Click-evoked otoacoustic emissions. *Proceedings of the National Academy of Sciences, 95,* 2709–2713.

McKenna, M. A. (1999). Caring for the older adult patient: Nursing challenges in a changing context. In M. M. Andrews & J. S. Boyle (Eds.), *Transcultural concepts in nursing care* (3rd ed., pp. 189–220). Philadelphia: Lippincott.

MacDonald, C. B., Bauer, P. W., Cox, L. C., & McMahon, L. (1999). Otologic findings in pediatric cohort with sickle cell disease. *International Journal of Pediatric Otorhinolaryngology, 47,* 23–28.

Margolis, R. H. (2004). Audiology information counseling —What do patients remember? *Audiology Today, 16*(2), 14–15.

Miller, G. A., Heise, G. A., & Lichten, W. (1951). The intelligibility of speech as a function of the context of the test materials. *Journal of Experimental Psychology, 41,* 329–340.

Mundy, L. (2002). *A world of their own.* The Washington Post, March 31, p. W22.

Nasr, S.H. (1981). *Islamic life and thought.* London: George Allen and Uwin.

National Institute on Deafness and Other Communication Disorders (NIDCD). (2003). *Fact sheet—Auditory neuropathy: Quick facts.* Bethesda, MD: NIDCD Information Clearinghouse.

Newman-Ryan, J. (2001). *Auditory brain stem evoked potentials: Laboratory exercises and clinical manual.* Boston: Allyn and Bacon.

Newman-Ryan, J. (2004). *Health literacy: Implications for working with adults who have hearing impairments.* Presentation to the Academy of Rehabilitative Audiology Summer Institute, June 12, Saratoga Springs, NY.

Newman-Ryan, J., Northrup, B. de L., & Villarreal-Emery, C. (1995). Testing balance function in Spanish-speaking patients: Guidelines for non- Spanish-speaking clinicians. *American Journal of Audiology, 4,* 15–23.

Newman-Ryan, J. (1999). *Race, age, and gender of both professionals and customers depicted in hearing health-care advertisements.* Presentation to the American Academy of Audiology Annual Convention. May 1, Miami, FL.

Norton, M. E. (1999). Ethics and culture: Contemporary challenges. In M. M. Andrews & J. S. Boyle (Eds.), *Transcultural concepts in nursing care* (3rd ed., pp. 444–470). Philadelphia: Lippincott.

Nuñez, A. E. (2000). Transforming cultural competence into cross-cultural efficacy in women's health education. *Academic Medicine, 75,* 1071–1080.

Oticon Useful Tips for Friends and Relatives *www.oticon.com* accessed 3 June, 2004.

Paige, R. M. (1986). Trainer competencies: The missing conceptual link in orientation. *International Journal of Intercultural Relations, 10*(3), 135–158.

Paniagua, F. A. (1994). *Assessing and treating culturally diverse clients: A practical guide.* Thousand Oaks, CA: Sage.

Parikh, N. S., Parker, R. M., Nurss, J. R., Baker, D. W., & Williams, M. V. (1996). Shame and health literacy: The unspoken connection. *Patient Education and Counseling, 27,* 33–39.

Ramkissoon, I., Bilger, R. C., & Proctor, A. (2000). Digit-speech recognition thresholds among nonnative speakers of English. *ASHA Leader, 5*(16), 72.

Ramsey, C. (2000). Ethics and culture in the Deaf community: Response to cochlear implants. *Seminars in Hearing, 21,* 75–86.

Randall-David, E. (1989). *Strategies for working with culturally diverse communities and clients.* (Monograph). Bethesda, MD: The Association for the Care of Children's Health.

Robins, L. S., Fantone, J. C., Hermann, J., Alexander, G. L., & Zweifer, A. J. (1998). Improving cultural awareness and sensitivity training in medical school. *Academic Medicine, 73*(10 suppl.): S31–S34.

Roup, C. M., Wiley, T. L., Safady, S. H., & Stoppenbach, D. T. (1998). Tympanometric screening norms for adults. *American Journal of Audiology, 7,* 55–60.

Royster, L. H., & Thomas, W. G. (1979). Age effect hearing levels for a white nonindustrial noise-exposed population (NINEP) and their use in evaluating industrial hearing conservation programs. *American Industrial Hygiene Association Journal, 40,* 504–511.

Rudmin, F. (1987). Speech reception threshold for digits. *Journal of Auditory Research, 27,* 15–21.

Schoenberg, N. E. (1997). A convergence of health beliefs: An "ethnography of adherence" of African-American rural elders with hypertension. *Human Organization, 56*(2), 174–181.

Scott, D. M. (2002). Multicultural aspects of hearing disorders and audiology. In D. E. Battle (Ed.), *Communication disorders in multicultural populations* (3rd ed., pp. 335–360). Boston: Butterworth-Heinemann.

Shapiro, J., & Lenahan, P. (1996). Family medicine in a culturally diverse world: A solution-oriented approach to common cross-cultural problems in medical encounters. *Family Medicine, 28,* 249–255.

Shaw, J. R., Todd, N. W., Goodwin, M.., & Feldman, C. M. (1981). Observations on the relation of environmental and behavioral factors to the occurrence of otitis media among Indian children. *Public Health Reports, 96*(4), 342–349.

Silverman, F. H. (1999). *Essentials of professional issues in speech-pathology and audiology.* Boston: Allyn and Bacon.

Swarns, R. L. (2004). *"African-American" becomes a term for debate*. The New York Times, *August 29.*

Szasz, T. S., & Hollender, M. H. (1956). A contribution to the philosophy of medicine: The basic models of the doctor-patient relationship. *Archives of Internal Medicine, 97,* 585–592.

Talabere, L. R. (1996). Meeting the challenge of culture care in nursing: Diversity, sensitivity, and congruence. *Journal of Cultural Diversity, 3*(2), 53–61.

van Ryn, M., & Burke, J. (2000). The effect of patient race and socio-economic status on physician's perceptions of patients. *Social Science and Medicine, 50,* 813–828.

Viafora, C. (1996). Ethics today: An historic and systematic account. In R. Dell'oro & C. Viafora (Eds.) *History of bioethics: International perspectives* (p. 11). San Francisco: International Scholars Publication.

vos Savant, M. (2004). *Ask Marilyn.* Parade, April 11, p. 13.

Wallach, C. (2004). *Letter to the editor in response to "African-American" becomes a term for debate.* The New York Times, September 5.

Wan, I. K. K., & Wong, L. L. N. (2002). Tympanometric norms for Chinese young adults. *Ear and Hearing, 23,* 416–421.

Weiss, B. D. (2003). *Health literacy: A manual for clinicians.* Chicago: American Medical Association.

Wenger, A. F. (1993). Cultural meaning of symptoms. *Holistic Nursing Practice, 7*(2), 22–35.

Westby, C. (1995). Language, culture, and education: Learning to live in two worlds. Presented to the Illinois Speech-Language-Hearing Association convention, February, Arlington Heights, IL.

Widex Maintenance *www.widexusa.com* accessed 3 June, 2004.

Wiley, T. L., Cruickshanks, K. J., Nondahl, D. M., Tweed, T. S., Klein, R., & Klein, B. E. K. (1996). Tympanometric measures in older adults. *Journal of the American Academy of Audiology, 7,* 260–268.

Will, G. F. (1994). A kind of compulsory chapel: Multiculturalism is a campaign to lower America's moral status. *Newsweek*, November 14, p. 84.

Wilson, H. S. & Kneisl, C. R. (1983). *Psychiatric nursing.* Reading, MA: Adison-Wesley.

Wolf, K. E., & Hewitt, E. C. (1999). Hearing impairment in elderly minorities. *Clinical Geriatrics, 7,* 56–66.

Wood, J. B. (1989). Communicating with older adults in health care settings: Cultural and ethnic considerations. *Educational Gerontology, 15,* 351–362.

Wyatt, T. (2002). Assessing the communicative abilities of patients from diverse cultural and language backgrounds. In D. Battle (Ed.), *Communication disorders in multicultural populations* (3rd ed., pp. 415–459). Boston: Butterworth-Heinemann.

Zweifler, J., & Gonzalez, A. M. (1998). Teaching residents to care for culturally diverse populations. *Academic Medicine, 73,* 1056–1061.

APPENDIX

Definitions of Culture and Related Concepts

Bilingual/multilingual clinician: Native or near-native proficiency in the language(s) spoken or signed by patient (ASHA, 2004a).

Culture: The first record of the term *culture* as used today is credited to Sir Edward Tylor, a British anthropologist who wrote in 1871 that culture is "that complex whole which includes knowledge, belief, art, morals, law, custom and any other capabilities and habits acquired by man as a member of society." Modern definitions differ little from this initial definition: e.g., currently culture is defined as an integrated pattern of learned beliefs and behaviors that can be shared among groups and include thoughts, styles of communicating, ways of interacting, views of roles and relationships, values, practices, and customs (Robins, Fantone, Hermann, Alexander, & Zweifer, 1998; Donini-Lenhoff & Hedrick, 2000). Culture is learned and shared, both formally, as in class or religious instruction, and informally by observation and experience (Kavanagh, 1999). Culture is constantly changing yet not easily changed. It strongly influences, but does not determine, ideas and behavior. Culture does not involve biologic or personal characteristics but only those values, beliefs, and ideals that people share. Everyone has cultural affiliations, not only others who are "different." Culture is not always neat and orderly; various cultures and subcultures overlap. Values, attitudes, ideas, and patterns of behavior are shared in this time of instant and visual communication when many people are exposed to multiple cultures (Kavanagh, 1999).

Culture-specific refers to particular values, beliefs, and patterning of behavior that tend to be special or unique to a group and which do not tend to be shared with members of other cultures. *Culture-universal* refers to the commonly shared values, norms of behavior, and life patterns that are similarly held among cultures about human behavior and lifestyles (Leininger, 1978, 1995).

Cultural competence: Cultural competence is defined cultural competence as a set of behaviors, attitudes, and policies that enable a system, agency, or group of professionals to work effectively in cross-cultural situations (Cross, Bazron, Dennis, & Issacs, 1998); in health care, it is the ability of providers and organizations to effectively deliver health care services that meet the social, cultural, and linguistic needs of patients (Betancourt, Green, & Carrillo, 2002).

Dialect: A neutral term used to describe a language variation. Dialects are seen as applicable to all languages and all speakers. All languages are analyzed into a range of dialects, which reflect the regional and social background of their speakers (ASHA, 2004a).

Diversity: In its broadest sense, diversity refers to differences in race, ethnicity, national origin, religion, age, gender, sexual orientation, ability/disability, social and economic status or class, education, and related attributes of groups of people in society.

Interpreter: A person specially trained to translate oral communications or manual communication systems from one language to another (ASHA, 2004a).

Isms: The "Isms" (as described by Kavanagh, 1999, p. 237) are a variety of biases that could influence behavior towards others.

Egocentrism: the assumption that oneself is superior to others.

Ethnocentrism: the assumption that one's own cultural or ethnic group is superior to that of others. Ethnicity refers to cultural differences and should not be confused with race. Ethnocentrism occurs, for example, when everyone is expected to speak English and to know the rules (many of which are implicit) for living in a predominant English-speaking society.

Racism: the assumption that members of one race are superior to those of another.

Sexism: the assumption that members of one sex are superior to those of the other.

Heterosexism: the assumption that everyone is or should be heterosexual and that heterosexuality is superior and typical. It is only rather recently that homosexuality was redefined as a lifestyle rather than a disease.

Ageism: the assumption that members of one age group are superior to those of others. Note that according to this definition, ageism could occur in either direction, i.e., younger against older or older against younger.

Adultism: the assumption that adults are superior to youths and can or should control, direct, reprimand, reward, or deprive them of respect.

Sizism: the assumption that people of one body size are superior to or better than those of other shapes and sizes. Positions involving interaction with the public, for example, may be denied individuals whose weight fails to meet the standards of ideal appearance.

Classism/elitism: the assumption that certain people are superior because of their social and economic status or position in a group or organization.

Ableism: the assumption that the ablebodied and sound of mind are physically or developmentally superior to those who are disabled, mentally ill, mentally retarded, or otherwise different. An example of ableism is not offering patients choices owing to the assumption that they do not want to make, or cannot make, decisions themselves.

Personality: Personality is defined as the personal beliefs, expectations, desires, values, and behaviors that derive from the interaction between culture and the individual. It could be seen as the behaviors and techniques for solving problems that are used by an individual. Personality is to the individual as culture is to the group.

Subculture: Subculture refers to a large group of people who, although members of a larger cultural group, share characteristics that are not common to all members of the larger cultural group. Subcultures can be categorized by geographic region, religion, age, gender, social class, political party, ethnic, racial or cultural identity, occupational role, or isolation from the dominant society by choice, discrimination, or locale (Andrews, 1999a). Subcultural groups are distinguished from one another and from the dominant culture by such characteristics as speech patterns, dress, gestures, etiquette, and lifestyles. For the purposes of this chapter, consider subcultures of biomedicine, of clinics, of private practices, of school settings, etc. Behavior within those settings differs from behavior in other settings, thus establishing them as subcultures.

Translator: A person specially trained to translate written text from one language to another (ASHA, 2004a).

CHAPTER 17

Case Studies

Neil T. Shepherd
*University of Nebraska—Lincoln and
Boys Town National Research
Hospital*

Annette Mazevski and
Danielle Inverso
Gallaudet University

R. Steven Ackley
Gallaudet University

James W. Thelin
University of Tennessee

Jennifer Ratigan
Arizona Ear Center, Phoenix, Arizona

Kerri S. McDill
Wyoming Otolaryngology, Casper, WY

DIZZINESS AND BALANCE DISORDER CASES

Case 1. Male, 35 years of age seen for complaints of sudden onset vertigo, six months prior, with nausea and vomiting in a crisis event with continuous symptoms lasting 3 days, steadily showing slow improvement and no accompanying auditory symptoms. The continuous vertigo resolved into head movement provoked spells of lightheadedness with imbalance and occasional vertigo lasting seconds to a minute after a movement. All planes of motion were provocative. Symptoms had continued to improve but still occurred on an infrequent daily basis. He presented with no neurological focal complaints and past medical history was non-contributory. Audiometric evaluation was completely normal bilaterally as was his contrast MRI study of the head. His detailed vestibular examination both with and without visual fixation was remarkable for a positive head thrust test to the left, right beating post head-shake nystagmus, and spontaneous right beating nystagmus with visual fixation removed. The full neurological and ocular motor components of the examination together with Hallpike testing were normal. The history with the examination was strongly suggestive of uncompensated left peripheral vestibular hypo-function, secondary to vestibular neuritis. Laboratory vestibular function testing revealed spontaneous right beating nystagmus with visual fixation removed and a 76 percent left reduced vestibular response with ocular motor testing and postural control assessment normal. In this case the tests were, as is typical in most cases, confirmatory of the clinic suspicions from the history and direct examination. Management decisions made at the time of the office visit to initiate treatment with Vestibular and Balance Rehabilitation Therapy (VBRT) and to discontinue vestibular suppressive medication were not in any manner altered with the obtaining of the laboratory findings. The vestibular function and balance tests were well justified given the length of symptoms and the fact that the testing has better sensitivity for some ocular motor findings than the direct examination, specifically saccade velocity testing and quantification of smooth pursuit. Sensitivity to mild peripheral vestibular function asymmetry is also better with the laboratory testing. In this case the magnitude of the peripheral asymmetry made it detectable by both the direct examination and the caloric irrigation studies.

Case 2.   Male, 31 years of age with onset of head motion provoked vertigo with more or less constant imbalance with standing and walking. He denied any vestibular crisis event or auditory complaints. His symptoms were more concentrated in saggital plane movement and when rolling left or right from a supine position. These symptoms had been ongoing for over several years with intervals when the vertigo was resolved and the imbalance reduced but not absent. He reported an MRI from several years prior to this evaluation that was normal with a cervical MRI positive for mild disc abnormalities. Audiological examination was normal. Other than the development of mild paresthesia of the right hand and arm over the last year he had no other neurological complaints and his past medical history was non-contributory. His direct office examination was remarkable for anterior semi-circular canal Benign Paroxysmal Positional Vertigo (BPPV). The remainder of the examination was normal. He was treated in the office with a Canalith Repositioning Procedure and referred on for a formal vestibular and balance rehabilitation therapy (VBRT) program. Secondary to the length of time of the symptoms and the complaints of persistent imbalance (although this is a common report with BPPV) vestibular and balance function testing was requested. The laboratory studies continued to show anterior canal BPPV with no other indications of peripheral vestibular system involvement. Pursuit tracking tests were normal, but saccade testing was positive for mild right Internuclear Ophthalmoplegia. Postural control abnormalities were collectively consistent with that seen in demylinating disorders. Secondary to these findings and his report of paresthesia starting in the left foot a new MRI was obtained that showed multiple hyper-intense spots throughout the brain stem region. He was referred on to neurology and is being followed with a diagnosis of probable Multiple Sclerosis with BPPV. Unlike case 1 this case was driven strongly by the results of the vestibular and balance function tests. The test results revealed abnormalities too subtle to be detected in a direct examination. This is clearly the exception to the impact that the testing has on a more routine basis in the decisions regarding management of the dizzy patient.

Case 3. Male, 70 years of age reports with a working diagnosis of right side Meniere's disease.

Laboratory testing was to be used to establish a baseline against which to compare for monitoring his disorder and possible treatment. His history was classic with regard to Meniere's disease with spontaneous spells of true vertigo with nausea and emesis production lasting 1–4 hours. Spells had been ongoing for a year beginning with one event every 2 months increasing in frequency to 1–2 times per week at the time of his evaluation. Conservative treatment with a low sodium diet and diuretic were being used with no effect. He reported fluctuant hearing on the right with bilateral tinnitus and significant past noise exposure (Figure 17–1). Between the events he was free of dizziness symptoms. He did admit to increasing falls with his events but not between. The remainder of his past medical/surgical history was non-contributory. Results from his VNG showed ocular motor findings that were normal or consistent with his age. Spontaneous right-beating nystagmus with a slow component velocity of 1–3°/sec was noted in sitting with fixation removed. No exacerbation with headshake testing and no positional nystagmus were seen. His caloric irrigation test revealed a surprising bilateral reduction

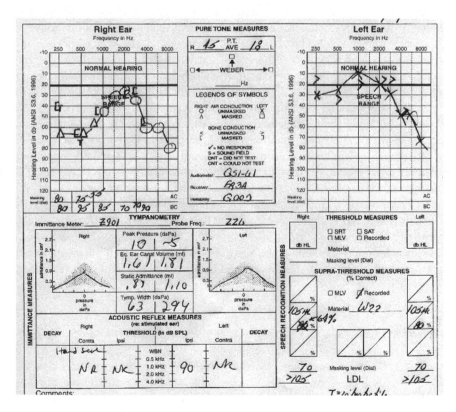

FIGURE 17–1. Audiograms for right and left ears showing low frequency sensorineural hearing loss for the right ear characteristic of Meniere's disease.

with warm, cool and ice water irrigations producing nystagmus with slow component velocity $< 4°/sec$ for both right and left stimulations. The immediate question that required an answer was what was the degree of his bilateral involvement? If this was significant it could limit more aggressive treatment options.

To attempt an answer to the issue of the degree of bilateral involvement rotational chair, the SOT of dynamic posturography and Dynamic Visual Acuity (DVA) testing were combined to provide a collective estimate of involvement. In summary the chair results demonstrated an abnormally high phase lead in the lower frequencies with a left greater than right slow component velocity asymmetry. These findings, given the negative ocular motor testing, would suggest peripheral involvement of either a left paretic or right irritative style lesion. Given his spontaneous right beating nystagmus and documented asymmetrical hearing loss worse on the right, the right irritative lesion would be considered more likely. Of importance was the overall gain values within normal limits although trending to the lower limit of normal as the test frequencies approached 0.01 Hz. This suggested that the extent of the bilateral involvement was minimal and restricted to the very low frequency region of the peripheral system. The magnitude of the phase lead at 0.01 Hz was also supportive of this impression. If this impression from rotary chair is correct then the functional impact of his bilateral involvement should also be minimal regarding maintenance of quiet up-right stance and his ability to maintain visual clarity with his head in motion. The results of the SOT while showing difficulty when he was forced to rely on vestibular system cues alone, demonstrates his ability with practice to maintain stance within a normal range for his age by the second or third trial of test conditions 5 and 6. This SOT result would be consistent functionally with minimal bilateral vestibular involvement. Lastly, the DVA test performed using the clinical office technique with horizontal reciprocal head movements at 2 Hz was within normal limits. Overall, the collective results of the laboratory studies demonstrated peripheral vestibular system involvement bilaterally, but mild in degree and restricted to the very low frequency region of function of the peripheral system with greater involvement on the right than the left. These findings including the SOT and DVA provided a firm baseline physiologically and functionally for monitoring of the patient's slowly titrated transtympanic gentamicin treatment for his right side Meniere's disease. This was successful in stopping the spontaneous events without causing him to experience any functional deficits of significance related to his bilateral peripheral system involvement.

HEARING LOSS CASES

Case 4. Normal cochlear sensitivity with tumor-filled cochlea.   The audiometric results are shown for a 23 year-old female with right glomus jugulare tumor and a right carotid body tumor. These tumors filled the middle ear cavity, caused conductive hearing loss, and affected the function of cranial nerves VII, IX, X, and XII.

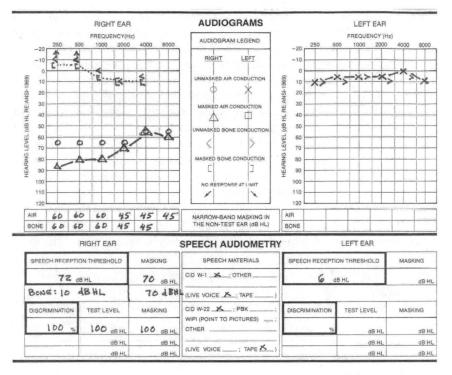

FIGURE 17–2.   Audiograms for right and left ears showing severe conductive hearing loss for the right ear and normal hearing for the left ear.

This case is rare because the glomus tumor invaded the cochlea (through the stapes footplate) and all of the semicircular canals of the vestibular mechanism. The labyrinth was sacrificed in the process of surgical removal of the tumor, resulting in total loss of hearing and vestibular function on the right.

Preoperatively, the surgeons believed that cochlear function should have been severely compromised. Audiometric results were obtained from the referring physician, and two preoperative audiograms were done in addition. All showed very similar results. The results of the second preoperative audiometric evaluation are shown here. They indicate the presence of a large conductive hearing loss in the right ear with cochlear sensitivity in the normal hearing range. Very high masking levels (levels that were even overmasking) were used to guarantee that there was no way that the responses were being obtained from the left ear when the right ear was being stimulated.

The results indicate that the right cochlea was functioning nearly normally despite that presence of extensive tumor in the cochlea. The explanations of these findings are (1) that the tumor functioned in a similar manner as the fluids of the cochlea and (2) that the tumor probably did not invade scala media and disrupt the function of the organ of Corti. Thus, despite the presence of extensive tumor tissue, cochlear function remained normal.

Case 5. 85 year-old patient with advanced otosclerosis and cochlear implant.   An 85 year-old patient has a 60 year history of bilateral advanced otosclerosis with cochlear involvement. Her family history revealed that both of her parents and one of her children have hearing loss. She first noticed hearing loss after the birth of her first child, and she had a fenestration operation about 50 years earlier in the left ear. She began wearing a power BTE hearing aid in her left ear one year after her fenestration surgery which she still wears regularly. Twenty years after her left ear sugery, the patient reported having a stapedectomy operation in her right ear. However, she has had a profound hearing loss in that ear for nearly 20 years, and she was advised not to wear a hearing aid in her right ear. The remainder of her past medical/surgical history was non-contributory.

The audiometric test results (Figure 17–3) show a profound mixed hearing loss bilaterally and word recognition scores were 0 percent bilaterally. As part of a pre-cochlear implant evaluation the Hearing in Noise Test (HINT) was performed with hearing aids. Her scores with an input of 60 dB HL were 0 percent bilaterally.

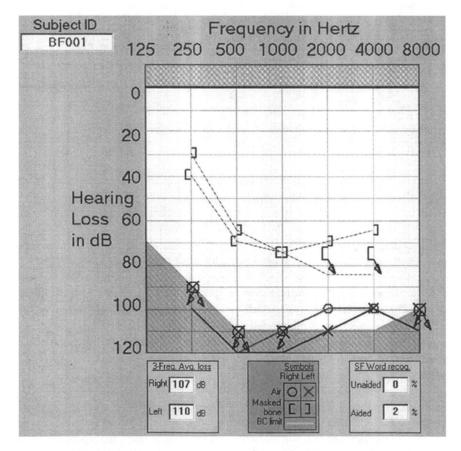

FIGURE 17–3.   Audiogram of right and left ears showing profound mixed hearing loss bilaterally.

As part of the standard Cochlear Implant candidacy evaluation at the Mayo Clinic, vestibular assessment is included in part to help determine and/or counsel regarding the decision of which ear to implant. Vestibular assessment was also done to help with this decision, and results of bithermal caloric irrigation showed better responses for the right ear than the left ear, which were well below normal.

Cochlear Implant Ear Selection

Choosing which ear to implant proved to be difficult. The left ear would require a complicated two-stage surgical reconstruction due to the patient's enlarged mastoid cavity following her fenestration surgery. The first stage would consist of closing the ear canal and removing excess skin. Nine to twelve months later, a second stage would be performed to check for residual cholesteatoma, and possible cavity obliteration using fat. In addition, she had poor word recognition ability when using conventional amplification on the left ear, indicating possible poor performance with a cochlear implant. However, the right ear had the risk of vestibular loss, leaving the patient with bilateral hypofunction if implanted, and the right ear performed better than the left with conventional amplification, which might indicate more success with implantation.

Because of a vestibular weakness in the left ear the decision to retain balance capability of the right ear needed to be taken into consideration. Vestibular test results were imperative in this situation in order to counsel the patient regarding the possibility of balance problems post surgery. Ultimately, due to the audiometric and surgical implications, the decision was made by the implant surgeon to perform the implant operation on the right ear. The patient was counseled extensively regarding the possibility of balance dysfunction due to the results of the vestibular test findings. The patient understood the risks and decided to move forward with the procedure regardless.

Post Cochlear Implant Performance

Three months after activation, speech perception greatly improved for the patient. Scores from the Overlearned Sentence Test, HINT in Quiet, and HINT with a signal-to-noise ratio of +10dB were 95 percent, 80 percent, and 57 percent, respectively. Additionally, though residual balance function was a pre-surgical concern, the patient also reported no disruption of equilibrium or balance.

CONCLUSION

Cochlear implantation for patients with mixed hearing loss secondary to advanced otosclerosis is a viable option after careful consideration of medical and audiological factors. Benefits for this patient include restored auditory sensitivity to a level not possible with conventional amplification; preserved vestibular function in her right ear; improved word recognition and communication function; and finally an overall improvement in quality of life.

Case 6. Sudden sensorineural hearing loss: Auditory neuropathy.   The subject, a 23 year old female from West Africa, developed a sudden severe to profound hearing loss at the age of 16. Her symptoms began with sharp pain and dryness to her eyes, followed by a decrease in vision. Within days, her hearing was gone, her vision remained blurred, her gait was disordered and a burning sensation in her lower extremities caused a severe pain. Her initial intervention included various Eastern medicinal theories. The subject and her tribe moved often throughout the country which was involved in a civil war. She was exposed to harsh chemicals in the air and soil brought on from the attacks of the war. She and her family went through a period of starvation, with only a diet of raw cassava, a hard fiber and a main crop in parts of West Africa.

After arriving in the United States, two years after symptoms began, the subject completed an audiologic assessment, consisting of only pure tone thresholds and word recognition results. A brief medical exam was conducted including an MRI and blood tests, both of which resulted negative. The subject's visual, vestibular, and somatosensory symptoms were not assessed at this time, and there was not a record of any neurological consult or referral. Audiologic records reported the subject as a malingerer on several occasions, and finally with a profound sensorineural hearing loss, although an evaluation of immittance, otoacoustic emissions, auditory evoked potentials or bone conduction was never assessed. She purchased hearing aids, saw two optometrists, purchased three sets of eye glasses, and tried her best to compensate for the imbalance.

Test Results

Figures 17–4 and 17–5 show hearing test results for right and left ears using narrow-band-noise (NBN) and pure tone stimuli. The subject reported that her auditory ability would range from not being able to perceive the telephone ringing, to

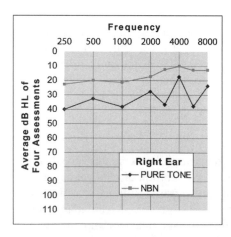
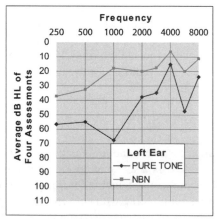

FIGURE 17–4a & b.   Audiograms for right and left ears showing discrepancy between hearing for narrow bands of noise (NBN) and pure tones.

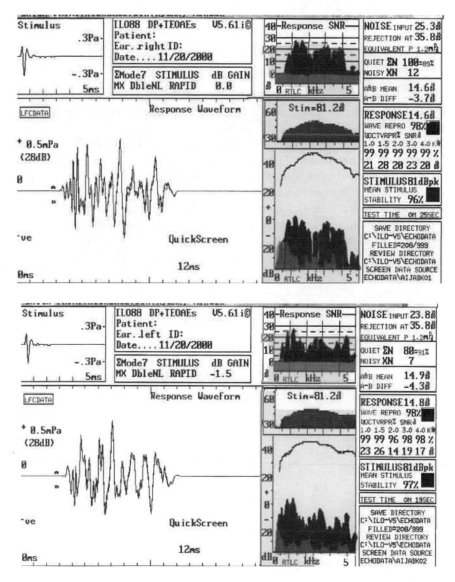

FIGURE 17–5a & b.   Normal otoacoustic emissions for right (Fig. 3) and left (Fig. 4) ears.

being able to hear the dial tone and speaker on the phone. She would comment that her hearing would fluctuate often and unexpectedly.

Otoacoustic Emissions

Transient evoked otoacoustic emissions show between a 96 percent–99 percent response at all tested frequencies for both the right ear (Fig. C) and the left ear, (Fig. D). Measurable dB levels ranged from 14dB to as high as 28dBpk. This measurement of robust emissions reveals normal outer hair cell function of the cochlea.

Auditory Brainstem Responses

The ABR waves show questionable responses bilaterally indicating very poor VI-IIth cranial nerve and brainstem function. Square pulse ("click")-trains were delivered at 90 dB nHL monaurally to each ear.

The classical definition of 'auditory neuropathy' is normal cochlear function and abnormal or absent neural function. This patient meets this definition as indicated by her normal otoacoustic emissions and abnormal auditory brainstem responses. In addition she shows pure tone hearing fluctuation and variable word recognition ability. The patient was ultimately diagnosed with multiple neuropathies, including auditory neuropathy, secondary to chemical toxicity from

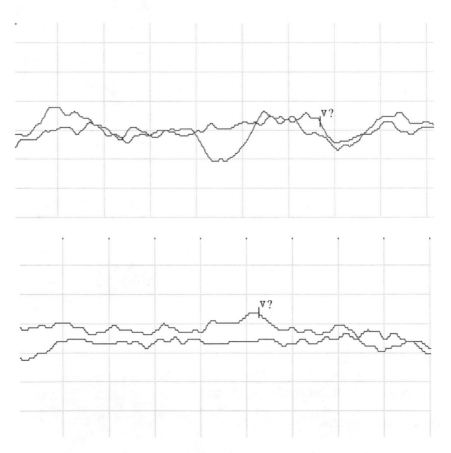

FIGURE 17–6a & b   Auditory Brainstem Responses for right (Fig. 5) and left (Fig. 6) ears show questionable results at 90 dB nHL.

food consumption in her native West Africa homeland. Her condition was undiagnosed for years while she was labeled erroneously as a 'malingerer'. Accurate diagnosis in such cases can help the patient to adjust to a set of puzzling and seemingly contradictory symptoms.

Case 7. Enlarged vestibular aqueduct syndrome.   A 12 year-old male with history of fluctuating hearing loss bilaterally was seen following traumatic head injury from a baseball. Patient was playing an outfielder position at a baseball game when he was struck on the left side of his head by a baseball from an adjacent field. Following the incident, he initially reported improved hearing; however, he was admitted to the hospital later that day due to severe vertigo, nausea, and vomiting. Patient remained in the hospital until the vertigo subsided. He could not raise his body greater than 30 degrees before becoming vertiginious and nauseated. A CT scan performed without contrast indicated bilateral enlarged vestibular aqueducts (EVA). Figure 17–7 shows an example of what EVA looks like on a CT scan.

Prior to this diagnosis, patient's doctors felt he had fluctuating conductive hearing loss, although he has no significant history of otitis media or other middle ear pathology. Medical records indicated that tympanometry was within normal limits bilaterally, except for one instance when he had negative pressure in

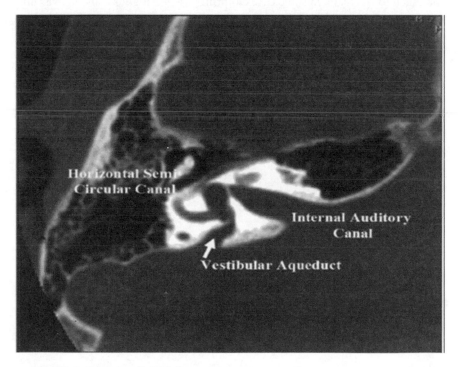

FIGURE 17–7.   Enlarged vestibular aqueduct.

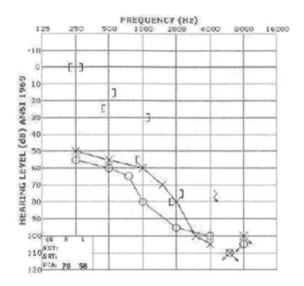

FIGURE 17–8.   Audiogram of patient prior to his head injury. The thresholds plotted here are essentially the same as those from 8 years prior.

both ears and subsequently had pressure equalization tubes placed. Hearing loss continued to fluctuate, in some cases to profound hearing loss, and he was ultimately fit with binaural amplification. A CT scan without contrast performed when he was 2 years of age came back unremarkable and showed properly pneumatized mastoids and normal inner ear structures. It could be suggested that the resolution was insufficient to identify the EVA that the patient had, but it is unclear whether contrast would have an effect on test results.

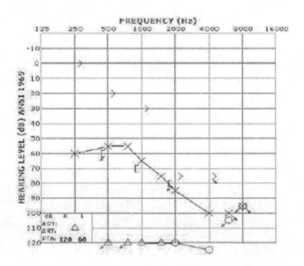

FIGURE 17–9.   Audiogram of patient five weeks after his head injury.

Figure 17–8 shows the hearing loss the patient had prior to being struck by the baseball. Patient had essentially the same hearing loss for 8 years beforehand. Figure 17–9 shows an audiogram after the patient was released from the hospital. Right ear thresholds are of significant interest here, as patient essentially had no measurable hearing. Figure 17–10 shows improvement in the patient's hearing and what his current hearing thresholds are bilaterally. Word recognition scores from the last audiogram were 86 percent for the left ear and 78 percent for the right ear.

Patient is now 15 years old and wears binaural amplification. He goes to a public high school where he is mainstreamed and he uses an FM system for improved signal-to-noise ratio while in class. He was originally seen at a school for the deaf close to his home to see if attending there would be more appropriate. While there, preliminary examinations indicated that he was performing at the average level for children his age without hearing loss, and above average for the cohort of children with his type of hearing loss. Patient is currently interested in playing football and continues to play baseball. He is aware of the risks associated with playing these sports to his hearing; however, he feels that he does not want his condition to affect his quality of life. The patient is aware of the option of a cochlear implant if he becomes profoundly hearing-impaired and if his hearing aids no longer provide him benefit.

Case 8. Goldenhar Syndrome.   Characteristics of Goldenhar syndrome may include: epibulbar dermoids, auricular appendages or fistulae, as well as vertebral,

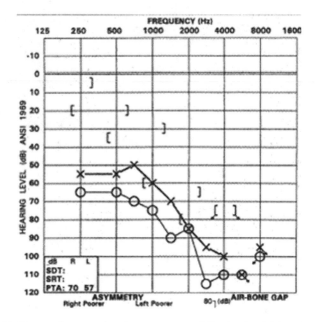

FIGURE 17–10.   Audiogram of patient three years following head injury. Hearing has remained stable since his injury.

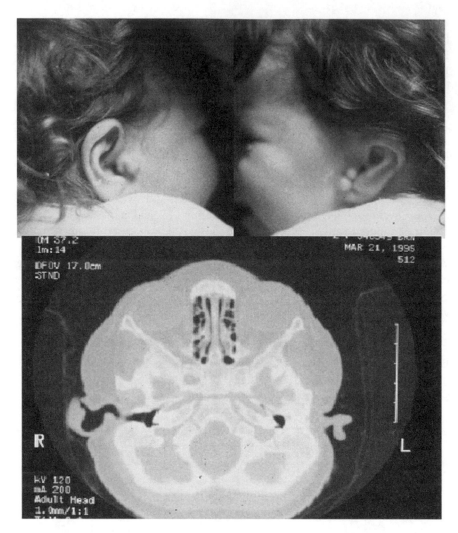

FIGURE 17–11.   Preauricular appendages are evident on right and left ears, although more prominent on the left side. Similarly, the right ear canal (R) evident on the CT scan below is more normal and shows a patent ear canal. The left ear canal (L) is not developed.

CNS, cardiac, pulmonary and/or renal anomalies. Because of the complexity of this disorder, Oculo-auriculo-vertebral spectrum (OAVS) better describes this defect involving the first and second branchial arches and is characterized by microtia, mandibular hypoplasia, vertebral anomalies, and epibulbar dermoids. When pre-auricular appendages are seen, a CT scan can determine external canal patency.

In addition, ABR assessment determined electrophysiological response of each ear showing normal hearing for the right ear, consistent with patent ear canal, and 60 dB hearing loss for the left, consistent with no developed ear canal.

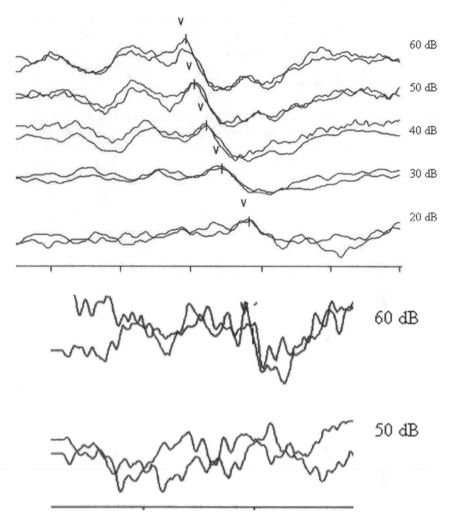

FIGURE 17–12a & b.   Auditory Brainstem Response (ABR) results showing normal results for the right ear and 60 dB threshold for the left ear.

Although the CT scan may show a patent ear canal, the ABR gives the 'gold standard' physiological work-up. This case illustrates that CT scans are vital but do not replace electrophysiological data. The ABR results confirm that the patent ear canal delivers sound to a functioning cochlea, while the atretic ear shows maximum conductive hearing loss.

CONCLUSION

These case studies illustrate the importance of thorough clinical assessment. Traditional audiometric testing is necessary in all cases, but it provides only a basis for further test procedures. The case history information also provides a foundation for the direction the testing should take. As test results are compiled yet another platform for test direction evolves and a final diagnosis is the end product.

ACKNOWLEDGMENTS

Danielle Inverso gratefully acknowledges the contributions to Case Study 5 from the Cochlear Implant Team at the Mayo Clinic in Scottsdale Arizona. Annette Mazevski gratefully acknowledges the contributions to Case Study 7 from the Audiology Department at the Massachusetts Eye and Ear Infirmary in Boston, Massachusetts.

Author Index

Lane, R. H., 159, 167
Lange-Nielsen, F., 91, 111
Langer, D. H., 245
Langer, E., 325, 349
Langlois, J., 346
Lapierre, E. D., 401, 419
Lapsley M. J., 315, 321
Larson, E., 335, 340, 349
Larson, T., 36, 40
Larunagaray, D., 246
Lasher, K. P., 339, 345
Laszig, R., 199, 200
Lau, C., 284
Lauderdale, J., 419,
Laufer, M. B., 325, 345
Lavigne-Rebillard, M., 289, 323
Lavizzo-Mourey, R., 408, 419
Lawson, D. T., 177, 193, 198, 201
Layton, K., 286
Lebacqz, K., 419
Lee, L. J., 403, 419
Lee, M. K., 84
Lee, M. P., 91, 112
Lee, W. W., 150, 168
Lee, W., 161, 166
Legros, D., 119, 135
Lehner, R., 201
Lehnhardt, E., 200
Leisti, J. T., 87, 112
Lenahan, P., 400, 420
Lenarz, T., 184, 191, 197, 198, 201
Lesner, S. A., 334–337, 345
Lesperance, M. M., 76, 84
Levin, B. W., 419
Levin, V. A., 119, 135
Levine, S. M., 144, 167
Lew, H. L., 163, 169
Lew, H., 284, 334, 344
Lewis, D. E., 244, 246, 247
Lewis, D. L., 225, 247
Lewis, D., 247, 277, 286
Lewis, S., 244
Lewis, W. R., 172, 173, 200
Leysieffer, H., 201
Li, L., 58, 64
Li, X. C., 112
Li, Y., 119, 135
Liang, Y., 84
Liberfarb, R. M., 111
Liberman, M. C., 310, 311, 321
Lichten, W., 410, 419
Lichtenstein, M., 262, 284
Lieu, T. L., 114

Lilly, D. J., 136, 144, 147, 167
Limb, C. J., 35, 39, 192, 198
Limberger, A., 201
Lin, K., 228, 245
Lindberg, P., 339, 342
Linder, T., 36, 39
Lindholm, P. K., 87, 112
Ling, D., 83
Linn, R., 329, 343
Linthicum, F. H. Jr., 25, 39
Linthicum, F. H., 181, 196
Lipman, A., 332, 342
Lipson, J. G., 400, 419
Lipton, A., 120, 135
Liskow, C., 244
Litterst, C. J., 136
Liu, C. C., 312, 321
Liu, J., 135
Liu, K. P., 243
Liu, R., 59, 63, 243
Liu, T., 228, 245
Liu, W., 135
Liu, X. Z., 67, 78, 84, 113
Lloyd, L., 347
Lock, M., 419
Loescher, L., 135
Logan, S., 262, 284
Logigian, E. L., 25, 39
Lohnstein, P., 199
Loizou, P. C., 177, 178, 180, 196, 198
Lombardo, P. A., 418
Lomranz, J., 333, 345
Long, D. M., 35, 39
Lonsbury-Martin, B. L., 130, 135, 136, 315, 321
Loth, D., 315, 320
Lous, J., 97, 112
Lousteau, R. J., 165
Love, R. R., 136
Lovegrove, R., 244
Lowder, M. W., 186, 197
Lowder, M., 197
Luban, L. L. C., 407, 418
Lubinski, R., 329, 331, 334, 335, 345
Lucks Mendel, L., 244
Ludvigsen, C., 275, 284
Ludwig-Beymer, P., 419
Luey, H. S., 338, 341, 345, 346
Luk, G. D., 133
Lundh, P., 272, 285
Luntz, M., 184, 185, 198
Lustig, L. R., 30, 32, 39, 107, 112, 113
Lustig, L., 108, 113, 198
Luxford, W. M., 184, 197

Subject Index